# Memory disorders in psychiatric pra

Memory complaints are a frequent feature of psychiatric disorder, even in the absence of organic disease. In this book, German Berrios and John Hodges lead an international team of eminent clinicians to focus on the psychiatric, as well as the organic, aspects of memory disorder from the perspective of the multidisciplinary memory clinic.

This is a practical reference for the clinician. Psychiatrists, behavioural neurologists and clinical psychologists will share an interest in the historical and neurobiological accounts of memory and its disorders, which precede detailed accounts of the main memory syndromes seen in practice. These include organic syndromes such as the dementias, the amnesic syndrome and transient amnestic states, and also psychiatric aspects of memory disorders in the functional psychoses. Among the specific topics reviewed are the paramnesias, déjà vu, flashbulb and flashback memories, and the problems of recovered, false and feigned memories.

Throwing new light on established conditions, and also introducing two new syndromes, this book makes a major contribution to the understanding and clinical management of memory disorders in psychiatry, neuropsychology and other disciplines.

**German E. Berrios** is Consultant and University Lecturer in Neuropsychiatry at Addenbrooke's Hospital at the University of Cambridge. He has published ten books, including *The History of Mental Symptoms*, Cambridge, 1996 (British Medical Association 1997, First Prize, Mental Health).

**John R. Hodges** is Professor of Behavioural Neurology at the University of Cambridge Clinical School and MRC Cognition and Brain Sciences Unit. He has published widely on memory, dementia and cognitive assessment, and in 1998 was elected chairman of the British Neuropsychiatric Association.

# Memory disorders
## in psychiatric practice

Edited by

## German E. Berrios
Department of Psychiatry, University of Cambridge, UK

and

## John R. Hodges
MRC Cognition and Brain Sciences Unit, Cambridge, UK

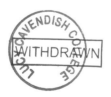

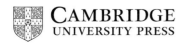

CAMBRIDGE
UNIVERSITY PRESS

PUBLISHED BY THE PRESS SYNDICATE OF THE UNIVERSITY OF CAMBRIDGE
The Pitt Building, Trumpington Street, Cambridge, United Kindom

CAMBRIDGE UNIVERSITY PRESS
The Edinburgh Building, Cambridge CB2 2RU, UK   http://www.cup.cam.ac.uk
40 West 20th Street, New York, NY 10011–4211, USA   http://www.cup.org
10 Stamford Road, Oakleigh, Melbourne 3166, Australia
Ruiz de Alarcón 13, 28014 Madrid, Spain

First published 2000

Printed in the United Kingdom at the University Press, Cambridge

*Typeface* Adobe Minion 10.5/14pt. *System* QuarkXPress™   [SE]

*A catalogue record for this book is available from the British Library*

*Library of Congress Cataloguing in Publication data*
Memory disorders in psychiatric practice
edited by German E. Berrios and John R. Hodges.
       p.      cm.
Includes index.
ISBN 0 521 57671 7 (pb)
1. Memory disorders. 2. Neuropsychiatry. I. Berrios, G.E.
II. Hodges, John R.
[DNLM:   1. Memory Disorders.   2. Amnesia.   3. Dementia.
4. Neuropsychology.   WM 173.7 M5326 2000]
RC394.M46M466   2000
616.8′4–dc21   99-32281 CIP
DNLM/DLC
for Library of Congress            5610207452

ISBN 0 521 57671 7 paperback

# Contents

# Contributors

David F. Allen
15 rue des Lions-St Paul, Paris 75004, France

Debra A. Bekerian
Department of Psychology, University of
East London, Romford Road, London
E15 4LZ, UK

German E. Berrios
Department of Psychiatry, University of
Cambridge, Box 189 Addenbrooke's
Hospital, Hills Road, Cambridge CB2 2QQ,
UK

Kristin Breen (deceased)
Department of Neurology, Addenbrooke's
Hospital, Hills Road, Cambridge CB2 2QQ,
UK

J. Douglas Bremner
Depart of Psychiatry, Yale University School
of Medicine, Yale Psychiatric Institute, Yale
Trauma Research Program, New Haven,
USA

Jennifer T. Coull
Wellcome Department of Cognitive
Neurology, Leopold Muller Functional
Imaging Laboratory, Institute of Neurology,
12 Queen Square, London WC1N 3BG, UK

Sally G. Cox
MRC Cognition and Brain Sciences Unit,
15 Chaucer Road, Cambridge CB2 2EF, UK

Tim Dalgleish
MRC Cognition and Brain Sciences Unit,
15 Chaucer Road, Cambridge CB2 2EF, UK

Ennio De Renzi
Clinica Neurologica, Via del Pozzo 71,
41100 Modena, Italy

Gabriel desRosiers
Oxford Memory Assessment Clinic, Radcliffe
Infirmary, University of Oxford, UK

Roger A. Dixon
Department of Psychology, University of
Victoria, Victoria, BC V8W 3P5, Canada

Jonathan J. Evans
Oliver Zangwill Centre for
Neuropsychological Rehabilitation, Ely,
Cambs, UK

Nestor Girala
L.A. de Herrera 272, Asuncion (CP1320),
Paraguay

Susan J. Goodrich
Department of Psychology, University of
East London, Romford Road, London
E15 4LZ, UK

John D.W. Greene
Neurology Department, Western General
Hospital, Crewe Road, Edinburgh RH4 2XU,
UK

**Adrian Grounds**
Forensic Psychiatry Service, Box 175, S3,
Psychiatric Outpatients, Addenbrooke's
Hospital, Cambridge CB2 2QQ, UK

**John R. Hodges**
MRC Cognition and Brain Sciences Unit, 15
Chaucer Road, Cambridge CB2 2EF, UK

**David G. Lamb**
Barrow Neurological Institute, 350 West
Thomas Road, Phoenix, AZ 85013, USA

**Keith Laws**
Department of Psychology, University of
Hertfordshire, Hatfield, Herts AL10 9AB, UK

**Ivana S. Marková**
Department of Psychiatry, University of Hull
HU10 6NS, UK

**Andrew R. Mayes**
University Department of Clinical
Neurology, Royal Hallamshire Hospital,
Glossop Road, Sheffield S10 2JF, UK

**A. Paula McKay**
Department of Psychiatry, The Adelaide
and Meath Hospital, Tallaght, Dublin 24,
Ireland

**Peter J. McKenna**
Fulbourn Hospital, Cambridge CB1 5EF, UK

**Jacques Postel**
8 rue de l'Alouette, 94160 Saint-Mandé,
France

**George P. Prigatano**
Barrow Neurological Institute, 350 West
Thomas Road, Phoenix, AZ 85013, USA

**Barbara J. Sahakian**
Department of Psychiatry, University of
Cambridge, Box 189, Addenbrooke's
Hospital, Hills Road, Cambridge CB2 2QQ,
UK

**Mauricio Sierra**
Robinson College, Grange Road, Cambridge
CB3 9AN, UK

**Herman N. Sno**
Department of Psychiatry, Ziekenhuis 'De
Heel', PO Box 210, 1500 EE Zaandam, The
Netherlands

**Bohdan Solomka**
Norvic Clinic, St Andrew's Business Park,
Thorpe, Norwich NR7 0HT, UK

**Eric Vermetten**
Department of Psychiatry, Yale University
School of Medicine, Yale Psychiatric
Institute, Yale Trauma Research Program,
184 Liberty Street, New Haven CT 06511,
USA

**Barbara A. Wilson, OBE**
MRC Cognition and Brain Sciences Unit,
Elsworth House, Box 58, Addenbrooke's
Hospital, Cambridge CB2 2QQ, UK

**Adam Zeman**
Neurology Department, Western General
Hospital, Crewe Road, Edinburgh RH4 2XU,
UK

# Preface

The recent appearance of many excellent books on memory (and its disorders) attests to the growing interest in this clinical field. Whether out of theoretical interest, or driven by shared social anxieties relating to a putative dementia 'epidemic', these publications concentrate on memory deficits arising in the context of brain disease. This emphasis may give the (wrong) impression that the investigation and management of patients complaining of poor memory are now the exclusive preserve of the neurologist and neuropsychologist.

Historical analysis helps us to understand how this state of affairs has come about. During the nineteenth century, memory complaints of all types (e.g. dysnomias, déjà vu, confabulation, the Ganserian state, paramnesias, etc.) were accepted at face value, i.e. regarded as genuine 'memory disorders'. However, after the 1880s the concept of memory (and its disorders) was narrowed down. Whilst undoubtedly benefiting the study of the 'organic' disorders of memory, this change cut asunder patients with a range of memory complaints including delusions and hallucinations of memory, déjà vu, the Ganserian state, etc. who, because they had 'negative investigations', were no longer considered as suffering from a 'memory problem'. Unfortunately, the concept of 'negative investigation' remains a relative one for it is determined by the sensitivity and specificity of the tests available in each historical period.

It is also the case that the (welcomed) collaboration between the new breed of cognitive neuropsychologists and clinicians has resulted in ever more refined clinical subgroups. Because some of these syndromes are dependent upon emerging concepts and complex psychometric profiles, their identification remains difficult, particularly in the busy environment of a neuropsychiatric clinic. Indeed, this may be one of the reasons for the reported increase in the number of 'Memory Clinics' that has taken place during the last 10 years.

The objective of this book is partly to redress the balance by taking the concept of 'memory complaint' seriously, irrespective of whether or not it is associated with dementia or other organic brain disorders. Hence, it dedicates much space to phenomena that until recently have been clinically disenfranchised. The idea has been to emphasize descriptive and conceptual aspects of a range of memory complaints and to reclaim for them a provisional place under the umbrella of the memory disorders. This has been done without prejudice to any future discoveries about their mechanisms as it is our hope that, in due course, *all* disorders of memory (whether the conventional 'organic ones' or those touched upon in this book) should be explained by the same mechanisms. This explains why we have also made sure that enough information on the 'organic disorders' has been included in this book.

The central message will be that there is also a 'psychiatric approach' to memory complaints. In this new domain the concepts, knowledge and therapeutic skills of psychiatrists and clinical psychologists should also play a central role. This view reflects our experience in running a Memory 'Complaints' Clinic rather than a Dementia Clinic. In this venue, we have examined many cases who, in spite of having 'normal' neurology and neuropsychology and being free from depression, still worry about their memory.

It is our view that these patients need as much clinical help as do the 'organic' patients. Treatment and management, however, depend upon their detailed study and on the identification of relevant subgroups; in this regard, two new clinical subgroups are reported here. This approach was also shared by Dr Kristin Breen, our neuropsychological partner in the Clinic. In January 1998, and at a young age, Kristin passed away and we still mourn her absence. Because this book is permeated by her views and spirit, we take the liberty of dedicating it to her.

G.E. Berrios and J.R. Hodges
Cambridge

# Part I

# Historical aspects of memory and its disorders

German E. Berrios

Historical analysis can contribute to the understanding of memory complaints and disorders (e.g. Burnham, 1888–89; Berrios, 1985a, 1990, 1992b, 1995; Bulbena & Berrios, 1986; Levin et al., 1983), particularly if it takes into account their *psychiatric dimension*. At a surface level, history may identify those current concepts that have developed out of the clinical observation of specific patients. At a deeper level, it can identify the theoretical and social frames within which those observations were made. In general, history will inform the memory researcher of the hidden conceptual stipulations (Edgell, 1924; Schacter, 1982; Simondon, 1982) governing the nosological status of phenomena such as fugues (Hacking, 1996), déjà vu (Berrios, 1995), and the 'memory failure' of schizophrenia (Rund, 1988; Kirkpatrick et al., 1986).

Using the criterion of 'amount of experimental work', Tulving (1983) called the period before Ebbinghaus the 'dark ages' in the history of memory.[1] In the same vein, Hacking (1995) proposed that 'the sciences of memory were new in the latter part of the nineteenth century' (p. 198) but as Murray (1976) has shown, memory and its disorders were in fact frequently discussed during and before this period.[2] Interestingly enough, these debates also focused on narratives style, laws of association, and content of memory,[3] features which until recently had been neglected. To be sure, 'models of memory' during these earlier periods are *different* from what Ebbinghaus (1885) was to propose towards the end of the century (e.g. Shakow, 1930; Postman, 1968; Caparrós, 1986), and from what Tulving (1983) would consider as 'scientific'.

In general, two approaches run parallel during this period: a quantitative one (as per Ebbinghaus) which has been well studied by historians and which, at the time, rarely influenced clinical practice; and a qualitative one, born out of (and used in) clinical observation. This chapter will only deal with the history of the latter, particularly with the contribution of nineteenth-century alienists.[4]

## Pre-nineteenth century

From earlier times, man's ability to conserve, retrieve (or lose!) information about himself and/or the world has been the subject of of wonder (Simondon, 1982; Carruthers, 1990; Geary, 1994). Classical writers identified two aspects of memory: 'conservation' and 'retrieval'. The former implied a 'three-dimensional space' associated with metaphors such as 'storing', 'containing', 'tracing' and 'engraving'. After Descartes, these spatial metaphors became grafted upon his concept of *res extensa* (extended substance) and therefrom the capacity to 'store or conserve' was explained in 'somatic or 'organic' rather than in psychological terms. On the other hand, the capacity to 'recollect' or 'retrieve' was figuratively described in terms of the action of 'looking for', 'searching' and 'recognizing'; from the start, this analogy demanded the associated presence of concepts such as self, intentionality, effortful activity, and duration.[5]

The metaphors of 'storing' and 'looking for' remain popular in Western writings on memory (Koriat & Goldsmith, 1996): for example, the 'sketch pad' analogy (Baddeley, 1986: p. 71) is a version of the space-metaphor; and the 'activity of the self' model is represented by the currently popular view that memory is about searching, reconstructing and 'narrating'.[6] A crucial question for the conceptual historian is whether these two ancient metaphors still retain some heuristic capacity (Hesse, 1966) or must be replaced.

## Classical models and metaphors

### Aristotle

References to aspects of 'memory' can be found in the Old Testament, the Babylonian Talmud, and Hesiod's Theogony.[7] However, it was Aristotle who, by distinguishing 'conservation' (*mneme*) from 'recollection' (*anamnesis*),[8] set the conceptual agenda:

Memory of the object of thought implies a mental picture. Hence it would seem to belong incidentally to the thinking faculty, but essentially to the primary sense-faculty. Hence memory (*mneme*) is found not only in man and beings which are capable of opinion and thought, but also in some other animals . . . (Aristotle, 1908: p. 293).

Recollection, on the other hand, can only be a human activity for it required awareness and logical thought.[9]

Some of Aristotle's assertions are clinically meaningful; for example, when dealing with the 'referential' aspects of the mental act involved in 'recollection', he states:

if there is in us something like an impression or picture, why should the perception of just this be memory of something else and not of itself? For when one exercises his memory this affection is what he considers and perceives. How then does he remember what is not present? This would imply that one can also see and hear what is not present. But surely in a sense this can and does occur. Just as the picture painted on the panel is at once a picture and a portrait, and though one and the same, is both, yet the essence of the two is not the same, and it is possible to think of it both as a picture and as a portrait, so in the same way we must regard the mental picture within us both as an object of contemplation in itself and as a mental picture of something else . . . (p. 297).

Aristotle also analysed the 'awareness' involved in the recollection process, i.e. how does one know that a given mental content is a memory and not something experienced for the first time?:

sometimes we do not know, when such stimuli occur in our soul from an earlier sensation, and we are in doubt whether it is memory or not. But sometimes it happens that we reflect and remember that we have heard or seen this something before. Now, this occurs whenever we first think of it as itself, and then change and think of it as referring to something else . . . (p. 297).

Aristotle's effort to differentiate between the experience itself and the factors required to convert it into a memory, is reflected in the popular nineteenth-century view that déjà vu and confabulation were 'first-time experiences' which, due to the presence of an anomalous 'memory-converting' factor, were mistaken for 'real' memories.[10] Aristotle (1908) might have been partially based on clinical observation:

The opposite also occurs, as happened to Antiphenon of Oreus, and other deranged people (*egistamenois*); for they spoke of their mental pictures (*fantasmata*) as if they had actually taken place, and as if they actually remembered them . . . (p. 297).

Whether Aristotle is referring here to hallucinatory experiences or to delusions of memory (déjà vu) is difficult to tell, although the drift of the text suggests that it was the latter. Lastly, the Greek philosopher also dealt with the mechanisms that facilitate recollection, and in doing so he managed to formulate the 'laws of association'.

## Augustine and medieval views

Together with *Intellectus* and *Voluntas*, *Memoria* was for Augustine,[11] a 'faculty of the soul'. It also was the repository of archetypal ideas and information that made man the carrier of divine truths. In fact, it contained all the ordinary data of experience including the epistemological matrix of all knowledge. Echoes of this Platonic view reappeared in Descartes, and later in Jung.

There were three Medieval concerns on the nature of memory: was it a *sense* or a faculty? How valid was its division into intellective and sensitive? Where was it located in the brain? The first two questions intended to reconcile Platonic and Aristotelian views. For example, St Bonaventure's solution is typical for the period:

Memory has three meanings: (a) faculty that receives and stores sensations from the past, (b) faculty that receives and stores intelligible things, and (c) it preserves intelligible things in an abstract manner which is independent from time markers, that is, it can be considered as a faculty dealing with innate intelligible forms (quoted in Wéber, 1990: p. 1591).

with regard to localization, Bernard of Gordon's views are representative: '[disorders of memory] result from corruption of the posterior part of the brain . . . and that forgetting sometimes occurs in madness' (Gordon, 1495: Chapter xiii, p. jiij). More than a century later, Father Thomas Wright (1630) was still asking:

How we remember? In what part of the braine resideth the formes fit for memory? How we forget? What helpeth and hindereth Memory, and by what manner? Why doth memory faile in old men? How can possibly be conserved, without confusion, such an infinite number of formes in the Soule . . .? (p. 304).

### Descartes

As Hall (1972) has rightly commented: 'Historically, Descartes's theory [of memory] may be understood as a corpuscularized version of explanations set forth by Scholastic philosophers and Renaissance anatomists who in turn had elaborated Greek ideas' (p. 88). The Cartesian version entailed a 'physiological' account in terms of which memory was a 'fifth' stage in cognition (the first four were 'object, retinal image, brain lining, and spirits leaving the gland'):

thus when the soul desires to recollect something, this desire causes the gland, by inclining successively to different sides, to thrust the spirits towards different parts of the brain until they come across that part where the traces left there by the object which we wish to recollect are found; for these traces are none other than the fact that the pores of the brain, by which the spirits have formerly followed their course because of the presence of this object, have by that means acquired a greater facility than the others in being once more opened by the animal spirits which come towards them in the same way . . .' (Descartes, 1967: p. 350).

Thus, for Descartes, the laying down of memory traces was *not* a passive act; hence recall could improve with repetition. As far as the traditional question of the relationship between memory and sensitive and intellective forms was concerned, Descartes distinguished between 'the recall of universals which is a function of intellectual memory, and the recall of particulars which is a function of corporeal memory' (Clarke, 1982: p. 29).

Locke

Returning to Aristotelian associationism, John Locke (1959) suggested mechanisms redolent of what is called 'semantic processing' and 'time-tagging': 'this laying down of our ideas in the repository of memory signifies no more than this, that the mind has a power in many cases to revive perceptions which it once had, with this additional perception annexed to them, that it has had them before' (Book II, Chapter X). Locke also felt that emotions helped to fix the ideas in the mind, but was ambivalent about the mechanisms involved in the laying down of memory traces. Indeed, on occasions it does seem as if he resorts to the Cartesian explanation.[12] English writers of the eighteenth century, such as David Hartley (1834), kept alive the physiological explanation, and it is by this channel that it arrived into the nineteenth century.

## The nineteenth century

During the early nineteenth century, French philosophy of mind is best represented in the work of Laromiguière[13] and Royer-Collard[14] who believed that memories had first to be entertained in consciousness: 'the objects of consciousness are the only objects of memory. Properly speaking, we never remember anything but the operations and diverse states of our minds . . .' (Janet & Séailles, 1902: p. 158). This view was taken up by Gratacap (1866) and Ravaisson (1885) who developed Laromiguière's 'active' model of the mind. Echoes of this view, combined with the English ideas that he so much admired, can be found in Ribot (Gasser, 1988).

Virey (1819) defined memory as: 'the faculty that conserves in the spirit the impressions and images of objects obtained via sensations, and that recollects these impressions in the absence of the object . . .' (p. 278); according to this French writer, amnesia resulted from drunkenness and sexual abuse. Louyer-Willermay (1819) subdivided both dysmnesia and amnesia into idiopathic (independent from any known cause) and symptomatic (secondary to another disease) (p. 303); most importantly, he described the 'law of regression', later attributed to Ribot,[15] and proposed that in the elderly the typical memory deficit was forgetting of recent events and a good recollection of remote ones (p. 307). His views survived in the work of Bouillaud (1829) and Falret (1865).

Views on memory in England were inspired by associationism, as can be seen in the work of Fearn, Mill and Bain. Fearn (1812) wrote:

if we remember a thing brought in by association, this affection is, notoriously, forced upon us; but, if we try to recollect a thing, we will to put ourselves in this and that mood, or posture of thought, until at length the thing strike us by the medium of association (p. 277).

Nonetheless, like Descartes he believed that an act of specific attention was needed for memories to be laid down in the first place (p. 274). James Mill (1869), in turn, wrote: 'In memory there are ideas, and those ideas both rise up singly, and are connected in trains by association' (p. 328). His once secretary, Alexander Bain (1874) expressed a more physiological view: 'for every act of memory, every exercise of bodily aptitude, every habit, recollection, train of ideas, there is a specific grouping, or co-ordination, of sensations and movements, by virtue of specific growths in the cell junctions' (p. 91). After the middle of the century, this mechanistic model was reinterpreted in evolutionary terms, first by Herbert Spencer (1890), and then Lewes (1877) and Hughlings Jackson.[16]

## Hering and 'organic memory'

Under the influence of Evolution theory, views on memory began to change after the 1870s. For example, this is the case of Hering (1870), who in his seminal lecture 'Memory as a universal function of organized matter' (delivered before the Imperial Academy of Science at Vienna in 1870) made two crucial points: (a) 'memory is a function of brain substance whose results, it is true, fall as regards one part of them into the domain of consciousness, while another part escapes unperceived as purely material processes . . .'; and (b) 'we have ample evidence of the fact that characteristics of an organism may descend to offspring which the organism did not inherit, but which it acquired owing to the special circumstances under which it lived . . . an organized being, therefore, stands before us a product of the unconscious memory of organized matter . . .'. These views influenced Ribot (Gasser, 1988), Freud (Otis, 1993), Semon (Schacter et al., 1978) and others interested in the concepts of 'engram' (Gomulicki, 1953; Schacter, 1982) and of organic memory (Augier, 1939). Thus, Hering not only developed the view that matter (brain sites) are important to memory but also introduced a Lamarckian mechanism (Lamarck, 1984; Jordanova, 1984).

The timing of the Vienna lecture was right: both evolutionary theory (Mayr, 1982) and degenerationism (Génil-Perrin, 1913; Saury, 1886; Talbot, 1898; Thompson, 1908) were in need of a mechanism to explain how new information might be incorporated into the genetic make-up of a species (Ribot, 1906). Hering's views were not lost to those working in the field of memory: nature had provided brain sites for memory, and these needed investigating. Encouraged by the view, popular at the time, that disease was a natural laboratory to investigate how healthy mechanisms break down, soon enough all manner of psychiatric patients were investigated for memory deficits.

In 1880, Samuel Butler published his 'Unconscious Memory' including a translation of Hering's lecture. Not everyone agreed, however, with the extrapolations he suggested and in a scathing review, Romanes (1880) said:

This view, in which Mr Butler was anticipated by Prof. Hering, is interesting if advanced merely as an illustration; but to imagine that it reveals any truth of profound significance, or that it can possibly be fraught with any benefit to science, is simply absurd.

### Ribot, Paulhan and Bergson

During the 1880s, two great French psychologists contributed to the development of the notion of 'organic' memory. In the first edition of his *Disorders of Memory*, Ribot (1882), the best known of the two, included a chapter on 'memory as a biological fact'.[17] He inspired many. For example, Richet's (1886) views on the origins and modalities of memory, on its organic basis, and on the distinction between memory of 'fixation' and 'evocation'; to these, van Biervliet (1902) added a third type, 'memory of identification'. The 'organic' view continued well into the twentieth century in the work of Piéron (1910), Dugas (1915, 1917), Semon (1908, 1909),[18] and Rignano (1926).

Criticizing the 'intellectualistic' approach, Frédéric Paulhan (1904) emphasized affectivity, as expressed in his great book on 'affective or emotional memory'. By the latter he meant traces or footprints 'left in the spirit by sentiments' (p. 5) for 'an emotion may leave on the spirit traces which will not show themselves as emotional acts but as phenomena which are unconscious, automatic, and intellectual ...' (p. 6). On this he was following Ribot's (1896) *Psychologie des Sentiments* where the great French psychologist had dedicated a chapter to 'la mémoire affective'. This was harshly criticized by Titchener (1895) who challenged Ribot to offer one example of 'pure' affective memory in which the emotion be revived 'as such'.[19]

Although not a psychologist, Henri Bergson's views on memory were important for a generation.[20] He distinguished two types: one consisting of sensory mechanisms or habits fixed in the body of the organism and common to all animals; the other, or 'pure memory' was only possessed by man, registering the multitude of images that was his life. Confronted with the argument that it would be uneconomical to store a separate image for each variation, he accepted the view that memory traces needed to be written onto the brain in a 'schematic form'. The brain was not a mechanism for remembering but for forgetting, for otherwise all memories would appear at the same time; in the human, the role of memory mechanisms was to direct him to the future (Bergson, 1911).

### Janet, Williams and Wundt

The latter part of the nineteenth century is well endowed with writers on memory.[21] For example, Pierre Janet (1889) suggested that studying memory changes in sleepwalkers threw light on psychological function in general (pp. 83–145). Events occurring during sleepwalking might not be recollected during wakefulness but were retrieved in the next sleepwalking episode. This was due to

the fact that memories were associated (as in state-dependent learning) to particular levels of awareness (Vincent & Boucharlat, 1989). Janet (1909) also dealt with
hysterical amnesia (pp. 39–63); and later with the relationship between time and
memory (Janet, 1928).

William James (Feinstein, 1984; Perry, 1936) differentiated between 'primary'
(or sensory) and 'secondary' or 'memory proper'. The latter was 'the knowledge of
a former state of mind after it has already once dropped from consciousness; or
rather it is the knowledge of an event, or fact, of which meantime we have not been
thinking, with the additional consciousness that we have thought or experienced
before' (James, 1890: p. 648). Memories were not only carried in a 'dating of the
fact in the past. It must be dated in my past' (p. 650). Both retention and reminiscence were based on the 'law of habit in the nervous system, working as it does in
the "association of ideas"' (p. 653). Hence 'being altogether conditioned on brain-
paths, its excellence in a given individual will depend partly on the number and
partly on the persistence of these paths' (p. 659). James agreed with Ebbinghaus'
efforts to measure verbal memory, and believed that aphasia was a good example
of memory loss.

Wilhelm Wundt (1897) considered memory as a 'complex intellectual function':
'various different functions connected with the process of recognition and
remembering are all included under the name "memory". This concept, of course,
does not refer to any unitary force, as faculty-psychology has assumed . . .' (pp.
224–47). Wundt used the term memory infrequently and his broader 'cognitive
approach' differed from that propounded by Ebbinghaus. As Scheerer (1980) has
stated: '[this] should [make] him more attractive to modern theorists'.

## Ebbinghaus and measurement

The evaluation of clinical cases required measuring instruments; the problem then
was that it was not altogether clear whether tests developed for the study of
memory in 'normal subjects' were of use in disease. In medicine, the view that the
normal and the pathological were discontinuous was already popular during the
middle of the nineteenth century (Canguilhem, 1966), and led to a 'two-tier'
psychometric tradition (Bondy, 1974), namely, special instruments were created
to measure certain functions in disease. However, Hering's view that in the field of
memory there seemed to be a continuity, led to the use of tests for normals in the
clinical population.

Testing subjects with 'memory' disorders, however, was a sobering experience
in that many simply did not fit into the then conventional 'one-storage' model of
memory put forward by Ebbinghaus and others. The understanding of paramnesia, false recognition, déjà vu, confabulation, delusions of memory, and some
specific amnesic syndromes (the sort of phenomena described by Kraepelin,

1886–87; Pick, 1903; Bernard-Leroy, 1898; Lalande, 1893; Dugas, 1894a, b; Korsakoff, 1889; Rouillard, 1885, etc.) required more than a 'retention mechanism'. Their irreducibility to simple memories caused, at the time, theoretical consternation.

On the other hand, there were also mnestic clinical phenomena amenable to conventional analysis, and one of these was the memory deficit of dementia. Noticing this, Ribot (1882) soon used dementia to illustrate the working of his 'law of dissolution' (first described, in fact, by Louyer-Willermay, 1819): 'to discover this law it is essential that the progress of dementia should be studied from a psychological viewpoint' (p. 117). Ribot decided to deal with dementia as a 'syndrome', regardless of aetiology: 'physicians distinguish between different kinds of dementia according to causes, classing them as senile, paralytic, epileptic, etc. These distinctions have no interest to us. The progress of mental dissolution is at bottom the same . . .' (p. 117). This view is typical for the period. In England, Shaw (1892) stated 'sometimes the existence of dementia is only shown by loss of memory or loss of energy and there are no positive signs of acute disturbance . . .' (p. 348). The testing of memory, however, depended upon the making of certain assumptions to be discussed presently.

Memory testing à la Ebbinghaus (1885), Bourdon (1894) or Jung (1905) was based on the assumption that quantification captured more information than qualification. That by the turn of the century this view felt reasonable, suggests that certain conceptual changes had already taken place; one such had been brought about by the psychophysical approach of Weber and Fechner, the measuring of audition by Hering, and of reaction times by Donders.[22] On the other hand, the quantification of psychological events was not welcomed by everyone, and it formed part of the célèbre debate between Dilthey[23] (1976) and Ebbinghaus (Caparrós, 1986: pp. 177–205).

In his history of mental testing, Kimball Young (1923) identified four quantificatory strands in nineteenth-century psychology: psychophysics, the study of difference limens, and mental and physiological measurement. As acknowledged by Ebbinghaus (1885), all strands are reflected in the measurement of memory:

in the realm of mental phenomena, experiment and measurement have hitherto been chiefly limited in application to sense perception and to the time relations of mental processes . . . we have tried to go a step further into the workings of the mind and to submit to an experimental and quantitative treatment the manifestations of memory . . ..

Analysis of the large arrays of numbers generated by the new measurements required the help of statistical techniques that were not available at the time. Ebbinghaus (1885) was aware of this and had to make do with using 'constant averages', 'the law of errors', and 'probable error'. He, in fact, believed that 'mental events' were beyond the reach of quantification: 'the persistent flux and change-ability of mental events do not admit of the establishment of stable experimental conditions' . . . 'psychological processes are not susceptible to measurement and enumeration'. Hence he used proxy variables such as 'time and number of repetitions' of nonsense syllables given to subjects to learn.

## Social frames

To a large extent, research into memory remains governed by the categories of 'mneme' and 'anamnesis'. During the late nineteenth century, the former encour-aged a quantitative and mechanistic approach whose testing techniques (e.g. the memorizing of nonsense syllables as per Ebbinghaus) became gradually discon-nected from real life situations. However, 'anamnesis' was meant to deal with 'rec-ollecting the past' and with what nowadays might be called 'every day or real world memories' (Cohen, 1996). The mnestic complaints on the basis of which nine-teenth-century alienists built the clinical sciences of memory pertained to failures of anamnesis. This explains why the clinical study of amnesia, hypermnesia, dysm-nesia and paramnesia often required that social and psychological context be taken into account. Psychoanalysis was to follow a similar approach which, by assuming that everything was stored, made memory disorders into problems of selective for-getting.

Fin de siècle redefinitions of concepts such as 'faculty', 'consciousness', and 'introspection', and of views on how thought and language were related, led to changes in the very notions of 'recollection' and 'memory'. A group of French writers working at Strasbourg was particularly creative in this respect, and their ideas, neglected for more than 50 years, have recently been rediscovered. There is space here only for the briefest of accounts of their achievements.

### Blondel, Halbwachs and 'La mémoire collective'

The view that remembering cannot take place, let alone be studied, independently from the social frames within which it occurs was developed by two great French scientists, Charles Blondel (1876–1939)[24] and Maurice Halbwachs (1877–1944).[25] Both *Normaliens*, their paths crossed again at the University of Strasbourg where they became professors of experimental psychology and sociology, respectively; and where they joined Marc Bloch, the historian. At their famous 'Saturday sem-inars', the group regularly exchanged ideas so that it is difficult to decide on the paternity of the latter. For example, with regard to the notion of 'collective memory' there seems to be no problem with the view that Halbwachs (1925) developed it first in his book *Les Cadres Sociaux de la Mémoire*.[26] However, if the view that consciousness itself is determined by social frames is taken to be the parent idea, then Blondel's (1914) early book *La Conscience Morbide* has a crucial role to play. And the same can be said of the very idea of *la conscience collective* which, although attributed to Durkheim, can be traced back to the beginning of the nineteenth century (Brunschvicq, 1927: pp. 565–81).[27]

Conceptual frames, determined by a common culture (expressed in language, images and other communication devices and social practices)[28] are internalized by members of the collective, so that their perception of the world becomes homogeneously shared, and their view of themselves tends to revolve around what is general to the culture inhibiting what is personal in their lives.[29] Memory, particularly the remembering of one's past (autobiographical memory), is the domain where this shaping influence is at its strongest. So much so that personal memories can be said to be a biased 'reconstruction':

The individual calls recollections to mind by relying on the frameworks of social memory. In other words, the various groups that compose society are capable at every moment of reconstructing their past. But, as we have seen, they most frequently distort the past in the act of reconstructing it. There are surely many facts, and many details of certain facts, that the individual would forget if others did not keep their memory alive for him' (Halbwachs, 1925: p. 391).

However, for the psychiatrist working in a memory clinic, the issue remains what does this all mean in regards to specific patients? Blondel, a clinician himself, developed a less *au outrance* version. Self-narratives about the past are constituted by 'memories proper' and by 'inferred knowledge'. The former included spontaneous recollections, usually accompanied by a feeling of participation and familiarity; the latter information about ourselves learned from all sources or inferred from the regularities of our lives (Blondel, 1928a: pp. 152–3). However, these two databases are inert without 'social frames', i.e. without the application of maps to determine their spatial organization, time sequencing, semantic hierarchization, etc.[30] These frames are borrowed mostly 'ready-made' from the culture we live in and carry fixed interpretations of events, calendars, etc. Furthermore, each period of our life is governed by different frames and these may well be stored together with the 'original pictures' of our experiences. But when as adults we are asked to narrate events from our childhood: which frame are we to use? The fact that often enough we reframe the 'original pictures' leads to interesting feelings of dissonance particularly when we revisit the haunts of childhood and feel strangely disappointed about the size and beauty of the original components of their landscape.[31]

Blondel's approach is also helpful with regard to patients who after losing a dominant relative seem unable to organize their own 'original pictures' in any meaningful sense, and who often perceive this failure as a 'memory problem'. It is likely that, in a subset of the latter, the pathology may not be in the storing or retrieval of 'the original pictures' but in the fact that they lack in 'social frames', or are unable to make use of those available.[32]

## Janet and Bartlett

Three years after Halbwachs' book, Pierre Janet (1928) published a set of lecture-notes[33] where he conceived of memory as a general mental function adapted to deal with 'remoteness and absence' (p. 233). The natural medium of memory was the *récit* (the narrative): 'in the description we have the illusion that objects continue to exist' (p. 245). [but] . . . 'the narrative does not guarantee that we will recover the object' (p. 247) . . . 'the first act of memory, its point of departure, is the moment when the act is fabricated' (p. 255) . . . 'I would like to say a word on one essential feature of remembering . . . its objective is that of getting the interlocutor to experience the feelings that he would have experienced had he been present at the original event' (p. 270). Janet sees this narrative capacity as the expression of a primitive fabulative function.[34] Although subscribing to a type of 'reconstruction hypothesis', Janet said little about the social frames of memory, and not uncharacteristically, he refrained from mentioning Halbwachs. If anything, he seemed to disagree with Blondel's view that psychosis results from the rebellion of the personal, idiosyncratic language of coenesthesia against the official language of collective consciousness (pp. 461–2).

In his chapter on 'requirements of a theory of social recall', Bartlett (1932) commented upon Janet's 'persuasive and attractive manner' but hastened to say that any similarity between that and his own views was coincidental for 'he had completed this part of [my] study before Janet's volumes appeared' (footnote, p. 293). In the same chapter, Bartlett seemed to accept Halbwachs's views 'certainly most of these remarks, in so far as it is possible to give them clear significance, seem both true and important' (p. 296). But then writes: 'yet [Halbwachs] is still treating only of memory in the group, and not of memory of the group. As to former, there need be no dispute whatsoever . . . but we need to go far beyond this if we are to show that the social group itself possesses a capacity to retain and recall its own past' (p. 296). It is not clear what the criticism is here for neither Halbwachs, Blondel nor Durkheim purported to reify the social object to the point that, by collective memory, they mean some external entity which has its own memory system.

Interesting is also the way in which Bartlett's notion of 'schemata' has been understood (or re-interpreted) by his followers. Whilst Bartlett (1932) himself seemed to admit that Halbwachs had been at least an inspiration: 'more over this persistent framework [the social frames] helps to provide those *schemata* which are a basis for the imaginative reconstruction called memory' (p. 296), Oldfield and Zangwill (1942) agonized over where Bartlett had got the idea from but surprisingly do not mention Blondel, Janet or Halbwachs. All they could say was: 'it is evident that Bartlett's conception [of schemata] differs from that of Head in a number of respects. Indeed, it might reasonably be said that little has been taken over from Head except the general principle' (p. 116).

## Clinical disorders of memory

### The early nineteenth century

A paucity of specific publications on memory disorders during this period suggests that they did not occupy the forefront of clinical interest. However, matter of fact descriptions can be found incorporated in clinical writings dealing with other diseases. Theorizing on what these cases meant or had in common started after the 1840s, when a theory of memory emerged out of clinical observation. This view, unsurprisingly, was not at one with what philosophical psychologists such as Mill, Hamilton, Cousin or Garnier thought of the nature of memory.

#### Landre-Beauvais and semiology

'Semiology', the science of the signs and symptoms of disease was born in medicine at the beginning of the century, and reached psychiatry (as a descriptive psychopathology) by the 1840s (Berrios, 1996). By 1813, the leading book on medical semiology already included commentaries on memory: 'amongst the early signs of delirium one finds agitation and lesions of memory' (Landre-Beauvais, 1813: p. 284). This author also referred to memory loss in the context of lethargy:

The suspension or abolition of the intellectual faculties is often manifested in a total or partial loss of memory . . . when this occurs during the acute stage of the disease, is a prodromal sign of delirium; but when delirium does not follow, the danger is even greater as the memory loss may herald a paralysis of some segment of the body . . . when after a serious disease, memory does not improve, the damage may become permanent (p. 294).

This is a good example of memory complaints becoming prima facie parts of a universe of medical signs; indeed, other mental symptoms such as hallucinations, anxiety, etc., were similarly handled during this period (Berrios, 1996).

#### Rush, Prichard and Holland

Influenced by his teacher William Cullen, Benjamin Rush (1812) considered 'Derangement of Memory' as a separate 'disease' that included the 'oblivion of names, vocables, sounds, mode of spelling, qualities or number of most familiar objects, and of events in time and space (often of the most recent)'. 'Corporeal' causes of oblivion included 'intemperance in eating and drinking, excess in venery, fevers, vertigo, apoplexy, brain lesions, and the use of snuff'; and 'grief, terror, oppressing the memory in early life with studies disproportionate to its strength, and undue exercise of memory or its neglect' were the main 'mental' causes. To improve memory, Rush recommended hygienic techniques based on association psychology (pp. 276–90).

Prichard (1835) distinguished four stages in the evolution of dementia: [loss of] memory, reasoning, comprehension and voluntary action. The first one was characterized by 'forgetfulness of recent impressions, while the memory retains comparative firm hold of ideas laid up in the recesses from times long past . . .' (p. 89). His contemporary Esquirol (1838), however, showed little interest in this field and only in passim, mentions memory deficits in mental handicap and dementia: 'many of those in dementia have lost their memories for information relevant to their lives. Particularly the faculty of recollecting impressions recently obtained . . .' (p. 220).

Sir Henry Holland (1852) put it differently:

the processes of memory, indeed, are performed by association, and depend on suggestion; but neither of these terms, in their ordinary use, express all that we mean even by simply memory, still less denote the higher power of recollection . . . for our present purpose we need nothing more than the simple expression of certain assured facts; – viz., that there is a faculty of our mental constitution, by which the successive states of mind passed through, whether of perception or thought, leave impressions behind of more or less clearness and persistence . . . (p. 150).

Holland also pointed out that, in insanity, there tends to be a loss of memory for the episode of illness, and that memory is affected by age, partly because it 'may arise from too feeble circulation through the brain' or excitement and fatigue; likewise 'the natural decay of memory in old age, though not in any obvious proportion to the decline of those powers which connect us more directly with the external world, must be admitted as a fact in our mental constitution . . .' In this age group 'the capacity for receiving and fixing impressions appears, indeed, to decline sooner than the power of recalling and using those formerly received . . .' (Holland, 1852: p. 165).

Holland's views were more organized than any expressed by Forbes Winslow (1861) who in five chapters on the psychology and pathology of memory in his book *On Obscure Diseases of the Brain and Disorders of the Mind* lists many cases of dementia, déjà vu, transient global amnesia, etc. without drawing any theoretical conclusions.

## Feuchtersleben and Griesinger

Quoting Kant, Feuchtersleben (1847) marvelled at the faculty of memory: 'the most wonderful of all powers of the human mind' (p. 121), and called into question Locke's memory mechanism: 'it is at once self-evident that the notion of a tabula rasa, which is by degrees written all over, is not tenable'. Likewise, influenced by phrenology, the Austrian nobleman believed that: '(a) Memory in man was in direct proportion to the size of the healthy brain, (b) memory increased and decreased with the consistency of the medullary substance [white matter] of the brain, from childhood to old age, and (c) memory was improved or impaired in proportion as the cerebral vitality is improved or impaired' (p. 121).

Feuchtersleben recognized four types of memory disorder: (a) 'unusually heightened memory (hypermnesia) . . .' (b) a morbidly weakened memory (dysmnesia) . . ., (c) an altered memory manifesting itself by the perverted manner of remembering . . . certain phantasms of the memory are to be referred to this head; for instance, when a person feels as if a situation in which he actually finds himself had already existed at some former time . . ., and (d) a relatively diseased memory, metaphorically called 'partially' diseased or lost' . . .' (p. 237). Amnesia and senile loss of memory were included under heading (b), and the aphasias under heading (c) which also contained all manner of 'psychiatric' memory disorders such as delusions of memory and déjà vu (thus baptised by the French towards the end of the nineteenth century).[35] Feuchtersleben also believed that the causes of 'diseased memory were psychical or physical'.

Far more theoretical was Griesinger (1867) who wrote: 'The more intimate proceedings of this process of reproduction are obscure, and quite incomprehensible; old ideas suddenly arise without any origin' . . . 'any disease of the brain may impair or destroy memory, consequently the state of memory, in many of the insane, indicates the severity of their malady' (p. 32). Griesinger made here the important point that memory was not specifically localized on any one part of the brain:

The examples of quite partial loss of memory, so frequently the result of wounds or diseases of the brain, in which one might infer the loss of the apparatus devoted to a particular class of ideas, appear in reality to be more general in their effects than might at first be supposed . . . (p. 32).

(This point was to be made repeatedly around this period, see Maury, 1878: p. 445.) Griesinger (1867) recognized the disorders of memory characteristic of dementia, insanity (melancholia and mania); and following the mood of his period also considered neologisms and language deficits as memory deficits (pp. 68–70).[36]

## The second half of the nineteenth century

### The concept of amnesia

The term *amnesia* is already present in the medical language of the early nineteenth century.[37] Throughout the century, clinicians were interested to know whether patients with 'vesania' (i.e. psychoses not accompanied by demonstrable brain lesions) did also suffer from memory impairment. For example, Baret (1887) concluded that only some severe forms of melancholia were accompanied by memory deficit. Kirchhoff (1893), on the other hand, suggested that 'the insane exhibit notable disturbances in the truth of their memories; as the mood of the moment exercises the greatest influence on the manner in which memory-pictures are conceived, a falsification of the previous impressions is thus produced' (p. 82). (For a historical study of the relationship between melancholia, mood and memory disorders see Berrios, 1985b.) The terms 'anterograde' and 'retrograde', however, only came into currency at the end of the nineteenth century.[38]

*Falret and Ribot*

Jules Falret (1865) was a well-known alienist. Written from a medical viewpoint, his work on amnesia offers one of the best accounts of the disorder available at the division of the century. There is no space here to summarize it in any detail. It shows, however, that even during this period the term and concept of 'amnesia' still had a descriptive function and made no assumptions as to duration, aetiology or reversibility. In very general terms, Falret distinguished between 'physical' and 'psychological' causes of amnesia, and between 'general' and 'partial' forms. He also offered a rich collection of clinical observations where the modern neuro-psychiatrist will find an antecedent for recently described syndromes including transient global amnesia (p. 729), acute intoxication with anti-cholinergics (p. 736), senile dementia (p. 733), and state-dependent learning (p. 735).

By the second half of the nineteenth century, 'disorders of memory' had become a popular topic of research. In this, Ribot (1882) played an important role although his oft-quoted book is not a straightforward one. After dwelling on Hering's ideas, Ribot divided mnestic disorders into 'amnesia', 'partial amnesia', and 'exaltations of memory'. He conceived of 'diseases of memory as morbid psychical states' dividable into those 'limited to a single category of recollections' [partial] and those affecting 'the entire memory in all its forms' [general] (p. 70). Whether general or partial, amnesia must be divided into temporary, periodical, progressive and congenital. Memory deficits were caused by all manner of things, for example, epilepsy gave rise to a 'typical form' of temporary amnesia; senile dementia and cerebral haemorrhage caused progressive forms of amnesia; congenital amnesias were seen in the idiot and cretin; and the so-called phenomenon of 'double consciousness' (à la Azam),[39] was his best example of 'periodic amnesia'. After Falret and Ribot, and towards the turn of the century, books on specific memory disorders such as the paramnesias began to appear.[40]

The paramnesias

> For a history of these disorders see Chapter 14: 'Paramnesias and delusions of memory', this volume.

> *Déjà vu*
>
> For the history of this disorder see Chapter 15, 'Déjà vu and jamais vu', this volume.

> *Confabulations*
>
> For the history of these disorders, see Chapter 16, 'Confabulations', this volume.

> *Fugues and other transient amnesias*
>
> Up to the division of the nineteenth century, it was assumed that memory disorders, including those that improved, had a general 'organic' basis. The view that some were, in fact, 'functional' resulted from conceptual changes that occurred after the 1880s, inter alia, the softening in the medical definition of 'lesion', Charcot's interest in the 'functional', the growing importance of hypnosis, and the acceptance of 'non-conscious' and 'automatic' psychological mechanisms.
>
> Odd behavioural phenomena such as 'multiple personalities' (Hacking, 1995), the 'wandering behaviour' of some vagrants (Meige, 1893), and cases of transient and total loss of autobiographical memory were also medicalized during this period, and soon enough discussed in the context of the memory disorders. By the 1890s, the latter or 'fugue states' had been subdivided, and their core symptoms actively sought for. [41] Psychoanalysis contributed to their understanding with the mechanisms of 'repression' and 'dissociation', and ensured their survival to the present (see interesting study by van der Hart, 1985). In this sense, the claim that 'vagrancy as an issue passed from view by 1910, and fugue with it' (Hacking, 1996: p. 448) is inaccurate. Indeed, fugue states are regularly seen in clinical practice, and still pose an aetiological conundrum.[42] In this regard, the historian must offer an account of the process by which 'fugue states' 'converged' as a medical entity.[43]

Early history

> Descriptions of behaviours redolent of 'fugue states' can be found since early in the medical literature of the nineteenth century. For example, Aubanel (1851) reported the case of a patient with neurosyphilis who used to escape in a 'bewildered state'. The term 'fugue' seems to have been first used by Lasègue (1868) to describe the dreamy, hallucinatory state of an alcoholic subject. In an important monograph, Foville (1875) reported 14 cases of psychotic subjects with a tendency to travel or wander away from home (les aliénés voyageurs ou migrateurs) (for this concept see also Tissié, 1887); chronically deluded and hallucinated, some also

exhibited depressive features which he classified as 'Lypémanie'. It would seem, however, that no one wandered off in a state of autobiographical amnesia. Foville made it clear that they did not constitute a separate group of psychotics but just a subset of psychotic depressives whose hallucinations and delusions caused their travelling. Luys (1881) reported a subject with a 'fugue-like state lasting four days'; and Motet (1886) another with similar behaviour after a fall. These, and other similar cases reported before 1888, concern patients who, in the wake of an organic disorder, and whilst confused, wandered off for varied periods of time. [44]

In his 'Tuesday Lectures', Charcot (1987) presented the case of a 37-year-old epileptic with 'wandering' behaviour. Calling it 'somnambulism', Charcot classified these behaviours into primary, post-hypnotic and 'hysterical', thereby suggesting that not all 'automatisms' were epileptic (comital). Charcot also described at length the case of Klein, a 23-year-old Hungarian Jew, who after criss-crossing Europe was admitted into La Salpêtrière on 11 December 1888, and four other cases of 'wandering Jews'.[45] A year later, Voisin (1889) reported a case of 'hysterical' (as opposed to epileptic) automatism; and in the year of Charcot's death, Meige (1893) published his famous monograph on the 'wandering Jew'.

Régis (1906) coined the term 'dromomanie' to refer to a 'general impulse to wandering' seen in various forms of mental illness. Therefore, Raymond (1896) was rightly to conclude in one of the volumes of his *Lectures at La Salpêtrière*, that 'fugue states constituted a syndrome' that could be seen in epilepsy, hysteria, and degeneration states. After firmly identifying amnesia and lack of insight (and occasionally multiple personality) as the core features, Raymond excluded all wandering behaviours that were 'consciously planned' (such as that of some of Régis's 'dromomanes').

### Fugue in the early twentieth century

The early twentieth century saw an explosion of publications on the fugue state. The magnificent thesis by Hamelin (1908) set the scene by offering an historical analysis, case reports, and a tripartite classification: (a) fugues (ambulatory automatisms) in epilepsy, hysteria, and somnambulism (12 cases); (b) fugues in 'dromomanes' affected by mental degeneration (7); and (c) fugues in psychotics, e.g. chronic hallucinatory states, paranoiacs, etc. (7). Hamelin assessed their prognosis and suggested specific therapeutic measures.

In a lecture before la Société Médico-Psychologique, Benon & Froissart (1908) proposed definitions for both 'fugue' and 'wandering behaviour' (vagabondage). The former they defined as 'a transient, paroxysmal and non-habitual disorder of action during which the patient will displace himself short or long distances under the influence of a psychological abnormal state' (p. 306); and 'vagabondage' as 'a habitual disorder of action that leads the subject to displace himself under the influence of an abnormal mental state' (p. 307). Given the 'clarity and richness of the French language', Collin called into question (during the exchanges that followed the lecture) the need of having definitions at all; and Lwoff and Vallon made the point that in many cases it could not be said that vagabonds were 'ill in any way'. Benon defended their position by saying that the whole point of the paper had been to establish a clear difference between fugue and vagabondage which were still confused by many authors. A year later, Benon and Froissart (1909) published a major review making the point that the mental state of the subject (whether or not he was in a state of 'absence', i.e. had temporarily lost his autobiographical memory) was more important to diagnosis than the objective features of the travelling itself. They also offered a classification, including sections on fugues in the military (Roue, 1967), the elderly (Commandeur et al., 1989), and in children (Yazmadjian, 1927; Lagache, 1979).

The detailed monograph by Joffroy and Dupouy (1909) appeared after the senior author, a great professor at St Anne, had already died. In a preface to this work, G. Deny made the point that in most cases vagabonds were neither criminal or mad. Joffroy and Dupouy proposed that, together with some 'automatisms' and obsessional disorders, fugues were disorders of the will (on the latter see Berrios & Gili, 1995).

The transient loss of autobiographical information (including personal identity) characteristic of the 'fugue states' was also highlighted by Abeles and Schilder (1935) in a classical paper on 'motivated amnesia' (defined as one in which a trigger or reason could usually be found). The authors reported 28 cases with 'temporary personal disorientation' who had retained the ability to learn information during the attack. Spontaneous recovery occurred in most cases, and 'behind the superficial conflicts which precipitated the amnesia [many had] deeper motives . . .' (p. 609). In his review on memory disorders, Gillespie (1937) included 'psychogenic amnesia' which he defined as a 'failure to recall . . . inhibition of recall may result from the activity of the ego itself' (p. 763).

Two years later, Stengel (1939), started his series of papers on the 'fugue state' (compulsive wandering or porimania). In a substantial second paper, Stengel (1941) reported 25 cases out of which 10 were related to epilepsy, one to schizophrenia, and the 'remaining were manic-depressives, hysterics and psychopaths' (p. 597). Most patients had a disturbed childhood, were prone to compulsive lying, and showed a tendency to periodic changes in mood and to developing 'twilight states'. A third paper added 11 cases concluding that 'fugues with an impulse to wander occur in a variety of conditions' and that 'the symbolic meaning of the fugue' was important (Stengel, 1943: p. 241).

A year later, and based on the examination of 30 patients, Parfitt and Gall (1944) concluded that: (a) both organic and hysterical factors contributed to the development of the fugue states, (b) 'personal recall' (their name for autobiographical memory) was more often affected than impersonal recall (semantic memory), (c) patients do not forget but refuse to remember, and (d) the difference between hysterical amnesia and malingering was only one of degree (pp. 526–7).

Berrington et al. (1956) re-evaluated Stengel's views and after studying 37 cases concluded that alcoholism, hysterical mechanisms and brain injury were more important causal factors than 'disturbed childhood'. The same year, Bergeron (1956) reasserted the French view that fugues (impulsive wandering accompanied by transitory amnesia) differed from the wandering behaviour of travellers, vagabonds and tramps whose mental state ranged from normality to severe psychosis, and in whom 'amnesia' and 'secondary gain' were conspicuous for their absence.

### 'Ictus amnésique' and transient global amnesia

By 1910, French alienists separated off from the large group of 'fugues' the condition called l'ictus amnésique (Benon, 1909) or 'l'éclipse mnésique' (Dromard, 1911) conceived of as a transient amnesia of 'organic' origin. The former author reported four cases with a mean age of 70, defining his syndrome as: a 'clinical disorder characterized by a sudden and short lived loss of retrograde memory; the deficit being dense and diffuse' (Benon, 1909: p. 207). Dromard (1911), in turn, suggested that this condition may follow a violent emotion. To this day, this syndrome, known in Anglo-Saxon medicine as 'Transient Global Amnesia' is referred to by the French as 'l'ictus amnésique' (Trillet, 1990).

As always, clinical reports redolent of 'l'ictus amnésique' can be found much earlier. For example, Forbes Winslow (1861) reported a case with 'sudden, transient, and paroxysmal attacks of forgetfulness, particularly if associated with an inability to articulate clearly . . . ought to be regarded as harbingers of fatal attacks of paralysis, softening, apoplexy and insanity' (p. 372) (for other historical cases see Markowitsch, 1990a).

In the 1950s, the syndrome was rediscovered by the Americans as 'Transient Global Amnesia' (TGA) (Fisher & Adams, 1958) and the view expressed that an 'organic' causation was always involved. For a time, confusion reigned as to whether, in addition to age and psychodynamic mechanisms, there were other differences between TGA and conventional fugues (Markowitsch, 1990b). In this regard, in a classical monograph, Hodges has concluded: 'it is increasingly likely that different mechanisms underlie the various components of the amnestic syndrome and that no single deficit can explain the anterograde and extensive retrograde amnesia observed in patients with permanent amnesia and in TGA' (Hodges, 1991: p. 100) (see Chapter 9, 'Transient global amnesia and transient epileptic amnesia', this volume).

## Conclusions

This chapter has dealt exclusively with the conceptual history of memory complaints and disorders relatable to psychiatric practice (delusions of memory, déjà vu, and confabulations have been dealt with in other chapters). To set the scene, the frames within which the concept of memory and its disorders developed during the nineteenth century were described. It then suggested that what we have nowadays is the result of an interaction between the models of memory impairment developed out of clinical observation and the experimental tradition started with Ebbinghaus. Lastly, the point was made that current interest in personal narratives, ecological tests, and autobiographical memory are not new, for these ideas achieved a high level of development during the 1920s in the school of Strasbourg.

## REFERENCES

Abeles, M. & Schilder, P. (1935). Psychogenic loss of personal identity. *Archives of Neurology and Psychiatry*, **34**, 587–604.

Akhtar, S. & Brenner, I. (1979). Differential diagnosis of fugue-like states. *Journal of Clinical Psychiatry*, **40**, 381–5.

Andral (no initial) (1829). *Dictionnaire de Médicine*, pp. 166–9. Paris: Gabon.

Anonymous (1946). Nécrologie: Maurice Halbwachs 1877–1944. *Revue Philosophique*, **84**, 127–8.

Aristotle (1908). De Memoria et Reminiscentia. In *Parva Naturalia* [Translation J.I. Beare], Oxford: Clarendon Press.

Arnaud, M. (1896). Un cas d'illusion de 'déjà vu' ou de 'false memory'. *Annales Médico-Psychologiques*, **54**, 455–71.

Aubanel (no initial) (1851). Rapport médico-légal sur un paralytique général. *Annales Médico-Psychologiques*, **I**, 445.

Augier, E. (1939). *La Mémoire et la Vie*. Paris: Alcan.

Azam, E. (1876). Amnésie périodique. *Annales Médico-Psychologiques*, **34**, 5–35.

Baddeley, A. (1986). *Working Memory*. Oxford: Clarendon Press.

Bain, A. (1864). *The Senses and the Intellect*. 2nd edn. London: Longman.

Bain, A. (1874). *Mind and Body*. London: Henry S. King.

Baret, L.J.E. (1887). *L'État de la Mémoire dans les Vesanies*. Paris: A. Davy.

Bartlett, C. (1932). *Remembering*. Cambridge: Cambridge University Press.

Behr, F., Croq, L. & Vauterin, C. (1985). Sémiologie des conduites de fugue. *Encyclopédie Médico-Chirurgicale* (Paris) Psychiatrie, 37113 A10, 2, Paris: Editions Techniques.

Benon, R. (1909). Les ictus amnésiques. *Annales Médico-Psychologiques*, **67**, 207–19.

Benon, R. & Froissart. P. (1908). Fugue et vagabondage. Définition et étude clinique. *Annales Médico-Psychologiques*, **66**, 305–12.

Benon, R. & Froissart, P. (1909). Les fugues en pathologie mentale. *Journal de Psychologie Normale et Pathologique*, **6**, 293–330.

Bergeron, M. (1956). Fugues. In *Encyclopédie Médico-Chirurgicale*. Psychiatrie, 37140 E10. Paris: Editions Techniques.

Bergson, H. (1911). *Matter and Memory* [Translated by N.M. Paul and W.S. Palmer]. London: George Allen & Unwin [1st edn in French 1896].

Bergson, H. (1914). *Essai sur les données immédiates de la conscience*. Paris: Alcan [1st edn 1889].

Berlyne, N. (1972). Confabulation. *British Journal of Psychiatry*, **120**, 31–9.

Bernard-Leroy E. (1898). *L'Illusion de Fausse Reconnaissance. Contribution à L'étude des Conditions Psychologiques de la Reconnaissance des Souvenirs*. Paris: Alcan.

Bernutz (no initial) (1865). *Noveau Dictionnaire de Médicine*. vol 2, pp. 52–6. Paris: Baillière.

Berrington, W.P., Liddell, D.W. & Foulds, G.A. (1956). A Re-evaluation of the fugue. *Journal of Mental Science*, **102**, 280–6.

Berrios, G.E. (1985a). Presbyophrenia: clinical aspects. *British Journal of Psychiatry*, **147**, 76–9.

Berrios, G.E. (1985b). 'Depressive pseudodementia' or 'melancholic dementia': a 19th century view. *Journal of Neurology, Neurosurgery and Psychiatry*, **48**, 393–400

Berrios, G.E. (1990). The cognitive paradigm of dementia. In *Lectures in the History of Psychiatry*, ed. R. Murray & T. Turner, pp. 194–211. London: Gaskell.

Berrios, G.E. (1992a). Phenomenology, Psychopathology, and Jaspers: a conceptual history. *History of Psychiatry*, **3**, 303–27.

Berrios, G.E. (1992b). Some disorders of memory during the 19th century: paramnesias and fugues. In *Trastornos de la Memoria*, ed. D. Barcia, pp. 33–46. Mallorca: Editorial MCR.

Berrios, G.E. (1995). Déjà vu and other disorders of memory during the nineteenth century. *Comprehensive Psychiatry*, **36**, 123–9.

Berrios, G.E. (1996). *The History of Mental Symptoms. Descriptive Psychopathology Since the 19th Century*. Cambridge: Cambridge University Press.

Berrios, G.E. & Gili, M. (1995). Will and its disorders: a conceptual history. *History of Psychiatry*, **6**, 87–104.

Biervliet, J.J. van (1894). Observations et documents sur les paramnésies. *Revue Philosophique*, **38**, 47–9.

Biervliet, J.J. van (1902). *La Mémoire*. Paris: Doin.

Bloch, M. (1925). Mémoire collective, tradition et coutume. A propos d'un livre récent. *Revue Synthese Historique*, **40**, 73–83.

Blondel, C. (1914). *La Conscience Morbide. Essai de Psycho-pathologie générale*. Paris: Alcan.

Blondel, C. (1926). Revue Critique. *Revue Philosophique*, **51**, 290–8.

Blondel, C. (1928a). *Introduction à la Psychologie Collective*. Paris: Colin.

Blondel, C. (1928b). *The Troubled Conscience and the Insane Mind*. London: Kegan Paul.

Bondy, M. (1974). Psychiatric antecedents on psychological testing (Before Binet). *Journal of the History of the Behavioral Sciences*, **10**, 180–94.

Boring, E.G. (1942). *Sensation and Perception in the History of Experimental Psychology*. New York: Irvington Publishers.

Boring, E.G. (1950). *A History of Experimental Psychology*. New York: Appleton–Century–Crofts.

Boring, E.G. (1961). The beginning and growth of measurement in psychology. *Isis*, **52**, 238–57.

Bouillaud, J. (1829). Amnésie. In ed. Andral, Bégin, Blandin et al. (no initials) *Dictionnaire de Médicine et de Chirurgie Pratiques*, vol 2, pp. 166–9. Paris: Gabon.

Bourdon, B. (1894), Influence de l'age sur la mémoire immédiate. *Revue Philosophique*, **38**, 148–67.

Bourgeois, M. & Geraud, M. (1990). Eugène Azam (1822–1899). *Annales Médico-Psychologiques*, **148**, 709–17.

Bruner, J. (1990). *Acts of Meaning*. Cambridge: Harvard University Press.

Bruner, J. (1994). The 'remembered self'. In *The Remembering Self. Construction and Accuracy in the Self-Narrative*, ed. U. Neisser & R. Fivush, pp. 41–54. Cambridge: Cambridge University Press.

Brunschvicq, L. (1927). *Le Progrès de la Conscience dans la Philosophie Occidental*, vol 2. Paris: Alcan.

Bulbena, A. & Berrios, G.E. (1986). Pseudodementia: facts and figures. *British Journal of Psychiatry*, **148**, 87–94.

Burke, P. (1989). History as social memory. In *Memory, History, Culture and the Mind*, ed. T. Butler, pp. 97–113. Oxford: Blackwell.

Burnham, W.H. (1888–9). Memory, historically and experimentally considered. *American Journal of Psychology*, **2**, 39–90; 225–70; 431–64; 568–622.

Butler, S. (1880). *Unconscious Memory*. London: David Bogue.

Callinicos, A. (1995). *Theories and Narratives*. Cambridge: Polity Press.

Canguilhem, G. (1966). *Le Normal et le Pathologique*. Paris: Presses Universitaires de France.

Caparrós, (1986). *H. Ebbinghaus*. Barcelona: Publicacions i Edicions de la Universitat de Barcelona.

Carruthers, M. (1990). *The Book of Memory. A Study of Memory in Medieval Culture*. Cambridge: Cambridge University Press.

Cassirer, E. (1945). *An Essay on Man*. Yale: Yale University Press.

Cattell, J.McK. (1890). Mental tests and measurements. *Mind*, **15**, 373–81.

Charcot, J.M. (1987). *The Tuesday Lessons* [Translated by C.G. Goetz]. New York: Raven Press [First edition, 1892].

Chevalier, J. (1928). *Henri Bergson* [Translated by L.A. Clare]. London: Rider.

Clarke, D.M. (1982). *Descartes' Philosophy of Science*. Manchester: Manchester University Press.

Claude, H. (1922). *Précis de Pathologie Interne. Maladies du Système Nerveux*. Vol 2, p. 52. Paris: Baillière.

Coady, C.A.J. (1992). *Testimony. A Philosophical Study*. Oxford: Clarendon Press.

Cohen, G. (1996). *Memory in the Real World*, 2nd edn. Hove: Psychology Press.

Commandeur, M.C., Bouckson, G. & Alcala, P. De (1989). La fugue de la personne âgée. *Psychologie Médicale*, **21**, 1098–101.

Conway, M.A., Rubin, D.C., Spinnler, H. & Wagenaar, W.A. (eds) (1992). *Theoretical Perspectives on Autobiographical Memory*. Dordrecht: Kluwer.

Coser, L.A. (1992). Introduction: Maurice Halbwachs 1877–1945. In *Maurice Halbwachs on Collective Memory*, pp. 1–34. Chicago: The University of Chicago Press.

Courbon, P. (1930). L'œvre de Charles Blondel. *Annales Médico-Psychologiques*, **97**, 365–81.

Delay, J. (1942). *Les Dissolutions de la Mémoire*. Paris: Presses Universitaires de France.

Descartes, (1967). The passions of the soul. In *The Philosophical Works of Descartes*. [Translated by E.S. Haldane & G.R.T. Ross], Vol 1. Cambridge: Cambridge University Press.

Dilthey, W. (1976). *Selected Writings*, pp. 87–97. Cambridge: Cambridge University Press.

Dromard (no initial) (1911). Mémoire et délire; éclipses mnésiques comme sources et comme conséquences de'idées délirantes. *Journal de Psychologie Normale et Pathologiques*, **8**, 252–60.

Dugas, L. (1894a). Observations sur la Fausse Mémoire. *Revue Philosophique*, **37**, 34–45.

Dugas, L. (1894b). L'Impression de 'l'entièrement noveau' et cella de 'déjà vu'. *Revue Philosophique*, **38**, 40–6.

Dugas, L. (1915). La Mémoire Organique. *Journal de Psychologie Normale et Pathologique*, **12**, 1–13.

Dugas, L (1917). *La Mémoire et L'Oubli*. Paris: Flammarion.

Ebbinghaus, H. (1885). *Über das Gedächtnis. Untersuchungen zur experimentellen Psychologie*. Leipzig: Duncker und Humblot. [English version: H. Ebbinghaus] (1964) *Memory. A Contribution to Experimental Psychology* [Translated by H.A. Ruger and C.E. Bussenius]. New York: Dover.

Edgell, B. (1924). *Theories of memory*. Oxford: Clarendon Press.

Edridge-Green. F.W. (1897). *Memory and Its Cultivation*. London: Kegan Paul, Trench, Trübner & Co.

Esquirol, E. (1838). *Des Maladies Mentales*, vol. 2. Paris: Baillière.

Ey, H. (1950). Les troubles de la Mémoire. Étude n°9 in *Études Psychiatriques*, vol. 2, pp. 9–68. Paris: Desclée de Brouwer.

Fabre (no initials) (1840). *Dictionnaire des Dictionnaires de Médicine*, vol. 2, pp. 221–5. Paris: Bureau de la Gazette des Hopitaux.

Falret, J. (1865). Amnésie. In *Dictionnaire Encyclopédique des Sciences Médicales*, ed. A. Dechambre, pp. 725–42. Paris: Asselin & Masson.

Fearn, J. (1812). *An Essay on Consciousness or a Series of Evidences of a Distinct Mind*, 2nd edn. London: Longman.

Feinstein, H.M. (1984). *Becoming William James*. Ithaca: Cornell University Press.

Feuchtersleben, E. (1847). *The Principles of Medical Psychology* [Translated by H.E. Lloyd and B.G. Babington]. London: Sydenham Society.

Fisher, C.M. & Adams, R.D. (1958). Transient Global Amnesia. *Transactions of the American Neurological Association*, **83**, 143–6.

Foville fils, A. (1875). Des aliénés voyageurs ou migrateurs. *Annales Médico-Psychologiques*, **33**, 5–45.

Galtier-Boissière (no initials) (1929). (ed.) *Larousse Médical Illustré*. Paris: Larousse.

Garnier, A. (1852). *Traité des Facultés de L'Ame. Comprenant L'Histoire des Principales Théories Psychologiques.* Paris: Hachette.

Garzón, A. (1992). Marcos sociales de la memoria. In *Trastornos de la Memoria*, ed. D. Barcia, pp. 79–101. Mallorca: Editorial MCR.

Gasser, J (1988). La notion de mémoire organique dans la oeuvre de T Ribot. *History and Philosophy of the Life Sciences*, **10**, 293–313.

Geary, P.J. (1994). *Phantoms of Remembrance, Memory and Oblivion et the End of the First Millennium.* Princeton: Princeton University Press.

Génil-Perrin, G. (1913). *Histoire des Origines et de l'Évolution de l'Ideé de Dégénérescence en Médicine Mentale.* Paris: Leclerc.

Gillespie, R.D. (1937). Amnesia. *Archives of Neurology and Psychiatry*, **37**, 748–64.

Gilson, E. (1940). Charles Blondel. *Annuaire de la Fondation Thiers* 1939–1940. Nouvelle Série, pp. 27–32. Paris: Gaignault.

Goldstein, J. (1985). The wandering Jew and the problem of psychiatric anti-semitism in fin-de-siècle France. *Journal of Contemporary History*, **20**, 521–32.

Gomulicki, B.R. (1953). The development and present status of the trace theory of memory. *The British Journal of Psychology Monograph Supplements*, vol. 14. Cambridge: Cambridge University Press.

Gordon, B. de. (1495). *Lilio de Medicina.* Sevilla: Ungut & S. Polonio.

Gratacap, A. (1866). *Théorie de la Mémoire.* Montpellier: Boehm & Fils.

Griesinger, W. (1867). *Mental Pathology and Therapeutics* [Translation of the 2nd German edn by C.L. Robertson & J Rutherford]. London: New Sydenham Society.

Hacking, I. (1995). *Rewriting the Soul.* Princeton: Princeton University Press.

Hacking, I. (1996). Les Aliénés voyageurs. *History of Psychiatry*, **7**, 425–49.

Halbwachs, M. (1925). *Les Cadres Sociaux de la Mémoire.* Paris: Alcan.

Hall, T.S. (1972). Commentary. In Descartes' *Treatise of Man*. [French Text with Translation & Commentary by Thomas Steel Hall]. Cambridge: Harvard University Press.

Hamelin, F.G. (1908). *Contribution à l'Étude des Fugues.* Lille: Le Bigot Frères.

Hamilton, Sir W. (1859). *Lectures on Metaphysics and Logic*, vol. 2, pp 205–58. Edinburgh: William Blackwood and Sons.

Hart van der, O.(1985). Metaphoric and symbolic imagery in the hypnotic treatment of an urge to wander: a case report. *Australian Journal of Clinical and Experimental Hypnosis*, **13**, 83–95.

Hartley, D. (1834). *Observations on Man. His Frame, His Duty and His Expectations.* London: Thomas Tegg and Son [1st edn, 1748].

Hering, E (1870). Über das Gedächtnis als eine allgemeine Funktion der organisierten Materie. Vortrag gehalten in der feierlichen Sitzung der Kaiserlichen Akademie der Wissenschaften in Wien, Wien.

Herrmann, D.J. & Chaffin. R. (1988). *Memory in Historical Perspective.* Berlin: Springer.

Hesse, M. (1966). *Models and Analogies in Science.* Indiana: University of Notre Dame Press.

Hodges, J.R. (1991). *Transient Amnesia. Clinical and Neuropsychological aspects.* London: Saunders.

Holland, H. (1852). *Chapters on Mental Physiology.* London: Longman, Brown, Green, and Longmans.

Hutton, P.H. (1987). The art of memory reconceived: from rhetoric to psychoanalysis. *Journal of the History of Ideas,* **48**, 371–92.

Hutton, P.H. (1993). *History as an Art of Memory.* Hanover: University Press of New England.

Jackson, J.H. (1931). *Selected Writings,* ed. J. Taylor. London: Hodder.

James, W. (1890). *The Principles of Psychology,* 2 vols. London: Macmillan.

Janet, P. (1889). *L'Automatisme Psychologique.* Paris: Alcan.

Janet, P. (1909). *Les Névroses.* Paris: Flammarion.

Janet, P. (1928). *L'Évolution de la Mémoire et de la Notion du Temps.* Paris: A. Chahine.

Janet, P. & Saillés, G. (1902). *A History of the Problems of Philosophy* [translated by A. Monahan and H. Jones], vol .1, pp. 145–65. London: MacMillan.

Jaspers, K. (1910). Die Methoden der Intelligenzprüfung und der Begriff der Demenz. *Zeitschrift für des gesamte Neurologie und Psychiatrie* [*Referate & Ergebnisse*] **1**, 402–52.

Joffroy, A. & Dupouy, R. (1909). *Fugues et Vagabondage.* Paris: Alcan.

Jordanova, L.J. (1984). *Lamarck.* Oxford: Oxford University Press.

Jung, C.G. (1905). Experimentelle Beobachtungen über das Erinnerungsvermögen. *Zentralblatt für Nervenheilkunde und Psychiatrie,* **28** [English version: 'Experimental observations on the Faculty of Memory']. In *The Collected Works,* vol. 2, pp. 272–87. London: Routledge & Kegan Paul.

Kay, D. (1902). *The Sciences of Memory.* London: Kegan, Paul, Trech, Trübner & Co.

Kelley, C.M. & Jacoby, L.L. (1990). The construction of subjective experience: memory attributions. *Mind and Language,* **5**, 49–68.

Kirchhoff, T. (1893). *Handbook of Insanity.* New York: William Wood.

Kirkpatrick, B., Johnson, M., McGuire, K. & Fletcher, R.H. (1986). Confounding and the dementia of schizophrenia. *Psychiatry Research,* **19**, 225–31.

Koriat, A. & Goldsmith, M. (1996). Memory metaphors and the real-life/laboratory controversy: correspondence versus storehouse conceptions of memory. *Behavioral and Brain Sciences,* **19**, 167–228.

Korsakoff, S. (1889). Étude médico-psychologique sur une forme des maladies de la mémoire. *Revue Philosophique,* **28**, 501–30.

Korsakoff, S.S. (1891). Erinnerungstäuchschungen (Pseudoreminiscenzen) bei polyneuritischer Psychose. *Allgemeine Zeitschrift für Psychiatrie,* **47**, 390–410.

Kraepelin, E. (1886–87). Über Erinnerungsfälschungen. *Archiv für Psychiatrie und Nervenkrankheiten,* **17**, 830–43; **18**, 199–239; 395–436.

Lagache, D. (1979). *Œuvres II (1947–1952),* Paris: Presses Universitaires de France.

Lalande, A. (1893). Des Paramnésies. *Revue Philosophique,* **36**, 485–7.

Lamarck, J.B. (1984). *Zoological Philosophy.* Chicago: University of Chicago Press.

Landre-Beauvais, A.J. (1813). *Séméiotique, ou Traité des Signes des Maladies.* 2nd edn. Paris: Brosson.

Lange, K. (1900). *Apperception.* Boston: Heath & Company.

Lapie, P. (1894). Note sur la Paramnésie. *Revue Philosophique*, **37**, 351–2.

Lasègue (no initial) (1868). Alcoolisme subaigu, fugue. *Archives Générales de Médicine*, **ii**, 159.

Le Goff, J. (1992). *History and Memory*. New York: Columbia University Press.

Levin, H.S., Peters. B.H. & Hulkonen, D.A. (1983). Early concepts of anterograde and retrograde amnesia. *Cortex*, **19**, 427–40.

Lewes, G.H. (1877). *The Physical Basis of Mind*. London: Trübner & Co.

Lieury, A. (1975). *La Mémoire, Résultats et Théories*. Brussels: Dessart et Mardaga.

Lloyd, G.E.R. (1990). *Demystifying Mentalities*. Cambridge: Cambridge University Press.

Locke, J. (1959). *An Essay Concerning Human Understanding*. A.C. Fraser edn, vol. 1. New York: Dover.

Loewenstein, R.J. (1996). Dissociative amnesia and dissociative fugue. In *Handbook of Dissociation: Theoretical, Empirical, and Clinical Perspectives*, ed. L.K. Michelson & W.J. Ray, pp. 307–36. New York: Plenum Press.

Loftus, E.F. (1979). *Eyewitness Testimony*. Cambridge: Harvard University Press.

Louyer-Willermay (no initials) (1819). Maladies de la Mémoire. In *Dictionnaire des Sciences Médicales*, vol. 32. Paris: Panckouke.

Luys (no initial) (1881). Obnubilation passagère de la concience des choses du monde extérieur, ayant duré plusieurs jours, chez un homme adulte, continuant à vivre de la vie commune. *L'Encephale*, **6**, 251.

Mairet, A & Piéron. H. (1915). Les Troubles de Mémoire D'origine Commotionnelle. *Journal de Psychologie Normale et Pathologique*, **12**, 300–28.

Markowitsch, H.J. (1990a). Early concepts of transient disorders with symptoms of amnesia. In *Transient Global Amnesia*, pp. 4–14. Berlin: Springer.

Markowitsch, H.J. (1990b). Transient psychogenic amnesic states. In *Transient Global Amnesia*, pp. 181–90. Berlin: Springer.

Maury, L.F.A. (1878). *Le Sommeil et les Rêves*. Paris: Didier.

Mayr, E. (1982). *The Growth of Biological Thought*. Cambridge: The Belknap Press of Harvard University Press.

Meige, H. (1893). *Études sur Certains Névropathes Voyageurs. Le Juiferrant à la Salpêtrière*. Paris: Bataille.

Meige, H. (1993). *Le juif-errant à la Salpêtrière*. Paris: Editions de Nouvel Object [first published in 1893].

Meletti, M. (1991). *Il Pensiero e la Memoria. Filosofia e Psicologia nella 'Revue Philosophique' di Théodule Ribot (1876–1916)*. Milano: Franco Angeli.

Mill, J. (1869). *Analysis of the Phenomena of the Human Mind*. London, Longmans: Green, Reader & Dyer.

Motet (no initial) (1886). Fugues de quatre et dix jours consécutives à une chute grave. *Annales Médico-Psychologiques*, **40**, 128.

Mouren, M.C., Rajaona, F.R., Thiébaux, M. & Tatossian, A. (1978). Le vagabondage: aspects psychologiques et psychopathologiques. *Annales Médico-Psychologiques*, **135**, 415–47.

Murray, D.J. (1976). Research on human memory in the nineteenth century. *Canadian Journal of Psychology*, **30**, 201–20.

Neisser, U. & Winograd, E. (eds.) (1988). *Remembering Reconsidered*. Cambridge: Cambridge University Press.

Neisser, U. & Fivush, R. (eds.) (1994). *The Remembering Self*. Cambridge: Cambridge University Press.

Offner, M. (1911). *Das Gedächnis*. Berlin: Reuther & Reichard.

Oldfield, R.C. & Zangwill, O.L. (1942). Head's concept of the schema and its application in contemporary British psychology. Part III. *British Journal of Psychology*, **33**, 113–29.

Otis, L. (1993). Organic Memory and Psychoanalysis. *History of Psychiatry*, **4**, 349–72.

Parfitt, D.N & Gall, C.C.C (1944). Psychogenic amnesia: the refusal to remember. *The Journal of Mental Science*, **90**, 511–31.

Paulhan, F. (1904). *La Fonction de la Mémoire et le Souvenir Affectif*. Paris: Alcan.

Perry, R.B. (1936). *The Thought and Character of William James: As Revealed in Unpublished Correspondence and Notes, Together with his Published Writings*, 2 vols. London: Oxford University Press.

Pick, A. (1903). Clinical studies. III. On reduplicative paramnesia. *Brain*, **26**, 260–7.

Piéron, H. (1910). *L'Évolution de la Mémoire*. Paris: Flammarion.

Postman, L. (1968). Hermann Ebbinghaus. *American Psychologist*, **23**, 149–57.

Prichard, J.C. (1835). *Treatise on Insanity and Other Disorders Affecting the Mind*. London: Sherwood, Gilbert, and Piper.

Ravaisson, F. (1885). *La Philosophie en France au XIXᵉ siècle*, 2nd edn. Paris: Hachette.

Raymond, F. (1896). *Leçons sur les Maladies du Système Nerveux. (Clinique de la Salpêtrière 1894–1895)* Paris: Doin, Lectures 31 & 32.

Régis, E. (1906). *Précis de Psychiatrie*. Paris: Doin.

Ribot, Th. (1880). Les désordres généraux de la mémoire. *Revue Philosophique*, **10**, 181–214; 485–516.

Ribot, Th. (1882). *Diseases of Memory* [translation of 1881 1st French edn] London: Kegan Paul, Trench & Co.

Ribot, Th. (1896). *Psychologie des Sentiments*. Paris: Alcan.

Ribot, Th. (1906). *L'Hérédité Psychologique*. Paris: Alcan.

Rice, E. & Fisher, C. (1976). Fugue states in sleep and wakefulness: a physiological study. *Journal of Nervous and Mental Disease*, **163**, 7–87.

Richet, C. (1886). Les Origines and les Modalités de la Mémoire. *Revue Philosophique*, **21**, 562–90.

Riether, A.M. & Stoudemire, A. (1988). Psychogenic fugue states: a review. *Southern Medical Journal*, **81**, 568–71.

Rignano, E. (1926). *Biological Memory*. London: Kegan Paul, Trench, Trubner & Co.

Robinson, J.A. (1986). Autobiographical Memory: a historical prologue. In *Autobiographical Memory*, ed. D.C. Rubin, pp. 19–24. Cambridge: Cambridge University Press.

Romanes, G. (1880). Review of 'Unconscious Memory'. *Nature*, **23**, 285–7.

Ross, J. (1891). On Memory. *Brain*, **14**, 35–50.

Ross, B.C. (1991). *Remembering the Personal Past*. New York: Oxford University Press.

Roue, R. (1967). *Les Conduites de Fugue en Milieu Militaire*. Université de Bordeaux: Thèse de Médecine.

Rouillard, T. (1885). *Essai sur les Amnésies. Etiologie des Troubles de la Mémoire*. Paris: Jules Leclerc.

Rouillard, T. (1888). Les Amnésies. *L'Encéphale*, **8**, 652–71.

Rubin, D.C. (ed.) (1986). *Autobiographical Memory*. Cambridge: Cambridge University Press.

Rubin, D.C. (ed.) (1996). *Remembering our Past*. Cambridge: Cambridge University Press.

Rund, B.R. (1988). Cognitive disturbances in schizophrenics: what are they, and what is their origin? *Acta Psychiatrica Scandinavica*, **77**, 113–23.

Rush, B. (1812). *Medical Inquiries and Observations upon the Diseases of the Mind*. Philadelphia: Kimber & Richardson.

Saint Augustine (1992). *Confessions* [A New Translation by Henry Chadwick]. Oxford: Oxford University Press.

Saury, H. (1886). *Étude clinique sur la Folie Héréditaire*. Paris: Delahaye & Lecrosnier.

Schachtel, E.G. (1947). On memory and childhood amnesia. *Psychiatry*, **10**, 1–26.

Schacter, D.L. (1982). *Stranger Behind the Engram*. Hillsdale: Erlbaum.

Schacter, D.L. (ed.) (1995). *Memory Distortion*. Cambridge: Harvard University Press.

Schacter, D.L., Eich, J.E. & Tulving, E. (1978). Richard Semon's theory of memory. *Journal of Verbal Learning and Verbal Behavior*, **17**, 721–43.

Schatzmann, J. (1968). *Richard Semon (1859–1918) und seine Mnemetheorie*. Zürich: Juris Druck.

Scheerer, E. (1980). Wilhelm Wundt's psychology of memory. *Psychological Research*, **42**, 135–55.

Schuman, H. & Scott, J. (1989). Generations and collective memories. *American Sociological Review*, **54**, 359–81.

Semon, R. (1908). *Mneme* 2nd edn. Leipzig: Wilhelm Engelmann [first edition 1904].

Semon, R. (1909). *Mnemische Empfindungen* [rendered into English in 1923 as *Mnemic Psychology*]. London: Allen & Unwin.

Shakow, D. (1930). Hermann Ebbinghaus. *American Journal of Psychology*, **42**, 505–18.

Shaw, T.C. (1892). Dementia. In *A Dictionary of Psychological Medicine*, ed. D.H. Tuke, vol. 1, pp. 348–351. London: Churchill.

Simondon, M. (1982). *La Mémoire et L'Oubli dans la pensée Grecque jusqu'a la fin du Vᵉ siècle avant J.C.* Paris: Les Belles Lettres.

Smith, W. (1870). *Dictionary of Greek and Roman Biography*, vol. 2. London: John Murray.

Sollier, P. (1892). *Les Troubles de la Mémoire*. Paris: Rueff.

Sorabji, R. (1972). *Aristotle on Memory*. London: Duckworth.

Spencer, H. (1890) *The Principles of Psychology*. London: William & Northgate [first edition 1855].

Sperber, D. (1996). *Explaining Culture. A Naturalistic Approach*. Oxford: Blackwell.

Stengel, E. (1939). Studies on the psychopathology of compulsive wandering. *British Journal of Medical Psychology*, **18**, 250–4.

Stengel, E. (1941). On the aetiology of the fugue states. *Journal of Mental Science*, **87**, 572–99.

Stengel, E. (1943). Further studies on pathological wandering (fugues with the impulse to wander). *Journal of Mental Science*, **89**, 224–41.

Talbot, E.S. (1898). *Degeneracy. Its Causes, Signs and Results*. London: Walter Scott.

Tannen, D. (1993). *Framing in Discourse*. New York: Oxford University Press.

Thompson, J.A. (1908). *Heredity*. London: Murray.

Tissié, Ph. (1887). *Les Aliénés voyageurs*. Paris: Doin.

Titchener, E.B. (1895). Affective memory. *Philosophical Review*, **4**, 65–77.

Treadway, M., McCloskey, M., Gordon, B. & Cohen, N.J. (1992). Landmark life events and the organization of memory: evidence from functional retrograde amnesia. In *The Handbook of Emotion and Memory. Research & Theory*, ed. S.-A. Christianson, pp. 389–410. Hillsdale: Erlbaum.

Trillet, M. (1990). L'ictus amnésique. *Concours Médicale*, **112**, 2370–3.

Tulving, E. (1983). *Elements of Episodic Memory*. Oxford: Clarendon Press.

Turner, S. (1994). *The Social Theory of Practices*. Cambridge: Polity Press.

Vega, L.S. & Palomo, T. (1995). Aspectos semiológicos y psicopatológicos de la fuga, el vagabundeo y la carencia de hogar. *Psiquiatría Pública*, **7**, 308–24.

Vincent, T. & Boucharlat, J. (1989). L'Oubli entre Freud et Janet. *Annales Médico-Psychologiques*, **147**, 990–1.

Virey (no initial) (1819). Mémoire. In *Dictionnaire des Sciences Médicales*, vol. 32. Paris: Panckouke.

Voisin, J. (1889). Automatisme ambulatoire chez une hystérique. *Annales Médico-Psychologiques*, **46**, 418.

Vovelle, M. (1990). *Ideologies and Mentalities. Translation E. O'Flaherty*. Cambridge: Polity Press.

Walker, C. (1988). Philosophical concepts and practice: the legacy of Karl Jaspers' psychopathology. *Current Opinion in Psychiatry*, **1**, 624–9.

Walser, H.H. (1974). Über Theorieen des Gedächtnisses in der letzen Dezenninen des 19. Jahrhunderts und ihre Bedeutung für die Entstehung der Psychoanalyse. *In Proceedings of the XXIII International Congress of the History of Medicine*, vol. 2, pp. 1227–32. London: Wellcome Institute of the History of Medicine.

Wéber, E. (1990). Memoria. In *Les Notions Philosophiques*, ed. S. Auroux, vol. 2. Paris: Presses Universitaires de France.

White, H. (1987). *The Content of the Form*. Baltimore: Johns Hopkins University Press.

Wigan, A.L. (1844). *The Duality of the Mind*. London: Longman, Brown, Green and Longmans.

Winslow, F. (1861). *On Obscure Diseases of the Brain and Disorders of the Mind*, 2nd edn. London: John W. Davies.

Wright, T. (1630). *The Passions of the Minde in Generall*. London: Flesher.

Wundt, W (1897). *Outlines of Psychology*. [Translated by C.H. Judd]. London: Williams & Norgate.

Yates, F.A. (1966). *The Art of Memory*. London: Routledge & Kegan Paul.

Yazmadjian H. (1927). *Essai de Psychopathologie Générale de la Fugue*. Paris: Le François.

Young, K. (1923). The history of mental testing. *The Pedagogical Seminar*, **31**, 1–48.

Young, M.N. (1961). *Bibliography of Memory*. Philadelphia: Chilton.

Zupan, M.L. (1976). The conceptual development of quantification in experimental psychology. *Journal of the History of the Behavioral Sciences*, **12**, 145–58.

# 2

# Mood and memory

Tim Dalgleish and Sally G. Cox

Mood disordered individuals who present at the clinic invariably complain of day-to-day problems with basic cognitive processes, particularly memory and concentration (Watts & Sharrock, 1985). The question for the clinician is whether these complaints reflect objective impairments in cognitive processes or whether they are merely a function of a self-report style biased towards the presentation of problems and difficulties.

Resolution of this question has important implications for assessment and treatment. Accurate knowledge about the types and degrees of cognitive impairment that can be attributed to the individual's mood disorder across a range of processes is often an important component in differential diagnosis, for example, between depression and senile dementia of the Alzheimer's type (SDAT) (e.g. Cummings, 1989). Furthermore, a number of intervention packages have been developed for problems with basic processes such as memory and concentration (e.g. Fogler & Stern, 1987), and the application of these to the mood disorders is dependent on a thorough understanding of the problems with which such individuals are grappling. Finally, a number of the talking therapies such as Cognitive Behaviour Therapy (e.g. Beck, 1976) involve large memory components both in the generation of material to work with in the therapeutic session and prospectively for remembering to carry out homework assignments.

Although the topic of mood and memory is a broad one, in terms of pragmatic clinical implications it can be narrowed down to the effect of negative mood states on memory performance. What is more, memory difficulties seem to be more clearly a problem for depressed individuals than for those presenting with anxiety disorders. Consequently, the prime focus of the present chapter will be on memory and depression. The effects of other mood states such as anxiety, and of positive emotions, such as happiness, on memory will only be highlighted and then, principally, for the purposes of comparison.

In the memory and depression literature two clear research themes can be identified. The first is concerned with the effects of depressed mood on general memory performance (see Burt et al., 1995; Ellis & Ashbrook, 1989; for reviews see

Watts, 1993). The second focuses on the effects of depressed mood on memory for emotional material which is either positive or negative in its hedonic tone (see Blaney, 1986; Dalgleish & Watts, 1990; Matt et al., 1992; Teasdale & Barnard, 1993; for reviews see Williams et al., 1988). These areas not only overlap but also have clinical implications regarding both assessment and treatment. Consequently, a consideration of these two strands of work forms the bulk of the chapter.

Researchers have generally embraced a number of methodologies. It has already been mentioned that self-report techniques invariably reveal a high level of perceived memory problems associated with depression. In parallel with these, a number of objective tests of memory have been applied, using either neutral material (e.g. Hertel & Hardin, 1990) or hedonically toned material (e.g. Bradley & Matthews, 1983). These methodologies have been applied to various subject groups; most commonly, clinically depressed subjects have been compared with non-clinically depressed controls (e.g. Watts et al., 1990). More rarely, a clinical control group has been included (e.g. Gotlib, 1981). In some studies, depressed individuals were tested again when they had recovered and thereby acted as their own controls (e.g. Stromgren, 1977). Finally, a host of studies has examined analogues of depression in the form of subclinically depressed individuals who have received some form of depressive mood induction. Each of these approaches has its own problems. Comparisons of depressed individuals with controls sheds little light on the specificity of any memory impairments to depression. The use of depressed subjects as their own controls runs the risk of practice effects and of statistical regression to the mean of an initially below-average group, clouding the true picture (Watts, 1993). The use of analogue groups raises the problem of the generalizability of the findings to the clinical population and, finally, all of the objective approaches potentially suffer from problems of ecological validity. How can we know if performance on a memory test is a valid reflection of day-to-day mnemonic experience. Subjects might be able to perform well for a short period of time or they may be able to summon up uncharacteristic levels of motivation for a test. All of these issues are important when it comes to translating results from the laboratory into practice in the clinic, and they will be returned to later.

## The effects of depressed mood on general memory performance

As was noted in the Introduction, depression seems strongly associated with self-reported memory problems. However, a series of studies has indicated that this association is far stronger than that between depression and objective memory performance (e.g. Kahn et al., 1975; O'Hara et al., 1986; O'Connor et al., 1990; Scogin, 1985; Scogin et al., 1985; West et al., 1984). For example, Kahn et al. (1975) studied subjects with differing degrees of depression and found a strong correlation between memory complaints and depression and no correlation between depression and memory performance on objective tests. Furthermore, neuropsychological tests, such as a mental status questionnaire, predicted memory performance but not the level of memory complaints. A related issue was investigated by Scogin et al. (1985) who demonstrated that a memory training package had a beneficial effect on memory performance but not on memory complaints or on levels of depression.

The finding of a discrepancy between self-reported memory problems and levels of performance on objective memory tests in depressed individuals does not mean that depression is unassociated with memory impairments. There is plenty of evidence which demonstrates impairments in general memory in depressed subjects relative to other groups (for a comprehensive listing, see Burt et al., 1995). For example, the seminal study by Cronholm and Ottosson (1961) compared depressed individuals with matched surgical patient controls on memory for word pairs, simple figures, and personal data about fictitious people using both immediate and delayed memory tests. The depressed subjects showed significantly poorer memory on all three tests at both occasions of testing, and these findings were replicated by Sternberg and Jarvik (1976).

In their meta-analytic review of depression and memory impairment on objective tests, Burt et al. (1995) concluded that the results of the meta-analysis indicate that depression and memory impairment are significantly associated . . . a great amount of research with results contrary to those of the studies reviewed would be required to alter this conclusion. As Watts (1993) notes, a disproportionate number of the studies, which do not show such an association, have involved a comparison of elderly depressives with normal elderly subjects – a control group in which the level of memory difficulties may already be quite high (e.g. Hart et al., 1987; Whitehead, 1973).

Burt et al. also include a number of moderator variables in their meta-analysis. The majority of these provide mixed findings which are difficult to interpret (e.g. depression subtype, medication status, stimulus type and retention interval on the memory task). However, there are clear effects of patient status, with inpatients exhibiting a greater association between depression and memory performance than outpatients, and of age, with a greater association in younger depressives than in older subjects. The former finding is perhaps unsurprising. However, the latter deserves some comment and again the residual level of memory problems associated with depression in older populations seems the most likely explanation (Watts, 1993).

It seems, then, that there is clear evidence of an association between depression and memory impairments. This raises the questions of why this should be the case? and what aspects of memory are impaired? Perhaps the most influential theory of general memory deficits in depression is the Resource Allocation Model (RAM; Ellis & Ashbrook, 1988). The thrust of Ellis and Ashbrook's argument is a simple one, affective states reduce the amount of processing resources available for allocation to a given task. Thus, in the memory domain, the suggestion is that less resources are available for the elaboration, organization, encoding and retrieval of material into and out of memory. Much of the support for this view is provided by studies with analogue populations (e.g. Ellis et al., 1984; Leight & Ellis, 1981). However, there are also a number of compelling studies with clinically depressed individuals. For example, Potts et al. (1989) replicated a previous study by Ellis et al. (1984). Both studies took advantage of a finding from earlier research that recall is greater for material presented in a context which requires high levels of elaboration at the encoding stage versus one which requires low levels of elaboration (Stein & Bransford, 1979). Potts et al. found that this elaboration advantage was eliminated in depressed patients suggesting that depression interferes with elaborative processing of neutral material. Other research which has sought to test the predications of resource allocation theory has generated more equivocal findings. For example, Weingartner et al. (1981) reported no differences between clinically depressed subjects and controls on recall of structured word lists but clear differences for the same material presented in an unstructured format, thus implying that depressed subjects may not have the resources to organize material at encoding. However, Levy and Maxwell (1968) using approximation to text as a method of structuring prose material found that depressed individuals benefited less from increased structure and Watts et al. (1990) found that depressed subjects performed optimally when the material was of medium text approximation.

It seems then that the RAM struggles to account for all of the data and this is perhaps not surprising as it is somewhat under specified. Ellis (1990) has proposed that the RAM is completely agnostic as to where the depressed mood states have their effect. It is also unclear what is the underlying reason for a reduction in available processing resources. Is it because resources are employed in processing task-irrelevant depressogenic thoughts? Or is it that there is simply a general resource depletion? These more specific issues are increasingly the subject of research; for example, Ellis et al. (1990) provide evidence for higher levels of task-irrelevant unfavourable thoughts associated with depressed mood.

A different take on the depression and general memory literature has been provided by Hertel and her colleagues (e.g. Hertel & Hardin, 1990; Hertel & Rude, 1991). She suggests that depressed individuals are exhibiting a deficit in initiative rather than simply resource allocation; that is, depressed individuals are less likely to instigate strategies or to generate relevant hypotheses when performing unstructured tasks. In a series of experiments to investigate this, Hertel and Hardin (1990) showed that, when depressed subjects are provided with instructions that enable them to structure a task appropriately, they show no performance deficits relative to controls, thus indicating that the resources to perform the task are available if the depressed individuals are guided to the right strategies. Perhaps not surprisingly, Ellis (1991) has suggested that such choice of strategy and initiative is itself resource dependent and that Hertel's findings present no problems for RAM.

In sum, there are clear general memory deficits associated with depression. The association is stronger for self-reports of memory difficulties but remains substantial even on objective memory tests with stronger effects being found in younger depressed subjects and in inpatients relative to outpatients. Theoretical accounts of these findings, such as Ellis and Ashbrook's Resource Allocation Model, have proved useful in pushing the research area forward. However, they now seem too catch all and the time has come for more tightly specified theoretical frameworks. There is some light on the horizon here with the advent of multi-representational theories of emotion such as Interacting Cognitive Subsystems (ICS; Teasdale & Barnard, 1993) and Schematic, Propositional, Associative and Analogue Representational Systems (SPAARS; Power & Dalgleish, 1997); however, the complex nature of these models precludes any detailed discussion in the present chapter.

## Memory for valenced material

And now a look at the effect of mood on memory for emotional material, that has a positive or negative valence. The intention is not to provide an exhaustive review of the literature, but again to focus on the basic ideas that have most relevance to clinical practice. As mentioned previously, the emphasis will be on depression.

Mood-congruence effects refer to a memory bias in which material which is affectively toned is more easily remembered if it is congruent with the individual's mood during retrieval as compared with material which is incongruent with the current mood state. Unlike state-dependent effects (i.e. when material which is learned in a particular mood is more likely to be recalled when in that same mood at retrieval), mood-congruency effects say nothing about mood at encoding. State-dependent effects have been difficult to demonstrate (Bower et al., 1978) and tend to be found only under very limited conditions (e.g. Schare et al., 1984). Empirically, however, these two phenomena are difficult to disentangle. This is particularly relevant if the researcher is unaware of mood at encoding, as is the case with recall of autobiographical memories. Hence, it is not realistic to rule out a possible role for state dependence with regard to mood-congruence effects and vice versa, and it is perhaps safer to assume that, in some studies, both of these processes may operate in combination. Mood-congruence is a phenomenon which has been studied in depth and has been demonstrated with a wide variety of cognitive tasks, materials and subject samples (including naturally occurring mood in clinically depressed and subclinically depressed populations and induced moods) and has produced 'relatively robust findings in clinical and experimental investigation' (Blaney, 1986).

The typical method of investigation in studies of mood-congruence involves exposing the subject to material with an affective valence and probing for memory of it in the same or different mood states. Memory is indexed through the speed and/or accuracy of recall and accuracy of recognition. The main finding of interest, with relevance to depression, is that a depressed mood leads to inhibited recall of positive material and in some cases a facilitative recall of negative material, although the latter is less common. In a day-to-day situation this material is most likely to be memories for events in the individual's life. In an attempt to see whether this emotional memory bias could be found under experimental conditions, Teasdale and Fogarty (1979) gave a sample of non-depressed subjects a list of neutral words to cue positive or negative memories and induced an elated mood in half of the subjects and a depressed mood in the remainder (Velten, 1968). They found that latencies to remember positive events were increased in the depressed group. Clark and Teasdale (1982) using a sample of clinically depressed individuals characterized by diurnal mood swings found that, when asked to retrieve positive or negative memories at different times in the daily cycle, negative memories were more probable than positive memories in the most depressed mood and the opposite was true when in the relatively positive mood. Finally, a biasing effect of mood (using various mood induction techniques, e.g. hypnosis, success vs. failure on a laboratory task, music and naturally occurring depressed mood) on autobiographical memories has been found to be robust and has been shown both with subjects in an induced mood and clinically depressed subjects (e.g. Lloyd & Lishman, 1975; Gilligan & Bower, 1984; Teasdale et al., 1980; Williams & Scott, 1988).

The main criticism of mood-congruence studies using autobiographical memories is that the mood at encoding is not known and hence one can not reliably distinguish between state-dependent and mood-congruent effects. Furthermore, the balance of positive and negative memories in a given subject is an unknown; it is therefore not possible to say whether memory effects represent a genuine bias or merely reflect the profile of the embedded material. A way of avoiding these confounds is to provide the to-be-learned material, for example, Bradley and Mathews (1983) gave clinically depressed and non-depressed subjects lists of affectively valenced (positive and negative) words. They found that depressed subjects showed lower recall of positive material when compared with controls. Memory bias effects using variations of this kind of paradigm have been shown in a large number of studies with subclinically depressed (e.g. Gotlib & McCann, 1984; Ingram et al., 1983), clinically depressed, and control subjects (e.g. Dunbar & Lishman, 1984;

McDowall, 1984, Study 1). The majority of these studies show that depressed subjects either remember less positive material or more negative material, compared with controls.

An important question concerns the relative contributions of mood at encoding and mood at retrieval, and mood induction studies have been used in an attempt to separate out the relative contributions of these two mnemonic operations. For example, Isen et al. (1978) gave subjects in a neutral mood a list of positive and negative personality trait words to learn. Subjects were then randomly allocated to one of two groups, and both groups played a game. By design, one group was bound to be successful and the other group was bound to fail. The subjects in the 'success' condition recalled more positive words, but subjects in the 'failure' condition did not recall more negative words. This suggests that it is mood-biasing effects occurring at retrieval that underlie the effect. However, Bower et al. (1981) suggested that mood-congruence effects also involve a bias at encoding. In their study, a story including an equal number of happy and sad statements, was read by subjects while in a hypnotically induced mood (happy or sad). Mood-congruence effects were shown, but there was no effect of mood at retrieval. Various reasons have been suggested for the lack of mood-congruent retrieval effects in Bower's study. It may have been due to associations being made between items of opposite valence within the story or because the fictional material was not self-referent as in other studies (Isen et al., 1978; Teasdale & Russel, 1983). Research tends to be consistent in suggesting that mood-congruence effects are obtainable only under self-referent conditions (Williams et al., 1988). It has been shown that if self-referencing is actively discouraged, mood-congruence effects are almost impossible to demonstrate (e.g. see Gotlib & Hammen, 1992).

There are a few studies which have failed to show mood-congruence effects and it has been suggested that this is due to problems in experimental design or with the material used. Ellis and Ashbrook (1989), for example, have suggested that highly structured material, such as narrative passages with the to-be-learned material embedded within them (e.g. Hasher et al., 1985), are impervious to mood-congruent effects. It has also been argued that mood-congruence effects may not involve only purely automatic processes. Thus individuals in a depressed mood may actively try to avoid negative material or retrieve happy memories thereby over-riding, to a greater or lesser extent, the automatic impact of mood-congruent accessibility thereby leading to mood-incongruent effects (Singer & Salovey, 1988). Matt et al. (1992) have pointed out that mood-congruence studies have failed to consider that mood-congruent memory effects may vary in magnitude. In their review of a subset of the published research, they suggested that failure to find a mood-congruent effect may have been due to a lack of statistical power.

One paradoxical finding by researchers has been that there is no correlation between the level of depressed mood and differential recall of congruent material within a particular mood (Mathews & Bradley, 1983; Riskind, 1983). It has been suggested that this is due to the complex nature of cognitive states and therefore it may not be mood per se that is responsible for mood-congruence effects, but perhaps processes involving priming of specific cognitive themes. Alternatively, mood states may be confounded with other characteristics of being in a particular mood, for example, certain personality traits (Mayer & Salovey, 1988), and it is these which influence processing of information.

As with the effects of depression on general memory, various models have attempted to explain mood-congruence effects. There are often variations on a theme, and the intention here is to provide a brief overview of the most widely recognized and most elaborately developed of these approaches. The most commonly used model to explain mood-congruence is Bower's Associative Network Theory of Affect (e.g. Bower, 1981). This theory describes an associative network of nodes. Each emotion is represented as a central node in this network and can be activated by physiological or symbolic verbal means, and is linked to all associated aspects of that emotion; that is, related ideas, events of corresponding valence, associated semantic material, autonomic activity and expressive behaviours. Bower suggests that mood-congruence effects occur owing to affectively valenced words being associated with the congruent emotion node; hence, at retrieval, when in a given mood the activated emotion node leads to a biased search and increased availability of mood-congruent materials due to spreading activation. However, this model is not able to explain many complex aspects of the data even with post hoc additions to the theory, and the major disadvantage of this model is that emotion is represented in the same network as semantic meaning (Dalgleish & Watts, 1990).

An alternative approach is based on Schema Theory as applied by Beck and colleagues to depression (e.g. Beck, 1976; Beck et al., 1979). Beck proposes that, when an individual is in a prevailing mood (e.g. a depressed mood), a schema which is consistent with that mood state, organizes and processes all new information in a biased schema-congruent way. In the case of depression the schema is purportedly concerned with negative aspects of the self, world, and future, and consequently influences the retrieval of specific memories congruent with those themes.

More sophisticated accounts of memory bias phenomena are offered by multi-representational models such as ICS (Teasdale & Barnard, 1993) and SPAARS (Power & Dalgleish, 1997). However, the predictions of these theories are broadly in line with the simpler models of Bower and Beck and no discussion of the details of their respective architectures and processing parameters will therefore be offered.

In sum, research on mood-congruence effects suggests that individuals in a depressed mood remember relatively more negative and relatively less positive material than controls.

In this chapter it has been argued that research reveals that depressed mood appears to lead not only to deficits in general memory performance, but also to mnemonic biases in favour of negative material and 'away from' positive material. What are the clinical implications of these issues? The first is diagnostic. Depressed individuals, because of the memory problems we have highlighted, may overlap in presentation with individuals with organic or neuropsychologically based memory difficulties. Care is therefore called for in differential diagnosis, especially in the elderly population (e.g. Cummings, 1989).

The second issue concerns day-to-day therapeutic management of mood disorders. The pattern of memory problems in, for example, depression suggests that work on timetabling and diary management would not only be pragmatically helpful but would also mitigate against further damage to self-esteem arising from the forgetting of important information. Similarly, cognitive therapy with mood-disordered individuals revolves around working with autobiographical material and using it to challenge core beliefs and assumptions about the self. If mnemonic access to this material is slanted in a negative direction in mood disordered individuals, then extra therapeutic work is indicated to generate positive memories for use in the cognitive therapy process.

The third issue relates to the research techniques themselves as much as to the findings they have generated. Cognitive psychology paradigms such as those described in the present chapter may provide a useful objective measure of mood disorder and may have potential applications in assessment and measurement of outcome. Admittedly, there is a long way to go from the sort of group effects that have been reviewed here to the development of cognitive tools which can be used reliably on an individual basis and the jury is still out on this issue.

To summarize, in this chapter there has been an endeavour to do justice to the wealth of literature on mood and memory. It has been possible to offer only the briefest of summaries of the many studies in this area. However, it is hoped that the spirit of the findings has been captured, if not the letter, in our conclusion that mood disorders, and by this is primarily meant depression, lead to both a general deficit in memory performance which is worse in older subjects and inpatients and also to biased memory in favour of negative material and away from positive material.

## REFERENCES

Beck, A.T. (1976). *Cognitive Therapy and the Emotional Disorders.* New York: Meridian.

Beck, A.T., Rush, A.J., Shaw, B.F. & Emery, G. (1979). *Cognitive Therapy of Depression.* New York: Guilford Press.

Blaney, P.H. (1986). Affect and memory: a review. *Psychological Bulletin*, **99**, 229–46.

Bower, G.H. (1981). Mood and memory. *American Psychologist*, **36**, 129–48.

Bower, G.H., Monteiro, K.P. & Gilligan, S.G. (1978). Emotional mood as a context for learning and recall. *Journal of Verbal Learning and Verbal Behaviour*, **17**, 573–87.

Bower, G.H., Gilligan, S.G. & Monteiro, K.P. (1981). Selectivity of learning caused by affective states. *Journal of Experimental Psychology: General*, **110**, 451–73.

Bradley, B. & Matthews, A. (1983). Negative self-schemata in clinical depression. *British Journal of Clinical Psychology*, **22**, 173–81.

Burt, D.B., Zembar, M.J. & Niederehe, G. (1995). Depression and memory impairment: a meta-analysis of the association, its pattern and specificity. *Psychological Bulletin*, **117**, 285–305.

Clark, D.M. & Teasdale, J.D. (1982). Diurnal variation in clinical depression and accessibility of memories of positive and negative experiences. *Journal of Abnormal Psychology*, **91**, 87–95.

Cronholm, B. & Ottosson, J.O. (1961). The experience of memory function after electroconvulsive therapy. *British Journal of Psychiatry*, **109**, 251–8.

Cummings, J.L. (1989). Dementia and depression: an evolving enigma. *Journal of Neuropsychiatry*, **1**, 236–42.

Dalgleish, T. & Watts, F. N. (1990). Biases of attention and memory in disorders of anxiety and depression. *Clinical Psychology Review*, **10**, 589–604.

Dunbar, G.C. & Lishman, W.A. (1984). Depression, recognition-memory and hedonic tone: a signal detection analysis. *British Journal of Psychiatry*, **144**, 376–82.

Ellis, H. C. (1990). Depressive deficits in memory: processing initiative and resource allocation. *Journal of Experimental Psychology: General*, **119**, 60–2.

Ellis, H.C. (1991, April 11–13). Mood, memories and cognition: data, theory, and applications. Invited keynote address to the annual meeting of the Southwestern Psychological Association, New Orleans.

Ellis, H.C. & Ashbrook, P.W. (1989). The 'state' of mood and memory research: a selective review. Special Issue: Mood and memory: theory, research and applications. *Journal of Social Behaviour and Personality*, **4**, 1–21.

Ellis, H.C., Thomas, R.L. & Rodriguez, I.A. (1984). Emotional mood states and memory: elaborative encoding, semantics processing, and cognitive effort. *Journal of Experimental Psychology: Learning, Memory and Cognition*, **10**, 470–82.

Ellis, H.C., Seibert, P.S. & Herbert, B.J. (1990). Mood state effects on thought listing. *Bulletin of the Psychonomic Society*, **28**, 147–50.

Fogler, J. & Stern, L. (1987). *Memory Improvement Programs for Older Adults: A Training Manual.* Ann Arbor, MI: University of Michigan Turner Geriatric Clinic.

Gilligan, S.G. & Bower, G.H. (1984). Cognitive consequences of emotional arousal. In *Emotions, Cognitions and Behaviour*, ed. C. Izard, J. Kagen & R. Zajonc, pp. 547–8. New York: Cambridge University Press.

Gotlib, I.H. (1981). Self-reinforcement and recall: differential deficits in depressed and non-depressed psychiatric inpatients. *Journal of Abnormal Psychology*, **90**, 521–30.

Gotlib, I.H. & McCann, C.D. (1984). Construct accessibility and depression: an examination of cognitive and affective factors. *Journal of Personality and Social Psychology*, **47**, 427–39.

Gotlib, I.H. & Hammen, C.L. (1992). *Psychological Aspects of Depression: Toward a Cognitive–Interpersonal Integration*. Chichester: Wiley.

Hart, R., Kwentus, A., Taylor, R. & Harkins, S.W. (1987). Rate of forgetting in dementia and depression. *Journal of Consulting and Clinical Psychology*, **55**, 101–5.

Hasher, L., Rose, K.C., Zacks, R.T., Samft, H. & Doren, B. (1985). Mood, recall, and selectivity in normal college students. *Journal of Experimental Psychology: General*, **114**, 104–18.

Hertel, P.T. & Hardin, T.S. (1990). Remembering with and without awareness in a depressed mood: evidence of deficits in initiative. *Journal of Experimental Psychology: General*, **119**, 45–59.

Hertel, P.T. & Rude, S.S. (1991). Recalling in a state of natural or experimental depression. *Cognitive Therapy and Research*, **15**, 103–27.

Ingram, R.E., Smith, T.W. & Brehm, S.S. (1983). Depression and information processing: self-schemata and the encoding of self-referent information. *Journal of Personality and Social Psychology*, **45**, 412–20.

Isen, A.M., Shalker, T.E., Clark, M. & Carp, L. (1978). Affect, accessibility of material in memory, and behaviour: a cognitive loop. *Journal of Personality and Social Psychology*, **36**, 1–12.

Kahn, R.L., Zarit, S.H., Hilbert, N.M. & Niederehe, G. (1975). Memory complaint and impairment in the aged: the effect of depression and altered brain function. *Archives of General Psychiatry*, **32**, 1569–73.

Leight, K.A. & Ellis, H.S. (1981). Emotional mood states, strategies and state-dependency in memory. *Journal of Verbal Learning and Verbal Behaviour*, **20**, 251–66.

Levy, R. & Maxwell, A.E. (1968). The effect of verbal context on the recall of schizophrenics and other psychiatric patients. *British Journal of Psychiatry*, **114**, 311–16.

Lloyd, G.G. & Lishman, W.A. (1975). Effect of depression on the speed of recall of pleasant and unpleasant experiences. *Psychological Medicine*, **5**, 173–80.

McDowall, J. (1984). Recall of pleasant and unpleasant words in depressed subjects. *Journal of Abnormal Psychology*, **93**, 401–7.

Mathews, A. & Bradley, B. (1983). Mood and the self-referenced bias in recall. *Behaviour, Research and Therapy*, **21**, 233–9.

Matt, G.E., Vázquez, C. & Campbell, W.K. (1992). Mood-congruent recall of affectively toned stimuli: a meta-analytic review. *Clinical Psychology Review*, **12**, 227–55.

Mayer, J.D. & Salovey, P. (1988). Personality moderates the interaction of mood and cognition. In *Affect, Cognition and Social Behaviour*, ed. K. Fiedler & J. Forgas, pp. 87–99. Toronto: Hogrefe.

O'Connor, D.W., Pollitt, P.A., Roth, M., Brook, P.B. & Reiss, B.B. (1990). Memory complaints and impairment in normal, depressed and demented elderly persons identified in a community survey. *Archives of General Psychiatry*, **47**, 224–7.

O'Hara, M.W., Hinrichs, J.V., Kohout, F.J., Wallace, R.B. & Lemke, J.H. (1986). Memory complaint and memory performance in the depressed elderly. *Psychology and Aging*, 1, 208–14.

Potts, R., Camp, C. & Coyne, C. (1989). The relationship between naturally occuring dysphoric moods, elaborative encoding and recall performance. *Cognition and Emotion*, 3, 197–205.

Power, M. & Dalgleish, T. (1997). *Cognition and Emotion: From Order to Disorder*. Hove: Psychology Press.

Riskind, J.H. (1983). Nonverbal expressions and the accessibility of life experience memories: a congruency hypothesis. *Social Cognition*, 2, 62–86.

Schare, M.L., Lishman, S.A. & Spear, N.E. (1984). The effects of mood variation on state-dependent retention. *Cognitive Therapy and Research*, 8, 387–408.

Scogin, F. (1985). Memory complaints and memory performance: the relationship re-examined. Special Issue: Ageing and mental health. *Journal of Applied Gerontology*, 4, 79–89.

Scogin, F., Storandt, M. & Lott, L. (1985). Memory skills training, memory complaints, and depression in older adults. *Journal of Gerontology*, 40, 562–8.

Singer, J.A. & Salovey, P. (1988). Mood and memory: evaluating the network theory of affect. *Clinical Psychology Review*, 8, 211–51.

Sternberg, D.E. & Jarvik, M.E. (1976). Memory functions in depression. *Archives of General Psychiatry*, 33, 219–24.

Stromgren, L.S. (1977). The influence of depression on memory. *Acta Psychiatrica Scandinavica*, 56, 109–28.

Teasdale, J.D. & Fogarty S.J. (1979). Differential effects of induced mood on retrieval of pleasant and unpleasant events from episodic memory. *Journal of Abnormal Psychology*, 88, 248–57.

Teasdale, J.D. & Russel, M.L. (1983). Differential effects of induced mood on the recall of positive, negative and neutral words. *British Journal of Clinical Psychology*, 22, 163–71.

Teasdale, J.D. & Barnard, P.J. (1993). *Affect, Cognition and Change: Re-modelling Depressive Thought*. Hove: Lawrence Erlbaum Associates.

Teasdale, J.D., Taylor, R. & Fogarty, S.J. (1980). Effects of induced elation-depression on the accessibility of memories of happy and unhappy experiences. *Behaviour Research and Therapy*, 18, 339–46.

Velten, E. (1968). A laboratory task for induction of mood states. *Behaviour Research and Therapy*, 6, 473–82.

Watts, F.N. (1993). Problems of memory and concentration. In *Symptoms of Depression*, ed. C.G. Costello, New York: Wiley.

Watts, F.N. & Sharrok, R. (1985). Description and measurement of concentration problems in depressed patients. *Psychological Medicine*, 15, 317–26.

Watts, F.N., Dalgleish, T., Bourke, P. & Healy, D. (1990). Memory deficit in clinical depression: processing resources and the structure of materials. *Psychological Medicine*, 20, 345–9.

Weingartner, H., Cohen, R.M., Murphy, D.L., Martello, J.E. & Gerdt, C. (1981). Cognitive processes in depression. *Archives of General Psychiatry*, 38, 42–7.

West, R.L, Boatwright, L.K. & Schleser, R. (1984). The link between memory performance, self-assessment, and affective status. *Experimental Ageing Research*, 10, 197–200.

Whitehead, A. (1973). Verbal learning and memory in elderly depressives. *British Journal of Psychiatry*, **123**, 203–8.

Williams, J.M.G. & Scott, J. (1988). Autobiographical memory in depression. *Psychological Medicine*, **18**, 689–95.

Williams, J.M.G., Watts, F.N., MacLeod, C. & Mathews, A. (1988). *Cognitive Psychology and Emotional Disorders*. Chichester, UK: John Wiley.

# 3

# The concept of metamemory: cognitive, developmental, and clinical issues

Roger A. Dixon

In its most basic sense, the term 'metamemory' refers to cognition about memory – thinking about how, why and whether memory works. More elaborated views of metamemory include knowledge of memory functioning, awareness of current memory processes, beliefs about memory skills, and even memory-related affect. In this chapter, both an overview of an elaborated concept of metamemory and a brief review of literature pertaining to the assessment of it are provided. This elaborated view of metamemory is especially useful when considering developmental issues (e.g. how memory normally changes – grows and declines – across the lifespan) and clinical concerns (e.g. how memory disorders are developed, supported and remedied).

## Context of the concept of metamemory

In recent decades, the concept of metamemory has been the topic of considerable attention in a variety of neighbouring domains of psychological and psychiatric research and practice. The range of both the substantive interests and the theoretical perspectives of the researchers is notable, for it spans numerous 'disciplines' of the psychological sciences. Five such disciplines are noted here. First, cognitive psychologists have examined metacognition as bridging and reflecting such processes as self-monitoring, decision making, learning and memory, motivation, plans and strategies, and cognitive development (see Metcalfe & Shimamura, 1994). For example, Nelson and Narens (1990, 1994) have developed a framework of metamemory in which monitoring and control processes interact during the acquisition, retention, and retrieval phases of memory. Secondly, neuropsychologists have examined metacognition as it bridges cognitive psychology, neuroscience, and clinical neuropsychology. For example, researchers may be concerned with metacognitive impairment that has occurred as a function of brain injury, disease, or normal aging-related neurological changes (Dixon & Bäckman, 1999; Moscovitch & Winocur, 1992; Prigatano & Schacter, 1991; Shimamura, 1994).

Thirdly, some social and personality psychologists are interested in metamemory in so far as it reflects the principle that cognitive processes do not operate in isolation from personality and social cognitive processes. For example, researchers may examine the effects of self-concept, self-regulation, self-efficacy, and sense of mastery or control on cognitive performance in children or adults (Bandura, 1989; Berry & West, 1993; Lachman & Leff, 1989; Schunk, 1989). Fourthly, child developmental and educational psychologists have examined metamemory as it relates to the growth or improvement of basic cognitive skills in children (e.g. Brown, 1978; Cavanaugh & Perlmutter, 1982; Flavell & Wellman, 1977; Schneider & Pressley, 1989). An important pedagogical concern is when, and how, children learn and apply strategies that improve their learning performance in school and other settings. Fifthly, lifespan developmental psychologists have examined metamemory development in adulthood. From the beginning of research in this area (e.g. Perlmutter, 1978) the focus has been on multidimensional views of metamemory, how metamemory per se develops in adulthood, and whether metamemory failures may account for some aging-related declines in memory performance (Dixon, 1989; Gilewski & Zelinski, 1986; Hertzog & Dixon, 1994; Light, 1991; Lovelace, 1990). The latter view, which incorporates numerous perspectives from the other four 'disciplines' of metamemory research, is explicated further in the following section.

## A multidimensional concept of metamemory

### Four characteristics

What is the concept of metamemory emerging from this growing and variegated literature? Together with colleagues, Christopher Hertzog and David Hultsch, the author has emphasized an inclusive and multidimensional concept of metamemory (Dixon, 1989; Dixon & Hultsch, 1983b; Dixon et al., 1988; Hertzog & Dixon, 1994; Hertzog et al., 1990). Four important characteristics of the present concept are summarized. First, our definition is inclusive in that a wide variety of behaviours (knowledge, beliefs, evaluations, and estimates) are representative of the concept of metamemory and, when measured, may indicate the level, degree, or extent of an individual's metamemory performance or skill. Secondly, our definition is multidimensional and convergent, in that the multiple facets or behaviours are viewed as separate, but linked, dimensions of a coherent construct of metamemory.

Thirdly, our definition assumes not only that multiple operations and dimensions would converge on a higher-order construct of metamemory, but also that metamemory can be discriminated from related constructs. That is, metamemory is empirically and theoretically distinguishable from other related domains, such as social intelligence, crystallized intelligence, identity, general self-efficacy, and even other forms of metacognition. Fourthly, metamemory is a construct of interest in, and of, itself, but it may also have direct or indirect implications for normal or dysfunctional memory performance. That is, understanding metamemory may help researchers and clinicians to identify and understand (a) actual deficits or declines in memory performance and (b) the occasional gaps between hypothetical memory competence and actual memory performance.

## Definition and categories

Our definition was based on these characteristics, as derived from the research emphases of neighbouring disciplines. Specifically, according to our definition, metamemory is a term representing one's knowledge, awareness, and beliefs about the functioning, development, and capacities of one's own memory and human memory in general (Dixon, 1989; Dixon & Hultsch, 1983b; Hultsch et al., 1988). As such, metamemory includes three principal categories (Hertzog & Dixon, 1994). First, declarative knowledge about how memory functions includes knowledge of how the characteristics of memory tasks have an impact on memory performance, whether strategies are required, and which strategies may be usefully applied to particular situations. For example, knowledge that organized materials are easier to remember than unorganized materials is an example of memory knowledge, a practical implication of which is that the efficient rememberer might use such knowledge to organize disordered to-be-remembered information.

Secondly, self-referent beliefs about one's capability to use memory effectively in memory-demanding situations defines memory self-efficacy (Berry & West, 1993; Cavanaugh, 1996) and is related to memory controllability (Lachman et al., 1995). One's beliefs about one's ability to remember may determine (a) the extent to which one places oneself in memory demanding situations, (b) the degree of effort one applies to perform the memory task, (c) one's expectation regarding level of memory performance, and (d) one's actual memory performance. For example, if one believes that one is not good at remembering names and faces one may attempt to avoid circumstances in which such a demand will occur, apply little effort with little expected success when placed in such situations, and indeed fail to remember new names and faces. Notably, such a pattern would confirm the pre-existing low sense of memory self-efficacy.

Thirdly, awareness of the current state of one's ongoing memory performance is also known as memory monitoring. Effective rememberers are able to monitor actively and accurately their performance *vis-à-vis* the demands of the memory task. A high degree of accuracy in predictions of performance and on-line judgments of learning may indicate an effective and accomplished rememberer (Nelson & Narens, 1994). Clinically, an awareness of a deficit may be an important precursor to memory compensation (Dixon & Bäckman, 1995).

In our research a fourth possible category of metamemory has also been considered, namely, memory-related affect (Dixon & Hultsch, 1983b; Hultsch et al., 1988). For many people, memory-demanding situations may be associated with affect (such as anxiety and depression) and other aspects of personality (e.g. motivation). This affect may be produced by an evaluation that a given memory situation is too demanding (thus leading to memory anxiety). Affect may also produce an altered level of performance, such as when anxiety or depression lead to poorer memory performance (e.g. Burt et al., 1995) or when a high degree of achievement motivation is associated with a high level of effort, leading to higher performance. Investment of time and effort is one form of memory compensation (Bäckman & Dixon, 1992; Dixon & Bäckman, 1995). Affect – and knowledge of the role that affect may play in memory functioning – is an important part of metamemory and memory performance in many situations. Although it continues to be included in our research agenda, it is no longer actively proposed as a principal category of metamemory (Dixon 1989; Hertzog & Dixon, 1994).

## Some implications

These categories of metamemory are related to one another theoretically (Dixon, 1989; Hertzog & Dixon, 1994), empirically (Hertzog et al., 1990; Hultsch et al., 1988), and interwoven in determining everyday memory performance. Clarifying precisely how these categories of metamemory interweave to determine memory performance – as well as which categories are related to which performances on which memory tasks and for whom – is an abiding challenge to researchers and clinicians alike (Dixon & Hertzog, 1988; Lovelace, 1990). What are the logical and practical implications of the above categories of metamemory?

In principle, high performance on given memory tasks should be promoted by the following metamemory profile: (a) a well-structured declarative knowledge base about how memory functions in given tasks, (b) refined knowledge of one's own memory skills, (c) accurate and high memory self-efficacy, and (d) skill at the monitoring and control activities during acquisition, retention and retrieval. In addition, it could be useful to have (e) stable or low memory-related affect, such that the potential deleterious effects of memory-related anxiety or depression could be avoided. In contrast, some individuals with poorer – and perhaps impaired – performance could be experiencing some components of the following profile: (a) and (b) an ill-structured, incomplete, or erroneous knowledge base pertaining to general memory functioning or one's own memory skills, (c) inaccurate or low memory self-efficacy, (d) an inability to monitor and control the requisite activities of effective remembering, and (e) fluctuant, uncontrolled, or excessive memory-related anxiety or depression. These profiles define two hypothetical ends of a continuum.

Consider two clinical implications of these hypothetical profiles. First, can some non-organic memory disorders or impairments be remedied through clinical intervention designed to assess and improve selected categories of metamemory? In the case of normal aging-related memory decline, the evidence that selectively improving one component of one of these categories, e.g. a single aspect of memory self-efficacy, can lead to corresponding increments in memory performance, e.g. word list memory, is not persuasive. The clinical research on this matter, however, is not definitive. As yet, little effort has been made to effect change in multiple dimensions of metamemory simultaneously and to measure memory performance in appropriately selected, if not domain-specific, tasks. Thus, the extent to which intervention in metamemory may affect memory performance – improving performance from the normal to the superior or from the impaired to the normal – is an open and intriguing question for future researchers.

A second possible clinical implication: can the diagnosis of some organic memory disorders be advanced through the use of metamemory information? Although also not yet definitive, some recent clinical research suggests that at least one aspect of memory (i.e. memory complaints) should be explored further for its usefulness as an early or collateral indicator of dementia (e.g. Grut et al., 1993). A comprehensive multidimensional representation of metamemory has yet to be explored in this regard. One advantage of a multidimensional construct of metamemory is that the components of the profiles can be assessed and studied simultaneously. Therefore, the interactions among the components and the numerous possible relationships with memory performance and change (decline) can be evaluated. The next section reviews one way of accomplishing this multidimensional representation.

## Assessment of multiple dimensions of metamemory

Important theoretical and methodological advances have resulted from researchers programmatically investigating a single dimension of metamemory in normal, healthy, and (often) young adults. For example, the work of Nelson and Narens (1990, 1994) in judgments of learning and the work of Koriat (1994) in feelings of knowing have pushed cognitive metamemory research in important new directions. One goal of our research has been to investigate the extent to which metamemory not only plays a role in normal or skilled remembering, but also in deficits of remembering. Such deficits can derive from developmental differences, e.g. younger children, older adults, or a host of other causes. In addition, such memory deficits can be observed (a) for minute tasks under stringently controlled conditions in the experimental laboratory, (b) for more complex or ill-structured memory tasks in naturalistic settings, and (c) for standardized tasks reflecting memory dysfunction in the psychological or memory clinic.

The principle espoused is that the influence of metamemory on memory performance is multidetermined and interactive. Put simply, more than one dimension of metamemory may be involved in determining complex memory performance. Knowing about potential utilities of memory strategies may be necessary for everyday memory performance, but it is rarely sufficient. In addition, one must believe that one has the ability to select the correct strategy, monitor its implementation, and effectively perform the task. In order to examine metamemory from this perspective, a multidimensional representation is essential.

## The metamemory in adulthood instrument

Several multidimensional metamemory instruments are now available (for reviews see Dixon, 1989; Gilewski & Zelinski, 1986; Herrmann, 1982; Lovelace, 1990). The Metamemory in Adulthood (MIA) instrument was developed to reflect the definition, categories, and principles described above (Dixon & Hultsch, 1983a, b; Dixon et al., 1988). There are 108 items distributed among seven scales. These scales are defined as follows.

(i)   *Strategy*: Knowledge and use of information about one's remembering abilities such that performance in given instances is potentially improved.
(ii)  *Task*: Knowledge of basic memory processes, especially as evidenced by how most people perform.
(iii) *Capacity*: Beliefs about memory capacities as evidenced by predictive report of performance on given tasks.
(iv)  *Change*: Beliefs about memory abilities (including one's own) as generally stable, improving, or declining.
(v)   *Anxiety*: Feelings of stress related to memory performance.
(vi)  *Achievement*: Believed importance of performing well on memory tasks.
(vii) *Locus*: Perceived personal control over remembering abilities.

Further information on the MIA instrument, these seven scales, and the 108 items may be found in Dixon et al. (1988). (Please note, however, that there is a typographical error in the scoring key of this publication; please write to one of the principal authors for a corrected key.)

## Selected MIA research

Much research has been conducted with this instrument, as well as some shorter versions, in several languages (e.g. Dutch: Ponds & Jolles, 1996). Psychometric characteristics of the MIA are high and quite robust across samples varying in a number of dimensions. Among the psychometric characteristics investigated are

Cronbach's α (internal consistency of the scales), factorial validity of the scales, convergent validity, discriminant validity, and predictive validity (see Dixon, 1989; Dixon & Hultsch, 1983a, b; Dixon et al., 1988; Hertzog et al., 1987, 1989, 1990; Ponds & Jolles, 1996). The MIA has been administered to several thousand adults, rendering a plethora of data pertaining to developmental differences in performance, as well as (in longitudinal studies) developmental changes (e.g. Hultsch et al., 1987; McDonald-Miszczak et al., 1995). Recently, the MIA has also been investigated in conjunction with on-line indicators of metamemory awareness (e.g. Hertzog et al., 1994).

Some basic findings as related to the issues discussed above may be summarized. Because of space limitations, four issues are focused on. First, does the MIA represent a multidimensional construct of metamemory? Several studies have indicated that indeed it does and, furthermore, have replicated basic factor structures (e.g. Dixon & Hultsch, 1983b; Hertzog et al., 1987; Ponds & Jolles, 1996). Secondly, is there convergence on the principal metamemory category of beliefs? Studies have shown that three MIA scales – capacity, change, and locus – converge with other indicators to form a robust Memory Self-Efficacy dimension (e.g. Hertzog et al., 1989). In addition, researchers have shown that older adults indicate lower memory self-efficacy than do younger adults (e.g. Cavanaugh & Poon, 1989; Dixon & Hultsch, 1983b; Hultsch et al., 1987; Loewen et al., 1992; Ryan, 1992). The intriguing suggestion is that differences in metamemory between 'normal' and at-risk adults (in this case, older adults) may be due substantially to a beliefs component of metamemory.

Thirdly, is there convergence on the principal metamemory category of knowledge? The MIA Task scale effectively measures the knowledge component of metamemory. Related to this, the Strategy scale measures self-reported use of internal mnemonics, e.g. rehearsal, and external memory aids, e.g. making lists. Some researchers have found that this scale may be usefully divided into Internal and External subscales (e.g. Dixon & Hultsch, 1983b; Ponds & Jolles, 1996). A theoretically and clinically intriguing possibility is that older adults (and, perhaps, other at-risk adults) may compensate for memory impairment by using external memory aids rather than internal mnemonics. Some evidence suggests that older adults indeed report more such use of external aids than (i) they do internal mnemonics and (ii) do younger adults (Dixon & Hultsch, 1983b; Loewen et al., 1992). Because external aids are generally easier to acquire and maintain – and because they may have more task generality – than internal mnemonics they may be useful for ameliorating moderate memory impairment. Nevertheless, several clinical researchers have noted that, because they require memory for implementation, memory-impaired individuals may fail to use them optimally (e.g. Intons-Peterson & Newsome, 1992; Wilson, 1995; Wilson & Watson, 1996).

Fourthly, is there evidence that a multidimensional construct of metamemory may be empirically discriminated from neighbouring constructs? The salient criterion of discriminant validity – one form of construct validity – would establish that specific dimensions of metamemory would be correlated higher with theoretically related constructs than with less-theoretically related constructs. The correlations observed in the literature suggest that metamemory factors, e.g. memory self-efficacy, are predictably related to, but distinct from, such constructs as neuroticism, depressive affect, general self-efficacy, and anxiety (Dixon et al., 1988; Hultsch et al., 1988).

## Conclusions

Metamemory is a concept larger and more complex than that captured by many unidimensional definitions. It includes but is not limited to cognition about memory, memory complaints, memory control, memory self-efficacy, memory knowledge, memory affect, memory monitoring, and memory awareness. A theoretically coherent elaborated concept of metamemory includes at least four components: declarative knowledge of memory functioning, awareness (or monitoring) of current memory processes, beliefs about memory skills and change, and memory-related affect. An overview of the rationale and the empirical evidence that a multidimensional concept of metamemory is theoretically and clinically promising is provided.

The brief review of the Metamemory in Adulthood instrument and literature demonstrates that it is possible to obtain indicators of multiple dimensions of metamemory simultaneously. The simultaneous measurement of multiple dimensions of metamemory is especially useful when considering developmental issues, e.g. how memory normally changes – grows and declines – across the lifespan and clinical concerns, e.g. how memory disorders are developed, supported, and remedied. Important issues of current and future research include: (i) the extent to which dimensions of metamemory interact in determining memory performance, impairment, or decline; (ii) the extent to which dimensions of metamemory may serve as early indicators of progressive memory decline, such as that associated with organic diseases; and (iii) the extent to which intervention in dimensions of metamemory may have indirect influence on memory performance, maintenance, improvement, or recovery.

## ACKNOWLEDGEMENT

Continuing research grant support from the US National Institute on Aging (AG08235) is gratefully acknowledged.

## REFERENCES

Bäckman, L. & Dixon, R.A. (1992). Psychological compensation: a theoretical framework. *Psychological Bulletin*, **112**, 259–83.

Bandura, A. (1989). Regulation of cognitive processes through perceived self-efficacy. *Developmental Psychology*, **25**, 729–35.

Berry, J.M. & West, R.L. (1993). Cognitive self-efficacy in relation to personal mastery and goal setting across the life-span. *International Journal of Behavioral Development*, **16**, 351–79.

Brown, A.L. (1978). Knowing when, where, and how to remember: a problem in metacognition. In *Advances in Instructional Psychology*, ed. R. Glaser, pp. 77–165. Hillsdale, NJ: Erlbaum.

Burt, D.B., Zembar, M.J. & Niederehe, G. (1995). Depression and memory impairment: a meta-analysis of the association, its pattern and specificity. *Psychological Bulletin*, **117**, 285–305.

Cavanaugh, J.C. (1996). Memory self-efficacy as a moderator of memory change. In *Perspectives on Cognitive Change in Adulthood and Aging*, ed. F. Blanchard-Fields & T.M. Hess, pp. 488–507. New York: McGraw-Hill.

Cavanaugh, J.C. & Perlmutter, M. (1982). Metamemory: a critical examination. *Child Development*, **53**, 11–28.

Cavanaugh, J.C. & Poon, L.W. (1989). Metamemorial predictors of memory performance in young and old adults. *Psychology and Aging*, **4**, 365–8.

Dixon, R.A. (1989). Questionnaire research on metamemory and aging: Issues of structure and function. In *Everyday Cognition in Adulthood and Old Age*, ed. L.W. Poon, D.C. Rubin & B.A. Wilson, pp. 394–415. New York: Cambridge University Press.

Dixon, R.A. & Hultsch, D.F. (1983a). Metamemory and memory for text relationships in adulthood: a cross-validation study. *Journal of Gerontology*, **38**, 689–94.

Dixon, R.A. & Hultsch, D.F. (1983b). Structure and development of metamemory in adulthood. *Journal of Gerontology*, **38**, 682–8.

Dixon, R.A. & Hertzog, C. (1988). A functional approach to memory and metamemory development in adulthood. In *Memory Development:Universal Changes and Individual Differences*, ed. F.E. Weinert & M. Perlmutter, pp. 293–330. Hillsdale, NJ: Erlbaum.

Dixon, R.A. & Bäckman, L. (1995). Concepts of compensation: Integrated, differentiated, and Janus-faced. In *Compensating for Psychological Deficits and Declines: Managing Losses and Promoting Gains*, ed. R.A. Dixon & L. Bäckman, pp. 3–19. Mahwah, NJ: Erlbaum.

Dixon, R. A. & Bäckman, L. (1999). Principles of compensation in cognitive neurorehabilitation. In *Cognitive Neurorehabilitation: A Comprehensive Approach*, ed. D. T. Stuss, G. Winocur & I. H. Robertson, pp. 59–72. Cambridge: Cambridge University Press.

Dixon, R.A., Hultsch, D.F. & Hertzog, C. (1988). The Metamemory in Adulthood (MIA) questionnaire. *Psychopharmacology Bulletin*, **24**, 671–88.

Flavell, J.H. & Wellman, H.M. (1977). Metamemory. In *Perspectives on the Development of Memory and Cognition*, ed. R.V. Kail & J.W. Hagen. Hillsdale, NJ: Erlbaum.

Gilewski, M.J. & Zelinski, E.M. (1986). Questionnaire assessment of memory complaints. In *Handbook for Clinical Memory Assessment of Older Adults*, ed. L.W. Poon, pp. 93–107. Washington, DC: American Psychological Association.

Grut, M., Jorm, A.F., Fratiglioni, L., Forsell, Y., Viitanen, M. & Winblad, B. (1993). Memory complaints of elderly people in a population survey: variation according to dementia stage and depression. *Journal of the American Geriatrics Society*, **41**, 1295–300.

Herrmann, D.J. (1982). Know thy memory: the use of questionnaires to assess and study memory. *Psychological Bulletin*, **92**, 434–52.

Hertzog, C. & Dixon, R.A. (1994). Metacognitive development in adulthood and old age. In *Metacognition: Knowing About Knowing*, ed. J. Metcalfe & A.P. Shimamura, pp. 227–251. Cambridge, MA: MIT Press.

Hertzog, C., Dixon, R.A., Schulenberg, J.E. & Hultsch, D.F. (1987). On the differentiation of memory beliefs from memory knowledge: the factor structure of the Metamemory in Adulthood scale. *Experimental Aging Research*, **13**, 101–7.

Hertzog, C., Hultsch, D.F. & Dixon, R.A. (1989). Evidence for the convergent validity of two self-report metamemory questionnaires. *Developmental Psychology*, **25**, 687–700.

Hertzog, C., Dixon, R.A. & Hultsch, D.F. (1990). Metamemory in adulthood: Differentiating knowledge, belief, and behavior. In *Aging and Cognition: Knowledge Organization and Utilization*, ed. T.M. Hess, pp. 161–212. Amsterdam: Elsevier.

Hertzog, C., Saylor, L.L., Fleece, A.M. & Dixon, R.A. (1994). Metamemory and aging: Relations between predicted, actual, and perceived memory task performance. *Aging and Cognition*, **1**, 203–37.

Hultsch, D.F., Hertzog, C. & Dixon, R.A. (1987). Age differences in metamemory: Resolving the inconsistencies. *Canadian Journal of Psychology*, **41**, 193–208.

Hultsch, D.F., Hertzog, C., Dixon, R.A. & Davidson, H. (1988). Memory self-knowledge and self-efficacy in the aged. In *Cognitive Development in Adulthood: Progress in Cognitive Development Research*, ed. M.L. Howe & C.J. Brainerd, pp. 65–92. New York: Springer.

Intons-Peterson, M.J. & Newsome, G.I. (1992). External memory aids: Effects and effectiveness. In *Memory Improvement: Implications for Memory Theory*, ed. D.J. Herrmann, H. Weingartner, A. Searleman & C. McEvoy, pp. 101–21. New York: Springer-Verlag.

Koriat, A. (1994). Memory's knowledge of its own knowledge: the accessibility account of the feeling of knowing. In *Metacognition: Knowing about Knowing*, ed. J. Metcalfe & A.P. Shimamura, pp. 115–35. Cambridge, MA: MIT Press.

Lachman, M.E. & Leff, R. (1989). Perceived control and intellectual functioning in the elderly: a 5-year longitudinal study. *Developmental Psychology*, **25**, 722–8.

Lachman, M.E., Bandura, M., Weaver, S.L. & Elliott, E. (1995). Assessing memory control beliefs: the Memory Controllability Inventory. *Aging and Cognition*, **2**, 67–84.

Light, L.L. (1991). Memory and aging: four hypotheses in search of data. *Annual Review of Psychology*, **42**, 333–76.

Loewen, E.R., Shaw, R.J. & Craik, F.I.M. (1992). Age differences in components of metamemory. *Experimental Aging Research*, **16**, 43–8.

Lovelace, E.A. (ed.) (1990). *Aging and Cognition: Mental Processes, Self-Awareness, and Interventions*. Amsterdam: North-Holland.

McDonald-Miszczak, L., Hertzog, C. & Hultsch, D.F. (1995). Stability and accuracy of metamemory in adulthood and aging: a longitudinal analysis. *Psychology and Aging*, **10**, 553–64.

Metcalfe, J. & Shimamura, A.P. (eds.) (1994). *Metacognition: Knowing about Knowing*. Cambridge, MA: MIT Press.

Moscovitch, M. & Winocur, G. (1992). The neuropsychology of memory and aging. In *The Handbook of Aging and Cognition*, ed. F.I.M. Craik & T.A. Salthouse, pp. 315–72. Hillsdale, NJ: Erlbaum.

Nelson, T.O. & Narens, L. (1990). Metamemory: a theoretical framework and new findings. In *The Psychology of Learning and Motivation*, ed. G. Bower, vol. 26. New York: Academic Press.

Nelson, T.O. & Narens, L. (1994). Why investigate metacognition? In *Metacognition: Knowing about Knowing*, ed. J. Metcalfe & A.P. Shimamura, pp. 1–25. Cambridge, MA: MIT Press.

Perlmutter, M. (1978). What is memory aging the aging of? *Developmental Psychology*, **14**, 330–45.

Ponds, R.W.H.M. & Jolles, J. (1996). The abridged Dutch Metamemory in Adulthood (MIA) questionnaire: structure and effects of age, sex, and education. *Psychology and Aging*, **11**, 324–32.

Prigatano, G.P. & Schacter, D.L. (eds.) (1991). *Awareness of Deficit after Brain Injury: Clinical and Theoretical Issues*. New York: Oxford University Press.

Ryan, E.B. (1992). Beliefs about memory changes across adulthood. *Journal of Gerontology: Psychological Sciences*, **47**, P41–6.

Schneider, W. & Pressley, M. (1989). *Memory Development Between 2 and 20*. New York: Springer.

Schunk, D.H. (1989). Social cognitive theory and self-regulated learning. In *Self-regulated Learning and Academic Achievement: Theory, Research, and Practice*, ed. B.J. Zimmerman & D.H. Schunk, pp. 83–110. New York: Springer.

Shimamura, A.P. (1994). The neuropsychology of metacognition. In *Metacognition: Knowing about Knowing*, ed. J. Metcalfe & A.P. Shimamura, pp. 253–76. Cambridge, MA: MIT Press.

Wilson, B.A. (1995). Memory rehabilitation: compensating for memory problems. In *Compensating for Psychological Deficits and Declines: Managing Losses and Promoting Gains*, ed. R.A. Dixon & L. Bäckman, pp. 171–90. Mahwah, NJ: Erlbaum.

Wilson, B.A. & Watson, P.C. (1996). A practical framework for understanding compensatory behaviour in people with organic memory impairment. *Memory*, **4**, 456–86.

# 4

# The neuropsychology of memory

Andrew R. Mayes

## Introduction

The human brain is not only a machine that processes many kinds of information, it is also an information storage system. The plasticity of the brain indicated by its ability to alter the synaptic connections between its neurons in several ways (see Rose, 1992) suggests that most regions of the brain, if not all, are capable of storing memories. There is a view, widely held by neuroscientists, that information is stored where it is processed, or, more precisely, represented, by the brain (for example, see Squire, 1987). Although there is relatively little direct evidence for this view, it is plausible to believe that, when a neuronal system is active because it is representing information, this activity will give rise to synaptic changes selectively within the neuronal system so that this information can be more readily re-represented from appropriate cues on future occasions. There is also overwhelming evidence that different brain regions process and represent different kinds of information (for example, see Kolb & Whishaw, 1990 *passim*), which implies that different kinds of information will be stored in different parts of the brain rather than in the same specialized 'memory storage system'. As there is good evidence for this implication (see Squire, 1987; Mayes, 1988), the view that information is stored where it is represented has considerable indirect support.

Until about 20 years ago most people assumed that memory (at least long-term memory) was a monolithic system, so that there was only one kind of memory that needed to be understood. All one needed to do was to find out how information was processed and represented at input (encoding), what processes were required to retain the encoded information (storage), and what processes were involved in reactivating the information from its latent form (retrieval). The problem only needed to be solved once. One of the striking changes of the past 20 years has been the disintegration of this view (see Squire, 1987; Mayes, 1988). For example, in a recent paper, Nyberg and Tulving (1996) argued for the existence of different long-term memory systems for episodic information, semantic information, procedural information (related to things like memory for skills and various forms of

58

conditioning), and implicit or unaware memory for specific items of information on the basis of functional or psychological, developmental, pharmacological, and neuropsychological dissociations between the four putative kinds of memory. Manipulations in these four domains produce double dissociations, i.e. one manipulation affects one of the putatively different kinds of memory, but does not affect any of the other three, whereas another manipulation does not affect the kind of memory affected by the first manipulation, but does affect one or more of the three other kinds of memory. On the basis of these kinds of dissociation, it might also be argued that short-term memory or its modern instantiation, working memory, is a different kind of memory system from these four long-term memory systems.

The concept of a memory system is unfortunately not a clearly defined one, however. It seems sometimes to mean only that different brain regions are concerned with encoding, storing and retrieving the kinds of information held by different brain systems (this seems to correspond to the sense in which Nyberg and Tulving use the concept). If the concept is used in this sense, then it will be necessary to postulate many more memory systems unless it is required that there be no overlap at all between the brain regions underlying distinct systems. For example, memory for faces and words can be dissociably disturbed by brain lesions (see Ellis & Young, 1988) and there is much other evidence to suggest that the two forms of memory are stored in distinct neocortical regions. There is even some evidence for neuropsychological dissociations between disturbances of semantic memory for inanimate and animate objects, which can be interpreted as support for the view that these kinds of information are stored in partially non-overlapping cortical regions (see Mayes, 1988).

It remains possible, however, that memory for different kinds of information depends on largely distinct brain regions, but nevertheless the algorithms that describe how the information is encoded, stored, and retrieved in the distinct regions are identical. This possibility is important because the other sense in which the concept of a memory system is used depends on the algorithms that drive encoding, storage, and retrieval such that different systems must use different algorithms (see Sherry & Schacter, 1987). As with the other sense, it needs to be specified whether different systems need to differ completely from each other or whether they can share some algorithmically identical processes. For this reason, it may be less confusing to talk about whether memory processes rather than systems differ either with respect to the brain regions that mediate them or the algorithms to which they conform. Also, if the algorithmic rather than brain region/type of information sense is adopted, it has to be accepted that, at present, there are only heuristic guidelines that can be used to decide whether different ways of encoding, storing, or retrieving information are being used. One of these is that the processes or systems depend on brain regions with radically different structural organizations of preferably different kinds of neuron. Another is to try and get hints about the underlying processes from psychological experiments. For example, if retrieving one kind of memory was always or, at least, often effortful whereas retrieving another kind never was, this would suggest that the retrieval processes may work in different ways.

Classification schemes for memory are hierarchical. Possibly the most widely known is that of Squire (for example, see Squire et al., 1993). At the top level, this scheme distinguishes between short-term and long-term memory. As Squire (1987) acknowledges and as will be made clear in the next section, there is good evidence that there are several distinct kinds of short-term memory. He focuses to a greater extent, however, on long-term memory, which he subdivides initially into declarative and procedural memory. Declarative memory is also referred to as explicit memory or, less commonly, relational memory, and procedural memory is also referred to as non-declarative or implicit memory. Declarative memory is sub-divided into episodic and semantic memory whereas procedural memory is subdi-vided into skills and habits; conditioning; non-associative forms of memory such as habituation; and priming or item-specific implicit memory.

Squire and his co-workers argue that these are different forms of memory because they are mediated by at least partially non-overlapping brain regions. The major evidence for this is that the putatively different forms of memory are differentially affected by damage to the brain. There is now also evidence for this claim from positron emission tomography (PET) and functional magnetic reso-nance imaging (fMRI) challenge studies. These studies compare the patterns of cerebral blood flow to, or blood oxygenation (measures which correlate with levels of neuronal activity) in, different brain regions in two or more states that ideally only differ with respect to the cognitive process of interest. Thus, it has been shown that when people engage in the different forms of memory they activate partially non-overlapping brain regions (for example, see Paulesu et al., 1993; Tulving et al., 1994). Much less can be said about whether the putatively different kinds of memory depend on encoding, storage and retrieval processes that are qualitatively distinct.

The following sections will consider short-term or working memory; declarative or explicit memory with a focus on whether the distinction between semantic and episodic memory is valid; priming or item-specific implicit memory; and skills, habits and conditioning. Each section will briefly define the terms and indicate how they are measured before considering in more detail on what brain regions and kinds of process they depend. In the final section, a new way of organizing think-ing about some of the memory processes will be suggested.

## Short-term or working memory

Complex mental operations require the ability to hold information of various kinds for brief periods of time. That short-term memory is distinct from long-term memory has been a dominant view since Atkinson and Shiffrin (1968) proposed that information is first held for around one second in a sensory store, e.g. iconic or echoic before some of it is passed to a short-term store in which it can only be retained for a few seconds unless rehearsed. They proposed that only a small amount of information is likely to be passed into long-term storage. The modern development of this view is the working memory hypothesis of Baddeley and Hitch (1977). Their hypothesis differed from earlier accounts of short-term memory in that they subdivided short-term memory into one storage system for verbal, or, more specifically, phonological information and one for visuospatial information. These storage systems, at least the phonological one, maintain information in store in conjunction with a dedicated rehearsal system, such as the articulatory loop. Working memory also includes a central executive system that guides and controls the operations that are performed on the contents of these short-term storage systems.

The capacity of the phonological short-term store is typically tested by seeing how many digits a subject can repeat back in the correct order immediately after hearing them spoken. Digit span depends not only on the efficiency of a passive phonological store, but also on the rehearsal of the stored material through the offices of the articulatory loop, which might be understood as a kind of inner speech system. When articulation is suppressed by getting subjects to repeat words like 'the' aloud, digit span is reduced. The capacity of the less researched visuospatial short-term store is typically tested by seeing how many randomly placed squares a subject can point to in the correct order immediately after seeing an examiner pointing in a particular sequence (the Corsi Blocks Test). If patients have impaired short-term storage, it is also important to show whether their encoding of the stored information is normal, e.g. by using a phonological matching task with minimal loading on memory for the phonological store and whether their rehearsal mechanism is normal, e.g. by seeing whether blocking it has a normal effect.

The central executive can also be examined. This system is best viewed as a set of executive processes such as shifting attention from one operation to another, and inhibiting operations which are not currently appropriate. These executive processes are primarily mediated by the prefrontal cortex and there is growing evidence that there are several of them. They are best assessed with tests sensitive to frontal lobe lesions such as the Cognitive Estimates Test (Shallice & Evans, 1978). They guide the specific operations, such as arithmetical calculations, that are performed on the contents of short-term memory. The specific operations are not regarded as part of working memory.

Short-term memory is distinguished from long-term memory on the grounds that the physiological processes underlying the two forms of memory are distinct. This means not only that the storage processes underlying short- and long-term memory at the neuronal level are different (see Rose, 1992), but, in recent times, it has also come to mean that the brain systems concerned with short- and long-term memory are partially distinct. This is a strong claim because the phonological and visuospatial information held in short-term storage can presumably also be held in long-term storage. If information is stored in the same brain regions in which it is represented, then this should apply equally whether the storage is short or long term. Nevertheless, there is good evidence that short- and long-term memory deficits can be dissociated from each other. Thus, organic amnesics have impaired long-term memory for all kinds of explicit memory, but preserved phonological and visuospatial working memories as shown, for example, by their normal digit and Corsi Blocks spans. In contrast, patients have been reported with relatively selective disorders of phonological short-term memory (see Shallice, 1988) or visuospatial short-term memory (Hanley et al., 1991). Some patients with severe phonological short-term deficits, as shown by their digit spans of around two items compared with a normal level of seven plus or minus two, seem to be able to process phonological information relatively normally and to be able to rehearse such information normally if they so wished so their deficit is presumably a selective one of short-term phonological storage. Nevertheless, they may have completely normal ability to acquire long-term memories of spoken verbal material such as stories or word lists.

The apparent normality of long-term memory in patients with phonological short-term memory deficits is, however, misleading. Thus, Baddeley et al. (1988) have shown that patient P.V., who has a severe deficit in phonological short-term memory, was totally unable to learn associations with spoken Russian words that had been transliterated into her native Italian. Long-term memory is only normal to the extent that incoming information can be transformed into other codes such as semantic ones. The likelihood is that, if short-term memory for specific information is impaired, then long-term memory for that information will also be devastated unless the information can be rapidly recoded by the patient. Long-term memory for the information depends on other processes that transform short-term into long-term memory and which are impaired in patients with organic amnesia. It remains likely, therefore, that information is stored in the same brain region whether the storage is short or long term. What remains a serious puzzle is how short-term storage can be impaired without processing being apparently affected if information is stored exactly where it is represented.

Three more points should be made about short-term memory. First, it can now also be investigated by PET and fMRI challenge studies. For example, Paulesu et al. (1993) have found evidence that use of the articulatory loop activates the left premotor area whereas short-term phonological storage activates the left supramarginal gyrus. This is consistent with the lesion evidence that lesions in this part of the parietal cortex most reliably cause deficits in the short-term phonological store without affecting rehearsal.

Secondly, it is very probable that there are short-term storage systems beyond the two originally postulated. There is already good evidence for separate verbal, spatial, and visual object short-term stores, which are disrupted by lesions in slightly different posterior cortical regions (see Vallar & Papagno, 1995). For example, spatial short-term memory activates the right parietal cortex more than the left (Jonides et al., 1993) and is more disrupted by such lesions (see Vallar & Papagno, 1995). In addition, there may be short-term stores for each sensory system and for motor representations, but it is probably also necessary to postulate a more abstract, store that briefly holds semantic information in tasks such as problem solving and understanding stories. Evidence for such a store is the role played by semantic factors in interference in short-term memory tasks (Dale & Gregory, 1966).

Thirdly, the brain regions involved in rehearsal of information from the specific stores as well as the stores themselves should be explored by both lesion and PET/fMRI studies. The same approach should be used with locating the regions responsible for controlling the different processes of the central executive. For example, Cohen et al. (1994) found, in an fMRI study, that a working memory task, which particularly called on executive processes, activated the dorsolateral prefrontal cortex. This is consistent with the view that the executive processes of the central executive primarily rely on the prefrontal cortex.

## Declarative/explicit memory: semantic and episodic memory

Declarative and explicit memory are synonymous names for long-term memories of which rememberers are aware in the sense that they know they have encountered the remembered information before in some capacity, however vague this knowledge may be. Aware memory can be divided into episodic and semantic memory. Episodic memory is aware memory for episodes that have been personally experienced by the rememberer. In contrast, semantic memory was originally defined as aware memory for the kinds of factual information that make up people's mental dictionaries and encyclopaedias (Tulving, 1972). According to this dichotomy, both forms of memory may involve retrieval of what could be called facts, but with episodic memory these are associated with personal experiences. There is, therefore, a big overlap in the kinds of information retrieved in the two kinds of memory. This was made more apparent in a later account by Tulving (1985), who allowed that there could be semantic memories about personally experienced events, but that these would not include retrieval of information directly related to the experience. Thus, one could know (semantic memory) that something had happened in one's past or one could recollect things about the personal experience of this same thing happening to one.

Episodic memory can not only be assessed by determining how good individuals' memories are for their recent and remote autobiographical experiences, but also by examining how well they can recall or recognize verbal or non-verbal materials to which they are exposed under controlled conditions. Their episodic memory is probably being tapped provided they are asked to remember what the examiner presented to them in a specific study context, which they personally experienced. Semantic memory is more likely to be being tapped when they are asked to remember verbal or non-verbal facts with no specific reference to the contexts in which the facts may have been previously encountered. Unfortunately, however, it is possible for people to remember personally experienced episodes by merely retrieving information that they would have had if they had never experienced the episode, i.e. by using semantic memory, or to remember facts by making use of memories of personal experiences, i.e. episodic memory. These two possibilities have caused a great deal of confusion and may be one reason that led Tulving (1983) to develop the Remember/Know procedure in which subjects are asked to indicate whether they recognized something either because they recollected experiencing it or because they merely felt that they knew it had occurred. It is not clear, however, whether this attempt to separate episodic and semantic memory works.

In patients who have impaired episodic or semantic memory, it is important to see whether their problems may arise in part from poor encoding. If they do not encode information they cannot store and later retrieve it. Intelligence should be assessed preferably using a test that puts time pressure on the subject, but those with reduced intelligence do not encode so fast and so richly. This is one explanation of the impaired explicit memory of Alzheimer patients. The ability to focus and maintain attention in the face of distraction should also be assessed because there is some reason to suppose that the memory deficits of some patients with closed head injury are caused by their reduced attentional capacity.

Nyberg and Tulving (1996) have argued that episodic and semantic memory are different memory systems on the basis of functional (or psychological), developmental, pharmacological, and neuropsychological dissociations between them, but this view is not shared by everyone. This dispute can be illustrated by the case of organic amnesia. Organic amnesia is a syndrome in which patients typically show preserved intelligence and short-term memory. These areas of preservation make it unlikely that amnesics' poor memory is caused by poor encoding, a view that is also supported by their typically preserved attentional capacity. They show two kinds of memory deficit: anterograde and retrograde amnesia. In anterograde amnesia, there is an impairment in acquiring and recalling and recognizing not only information about personal episodes, but also about new facts. So, amnesics not only have problems remembering what they did yesterday, but are also worse than normal people at picking up new facts and the meanings of new words. However, whereas personal episodes occur only once, new facts may be presented many times and so are eventually learnt by some amnesics although much more slowly than they would have been before their brain injury. In retrograde amnesia, there is impairment in the ability to recall and recognize personal episodes that were experienced pre-morbidly. Knowledge of language and very well learnt factual information is usually unaffected. However, there is good evidence that memory for less overlearnt facts about public events and people is just as disrupted as is memory for personal episodes (for example, see Mayes et al., 1994).

It is likely therefore, that organic amnesics generally show comparable pre- and postmorbid explicit memory deficits for semantic and episodic memory when amount of learning is equivalent between the two kinds of memory. When level of learning is not equated, neuropsychological dissociations between the two kinds of memory appear. Not only do amnesics show preservation of overlearnt semantic memories in the face of episodic memory deficits, but other organic patients show deficits that primarily affect semantic memory. In recent years, many such patients have been described who have great difficulty in accessing memories about words and facts that had been exposed to a great deal of overlearning. For example, these patients may have great difficulty in identifying pictures of animals or artificial objects even though their vision and intelligence may otherwise be relatively intact. Similarly, they may have difficulty in giving the definitions of words that refer to either animate things or artificial objects (see Mayes, 1988; Patterson & Hodges, 1995). Some of these patients may show relative preservation of the ability to acquire episodic memories.

One particularly interesting group of patients has been described as having semantic dementia because they suffer from a progressively worsening problem with accessing semantic information in the face of the relative preservation of most other cognitive abilities (see Patterson & Hodges, 1995). In particular, such patients may have good preservation of their memory for recent personal episodes in so far as their memory for these episodes does not depend on semantic information to which they have lost access. For example, a patient with semantic dementia might remember normally a game of hockey if this concept was still intact, but have a problem remembering an experience involving animals because nearly all knowledge about animals has been lost.

Semantic dementia is particularly associated with damage to the anterolateral regions of the temporal lobes predominantly on the left or bilaterally, and similarly located lesions are found in patients with other aetiologies who have relatively selective semantic memory deficits (see Patterson & Hodges, 1995). In contrast, organic amnesia is caused by lesions of various aetiologies that either affect medial temporal lobe structures such as the hippocampus, parahippocampal and perirhinal cortices; midline diencephalic structures such as the mammillary bodies, the anterior thalamic nucleus, and the dorsomedial nucleus of the thalamus; basal forebrain structures such as the septum; or the fibre pathways such as the fornix that interconnect these regions (see Mayes, 1988; Zola-Morgan & Squire, 1993).

Although the neuroanatomical evidence seems to indicate that the brain regions mediating episodic and semantic memory are partially distinct, another interpretation of existing data is highly plausible. Amnesia is probably a syndrome comprising several distinct processing disorders related to differently located lesions. Within this framework, a currently influential view is that the memory problems caused by lesions of the hippocampus and structures such as the fornix, mammillary bodies, and mammillothalamic tract, and anterior thalamic nucleus in the hippocampal circuit of Papez disrupt explicit memory acquisition for both facts and personally experienced episodes when these involve associating items, particularly those items represented by different neocortical regions (Cohen et al., 1997). Explicit memory for these facts and events initially depends on storage and retrieval processes driven by the hippocampus, but as time passes and the memories are rehearsed, they are reorganized and transferred to storage sites in the association neocortex that probably centrally include the anterolateral temporal cortex (Alvarez & Squire, 1994). Damage to these neocortical sites will disrupt the storage of both semantic and episodic memories that are older and have been considerably rehearsed and transferred from their initial dependency on hippocampal storage. There is some evidence for this as autobiographical as well as semantic memories are disturbed in patients with semantic dementia. Also, unlike organic amnesics who tend to show a diminishing impairment as episodic and semantic memories become older, semantic dementia patients show worse deficits for older episodic as well as factual memories and relative preservation of younger ones (Graham & Hodges, 1997; Hodges & Graham, 1998; and see Graham, 1999).

The view that the neuropsychological double dissociation between semantic dementia and organic amnesia is caused by a dissociation between semantic and episodic memory may therefore be wrong. The dissociation is more likely to be produced by damage to the hippocampal and medial temporal lobe brain system that mediates the storage (including acquisition) and perhaps retrieval of semantic and episodic information for a period of perhaps up to a year or so and damage to the temporal association system that stores older and much more rehearsed memories of the same kind. This view may turn out to be wrong, although it is plausible. First, it may prove to be wrong if the retrograde amnesia shown by some organic amnesics can be shown to differentially affect premorbid and equally rehearsed semantic and episodic memories as is implied by some case studies (for example, see De Renzi et al., 1987). Such case studies need to be replicated, however, and it must be shown that selective deficits of episodic memory are caused by different lesions from selective deficits of semantic memory. Secondly, in the future, fMRI challenge studies may show that memories do not reorganize in the way postulated by Alvarez and Squire (1994). In the author's view, episodic memory is likely to require all the brain regions needed for semantic memory if irrelevant factors like rehearsal and age of memory are controlled, but may require some additional regions itself because it involves storage of associations to personal experiences that are excluded by definition from semantic memory.

One final comment should be made about the retrieval of episodic and semantic memories. On the basis of recent PET challenge studies, Tulving and his colleagues (Tulving et al., 1994; Kapur et al., 1994) have argued that the prefrontal association neocortex is more activated on the right by retrieving episodic information and more activated on the left by encoding such information. They interpreted this to argue that episodic encoding depends, in part, on semantic encoding so that the semantic retrieval depends more on activity in the left prefrontal cortex, whereas episodic retrieval depends more on activity in the right prefrontal cortex. It is probable that the prefrontal cortex's role in retrieval relates to guiding and planning more complex retrieval search and checking operations. It also probably subserves a similar role with the encoding of these kinds of information. This is supported by considerable evidence that lesions to this system cause long-term memory deficits, which are different from those seen in either organic amnesia or selective semantic memory deficits in that they are likely results of poor planning of encoding and/or retrieval operations. For example, frontal lobe lesions cause deficits that are primarily of free recall of organizable information whereas recognition, which is much less dependent on organizational processes working during encoding and retrieval, is often not affected at all (see Mayes, 1988). If the hypothesis of Tulving and his colleagues is correct, then semantic and episodic memory deficits should be dissociable with frontal lobe lesions, but this has not yet been convincingly demonstrated. The hypothesis may be wrong because episodic and semantic retrieval differ in many irrelevant ways which could explain the PET dissociations. For example, episodic retrievals often involve more complex associations and are more effortful. Future studies need to control for these irrelevant factors.

## Item-specific implicit memory (ISIM)

People can show evidence of memory not only by recalling or recognizing specific kinds of information (explicit or aware memory), but also by processing remembered kinds of information more fluently than they would have if the information had not been remembered (ISIM or unaware memory for specific information). ISIM is probably indicated by an increase in the fluency with which representations are activated from cues because of a strengthening of the storage processes. Some evidence for this is found with PET challenge studies in which reduced signs of neural activation are found in the brain regions where the representation of the information for which ISIM is shown, is likely to be made (see Ungerleider, 1995). This suggests that the neural representation may be retrieved more easily.

ISIM is typically tested by what are known as indirect memory tasks in which no reference is made to the fact that memory is being tapped. For example, subjects may be presented with a list of words and later either be shown the first three letters of the words and similar foils and asked to produce the first word that comes to mind beginning with these three letters (stem completion) or briefly presented with these words or similar foils and asked to identify them. ISIM is shown by an increased ability to generate or identify previously studied words (see Squire et al., 1993). Some indirect memory tests indicate unaware memory not only by an increase in the fluency with which representations are activated from cues, but by the tendency to attribute these changes in fluency to perceptual qualities of the remembered items. For example, studied words are judged as being presented for longer than foil words shown for equivalent periods of time (Witherspoon & Allan, 1985). In such cases, therefore, unaware memory is indicated by two different kinds of process: ISIM or an increase in the fluency with which representations are activated from cues because of a strengthening of storage processes and an attribution process. Both these kinds of process are probably automatic.

ISIM can be indicated for verbal and non-verbal items that were either novel or familiar prior to study (see Mayes, 1988; Squire et al., 1993). There is also good evidence that ISIM exists for both perceptual and semantic representations, and for associations between items as well as for individual items (see Mayes, 1992). The kinds of information that are retrieved for ISIM and explicit memory are relevant for determining the relationship between the two kinds of memory because a different pattern of dissociations might be expected depending on whether this information was the same or different. If the two kinds of memory involve retrieving the same kind of information, then they may depend on the same memory representation whereas when they involve retrieving different information they will depend on different memory representations. The likelihood of obtaining double dissociations between the two kinds of memory may depend on this. For example, perceptual kinds of ISIM are not enhanced by semantic orienting tasks at encoding whereas explicit memory, which often depends primarily on semantic representations, is. The opposite pattern of results is found with perceptual orienting tasks (see Graf & Masson, 1993 passim).

Recently, it has been argued that there is a neuropsychological dissociation between the amnesic patient, H.M., and a patient with damage focused primarily on the right posterior neocortex. Whereas H.M. showed impaired recognition memory and preserved ISIM for perceptual information, the other patient showed the reverse pattern of impairment (Keane et al., 1995). This dissociation may arise because the patient with posterior neocortical damage may be impaired at storing perceptual representations whereas amnesics may be impaired at storing associative semantic representations on which recognition is primarily dependent. There is certainly evidence that whereas organic amnesics show preserved ISIM for simple perceptual representations, they may be impaired at ISIM for associative representations particularly when these are of a semantic kind (Curran & Schacter, 1997). If organic amnesics with hippocampal system damage are impaired at storing associative representations, particularly of a semantic nature, then one would predict that their ISIM as well as their explicit memory for such representations should be poor. Meta-analysis supports this suggestion because, although global amnesics perform normally on tests of ISIM for information that was already familiar prior to study, they do not do so on tests of ISIM for novel associations (see Gooding et al., in press). Conversely, patients with impaired ability to store perceptual representations should be impaired not only at ISIM for these representations, but also at explicit memory when it is made heavily dependent on retrieving such perceptual information (for example, by using a recognition test with foils that are perceptually similar to targets). Initial evidence does not support this, since the patient with impaired ISIM for perceptual information was found to have intact perceptual recognition albeit for somewhat different perceptual features (Fleischman et al., 1997).

## Other kinds of procedural or implicit memory: skills and conditioning

Just as ISIM is a form of unaware memory, skills and conditioning do not depend on aware memory although they may be incidentally accompanied by it. Skills are motor, perceptual or cognitive procedures for operating in the world. In general, they depend on developing procedures that can be applied to classes of stimuli, particular instances of which may not have been encountered before. For example, one may become skilled at using the procedures for serving tennis balls even though one may throw the ball in a different way each time. There is considerable evidence that motor, perceptual, and cognitive skills may be acquired normally in organic amnesics provided that their acquisition does not depend significantly on the use of explicit memory in normal subjects. For example, the amnesic patients are able to acquire a mirror drawing motor skill normally (see Mayes, 1988; Squire et al., 1993), and other amnesics have been shown to acquire the perceptual skill of reading mirror reversed words normally (Cohen & Squire, 1980). Squire and

Frambach (1990) also found that amnesics could acquire a cognitive skill that depended on intuitively identifying the relationship between variables to achieve a target value provided normal subjects did not become aware of what the relationship between the variables was.

In contrast to amnesics, patients with Huntington's disease, who have damage to the neostriatum, have been reported to be impaired at the acquisition and retention of skills such as reading mirror reversed words and relatively normal at recognition tasks (Martone et al., 1984). Similarly, patients with Parkinson's disease, whose primary pathology is to the substantia nigra pars compacta have been shown to be impaired at cognitive skills, but normal at some explicit memory tasks (Saint-Cyr et al., 1988). Work with animals also suggests that the acquisition and retention of skills depend primarily on the structures of the basal ganglia or perhaps on the formation of connections between sensory processing regions of the neocortex and the basal ganglia (see Squire et al., 1993). The extent to which skill acquisition depends on the formation of links between neocortex and cerebellum also requires further exploration.

The acquisition and retention of motoric forms of classical conditioning has, however, been shown both by animal and human studies to depend strongly on the cerebellum (see Squire et al., 1993). For example, subjects may show a conditioned eye blink response to a tone only when this has been preceded for a number of trials by a puff of air into the eye. Just as there is some evidence for a double dissociation between explicit memory and skill memory, there is evidence for a similar dissociation between motoric classical conditioning and explicit memory. Whereas cerebellar lesions disrupt the acquisition of eye blink conditioning and leave explicit memory unaffected (Daum et al., 1993), there is evidence that some amnesics show preserved eye blink conditioning in the face of impaired explicit memory (Daum & Ackerman, 1994). It is not surprising that motoric classical conditioning probably depends on storage changes in a different brain region from those that underlie explicit memory for facts and episodes because these forms of memory almost certainly depend on storing very different kinds of memory representations. As the organization of the cerebellum is very different from the limbic–neocortical regions that underlie explicit memory, it is quite likely that these forms of memory depend on distinct encoding, storage and retrieval algorithms. A similar point may be made for the mechanisms underlying explicit memory and skill memory.

## Conclusions

There is then some evidence that short-term memory, explicit memory, skill memory and classical conditioning depend on partially non-overlapping regions of the brain. It is also likely that other less studied simple forms of memory such as habituation depend on partially distinct brain regions from the above kinds of memory. It is less clear to what extent ISIM and explicit memory depend on non-overlapping memory systems. There are two reasons for this. First, if the appropriate tests are used, it should be possible to make the two forms of memory dependent on retrieving the same information, and, therefore, probably depending on the same memory representation. So the encoding and storage processes underlying ISIM and explicit memory may depend on the same brain structures provided ISIM can be shown for complex associations including those involving personal experiences. If aware memory depends on using a different retrieval process from ISIM, then the two forms of memory should also depend on partially non-overlapping brain regions. There is some evidence that this is true to the extent that explicit memory depends on effortful retrieval whereas ISIM does not (Jacoby & Kelley, 1992). However, this may not be an essential characteristic of explicit memory when retrieval is unintentional.

Secondly, if explicit memory does not essentially depend on effortful retrieval, how is aware memory achieved? Retrieval of a memory representation is not sufficient because it might have arisen from imagination and/or have remained in ISIM. Jacoby et al. (1989) have suggested that explicit memory depends on making an attribution of pastness, i.e. aware memory on the basis of the increased fluency with which the representation is accessed (ISIM). If this account is correct and it is plausible, then it might be argued that explicit memory will depend on brain regions that mediate such memory attributions whereas ISIM will not. This distinction may not, however, apply to those forms of unaware memory that depend on making perceptual attributions (such as judging that an item has been displayed for longer) on the basis of the increased fluency with which its representation has been accessed. Much more work needs to be done comparing the neural bases of explicit memory and ISIM, which will depend on matching the kinds of information retrieved as well as exploring the brain regions underlying effortful retrieval processes and both mnemonic and perceptual forms of attribution.

A final comment is warranted on disorders of the kinds of memory outlined in this chapter. If it is true that information is stored in the brain region in which it is represented, then it becomes difficult to see how selective memory disorders can exist at all because one would expect encoding (and often retrieval) of the information to be just as badly affected as its storage. As far as can be told, this does not happen, except incidentally. Either the underlying assumption is false or kinds of incomplete lesion are possible that disrupt storage, but not encoding. Whatever is the case, this issue requires investigation.

# REFERENCES

Alvarez, R. & Squire, L.R. (1994). Memory consolidation and the medial temporal lobe: a simple network model. *Proceedings of the National Academy of Sciences, USA*, **91**, 7041–5.

Atkinson, R.C. & Shiffrin, R.M. (1968). Human memory: a proposed system and its control processes. In *The Psychology of Learning and Motivation: Advances in Research and Theory*, ed. K.W. Spence, vol. 2, pp. 89–195.

Baddeley, A.D. & Hitch, G. (1977). Working memory. In *Recent Advances in Learning and Motivation*, ed. G.A. Bower, vol. 8, pp. 647–67.

Baddeley, A.D., Papagno, C. & Vallar, G. (1988) When long-term learning depends on short-term storage. *Journal of Memory and Language*, **27**, 586–95.

Cohen, N.J. & Squire, L.R. (1980). Preserved learning and retention of pattern analysing skill in amnesia: dissociation of knowing how and knowing that. *Science*, **210**, 207–10.

Cohen, J.D., Forman, S.D., Braver, T.S., Casey, B.J., Servan-Schieber, D. & Noll, D.C. (1994). Activation of prefrontal cortex in a non-spatial working memory task with functional MRI. *Human Brain Mapping*, **1**, 293–304.

Curran, T. & Schacter, D.L. (1997). Implicit memory: what must theories of amnesia explain. *Memory*, **5**, 37–48.

Dale, H.C.A. & Gregory, M. (1966). Evidence of semantic encoding in short-term memory. *Psychonomic Science*, **5**, 153–4.

Daum, I. & Ackerman, H. (1994). Dissociation of declarative and nondeclarative memory after bilateral thalamic lesions: a case report. *International Journal of Neuroscience*, **75**, 151–65.

Daum, I., Schugens, M.M., Ackerman, H., Lutzenberger, W., Dichgans, J. & Birbaumer, N. (1993). Classical conditioning after cerebellar lesions in humans. *Behavioral Neuroscience*, **105**, 748–56.

De Renzi, E., Liotti, M. & Nichelli, P. (1987). Semantic amnesia with preservation of autobiographical memory: a case report. *Cortex*, **23**, 575–97.

Ellis, A.W. & Young, A.W. (1988). *Human Cognitive Neuropsychology*. Hove: Lawrence Erlbaum Associates.

Fleischman, D.A., Vaidya, C.J., Lange, K.L. & Gabrieli, J.D.E. (1997). A dissociation between perceptual explicit and implicit memory processes. *Brain and Cognition*, **35**, 42–57.

Graf, P. & Masson, M.E.J. (1993). *Implicit Memory: New Directions in Cognition, Development, and Neuropsychology*. Hillsdale, N.J.: Lawrence Erlbaum Associates.

Gooding, P.A., Mayes, A.R. & van Eyk, R. (in press). A meta-analysis of indirect memory tests for novel material in organic amnesics. *Neuropsychologia*.

Graham, K.S. (1999) Semantic dementia: a challenge to the multiple-trace theory? *Trends in Cognitive Sciences*, **3**, 85–7.

Graham, K.S. & Hodges, J.R. (1997). Differentiating the roles of the hippocampal complex and the neocortex in long-term storage: evidence from the study of semantic dementia. *Neuropsychology*, **11**, 77–89.

Hanley, J.R., Young, A.W. & Pearson, N.A. (1991). Impairment of the visuospatial sketch pad. *Quarterly Journal of Experimental Psychology: Human Experimental Psychology*, **43A**, 101–25.

Hodges, J.R. & Graham, K.S. (1998). A reversal of the temporal gradient for famous person knowledge in semantic dementia: implications for the neural organization of long-term mamory. *Neuropsychologia*, 36, 803–25.

Jacoby, L.L. & Kelley, C. (1992). Unconscious influences of memory: dissociations and automaticity. In *The Neuropsychology of Consciousness*, ed. A.D. Milner & M.D. Rugg, pp. 201–34. London: Academic Press.

Jacoby, L.L., Kelley, C.M. & Dywan, J. (1989). Memory attributions. In *Varieties of Memory and Consciousness*, ed. H.L. Roediger & F.I.M. Craik, pp. 391–422. Hillsdale, N.J.: Lawrence Erlbaum Associates.

Jonides, J., Smith, E.E., Koeppe, R.A., Awh, E., Minoshima, S. & Mintun, M.A. (1993). Spatial working memory in humans as revealed by PET. *Nature*, 363, 623–5.

Kapur, S., Craik, F.I.M., Tulving, E., Wilson, A.A., Houle, S. & Brown, G.M. (1994). Neuroanatomical correlates of encoding in episodic memory: levels of processing effect. *Proceedings of the National Academy of Sciences, USA*, 91, 2008–11.

Keane, M.M., Gabrieli, J.D.E., Mapstone, H.C., Johnson, K.A. & Corkin, S. (1995). Double dissociation of memory capacities after bilateral occipital-lobe or medial temporal lobe lesions. *Brain*, 118, 1129–48.

Kolb, B. & Whishaw, I.Q. (1990). *Fundamentals of Human Neuropsychology*. 3rd edn. New York: Freeman & Company.

Martone, M., Butters, N. & Payne, P. (1984). Dissociations between skill learning and verbal recognition in amnesia and dementia. *Archives of Neurology*, 41, 965–70.

Mayes, A.R. (1988). *Human Organic Memory Disorders*. Cambridge: Cambridge University Press.

Mayes, A.R. (1992) Automatic processes in memory: how are they mediated? In *The Neuropsychology of Consciousness*, ed. A.D. Milner & M.D. Rugg, pp. 235–62. London: Academic Press.

Mayes, A.R., Downes, J.J., McDonald, C., Poole, V., Rooke, S., Sagar, H.J. & Meudell, P.R. (1994). Two tests for assessing remote public knowledge: a tool for assessing retrograde amnesia. *Memory*, 2, 183–210.

Nyberg, L. & Tulving, E. (1996). Classifying human long-term memory: evidence from converging dissociations. *European Journal of Cognitive Psychology*, 8, 163–84.

Patterson, K. & Hodges, J. (1995). Disorders of semantic memory. In *Handbook of Memory Disorders*, ed. A.D Baddeley, B. Wilson & Watts, F.N., pp. 167–86. Chichester: John Wiley.

Paulesu, E., Frith, C.D. & Fractcowiak, R.S.J. (1993). The neural correlates of the verbal component of working memory. *Nature*, 362, 342–4.

Rose, S. (1992). *The Making of Memory*. London: Bantam Press.

Saint-Cyr, J.A., Taylor, A.E. & Lang, A.E. (1988). Procedural learning and neostriatal dysfunction in man. *Brain*, 111, 941–59.

Shallice, T. (1988). *From Neuropsychology to Mental Structure*. Cambridge: Cambridge University Press.

Shallice, T. & Evans, M.E. (1978). The involvement of the frontal lobes in cognitive estimation. *Cortex*, 14, 294–303.

Sherry, D.F. & Schacter, D.L. (1987). The evolution of multiple memory systems. *Psychological Review*, 94, 439–54.

Squire, L.R. (1987). *Memory and the Brain*. New York: Oxford University Press.

Squire, L.R. & Frambach, M. (1990). Cognitive skill learning in amnesia. *Psychobiology*, **18**, 109–17.

Squire, L.R., Knowlton, B. & Musen, G. (1993). The structure and organization of memory. *Annual Review of Psychology*, **44**, 453–95.

Tulving, E. (1972). Episodic and semantic memory. In *The Organization of Memory*, ed. E. Tulving & W. Donaldson, pp. 382–404. New York: Academic Press.

Tulving, E. (1983). *Elements of Episodic Memory*. Oxford: Oxford University Press.

Tulving, E. (1985). How many memory systems are there? *American Psychologist*, **40**, 385–98.

Tulving, E., Kapur, S., Markowitsch, H.J., Craik, F.I.M., Habib, R. & Houle, S. (1994). Neuroanatomicical correlates of retrieval in episodic memory: auditory sentence recognition. *Proceedings of the National Academy of Sciences, USA*, **91**, 2012–15.

Ungerleider, L.G. (1995). Functional brain imaging: studies of cortical mechanisms for memory. *Science*, **270**, 769–75.

Vallar, G. & Papagno, C. (1995). Neuropsychological impairments of short-term memory. In *Handbook of Memory Disorders*, ed. A.D. Baddeley, B. Wilson, & Watts, F.N., pp. 135–66. Chichester, UK: John Wiley.

Witherspoon, D. & Allan, L.G. (1985). The effects of a prior presentation on temporal judgements in a perceptual identification task. *Memory and Cognition*, **13**, 101–11.

Zola-Morgan, S. & Squire, L.R. (1993). Neuroanatomy of memory. *Annual Review of Neuroscience*, **16**, 547–63.

# 5

# Psychopharmacology of memory

Jennifer T. Coull and Barbara J. Sahakian

## Introduction

Since the rise of neuropsychological studies in brain-damaged patients, to the now current popularity of functional neuroimaging, neuroscientists have endeavoured to localize the elusive engram. Localizationist theories of cognitive function have now diminished, however, and neural network explanations are currently in vogue. Almost in parallel to this, an increasing interest in the influence of neurotransmitter systems on cognition has emerged. The study of the neurochemical modulation of memory has dominated the cognitive psychopharmacological literature, in both humans and animals, in recent years. Although this chapter does not provide an exhaustive review of this literature, it does introduce the reader to the more widely researched hypotheses concerning the modulation of this most enigmatic, yet most tangible, of cognitive processes. In addition, some pertinent data are included. While it is of obvious clinical import to treat memory dysfunction in patient populations, drugs which are shown to enhance memory in patients, healthy volunteers or experimental animals may additionally inform us as to the neurochemical basis of normal memory function.

Although the various manifestations of dementia are the most obvious form of clinical memory disorder (see Chapter 7, this volume), patients suffering from functional psychiatric disorders may also show signs of mnemonic dysfunction. This chapter will concentrate on drug treatments for dementia, since these have been the driving force behind the search for cognitive enhancers. For the more functional psychiatric disorders, such as depression and anxiety, psychoactive agents are generally used to treat the primary behavioural and affective symptoms, rather than any cognitive dysfunction. However, using depression as an example, it will be discussed how psychopharmacological agents may also alleviate the cognitive symptoms of psychiatric disorder, and potentially provide some clues as to the aetiology of the disease process.

A final important point concerns the psychological specificity of the memory dysfunction in psychiatric disorder. Attention and memory are inextricably linked, although they are very different cognitive processes. Neither attention nor memory are unitary processes: selective attention can be distinguished from divided attention or sustained attention, just as procedural, episodic or semantic memory are distinguished between. Reports of psychopharmacological memory enhancement may often be confounded by neurochemical modulation of attentional, rather than mnemonic processes, and it is therefore crucial to distinguish the effects of a putative cognitive enhancer on attentional vs. mnemonic components of a cognitive task. So, while this chapter has the psychopharmacology of memory as its focus, discussion of attentional factors is sometimes unavoidable, and indeed essential.

## Neurochemical substrates of memory function: psychopharmacological studies in humans and animals

### Acetylcholine

From the results of studies in both animals and humans, the cholinergic system has been the neurotransitter system most traditionally associated with the processes of memory and learning. The administration of the cholinergic (muscarinic receptor) antagonist scopolamine to healthy volunteers has been thought to provide a human model of the memory loss associated with Alzheimer's disease (AD). However, this proposal has recently been challenged (Kopelman, 1986; Rusted, 1994), and experimental evidence will be reviewed to determine whether cholinergic agents are associated with mnemonic function.

The consensus of studies over the past 20 years or so is that, while scopolamine spares performance on tests of immediate (or 'short-term' or 'primary') memory, it impairs the acquisition of memories into a more permanent 'long-term' store (for reviews, see Kopelman, 1986; Warburton & Rusted, 1991; Hart & Semple, 1990). For example, scopolamine has no effect on simple digit or spatial span (Drachman & Leavitt, 1974; Kopelman & Corn, 1988; Broks et al., 1988). Similarly, while having no effect on the recall of items presented at the end of a to-be-remembered list, the drug has been shown to impair the free recall of earlier items (Crow & Grove-White, 1973; Drachman & Leavitt, 1974; Ghonheim & Mewaldt, 1975; Mewaldt & Ghonheim, 1979; Frith et al., 1984). This effect on the primacy, rather than the recency, component of the serial position curve, is evidence for a selective impairment of encoding (or acquisition) rather than retrieval (Crow, 1979). Furthermore, while administration of scopolamine *before* word-list learning impaired subsequent recall, administration *after* learning had no such effect on recall (Ghonheim & Mewhaldt, 1975, 1977; Mewaldt & Ghonheim, 1979; Petersen, 1977). However, this apparent dissociation has been called into question by the scopolamine-induced impairment of performance in the Brown–Petersen paradigm (Caine et al., 1981; Kopelman & Corn, 1988). This task requires the subject to perform a distracting task between learning and recall of a word-list, and is thought to provide an index of the effect of proactive interference on the rate of forgetting from immediate memory. To use these findings to refute the sparing of immediate memory by cholinergic agents would be premature, however. These results could alternatively reflect an effect of scopolamine on working memory and the allocation of processing resources (as suggested by Warburton & Rusted, 1991; Rusted, 1994), or perhaps an effect on distractability and attention.

Support for the idea that the basal forebrain cholinergic system is crucially involved in the control of attentional processes has recently been reviewed (see Sahakian & Coull, 1994; Everitt & Robbins, 1996). For example, Drachman and Sahakian (1979) postulated that the cholinergic system boosted the 'signal to noise' ratio for information processing in the cerebral cortex. Furthermore, nicotine has been shown to increase the speed and accuracy of sustained attention performance, as measured by the Rapid Visual Information Processing task, whereas scopolamine has been shown to reduce accuracy (Wesnes & Warburton, 1984; Wesnes & Revell, 1984). This particular paradigm has been taken into the clinical setting with promising results (Sahakian et al., 1989, 1994; Jones et al., 1992; Coull et al., 1996a), and will be discussed further later in the chapter. Furthermore, Broks et al. (1988) report scopolamine-induced deficits in attentional function in healthy volunteers, as well as the expected deficits in learning. It is interesting to note that the errors made on a verbal learning task included an increased number of non-presented intrusions, as well as a reduced number of correctly recalled items. The former may represent increased drug-induced distractability (or a reduction in the signal to noise ratio), which has the net effect of impairing performance on a test ostensibly used to measure learning. Dunne and Hartley (1985) have suggested that attentional deficits can actually contribute to the mnemonic deficits produced by scopolamine. Subjects performing a dichotic listening task showed the expected attended ear advantage in the number of items reported under placebo conditions, but following the administration of scopolamine the number of items reported from the attended ear was significantly reduced. Importantly, scopolamine had no effect on the total number of items recalled (from both ears), but did reduce the number of items from the attended channel. Cholinergic manipulations are now regarded as influencing both memory and attention (Drachman & Sahakian, 1979; Sahakian, 1988; Warburton et al., 1992; Rusted, 1994), as indexed by studies in healthy volunteers, animals (see p. 80) and patients with AD (see p. 83). While scopolamine may not be a perfect pharmacological model for the mnemonic deficits of AD, it may provide an adequate model for the general cognitive dysfunction in this patient group, which includes deficits of attention as well as memory (Sahakian et al., 1989, 1990; Parasuraman & Haxby, 1993).

## Serotonin (5-HT)

Over the past five years or so, the serontonergic system has been widely publicised as a 'mood-modulator' in both the academic and general press. In addition, the neuroscientific community has been examining the role of serotonin in the cognitive processes of learning and memory. Although evidence from the animal literature for a specific role of serotonin in these cognitive processes is rather inconsistent (for reviews see Altman & Normile, 1988; McEntee & Crook, 1991; Gower, 1992), a general consensus appears to be that, while stimulation of serotonergic activity often impairs memory and learning (McEntee & Crook, 1991), a reduction in serotonergic function does not always facilitate memory or learning (Gower, 1992). For example, depletion of brain serotonin levels using the serotonin synthesis inhibitor, $p$-chlorophenylalanine (PCPA), has either no effect on water maze acquisition (Richter-Levin & Segal, 1989), or produces mild impairment in performance (Vanderwolf, 1987). Similarly, specific lesions to the serotonergic pathways using 5,7-dihydroxytryptamine (5,7-DHT), has either no effect on performance of the radial arm maze (Asin et al., 1985; Nilsson et al., 1988), or actually impairs learning (Wenk et al., 1987).

In humans, the effect of serotonergic agents on cognitive function has been less extensively researched. A study conducted by the authors' group has reported impairments in learning with administration of a low-tryptophan (LoTRP) drink to healthy volunteers (Park et al., 1993). This drink reduced levels of plasma tryptophan, the precursor to serotonin, and impaired reversal learning in a visual discrimination task, while having no effect on the ability to shift attention to a new stimulus dimension in the same task. Deficits in reversal learning using a parallel version of this task in primates have been observed in animals with cholinergic lesions to the frontal cortex (Roberts et al., 1990), suggesting perhaps a common mode of action of serotonin and acetylcholine in regard to this function. It is germane at this point to direct the reader's attention to the interaction between the cholinergic and 5-HT$_3$ receptor systems (Barnes et al., 1989), which has been suggested as a possible target for the search for effective cognitive enhancers. A LoTRP drink has also been found to selectively impair long-term memory consolidation in healthy volunteers, while having no affect on short-term immediate recall (Riedel et al., 1999).

Both animal and human studies have pointed to a role for the hippocampus in the serotonergic modulation of memory and learning (Altman et al., 1990; Grasby et al., 1992). Using Positron Emission Tomography (PET), the 5-HT$_{1A}$ agonist buspirone has been found to attenuate regional cerebral blood flow (rCBF) in the retrosplenial brain areas of healthy volunteers performing a supra-span word-list learning task (Grasby et al., 1992). Conversely, and in the same study, the dopaminergic agonist, apomorphine, was found to attenuate task-induced increases in rCBF in the left dorsolateral prefrontal cortex. Since the retrosplenial area is densely connected to the hippocampus (Goldman-Rakic et al., 1984), these results suggest serotonin may be involved in human mnemonic function subserved by parahippo-campal, rather than frontal, brain areas. It is pertinent to note here that lesions of the retrosplenial cortex have been reported to produce deficits in reversal learning of the rabbit nictitating membrane response (Berger et al., 1986). If serotonergic activity is important in this brain area, as Grasby et al. (1992) suggest, then the results of Berger et al. (1986) support the authors' findings of a LoTRP-induced reversal learning deficit in humans.

## GABA (and the benzodiazepines)

Like serotonergic drugs, the benzodiazepines (BZs) are reputed to have effects both on mood (they are widely prescribed as anxiolytics) and also on memory (Curran, 1991). The actions of BZs are closely linked to those of the inhibitory neurotrans-mitter GABA ($\gamma$-aminobutyric acid), since BZ binding sites are located on the $GABA_A$ receptor complex. This results in the existence of a synergistic relationship between GABA and BZs such that BZ agonists (such as diazepam (DZP)) poten-tiate GABA-mediated post-synaptic inhibition. In humans, BZ binding is highest in the cerebral cortex, hippocampus and cerebellum (Braestrup et al., 1977), where enhancement of GABA-mediated inhibition can lead to behavioural, cognitive or emotional effects, such as memory impairment or anxiolysis.

There are well-documented acquisition deficits seen following BZ administra-tion (e.g. Ghonheim et al., 1984; Rodrigo & Lusiardo, 1988; Hennessey et al., 1991), which are thought to underlie the BZ-induced anterograde amnesic state, whereby conversion of memories from short-term memory to long-term memory is impaired (for reviews see Curran, 1986, 1991). For example, Ghonheim et al. (1984) found a dose-dependent (0.1, 0.2 and 0.3 mg/kg DZP) decrease in the recall of early items in a free recall task, while later items, that could be maintained in short-term memory by rehearsal, were less affected. On the other hand, DZP-induced memory impairments have also been interpreted according to Baddeley's model of working memory (Baddeley, 1986). Rusted et al. (1991) reported that, while both 5 mg and 10 mg doses of diazepam produced selective deficits on tests of supra-span free recall and the Baddeley logic test (purported to be a measure of central executive function), performance on simple tests of digit span (demands on the phonologi-cal loop) or mental rotation (demands on the visuo-spatial sketchpad) was spared.

Two author studies have shown evidence to support both of these interpretations however. Diazepam was found to impair performance on tests of 'executive' func-tion in a manner strongly reminiscent of neurosurgical patients with frontal lobe excisions (Coull et al., 1995a), whilst also producing profound deficits on perfor-mance of a visuo-spatial paired-associates learning task (Coull et al., 1995b). These results are unlikely to be explained solely by sedative effects of the drug, since double dissociations in performance of the latter learning task and a task of sustained attention were noted with the noradrenergic α-receptor agonist, cloni-dine (Coull et al., 1995b). In addition, a more recent functional neuroimaging study using PET has demonstrated dissociable neuroanatomical bases for the mod-ulation of encoding vs. executive function by diazepam (Coull et al., 1999). This finding supports the notion that these represent distinct functional; effects of the drug. Thus, support has been provided for the well-established claims for a role for BZ receptors in memory, and in addition they have demonstrated a role for BZ receptors in frontal lobe function.

## Animal models of cognitive dysfunction: lesion studies in experimental animals

### Alzheimer's disease

One of the most important problems in interpreting psychopharmacological studies is that the systemic administration of psychoactive drugs produces indiscriminate effects on the entire system under investigation (both at the pharmacological and behavioural level) and so precludes analysis of a specific neurotransmitter pathway. The cholinergic system, for example, has separate pathways from the nucleus basalis of Meynert (nbM) to the cortex, and from the medial septum (MS) and the nucleus of the diagonal band of Broca (DBB) to the hippocampus (Woolf, 1991). The use of neurotoxic lesions in experimental animals allows the researcher a more detailed level of interrogation than is available with systemically administered drugs. Lesions of the nBM in the basal forebrain area have been used as animal models of AD, fol-lowing the findings of both nbM cell atrophy in patients with AD (Whitehouse et al., 1982; Candy et al., 1983) as well as impairments in memory and learning following lesions of this area in animals (for reviews see Price, 1986; Smith, 1988; Wenk & Olton, 1987; Hagan & Morris, 1988; Fibiger, 1991; Dunnett et al., 1991).

However, recent evidence has been accumulating to suggest that such selective neurotoxic lesions of the nBM affect attentional function, rather than having a direct action on memory (Robbins et al., 1989; Dunnett et al., 1991; Muir et al., 1992, 1993, 1994, 1995; Voytko et al., 1994; Wenk et al., 1994). Similarly, animal models of AD employing the cholinergic agonist nicotine have suggested that mod-ulation of attentional, rather than mnemonic, function by cholinergic manipula-tions may provide a better explanation of their findings (Gray et al., 1994; Widzowski et al., 1994; but see Levin, 1992). Conversely, it has been suggested that the learning and memory deficits, which are certainly produced by neurotoxins (e.g. ibotenic acid), are actually attributable to destruction of cortico-striatal pathways rather than neocortical pathways as was previously supposed (Dunnett et al., 1991). These findings advocate a greater emphasis on clinical and therapeutic studies of the attentional dysfunction in AD (Sahakian et al., 1987, 1989; Parasuraman & Haxby, 1993; Sahakian & Coull, 1994), in addition to the more obvious memory deficits.

## Parkinson's disease

Evidence of 'subcortical' dementia is often noted in patients with Parkinson's disease (PD), where the principal lesion appears to be in the substantia nigra, leading to degeneration of the nigrostriatal dopamine system and consequently profound dopamine loss in the dorsal striatum (caudate–putamen). While many animal models of PD focus on its motor symptoms (Brown & Robbins, 1991), a recent study has shown that some of the cognitive deficits seen in PD may also be modelled in the primate brain. Roberts et al. (1994) have examined the performance of monkeys with 6-hydroxydopamine (6-OHDA) lesions to the prefrontal cortex on an analogue of a traditional clinical test of frontal lobe function, the Wisconsin Card Sort Test (WCST) and on a spatial delayed response (DR) test also known to be sensitive to lesions of the frontal cortex (Goldman-Rakic, 1987). These authors found impairments in spatial DR performance, equivalent to those reported previously with this lesion (Brozoski et al., 1979), but improvements in attentional set-shifting ability. These findings were interpreted within the context of the observed increases in striatal dopamine in monkeys with depletions of prefrontal dopamine (Pycock et al., 1980), and it was suggested that reductions in dopamine activity in the prefrontal cortex leads to impaired working memory (DR) performance, while low levels of dopamine in the striatum impairs attentional set-shifting. Performance of directly analogous computerised tests (Roberts & Sahakian, 1993) are known to be impaired in PD (Downes et al., 1989; Owen et al., 1992, 1993), suggesting that fronto-striatal dopaminergic dysfunction most probably contributes to the cognitive, as well as the motor, symptomatology of this disease (see also Leenders et al., 1986, 1990), a finding supported by results from studies of PD patients when on and off L-Dopa (Lange et al., 1992).

## Frontal lobe dysfunction

While much of this chapter has reviewed the neurochemical correlates of (long-term) episodic memory, (short-term) working memory is yet to be discussed (Baddeley, 1986). The crucial difference between concepts of working memory (WM) and the original conception of short-term memory (STM) is that information can be held on-line in the WM store for further processing and manipulation, while that in a traditional STM store is passed on for further processing essentially unchanged. Based on neuropsychological reports of patients with frontal lobe damage, both Shallice (1988) and Baddeley (1986) suggest that the central executive (a central component of WM) depends on efficient functioning of the frontal cortex. Using the delayed response (DR) task (an index of WM function) in surgically or neuropharmacologically lesioned primates, Goldman-Rakic and her colleagues have documented a substantial, and quite compelling, body of work suggesting that working memory is indeed dependent on the functioning of the prefrontal cortex (PFC) (Goldman-Rakic, 1987, 1994). In particular, the role of the catecholamines, dopamine and noradrenaline, are emphasized (Arnsten & Goldman-Rakic, 1985; Arnsten & Contant, 1992; Sawaguchi & Goldman-Rakic, 1994).

A paradigm used by Goldman-Rakic and colleagues on several occasions involves the use of catecholaminergic compounds to remediate naturally occurring age-related deficits in DR performance. Arnsten and Goldman-Rakic (1985) found evidence of selective improvements in DR performance following administration of relatively high doses of the mixed $\alpha1/\alpha2$ adrenoceptor agonist clonidine to aged monkeys, which were subsequently blocked by administration of the more selective $\alpha2$ receptor antagonist yohimbine. This study further suggests these effects are mediated by $\alpha2$ receptors specifically in the principal sulcus of the PFC, since destruction of noradrenergic terminals in the principal sulcus by 6-OHDA lesions resulted in supersensitive $\alpha2$ receptors. However, this effect may not be selective to the noradrenergic system. Sawaguchi and Goldman-Rakic (1994) have recently found that local injection of dopamine receptor D1 antagonists into the monkey PFC produced deficits in an oculo-motor version of the DR task, while injections of D2 antagonists were without effect (although Luciana et al. (1992) have found D2 agonist-induced WM improvements in human volunteers). It is important to note at this point that the apparent dopaminergic modulation of WM is not irreconcilable with the effects found by Arnsten and Goldman-Rakic (1985) using noradrenergic $\alpha2$ agents. The central executive and WM are not unitary systems, but comprise several components which could be differentially modulated by separate neurotransmitter systems. For example, noradrenaline may modulate WM by preventing distraction from irrelevant stimuli, whereas DA may be involved in maintaining representations of stimulus-response contingencies across the delay period.

Animal models of WM function are critical in our understanding of the neurochemical basis of memory function, and may additionally suggest putative drug treatments for patients who have difficulties with such tasks.

## Pharmacological strategies for cognitive enhancement

### Cholinergic system

The cholinergic hypothesis of Alzheimer's disease (Drachman & Sahakian, 1980; Bartus et al., 1982) is probably one of the most enduring and resilient theories of cognitive psychopharmacology. It is a two-fold theory, stemming both from the psychopharmacological literature implicating a role for the cholinergic system in memory and learning (see pp. 76–7), and also, and perhaps primarily, from post-mortem biochemical studies of AD patients. The degree of cognitive impairment in these patients is positively correlated with reductions in choline acetyltransferase, and a reduction in acetylcholine (Ach) synthesis in the brain (Francis et al.,

1985; Perry et al., 1978), and patients suffering from AD have been shown to have large reductions of nicotinic receptors, in both the neocortex and hippocampus (Perry et al., 1986, 1987). It has further been shown that AD patients display severe neuronal degeneration in the nucleus basalis of Meynert (Whitehouse et al., 1982), the major cholinergic innervation to the cortex. While consideration of these findings suggests a cholinergic replacement therapy for AD, the past decade has borne little witness to any singularly successful treatment, and indeed a shadow of doubt has been cast upon the validity of the cholinergic hypothesis of AD.

There have been three general strategies for enhancement of cholinergic function in patients with AD: precursor loading, prevention of Ach breakdown, and post-synaptic agonism. The first of these was almost unanimously unsuccessful (Mohs et al., 1979; Peters & Levin, 1979; Little et al., 1985), possibly due to degeneration of the pre-synaptic neurones in AD where precursors synthesise Ach (Johns et al., 1983; Kopelman, 1986). The second of the treatment strategies has proven more successful, although inconsistencies in clinical findings are still reported. Acetylcholine is broken down by the enzyme acetylcholinesterase, and the therapeutic utility of the acetylcholinesterase inhibitors (CAT Is), especially physostigmine and tetrahydroaminoacridine (THA), have been extensively tested and reviewed (for reviews see Thal, 1992; Adem, 1993; Mohammed, 1993; Whitehouse, 1993; Muramoto et al., 1984; Sahakian et al., 1987, 1993; Eagger et al., 1991; Davis et al., 1992; Farlow et al., 1992). THA is the more promising due to its longer duration of action and improved bioavailability, and clinical trials have demonstrated varying degrees of cognitive improvement in AD patients. While most studies have concentrated on the effects of CAT Is on memory, a study of the authors has emphasized the effects of THA on attentional processes (Sahakian et al., 1994; see also Sahakian & Coull, 1994; Lawrence & Sahakian, 1995). In a placebo-controlled THA-with-lecithin therapeutic trial, patients with mild to moderate AD demonstrated drug-induced improvements on a choice reaction time attentional task, but showed no drug effect on mnemonic function as measured by a visual delayed matching to sample task. A similar task for use in rats has previously been shown to be sensitive to lesions of the nBM (see p. 80), and lesion-induced deficits of its performance can be ameliorated with cholinergic-rich grafts, physostigmine or nicotine (Muir et al., 1992, 1993, 1995). Velnacrine, another CAT I, has recently been reported to improve both mnemonic and attentional function in patients with AD, and also to increase tracer uptake (as measured by SPECT) in left frontal and right parietal brain areas of AD patients (Siegfried, 1993). These brain areas are known to be associated with verbal memory and visual attention, respectively (Grasby et al., 1993; Fletcher et al., 1995; Pardo et al., 1991; Corbetta et al., 1993).

Changes in attentional performance following cholinergic manipulation have also been noted in another of our studies which examined the therapeutic efficacy of the cholinergic receptor agonist nicotine. This study pertains to the third of the treatment strategies listed earlier. In the authors' own study (Sahakian et al., 1989; Jones et al., 1992), patients with mild to moderate AD showed nicotine-induced enhancement of attentional function, as measured by the Rapid Visual Information Processing (RVIP) task, but failed to demonstrate any improvement in performance of a delayed matching to location order task. Recently, the authors (Coull et al., 1996b) have shown a bilateral fronto-parietal network of activation associated with performance of the RVIP task in a Positron Emission Tomography (PET) study of normal volunteers, a neural network which is consistent with neuropsychological theories of attention (Mesulum, 1981; Posner & Petersen, 1990). The RVIP task was originally used to demonstrate impairments in attentional function in normal volunteers following administration of the muscarinic receptor antagonist scopolamine, and the amelioration of this deficit by nicotine (Wesnes & Warburton, 1984; Wesnes & Revell, 1984). Using a memory task, a preliminary study, Newhouse et al. (1988) failed to find any mnemonic improvements with nicotine in AD patients, but did note a reduction in intrusion errors, consistent with an effect on attentional processes (see also discussion of Broks et al., 1988 on p. 77). While these, and other, studies are suggestive of a cholinergic modulation of attentional function, it is clear that an effect on mnemonic processes cannot be ruled out. What is not so clear, however, is how greatly attentional deficits contribute to the memory dysfunction seen in AD, and whether cholinergic agents are ameliorating attentional processes, rather than mnemonic ones.

Treatment of symptoms, whatever their root cause, is still of obvious clinical benefit however, and the search must continue for more effective cognitive enhancers using a theory-driven cognitive psychopharmacological approach. An alternative therapeutic strategy is to increase cholinergic activity in the basal forebrain pre-synaptically via the $\beta$-carbolines (benzodiazepine receptor inverse agonists) (Sarter et al., 1988; Sarter & Bruno, 1994), or perhaps even via 5-HT$_3$ receptor antagonists such as ondansetron (see next section) (Barnes et al., 1989). However, the clinical utility of these agents is still uncertain.

Positron Emission Tomography (PET) has been used to localize neuroanatomical networks of memory function in the living human brain (Squire et al., 1992; Grasby et al., 1993; Fletcher et al., 1995). In addition, the introduction of psychoactive drugs into the PET paradigm enables observation of the neurochemical modulation of these networks (Grasby et al., 1992; Friston et al., 1991). Knowledge from psychopharmacological studies can be combined with that from imaging studies, to generate hypotheses about the brain areas implicated in the neurochemical modulation of memory. For example, scopolamine-induced encoding deficits are well known, and a recent PET study has shown a lateralization of encoding to the left prefrontal cortex (Shallice et al., 1994; Fletcher et al., 1995). This suggests that the effects of scopolamine on encoding may be modulated by left hemisphere activity more than by right, and may have practical implications for treatment of patients who have cognitive deficits associated with unilateral lesions.

## Serotonergic system

There is accumulating evidence that the serotonergic system is compromised in patients with DAT. For example, DAT patients have been reported to show cell loss in the raphe nuclei (Yamamoto & Hirano, 1985), a reduced density of 5-HT binding sites, and a reduction in levels of the 5-HT metabolite 5-hydroxy-2-indolacetic acid (5-HIAA) (Bowen et al., 1983). Lawlor et al. (1989) have reported a greater degree of menemonic impairment in DAT patients as compared to controls, following administration of the 5-HT agonist m-chlorophenylpiperazine (mCPP), suggesting the use of 5-HT antagonists as a possible treatment strategy for DAT. Ondansetron is a $5\text{-}HT_3$ receptor antagonist which is thought to act as a cognitive enhanceer in both rats and monkeys (Domeney et al., 1991; Carey et al., 1992; Muir et al., 1995; Costall & Naylor, 1992), although it may be exerting its therapeutic effects through a modulatory action on the cholinergic system, rather than a direct effect on the serotonergic system (Barnes et al., 1989). It is also important to note that the effects of depleting brain serotonin depend very much on the paradigm in question and the time of administration of the drug (pre- or post-training) (for a review see Gower, 1992). Therefore, while studies employing acute drug-dosing schedules may provide a *theoretical* model of the role of 5-HT in memory and learning, longitudinal studies which use chronic drug doses would be of more benefit in determining the *therapeutic* utility of 5-HT agents in DAT.

In addition to its putative role in memory and learning, serotonin has also been implicated in both the treatment and underlying pathology of depression. In neuropsychological studies, patients with depression have been shown to demonstrate an oversensitivity to negative feedback (Elliott et al., 1996) and to show two types of memory deficit: general impairments in episodic memory recall (Abas et al., 1990; Robbins et al., 1992; O'Brien et al., 1993), or memory biases for sad or negative stimuli (Lloyd & Lishman, 1975; Clark & Teasdale, 1982). Teasdale (1985) has proposed an influential cognitive theory of depression, based on differential activation of negative, as opposed to positive, memories during the depressed state. These negatively valenced memories then, in turn, produce symptoms of depression, culminating in a vicious cycle capable of maintaining the depressed state. In parallel to this, Deakin and Graeff (1991) suggest that an ineffective $5\text{-}HT_{1A}$ receptor system in depression leads to a breakdown in the human defence mechanism which allows us to cope with chronic aversive events. This receptor system is thought normally to interfere with new learning or consolidation, especially when aversive events are involved, thereby preventing (and therefore protecting) subjects from making negative associations between aversive events and their own behaviours. It is tempting to amalgamate these two theories – one psychological, the other neuropharmacological – and suggest that, in depressed patients, the dysfunctional 5-HT$_{1A}$ receptor system renders patients more likely to associate negative events with their depressive behaviours. This association is then laid down in memory and may be activated during a depressed state, leading to the vicious cycle described by Teasdale (1985). The use of antidepressants acting on the serotonergic system (e.g. the 5-HT reuptake inhibitor, fluoxetine) may actually help treat the emotional symptoms of depression indirectly through an action on cognitive processes. Stimulating the serotonergic system may prevent (and so protect) patients from making such aversive stimulus–response associations. However, this is somewhat speculative at the moment and the generation of clear predictions and their testing in a systematic manner are needed to substantiate this hypothesis.

### Noradrenergic α2 adrenoceptor system

While the $\alpha 2$ adrenoceptor system has generally been implicated in attentional processing (Clark et al., 1987, 1989; Arnsten & Contant, 1992; Coull, 1994; Coull et al., 1995b; Robbins & Everitt, 1994), there have been various reports of therapeutic effects of both $\alpha 2$ agonists and antagonists in patients generally believed to suffer from memory dysfunction (for a review see Coull, 1996). The initial report came from McEntee and Mair (1980), suggesting that an acute dose of the $\alpha 2$ receptor agonist clonidine (CLO) attenuated cognitive dysfunction in patients with Korsakoff's disease, and was followed up by a series of investigations demonstrating that the patients showing the greatest loss of noradrenaline (NA), as measured by levels of the NA metabolite 3-methoxy-4-hydroxyphenylglycol (MHPG), showed the greatest impairment in memory (Mair et al., 1985; McEntee et al., 1987), and also the most favourable response to clonidine (Mair & McEntee, 1986). Similarly, Fields et al. (1988) looked at the effects of clonidine on the cognitive symptoms of chronic schizophrenia, and found CLO-induced improvements in both immediate and delayed memory, and in the more difficult of two sustained attention tasks from the Wechsler Memory Scale. Importantly, these changes were independent of a drug effect on ratings of psychosis.

The authors have recently reported a putative clinical use for the $\alpha 2$ antagonist idazoxan, in the remediation of the cognitive symptomatology of dementia of frontal type (DFT) (Sahakian et al., 1994; Coull et al., 1996a). These patients suffer from a neurodegenerative disorder of the fronto-temporal areas of the brain, and show a cognitive profile of performance similar to patients with surgical excisions of the frontal lobes (Gregory & Hodges, 1993). Idazoxan was found to produce dose-dependent improvements in performance, particularly on tests of planning, verbal fluency, episodic memory, and on the same test of rapid visual information processing and sustained attention used in earlier studies of nicotine in patients with DAT. However, drug-induced deficits in performance on a test of spatial working memory were also evident. These results suggest that idazoxan may be useful as a putative cognitive enhancer, although the drug is thought to exert its effect via an attentional, rather than a mnemonic, mode of action (Coull et al., 1996a; Coull, 1996).

The $\alpha2$ adrenoceptor has also been implicated in behavioural symptoms of Parkinson's disease (PD) in both rat and monkey models of PD (Colpaert, 1987; Colpaert et al., 1991), and prompts speculation as to the therapeutic utility of $\alpha2$ receptor agents on the cognitive symptomatology of this disease. A preliminary report has demonstrated dose-dependent changes in memory performance following administration of guanfacine to a subset of patients with PD (Tidswell et al., 1992), suggesting the possible therapeutic utility of an $\alpha2$ agent for some of the cognitive symptoms of PD.

However, all of these studies administered the drug to the patients in acute doses, and the results of a study by O'Carroll et al. (1993) should illustrate that it may not always be possible to extrapolate directly from results obtained in the laboratory to the clinic. O'Carroll et al. (1993) attempted to replicate the original findings of McEntee and Mair (1980) in a study of eighteen patients with Korsakoff's disease (the original study contained only eight patients), given clonidine as part of a chronic dosing schedule and tested on exactly the same battery of neuropsychological tests as was used in the acute dosing regime study of McEntee and Mair (1980). O'Carroll et al. (1993) failed to find improvements on any of the cognitive measures employed, highlighting possible diagnostic differences, and the difficulty in extrapolating from acute to chronic dose studies.

## Conclusions

This review has made two main points: first, advances are being made in the understanding of the neurochemical basis of various forms of attention and memory. Secondly, it is necessary to be cautious in the interpretation of drug effects on tests which contain many cognitive components. If any real progress is to be made in understanding the neurochemical basis of memory, the constituent components of cognitive tasks should be delineated rather than assuming that a drug is affecting the predominant process involved in performance of the task. For example, the effects of cholinergic drugs on the Brown–Petersen paradigm (see pp. 76–7) make this point quite well. Scopolamine-induced deficits on performance of this task may reflect cholinergic modulation of the phonological loop component of working memory, allocation of processing resources, or even attentional distractibility. There is a fine line between attention and memory, particularly working memory which is thought to last only a few seconds, and Baddeley himself has suggested that a more fitting name for working memory could be working attention (Baddeley, 1993). One potentially useful approach may be a meta-analysis of the results of many different studies, with the crucial factor being the cognitive process which is common to all tasks sharing a specified drug effect. Another, is that advocated by Robbins and Everitt (1994) i.e. a single experimental paradigm being used in conjunction with a variety of neurotoxic lesions in experimental rodents, in order to outline the selectivity of function mediated by various neurotransmitter systems. A similar approach has been adopted by the authors (Coull et al., 1995a, b, c; Park et al., 1993) for studies in human cognitive psychopharmacology, with the same neuropsychological tasks being used with drugs affecting different neurotransmitter systems. This helps to elucidate the role of a particular neurotransmitter in a particular cognitive process, and in addition any double dissociations noted serve to demonstrate the selectivity of the psychopharmacological effects obtained. This latter strategy, of combining objective computerized neuropsychological testing with theory-driven cognitive psychopharmacology, provides a promising approach to the development of new treatments for the cognitive symptomatology of various forms of dementing disorders.

## ACKNOWLEDGEMENTS

This work was funded by a Wellcome Trust Programme Grant awarded to Drs T.W. Robbins, B.J. Everitt, A.C. Roberts and B.J. Sahakian. Dr J.T. Coull held an MRC Training Fellowship.

## REFERENCES

Abas, M.A., Sahakian, B.J. & Levy, R. (1990). Neuropsychological deficits and CT scan changes in elderly depressives. *Psychological Medicine*, **20**, 507–20.

Adem, A. (1993). The next generation of cholinesterase inhibitors. *Acta Neurologica Scandinavica, Supplement*, **149**, 10–12.

Altman, H.J. & Normile, H.J. (1988). What is the nature of the role of the serotonergic nervous system in learning and memory: prospects for development of an effective treatment strategy for senile dementia. *Neurobiology of Aging*, **9**, 627–38.

Altman, H.J., Normile, H.J., Galloway, M.P., Ramirez, A. & Azmitia, E.C. (1990). Enhanced spatial discrimination learning in rats following 5,7-DHT-induced serotonergic deafferation of the hippocampus. *Brain Research*, **518**, 61–6.

Arnsten, A.F.T. & Contant, T.A. (1992). Alpha-2 adrenergic agonists decrease distractability in aged monkeys performing the delayed response task. *Psychopharmacology*, **108**, 159–69.

Arnsten, A.F.T. & Goldman-Rakic, P.S. (1985). Alpha-2 adrenergic mechanisms in prefrontal cortex associated with cognitive decline in aged nonhuman primates. *Science*, **230**, 1273–6.

Asin, K.E., Wirtshafter, D. & Fibiger, H.C. (1985). Electrolytic, but not 5,7-dihydroxytryptamine lesions of the nucleus medianus raphe impair acquisition of a radial maze task. *Behavioural Neural Biology*, **44**, 415–24.

Baddeley, A. (1986). *Working Memory*. Oxford: Clarendon Press.

Baddeley, A. (1993). Working memory or working attention. In *Attention, Selection, Awareness and Control: A Tribute to Donald Broadbent*, ed. A. Baddeley & L. Weiskrantz, pp. 152–71. Oxford: Clarendon Press.

Barnes, J.M., Barnes, N.M., Costall, B., Naylor, R.J. & Tyers, M.B. (1989). 5-HT3 receptors mediate inhibition of acetylcholine release in cortical tissue. *Nature*, **338**, 762–3.

Bartus, R.T., Dean, R.L., Beer, B. & Lippa, A. (1982). The cholinergic hypothesis of geriatric memory dysfunction. *Science*, **217**, 408–17.

Berger, T.W., Weikart, C.L., Bassett, J.L. & Orr, W.B. (1986). Lesions of the retrosplenial cortex produce deficits in reversal learning of the rabbit nictitating membrane response: implications for potential interactions between hippocampal and cerebellar brain systems. *Behavioural Neuroscience*, **100**, 802–9.

Bowen, D.M.S., Allen, S.J., Bento, J.S., Goodhardt, M.J., Haan, E.A., Palmer, A.M., Sims, N.R., Smoth, C.C.T., Spillane, J.A., Esira, G.K., Neary, D., Snowden, J.S., Wilcock, G.K. & Davidson, A.N. (1983). Biochemical assessment of serotonergic and cholinergic dysfunction and cerebral atrophy in Alzheimer's disease. *Journal of Neurochemistry*, **41**, 266–72.

Braestrup, C., Albrechtsen, R. & Squires, R.F. (1977). High densities of benzodiazepine receptors in human cortical areas. *Nature*, **269**, 702–4.

Broks, P., Preston, G.C., Traub, M., Poppleton, P., Ward, C. & Stahl, S.M. (1988). Modelling dementia: effects of scopolamine on memory and attention. *Neuropsychologia*, **26**, 685–700.

Brown, V.J. & Robbins, T.W. (1991). Simple and choice reaction time performance following unilateral striatal dopamine depletion in the rat. *Brain*, **114**, 513–25.

Brozoski, T.J., Brown, R., Rosvold, H.E. & Goldman, P.S. (1979). Cognitive deficit caused by regional depletion of dopamine in prefrontal cortex of rhesus monkeys. *Science*, **205**, 929–31.

Caine, E.D., Wiengartner, H., Ludlow, C.L., Cudahy, E.A. & Wehry, S. (1981). Qualitative analysis of scopolamine-induced amnesia. *Psychopharmacology*, **74**, 74–80.

Candy, J.M., Perry, R.H., Perry, E.K., Irving, D., Blessed, G., Fairbairn, A.F. & Tomlinson, B.E. (1983). Pathological changes in the nucleus of Meynert in Alzheimer's and Parkinson's diseases. *Journal of Neurological Science*, **59**, 277–89.

Carey, G.J., Costall, B., Domeney, A.M., Gerrard, P.A., Jones, D.N., Naylor, R.J. & Tyers, M.B. (1992). Ondansetron and arecoline prevent scopolamine-induced cognitive deficits in the marmoset. *Pharmacology, Biochemistry and Behavior*, **42**, 75–83.

Clark, C.R., Geffen, G.M. & Geffen, L.B. (1987). Catecholamines and attention II: pharmacological studies in normal humans. *Neuroscience and Biobehavioural Reviews*, **11**, 353–64.

Clark, C.R., Geffen, G.M. & Geffen, L.B. (1989). Catecholamines and the covert orientation of attention in humans. *Neuropsychologia*, **27**, 131–9.

Clark, D.M. & Teasdale, J.D. (1982). Diurnal variation in clinical depression and accessibility of memories of positive and negative experiences. *Journal of Abnormal Psychology*, **91**, 87–95.

Colpaert, F.C. (1987). Pharmacological characteristics of tremor, rigidity and hypokinesia induced by reserpine in rat. *Neuropharmacology*, **26**, 1431–40.

Colpaert, F.C., Degryse, A.D. & Van Craenendonck, H. (1991). Effects of an $\alpha$2 antagonist in a 20 year old Java monkey with MPTP-induced parkinsonian signs. *Brain Research Bulletin*, **26**, 627–31.

Corbetta, M., Miezin, F.M., Shulman, G.L. & Petersen, S.E. (1993). A PET study of visuospatial attention. *Journal of Neuroscience*, **13**, 1202–26.

Costall, B. & Naylor, R.J. (1992). Astra Award Lecture. The psychopharmacology of 5-HT3 receptors. *Pharmacology and Toxicology*, **71**, 401–15.

Coull, J.T. (1994). Pharmacological manipulations of the $\alpha$2 noradrenergic system: effects on cognition. *Drugs and Aging*, **5**, 116–26.

Coull, J.T. (1996). $\alpha$2 adrenoceptors in the treatment of dementia: an attentional mechanism? *Journal of Psychopharmacology*, **10** (Suppl. 2), 44–9.

Coull, J.T., Middleton, H.C., Robbins, T.W. & Sahakian, B.J. (1995a). Contrasting effects of clonidine and diazepam on tests of working memory and planning. *Psychopharmacology*, **120**, 311–21.

Coull, J.T., Middleton, H.C., Robbins, T.W. & Sahakian, B.J. (1995b). Clonidine and diazepam have differential effects on tests of attention and learning. *Psychopharmacology*, **120**, 322–32.

Coull, J.T., Sahakian, B.J., Middleton, H.C., Young, A.H., Park, S.B., McShane, R.H., Cowen, P.J. & Robbins, T.W. (1995c). Differential effects of clonidine, haloperidol, diazepam and tryptophan depletion on focused attention and attentional search. *Psychopharmacology*, **121**, 222–30.

Coull, J.T., Sahakian, B.J. & Hodges, J.R. (1996a). The $\alpha$2-antagonist idazoxan remediates certain attentional and executive dysfunction in patients with dementia of frontal type. *Psychopharmacology*, **123**, 239–49.

Coull, J.T., Frith, C.D., Frackowiak, R.S.J. & Grasby, P.M. (1996b). A fronto-parietal network for Rapid Visual Information Processing: a PET study of sustained attention and working memory *Neuropsychologia*, **34**, 1085–95.

Coull, J.T., Frith, C.D. & Dolan, R.J. (1999). Dissociating neuromodulatory effects of diazepam on episodic memory encoding and executive function. *Psychopharmacology*, **145**, 213–22.

Crow, T.J. (1979). Action of hyoscine on verbal learning in man: evidence for a cholinergic link in the transition from primary to secondary memory? In *Brain Mechanisms in Memory and Learning: From Single Neuron to Man*, ed. M.A.B. Brazier. New York: Raven Press.

Crow, T.J. & Grove-White, I.G. (1973). An analysis of the learning deficit following hyoscine administration to man. *British Journal of Pharmacology*, **49**, 322–7.

Curran, H.V. (1986). Tranquilising memories: a review of the effects of benzodiazepines on human memory. *Biological Psychology*, **23**, 179–213.

Curran, H.V. (1991). Benzodiazepines, memory and mood: a review. *Psychopharmacology*, **105**, 1–8.

Davis, K., Thal, L., Gamzu, E. et al. (1992). A double-blind, placebo-controlled multicentre study of tacrine for Alzheimer's disease. *New England Journal of Medicine*, **327**, 1253–9.

Deakin, J.F.W. & Graeff, F.G. (1991). 5-HT and the mechanisms of defence. *Journal of Psychopharmacology*, **5**, 305–15.

Domeney, A.M., Costall, B., Gerrard, P.A., Jones, D.N.C., Naylor, R.J. & Tyers, M.B. (1991). The effect of ondansetron on cognitive performance in the marmoset. *Pharmacology, Biochemistry and Behavior*, **38**, 169–75.

Downes, J.J., Roberts, A.C., Sahakian, B.J., Evenden, J.L., Morris, R.G. & Robbins, T.W. (1989). Impaired extradimensional shift performance in medicated and unmedicated Parkinson's disease: evidence for a specific attentional dysfunction. *Neuropsychologia*, **27**, 1329–44.

Drachman, D.A. & Leavitt, J. (1974). Human memory and the cholinergic system: a relationship to aging? *Archives of Neurology*, **30**, 113–21.

Drachman, D.A. & Sahakian, B.J. (1979). The effects of cholinergic agents on human learning and memory. In *Nutrition and the Brain*, ed. A. Barbeau, J. Growden & R.J. Wurtman, vol. 5. New York: Raven Press.

Drachman, D.A. & Sahakian, B.J. (1980). Memory and cognitive function in the elderly: a preliminary trial of physostigmine. *Archives of Neurology*, **37**, 674–5.

Dunne, M.P. & Hartley, L.R. (1985). The effects of scopolamine on verbal memory: evidence for an attentional hypothesis. *Acta Psychologica*, **58**, 205–17.

Dunnett, S.B., Everitt, B.J. & Robbins, T.W. (1991). The basal forebrain-cortical cholinergic system: interpreting the functional consequences of excitotoxic lesions. *Trends in Neurosciences*, **14**, 494–501.

Eagger, S.A., Levy, R. & Sahakian, B.J. (1991). Tacrine in Alzheimer's disease. *Lancet*, **337**, 989–92.

Elliott, R., Sahakian, B.J., McKay, A.P., Herrod, J.J., Robbins, T.W. & Paykel, E.S. (1996). Neuropsychological impairments in unipolar depression: the influence of perceived failure on subsequent performance. *Psychological Medicine*, **26**, 975–89.

Everitt, B.J. & Robbins, T.W. (1996). Central cholinergic systems and cognition. *Annual Review of Psychology*, **48**, 649–84.

Farlow, M., Gracon, S.I., Hershey, L.A., Lewis, K.W., Sadowsky, C.H. & Dolan-Ureno, J. (1992). A controlled trial of tacrine in Alzheimer's disease. *Journal of the American Medical Association*, **268**, 2523–9.

Fibiger, H.C. (1991). Cholinergic mechanisms in learning, memory and dementia: a review of recent evidence. *Trends in Neurosciences*, **14**, 220–3.

Fields, R.B., van Kammen, D.P., Peters, J.L., Rosen, J., Van Kammen, W.B., Nugent, A., Stipetic, M. & Linnoila, M. (1988). Clonidine improves memory function in schizophrenia independently from change in psychosis: preliminary findings. *Schizophrenia Research*, **1**, 417–23.

Fletcher, P.C., Frith, C.D., Grasby, P.M., Shallice, T., Frackowiak, R.S.J. & Dolan, R.J. (1995). Brain systems for encoding and retrieval of auditory–verbal memory: an in vivo study in humans. *Brain*, **118**, 401–16.

Francis, P.T., Palmer, A.M., Sims, N.R., Bowen, D.M., Davison, A.N., Esiri, M.M., Neary, D., Snowden, J.S. & Wilcock, G.K. (1985). Neurochemical studies of early onset Alzheimer's disease: possible influence on treatment. *New England Journal of Medicine*, **313**, 7–11.

Friston, K.J., Grasby, P.M., Frith, C.D., Bench, C.J., Dolan, R.J., Cowen, P.J., Liddle, P.F. & Frackowiak, R.S.J. (1991). The neurotransmitter basis of cognition: psychopharmacological activation studies using positron emission tomography. In *Exploring Brain Functional*

*Anatomy with Positron Tomograhy*, ed. D.J. Chadwick & J. Whelan, pp. 76–92. Chichester: Wiley (Ciba Foundation Symposium 163).

Frith, C.D., Richardson, J.T.E., Samuel, M., Crow, T.J. & McKenna, P.J. (1984). The effects of intravenous hyoscine and diazepam upon human memory. *Quarterly Journal of Experimental Psychology*, **36A**, 133–44.

Ghonheim, M.M. & Mewaldt, S.P. (1975). Effects of diazepam and scopolamine on storage, retrieval and organizational processes in memory. *Psychopharmacologica*, **44**, 257–62.

Ghonheim, M.M. & Mewaldt, S.P. (1977). Studies on human memory: the interaction of diazepam, scopolamine and physostigmine. *Psychopharmacology*, **52**, 1–6.

Ghonheim, M.M., Hinrichs, J.V. & Mewaldt, S.P. (1984). Dose–response analysis of the behavioural effects of diazepam: I. Learning and Memory. *Psychopharmacology*, **82**, 291–5.

Goldman-Rakic, P.S. (1987). Circuitry of the primate prefrontal cortex and the regulation of behaviour by representational memory. In *Handbook of Physiology: The Nervous System of the Brain, Higher Functions of the Brain*, ed. F. Plum, Section 1, vol. V, Part 1. Bethesda, MD: American Physiological Society.

Goldman-Rakic, P.S. (1994). The issue of memory in the study of prefrontal function. In *Motor and Cognitive Functions of the Prefrontal Cortex*, ed. A.M. Thierry, J. Glowinski, P.S. Goldman-Rakic & Y. Christen, pp. 112–21. Berlin, Heidelberg: Springer-Verlag.

Goldman-Rakic, P.S., Selemon, L.D. & Schwartz, M.L. (1984). Dual pathways connecting the dorsolateral prefrontal cortex with the hippocampal formation and parahippocampal cortex in the rhesus monkey. *Neuroscience*, **12**, 719–43.

Gower, A.J. (1992). 5-HT receptors and cognitive function. In *Central 5-HT Receptors and Psychotropic Drugs*, ed. C.A. Marsden & D.J. Heal, pp. 239–59. Oxford: Blackwell Scientific.

Grasby, P.M., Friston, K.J., Bench, C.J., Frith, C.D., Paulesu, E., Cowen, P.J., Liddle, P.F., Frackowiak, R.S.J. & Dolan, R. (1992). The effect of apomorphine and buspirone on regional cerebral blood flow during the performance of a cognitive task – measuring neuromodulatory effects of psychotropic drugs in man. *European Journal of Neuroscience*, **4**, 1203–12.

Grasby, P.M., Frith, C.D., Friston, K.J., Bench, C., Frackowiak, R.S.J. & Dolan, R.J. (1993). Functional mapping of brain areas implicated in auditory-verbal memory function. *Brain*, **116**, 1–20.

Gray, J.A., Mitchell, S.N., Joseph, M.H., Grigoryan, G.A., Dawe, S. & Hodges, H. (1994). Neurochemical mechanisms mediating the behavioural and cognitive effects of nicotine. *Drug Development Research*, **31**, 3–17.

Gregory, C.A. & Hodges, J.R. (1993). Dementia of frontal type and the focal lobar atrophies. *International Reviews of Psychiatry*, **5**, 397–406.

Hagan, J.J. & Morris, R.G.M. (1988). The cholinergic hypothesis of memory: a review of animal experiments. In *Handbook of Psychopharmacology*, ed. L.L. Iversen, S.D. Iversen & S.H. Snyder, pp. 237–323, vol. 20. New York: Plenum Press.

Hart, S. & Semple, J.M. (1990). *Neuropsychology and the Dementias*. pp. 66–74. London: Taylor and Francis.

Hennesey, M.J., Kirkby, K.C. & Montgomery, I.M. (1991). Comparison of the amnesic effects of midazolam and diazepam. *Psychopharmacology*, **103**, 545–50.

Johns, C,A., Greenwald, B.S., Mohs, R.C. & Davis, K.L. (1983). The Cholinergic Treatment strategy in aging and senile dementia. *Psychopharmacology Bulletin*, 19, 185–97.

Jones, G.M.M., Sahakian, B.J., Levy, R., Warburton, D.M. & Gray, J.A. (1992). Effects of acute subcutaneous nicotine on attention, information processing and short-term memory in Alzheimer's disease. *Psychopharmacology*, 108, 485–94.

Kopelman, M.D. (1986). The cholinergic neurotransmitter system in human memory and dementia: a review. *Quarterly Journal of Experimental Psychology*, 38A, 535–73.

Kopelman, M.D. & Corn, T.H. (1988). Cholinergic 'blockade' as a model for cholinergic depletion. A comparison of the memory deficits with those of Alzheimer-type dementia and the alcoholic Korsakoff syndrome. *Brain*, 111, 1079–110.

Lange, K.W., Robbins, T.W., Marsden, C.D., James, M., Owen, A.M. & Paul, G.M. (1992). L-Dopa withdrawal selectively impairs performance in tests of frontal lobe function in Parkinson's disease. *Psychopharmacology*, 107, 394–404.

Lawlor, B.A., Sunderland, T., Mellow, A.M., Hill, J.L., Molchan, S.E. & Murphy, D.L. (1989). Hyperresponsivity to the serotonin agonist *m*-chlorophenylpiperazine in Alzheimer's disease: a controlled study. *Archives of General Psychiatry*, 46, 542–9.

Lawrence, A.D. & Sahakian, B.J. (1995). Alzheimer's disease, attention and the cholinergic system. *Alzheimer's Disease and Associated Disorders*, 9, 43–9.

Leenders, K.L., Palmer, A.J., Quinn, N., Clark, J.C., Firnau, G., Garnett, E.S., Nahmias, C., Jones, T. & Marsden, C.D. (1986). Brain dopamine metabolism in patients with Parkinson's disease measured with positron emission tomography. *Journal of Neurology, Neurosurgery and Psychiatry*, 49, 853–60.

Leenders, K.L., Salmon, E.P., Tyrell, P., Perani, D., Brooks, D.J., Sagar, H., Jones, T., Marsden, C.D. & Frackowiak, R.S.J. (1990). The nigrostriatal dopaminergic system assessed in vivo by positron emission tomography in healthy volunteer subjects and patients with Parkinson's disease. *Archives of Neurology*, 47, 1290–8.

Levin, E.D. (1992). Nicotinic systems and cognitive function. *Psychopharmacology*, 108, 417–31.

Little, A., Levy, R., Chuaqui-Kidd, P. & Hand, P. (1985). A double-blind, placebo-controlled trial of high-dose lecithin in Alzheimer's disease. *Journal of Neurology, Neurosurgery and Psychiatry*, 48, 736–42.

Lloyd, G.G. & Lishman, W.A. (1975). Effect of depression on the speed of recall of pleasant and unpleasant experiences. *Psychological Medicine*, 5, 173–80.

Luciana, M., Depue, R.A., Arbisi, P. & Leon, A. (1992). Facilitation of working memory in humans by a D2 dopamine receptor agonist. *Journal of Cognitive Neuroscience*, 4, 58–68.

Mair, R.G. & McEntee, W.J. (1986). Cognitive enhancement in Korsakoff's psychosis by clonidine: a comparison with L-Dopa and ephedrine. *Psychopharmacology*, 88, 374–80.

Mair, R.G., McEntee, W.J. & Zatorre, R.J. (1985). Monoamine activity correlates with psychometric deficits in Korsakoff's disease. *Behavioural Brain Research*, 15, 247–54.

McEntee, W.J. & Mair, R.G. (1980). Memory enhancement in Korsakoff's psychosis by clonidine: further evidence for a noradrenergic deficit. *Annals of Neurology*, 7, 466–70.

McEntee, W.J. & Crook, T.H. (1991). Serotonin, memory, and the aging brain. *Psychopharmacology*, 103, 143–9.

McEntee, W.J., Mair, R.G. & Langlais, P.J. (1987). Neurochemical specificity of learning: dopamine and motor learning. *Yale Journal of Biological Medicine*, **60**, 187–93.

Mesulum, M.M. (1981). A cortical network for directed attention and unilateral neglect. *Annals of Neurology*, **10**, 309–25.

Mewaldt, S.P. & Ghonheim, M.M. (1979). The effects and interactions of scopolamine, physostigmine and methscopolamine on human memory. *Biochemistry and Behavior*, **10**, 205–10.

Mohammed, A.H. (1993). Effects of cholinesterase inhibitors on learning and memory in rats: a brief review with special reference to THA. *Acta Neurologica Scandinavica Supplement*, **149**, 13–15.

Mohs, R.C., Davis, K.L., Tinklenberg, J.R., Hollister, L.E., Yesavage, J.A. & Kopell, B.S. (1979). Choline chloride treatment of memory deficits in the elderly. *American Journal of Psychiatry*, **136**, 1275–7.

Muir, J.L., Robbins, T.W. & Everitt, B.J. (1992). Attentional functions of the forebrain cholinergic system: effects of intraventricular hemicholinium, physostigmine, basal forebrain lesions and intracortical grafts on a multiple-choice serial reaction time task. *Experimental Brain Research*, 89: 611–22.

Muir, J.L., Page, K.J., Sirinathsinghji, D.J.S., Robbins, T.W. & Everitt, B.J. (1993). Excitotoxic lesions of basal forebrain cholinergic neurons: effects on learning, memory and attention. *Behavioural Brain Research*, **57**, 123–31.

Muir, J.L., Everitt, B.J. & Robbins, T.W. (1994). AMPA-induced excitotoxic lesions of the basal forebrain: a significant role for the cortical cholinergic system in attentional function. *Journal of Neuroscience*, **14**, 2313–26.

Muir, J.L., Everitt, B.J. & Robbins, T.W. (1995). Reversal of visual attentional dysfunction following lesions of the cholinergic basal forebrain by physostigmine nad nicotine, but not by the 5-HT3 receptor antagonist ondansetron. *Psychopharmacology*, **118**, 82–92.

Muramoto, O., Sugishita, M. & Ando, K. (1984). Cholinergic system and constructional praxis: a further study of physostigmine in Alzheimer's disease. *Journal of Neurology, Neurosurgery and Psychiatry*, **47**, 485–91.

Newhouse, P., Sunderland, T., Tariot, P., Blumhardt, C., Weingartner, H. & Mellow, W. (1988). Intravenous nicotine in Alzheimer's disease: a pilot study. *Psychopharmacology*, **95**, 171–5.

Nilsson, O.G., Strecker, R.E., Daszuta, A. & Bjorklund, A. (1988). Combined cholinergic and serotonergic denervation of the forebrain produces severe deficits in a spatial learning task in the rat. *Brain Research*, **453**, 235–46.

O'Brien, J.T., Sahakian, B.J. & Checkley, S.A. (1993). Cognitive impairments in patients with seasonal affective disorder. *British Journal of Psychiatry*, **163**, 338–43.

O'Carroll, R.E., Moffoot, A., Ebmeier, K., Murray, C. & Goodwin, G.M. (1993). Korsakoff's syndrome, cognition and clonidine. *Psychogical Medicine*, **23**, 341–7.

Owen, A.M., James, M., Leigh, P.N., Summers, B.A., Marsden, C.D., Quinn, N.P., Lange, K.W. & Robbins, T.W. (1992). Fronto-striatal cognitive deficits at different stages of Parkinson's disease. *Brain*, **115**, 1727–51.

Owen, A.M., Roberts, A.C., Hodges, J.R., Summers, B.A., Polkey, C.E. & Robbins, T.W. (1993). Contrasting mechanisms of impaired attentional set-shifting in patients with frontal lobe damage or Parkinson's disease. *Brain*, **116**, 1159–79.

Parasuraman, R. & Haxby, J.V. (1993). Attention and brain function in Alzheimer's disease: a review. *Neuropsychology*, 7, 242–72.

Pardo, J.V., Fox, P.T. & Raichle, M.E. (1991). Localization of a human system for sustained attention by positron emission tomography. *Nature*, 349, 61–4.

Park, S.B., Coull, J.T., McShane, R.H., Young, A.H., Sahakian, B.J., Robbins, T.W. & Cowen, P.J. (1993). Tryptophan depletion in normal volunteers produces selective deficits in learning and memory. *Neuropharmacology*, 33, 575–88.

Perry, E.K., Tomlinson, B.E., Blessed, G., Bergman, K., Gibson, P.H. & Perry, R.H. (1978). Correlations of cholinergic abnormalities with senile plaques and mental test scores in senile dementia. *British Medical Journal*, 2, 1457–9.

Perry, E.K., Perry, R.H., Smith, C.J., Purohit, J., Bonham, P., Dick, D., Candy, J., Edwarson, J.A. & Fairburn, A. (1986). Cholinergic receptors in cognitive disorders. *Canadian Journal of Neurological Science*, 13, 521–7.

Perry, E.K., Perry, R.H., Smith, C.J., Dick, D., Candy, J.M., Edwardson, J.A., Fairburn, A. & Blessed, G. (1987). Nicotinic receptor abnormalities in Alzheimer's and Parkinson's diseases. *Journal of Neurology, Neurosurgery and Psychiatry*, 50, 806–9.

Peters, B.H. & Levin, H.S. (1979). Effects of physostigmine and lecithin on memory in Alzheimer disease. *Annals of Neurology*, 6, 219–21.

Petersen, R.C. (1977). Scopolamine-induced learning failures in man. *Psychopharmacology*, 52, 283–9.

Posner, M.I. & Petersen, S.E. (1990). The attention system of the human brain. *Annual review of Neuroscience*, 13, 25–42.

Price, D.L. (1986). New perspectives in Alzheimer's disease. *Annual Review of Neuroscience*, 9, 489–512.

Pycock, C.J., Kerwin, R.W. & Carter, C.J. (1980). Effect of lesion of cortical dopamine terminals on subcortical dopamine receptors in rats. *Nature*, 286, 74–7.

Richter-Levin, G. & Segal, M. (1989). Spatial performance is severely impaired in rats with combined reduction of serotonergic and cholinergic transmission. *Brain Research*, 477, 404–7.

Riedel, W.J., Klaassen, T., Deutz, N.E.P. van Someren, A. & van Pragg, H.M. (1999). Tryptophan depletion in normal volunteers produces selective impairment in memory consolidation. *Psychopharmacology*, 141, 362–9.

Robbins, T.W. & Everitt, B.J. (1994). Arousal systems and attention. In *The Cognitive Neurosciences*, ed. M.S. Gazzaniga, pp. 703–20. Cambridge, MA: MIT Press.

Robbins, T.W., Everitt, B.J., Marston, H.M., Wilkinson, L., Jones, G.H. & Page, K.J. (1989). Comparative effects of ibotenic acid and quisqualic acid induced lesions of the substantia innominata on attentional functions in the rat: further implications for the role of the cholinergic system of the nucleus basalis in cognitive processes. *Behavioural Brain Research*, 35, 221–40.

Robbins, T.W., Joyce, E.M. & Sahakian, B.J. (1992). Neuropsychology and imaging. In *Handbook of Affective Disorders*, ed. E.S. Paykel, pp. 289–309. Edinburgh: Churchill Livingstone.

Roberts, A.C. & Sahakian, B.J. (1993). Comparable tests of cognitive function in monkey and man. In *Behavioural Neuroscience: A Practical Approach*, ed. A. Sahgal, pp. 165–84. Oxford: IRL Press.

Roberts, A.C., Robbins, T.W., Everitt, B.J., Jones, G.H., Sirkia, T.E., Wilkinson, J. & Page, K. (1990). The effects of excitotoxic lesions of the basal forebrain on the acquisition, retention and serial reversal of visual discriminations in marmosets. *Neuroscience*, **34**, 311–29.

Roberts, A.C., De Salvia, M.A., Wilkinson, L.S., Collins, P., Muir, J.L. & Robbins, T.W. (1994). 6-Hydroxydopamine lesions of the prefrontal cortex in monkeys enhance performance on an analogue of the Wisconson Card Sort Test: possible interactions with subcortical dopamine. *Journal of Neuroscience*, **14**, 2531–44.

Rodrigo, G. & Lusiardo, M. (1988). Effects on memory following a single oral dose of diazepam. *Psychopharmacology*, **95**, 263–7.

Rusted, J. (1994). Cholinergic blockade and human information processing: are we asking the right questions? *Journal of Psychopharmacology*, **8**, 54–9.

Rusted, J.M., Eaton-Williams, P. & Warburton, D.M. (1991). A comparison of the effects of scopolamine and diazepam on working memory. *Psychopharmacology*, **105**, 442–5.

Sahakian, B.J. (1988). Cholinomimetics and human cognitive performance. In *Handbook of Psychopharmacology*, ed. L.L. Iversen, S.D. Iversen & S.H. Snyder, pp. 393–424, vol. 20. New York: Plenum Press.

Sahakian, B.J. & Coull, J.T. (1994). Nicotine and tetrahydroaminoacradine: evidence for improved attention in patients with dementia of the Alzheimer type. *Drug Developmental Research*, **31**, 80–8.

Sahakian, B.J., Joyce, E. & Lishman, W.A. (1987). Cholinergic effects on constructional abilities and on mnemonic processes: a case report. *Psychological Medicine*, **17**, 329–33.

Sahakian, B.J., Jones, G.M.M., Levy, R., Gray, J.A. & Warburton, D.M. (1989) .The effects of nicotine on attention, information processing, and short-term memory in patients with dementia of the Alzheimer type. *British Journal of Psychiatry*, **154**, 797–800.

Sahakian, B.J., Downes, J.J., Eagger, S., Evenden, J.L., Levy, R., Philpot, M.P., Roberts, A.C. & Robbins, T.W. (1990). Sparing of attentional relative to mnemonic function in a subgroup of patients with dementia of the Alzheimer type. *Neuropsychologia*, **28**, 1197–213.

Sahakian, B.J., Owen, A.M., Morant, N.J., Eagger, S.A., Boddington, S., Crayton, L., Crockford, H.A., Crooks, M. & Levy, R. (1993). Further ananlysis of the cognitive effects of tetrahydroaminoacradine (THA) in Alzheimer's disease: assessment of attentional and mnemonic function using CANTAB. *Psychopharmacology*, **110**, 395–401.

Sahakian, B.J., Coull, J.T. & Hodges, J.R. (1994). Selective enhancement of executive function by idazoxan in a patient with dementia of the frontal lobe type. *Journal of Neurology, Neurosurgery and Psychiatry*, **57**, 120–1.

Sarter, M.F. & Bruno, J.P. (1994). Cognitive functions of cortical acetylcholine: lessons from studies on trans-synaptic modulation of activated efflux. *Trends in Neurosciences*, **17**, 217–20.

Sarter, M., Schneider, H.H. & Stephens, D.N. (1988). Treatment strategies for senile dementia: antagonist $\beta$-carbolines. *Trends in Neurosciences*, **11**, 13–17.

Sawaguchi, T. & Goldman-Rakic, P.S. (1994). The role of D1-dopamine receptor in working memory: local injections of dopamine antagonists into the prefrontal cortex of rhesus monkeys performing an oculomotor delayed-response task. *Journal of Neurophysiology*, **71**, 515–28.

Shallice, T. (1988). *From Neuropsychology to Mental Structure.* Cambridge: Cambridge University Press.

Shallice, T., Fletcher, P., Frith, C.D., Grasby, P.M., Frackowiak, R.S.J. & Dolan, R.J. (1994). Brain regions associated with acquisition and retrieval of verbal episodic memory. *Nature,* **368**, 633–5.

Siegfried, K.C. (1993). Pharmacodynamic and early clinical studies with velnacrine. *Acta Neurologica Scandinavica Supplement,* **149**, 26–8.

Smith, G. (1988). Animal models of Alzheimer's disease: experimental cholinergic denervation. *Brain Research Review,* **13**, 103–18.

Squire, L.R., Ojemann, J.G., Miein, F.M., Petersen, S.E., Videen, T.O. & Raichle, M.E. (1992). Activation of the hippocampus in normal humans: a functional imaging study of memory. *Proceedings of the National Academy of Sciences, USA,* **89**, 1837–41.

Teasdale, J.D. (1985). Psychological treatments for depression: how do they work? *Behaviour Research and Therapy,* **23**, 157–65.

Thal, L.J. (1992). Cholinomimetic therapy in Alzheimer's disease. In *Neuropsychology of Memory,* ed. L.R. Squire & N. Butters, pp. 277–84. New York: Guilford Press.

Tidswell, P., Sagar, H.J. & Robbins, T.W. (1992). Noradrenergic modulation of cognition in Parkinson's disease using guanfacine. *Journal of Psychopharmacology, BAP Summer Meeting, Abstract Book,* **A23**, 92.

Vanderwolf, C.H. (1987). Near-total loss of learning and memory as a result of combined cholinergic and serotonergic blockade in the rat. *Behavioural Brain Research,* **23**, 43–57.

Voytko, M.L., Olton, D.S., Richardson, R.T., Gorman, L.K., Tobin, J.R. & Price, D.L. (1994). Basal forebrain lesions in monkeys disrupt attention but not learning and memory. *Journal of Neuroscience,* **14**, 167–86.

Warburton, D.M. & Rusted, J.M. (1991). Cholinergic systems and information processing capacity. In *Memory: Neurochemical and Abnormal Perspectives,* ed. J. Weinman & J. Hunter, pp. 65–86. London: Harwood Academic Press.

Warburton, D.M., Rusted, J.M. & Fowler, J. (1992). A comparison of the attentional and consolidation hypotheses for the facilitation of memory by nicotine. *Psychopharmacology,* **108**, 443–7.

Wenk, G.L. & Olton, D.S. (1987). Basal forebrain cholinergic neurons and Alzheimer's disease. In *Animal Models of Dementia,* ed. J.T. Coyle, pp. 81–101. New York: Alan R. Liss.

Wenk, G., Hughey, D., Boundy, V., Kim, A., Walker, K. & Olton, D. (1987). Neurotransmitters and memory: role of cholinergic, serotonergic and noradrenergic systems. *Behavioural Neuroscience,* **101**, 325–32.

Wenk, G.L., Stoehr, J.D., Quintana, G., Mobley, S. & Wiley, R.G. (1994). Behavioural, biochemical, histological and electrophysiological effects of 192 IgG-saporin injections into the basal forebrain of rats. *Journal of Neuroscience,* **14**, 5986–95.

Wesnes, K. & Revell, A. (1984). The separate and combined effects of scopolamine and nicotine on human information processing. *Psychopharmacology,* **84**, 5–11.

Wesnes, K. & Warburton, D.M. (1984). Effects of scopolamine and nicotine on human rapid information processing performance. *Psychopharmacology,* **82**, 147–50.

Whitehouse, P.J. (1993). Cholinergic therapy in dementia. *Acta Neurologica Scandinavica Supplerment*, **149**, 42–5.

Whitehouse, P.J., Price, D.L., Struble, R.G., Clark, A.W., Coyle, J.T. & DeLong, M.R. (1982). Alzheimer's disease and senile dementia: loss of neurons in the basal forebrain. *Science*, **215**, 1237–9.

Widzowski, D.V., Cregan, E. & Bialobok, P. (1994). Effects of nicotinic agonists and antagonists on spatial working memory in normal adult and aged rats. *Drug Developmental Research*, **31**, 24–31.

Woolf, N.J. (1991). Cholinergic systems in mammalian brain and spinal cord. *Progress in Neurobiology*, **37**, 475–524.

Yamamoto, T. & Hirano, A. (1985). Nucleus raphe dorsalis in Alzheimer's disease: neurofibrillary tangles and loss of large neurons. *Annals of Neurology*, **17**, 573–7.

**Part II**

# 6

# The multidisciplinary memory clinic approach

John R. Hodges, German E. Berrios and Kristin Breen

The aim of this chapter is to describe briefly the origins, principles and organization of the Cambridge Memory Clinic (CMC) which was started by the editors in 1990. Memory clinics vary a great deal in scope and services. In their useful paper on memory clinics in the British Isles, Wright and Lindesay (1995) surveyed 20 such facilities, reporting that in only 45% a psychiatric instrument was used as a routine to measure 'affective state'; and although psychiatrists seemed to participate in about 75% of clinics, their role and the comprehensiveness of their psychiatric assessment were unclear. Some clinics seem to have a wide scope: for example, in an excellent study, Verhey et al. (1995) assessed the DSM-III-R psychiatric status of 430 consecutive patients and in 61 subjects found depression, 39 dysthymia, 23 adjustment disorder, 18 personality disorder, 6 anxiety disorder and 2 somatoform disorder; the authors made the important point that the low rates of non-affective psychiatric disorder reported by some clinics is likely to result from a perfunctory psychiatric examination or the use of insensitive instruments. On the other hand, many such clinics do not include a routine neurological or formal neuropsychological assessment.

## The Cambridge Memory Clinic

The objective when founding this clinic was to establish a truly multidisciplinary service which combined behavioural neurology, neuropsychiatry and neuropsychology. From the start its main objective was to assess patients complaining of memory impairment and patients whose memory is considered as impaired by others, even when the patient has no awareness of deficit. Since it was thought desirable to encourage a broad range of referrals no age limit was set and we accepted cases referred directly from general practitioners and from other consultant colleagues. A relevant carer or relative is always asked to attend and together with the appointment, three questionnaires are sent for completion: a 'carer's questionnaire (assessing behavioural deficits), and two 'Insight into memory deficit' questionnaires (to be completed separately by patient and carer) (see Chapter 10, this volume).

All patients referred to the clinic are seen by members of all three teams independently. Thus patients are asked to attend the hospital for a whole day. During this time they undergo a neurological and neuropsychiatric assessment and are given a standardized battery of neuropsychological tests (described below). Each of these assessments takes between one and one and a half hours. The teams meet at 5pm to discuss the patients evaluated on the day. Notes are compared and a friendly rivalry has developed as to who finds more relevant historical and clinical clues. Although this approach may not be very time-efficient, it also means that the probability of missing important clinical data is reduced. The consultant to whom the referral has been made collates all the information to write the final report. The aim of the meeting is to reach a preliminary conclusion on whether the patient has an organic or a functional problem, a combination thereof, or neither, and to formulate a plan of investigation and management. A number of patients are followed up, and when doubts remain some are admitted into hospital (either to neurological or neuropsychiatric beds) for specialized studies and/or treatment.

Over the past eight years over 800 patients have been assessed, approximately two-thirds of whom had a primary diagnosis of organic brain disease (dementia, amnesia, etc.) and the other third presented with a psychiatric diagnosis which, in many instances, had not been recognized by the referring doctor. This single fact highlights the need for an integrated assessment.

## The neurological assessment

The principles underlying the neurological interview, examination and 'bedside' testing of cognitive function performed in the clinic have been described in detail elsewhere (Hodges, 1994). The assessment of the patient should aim to cover each of the major domains of cognition (memory, language, numerical skills, visuospatial abilities, etc.) and behaviour as outlined in Table 6.1.

When evaluating a patient's history it is essential to start with a clear theoretical framework. The complaint of 'poor memory' is fairly non-specific but can usually be fitted into one of the three following categories which derive from the model of memory described in a number of places in this book (see Chapter 4, this volume and below): – each category has clear cognitive, neuroanatomical and diagnostic implications: (i) poor concentration with lapses of attention and difficulty dealing with more than one stream of information denotes a deficit in working (short-term) memory; (ii) difficulty retaining new information from day to day with rapid forgetting and a tendency to repetitiveness points to impairment in episodic memory; or (iii) problems with word finding or a loss of vocabulary suggest either a breakdown in semantic memory or a more specific anomia.

As well as covering the areas of cognition outlined in Table 6.1, enquiry should

**Table 6.1.** Checklist for Interviewing patients and relatives

| | |
|---|---|
| 1. Memory | • anterograde: recall of new episodic information in day-to-day life (e.g. recalling messages and conversation, family news, TV programmes, etc.)<br>• retrograde: past personal and public event memory<br>• semantic: vocabulary, names and general factual knowledge (history, geography, politics, etc.) |
| 2. Language | • output: word finding, grammar, word errors (paraphasias)<br>• comprehension of words and grammar<br>• reading<br>• writing: spelling and motor components |
| 3. Numerical skills | • handling money, shopping, dealing with bills |
| 4. Visuospatial skills | • dressing<br>• constructional abilities<br>• spatial orientation and route finding |
| 5. Neglect phenomena | • neglect of extra-personal space<br>• bodily neglect |
| 6. Visual perception | • recognition and identification of people<br>• object and colour identification |
| 7. Hallucinations | • visual, auditory, tactile, olfactory |
| 8. Personality change and social conduct | • disinhibition, apathy, impulsiveness, eating habits, sexual behaviour |
| 9. Thinking and problem solving abilities | • coping with complex tasks, using electrical equipment, planning meals, hobbies, etc. |
| 10. Affect | • mood<br>• energy, concentration<br>• biological features (appetite, sleeping) |
| 11. Self-care | • dressing, grooming, bathing, toileting |

also be made about activities of daily living (self-care, cooking and housework, hobbies, driving, work, etc.) and behaviour in a range of social situations.

A separate interview with the accompanying family member or close friend is of paramount importance: many patients lack complete insight into the nature or extent of their deficits. In addition, it allows one to enquire about potentially embarrassing areas of behavioural change (eating habits, libido, social interactions, etc.). A thorough family history should be part of the routine history with specific enquiry regarding psychiatric and neurological events. Particular attention is paid to the very earliest deficits noted by the family and to the pattern of cognitive/behavioural change over time which contribute greatly to the differential diagnosis in the dementias (see Chapter 7, this volume).

Although all patients should have a full general medical and neurological examination, there are perhaps some aspects which are more essential than others and can all be incorporated into a '5-minute' screening assessment which includes:

(i)      blood pressure;
(ii)     cardiac auscultation and carotids for bruits;
(iii)    frontal release signs especially pout and grasp reflexes;
(iv)     fundal examination and visual fields including bilateral simultaneous extinction;
(v)      eye movements, both pursuit and saccades;
(vi)     bulbar signs: speech, tongue movements and jaw jerk;
(vii)    limb tone, tendon reflexes and plantars;
(viii)   maintenance of hands outstretched posture looking for drift, tremor and dyskinesias;
(ix)     ability to perform rapid alternating hand movements;
(x)      observation of gait to include initiation, walking and turning;
(xi)     balance standing and walking heel-to-toe.

In the clinic a brief cognitive test schedule has been evolved, which incorporates the MMSE and can be completed in 5 to 10 minutes. It attempts to sample the main areas of cognition with special emphasis on subdomains of memory. The full schedule is included as an Appendix to this chapter and the guiding principles are outlined in Table 6.2.

## The neuropsychiatric assessment

A consultant neuropsychiatrist (GEB) and team carry out a full clinical and computerized psychiatric assessment. In addition to the history taking and mental state assessment (about 50 minutes), the subject completes a set of 9 core computerized instruments (in about 40 minutes) (see Table 6.3). If the mental state examination suggests the presence of any other type of psychopathology, other relevant computerized tests are added to the core battery. When it is suspected that no organic or psychiatric aetiology is present, subjects are also asked to complete the Metamemory test (see Chapter 3, this volume). Psychiatric diagnosis is made in terms of ICD-10 and DSM nomenclatures.

The questionnaires were computerized in 1986 by means of the QFast system (1986), and their reliability has been checked against the pencil and paper forms of the same tests. All the instruments are very well known. The same battery is, in fact, used in another eight Neuropsychiatric Clinics run by GEB (thus comparison across a range of neurological diseases is available). Because of the additional

**Table 6.2.** Framework for bedside assessment of cognitive function (from Hodges, 1994)

**Distributed cognitive functions**

• Attention/Concentration

    Orientation in time and place

• Memory

    (a) Anterograde: registration and recall of name and address after three learning trials

    (b) Retrograde – public events

• Frontal executive function

    Verbal fluency (1 min per letter or category)

    (a) Letter (FAS)

    (b) Category (animals)

**Localized cognitive functions**

• Language

    (a) Spontaneous speech

    (b) Naming of ten pictures of medium frequency items

    (c) Comprehension – words and sentences

    (d) Repetition of multisyllabic words and phrases

    (e) Reading aloud regular and irregular words

    (f) Writing a sentence

• Neglect phenomena and visuospatial abilities

    Drawing of overlapping pentagons and 3D cube

    Freehand drawing of clock face and setting the hands

measuring facilities provided by the QFast system, it is even possible to measure reaction times to each question and to undertake detailed item analysis. The questionnaires are presented on a PC and are saved on diskette for later analysis. About 800 patients have been seen and a large computerized database has accumulated.

## The neuropsychological assessment

All patients attending the clinic undergo a formal standardized neuropsychological assessment performed by a senior clinical neuropsychologist (KB) or a deputy. Clinical neuropsychology is concerned with the evaluation of cognitive function in patients with known or suspected neurological disease. It is often used as a tool for monitoring a change in function, to provide guidelines for rehabilitation and it plays a major role in the differential diagnosis between neurological

**Table 6.3.** Cambridge computerized neuropsychiatry assessment for memory disorders clinic

(All core[a] tests must be applied)

Name: ..........................................................    Date: .........................    Short ID (3 characters):

|  | Computer code | Tick if applied |
|---|---|---|
| **General** | | |
| General health questionnaire: | GHQ[a] | ☐ |
| Insight | INS | ☐ |
| Personality deviance scale | PER[a] | ☐ |
| **Affective disorders** | | |
| Hamilton depression scale (observer rated) | HDS | ☐ |
| Profile of mood states | POMS | ☐ |
| Irritability scale | IRR[a] | ☐ |
| Hospital-anxiety depression scale | HAD | ☐ |
| Mania scale | MAN | ☐ |
| Beck depression inventory | BECK[a] | ☐ |
| Geriatric depression scale (for older than 65) | GDS[a] | ☐ |
| **Cognitive** | | |
| Attention test | ATT | ☐ |
| Signal detection memory test | SIGNAL[a] | ☐ |
| Metamemory test | MET | ☐ |
| Cognitive failures questionnaire | CFQ[a] | ☐ |
| **Neuroses** | | |
| Obsessions interference / resistance | OCD | ☐ |
| Obsessive-compulsive disorder | MOC[a] | ☐ |
| Hypochondria scale | HYP | ☐ |
| Zung anxiety scale | ZG[a] | ☐ |
| Phobias scale | PHO | ☐ |
| Dissociative behaviours questionnaire | DIS[a] | ☐ |
| Self-evaluation questionnaire (Form Y-1) | STAI | ☐ |
| Self-evaluation questionnaire (Form Y-2) | STAI2 | ☐ |

*Note:*
[a] (NB: please apply other relevant instruments according to findings in interview).

and psychiatric disorders. It is well known that anxiety, depression and other psychiatric symptoms can interfere with cognitive processes and many patients complain of poor memory, concentration difficulties and even word finding difficulties or mispronunciation of words in conversation. The purpose of this review is to focus on the CMC and not to provide an exhaustive review of neuropsychological measures. This is available from a number of other texts (Hodges, 1994; Lezak, 1995; McCarthy & Warrington, 1990; Walsh, 1987). Instead, the neuropsychological assessment procedures used in the clinic will be described in some detail and the rationale for choosing these particular tests.

Probably the majority of patients referred to the memory clinic fall into the category of queried neurological/ psychiatric involvement, and it is important for this to be reflected in the neuropsychological assessment schedule. In addition, the neuropsychological investigation should be comprehensive enough to give sufficient information to answer questions about alertness and concentration, general intellectual skills, executive and adaptive functions and to identify more specific or localized impairments involving memory, language, calculation, praxis, perceptual, visuospatial and constructional skills. However, although it is important to evaluate a wide range of skills, the assessment should not be too long as patients get tired and do not perform at their most optimal level. Normally it is not possible to cover every area in great detail and a balance has to be achieved between the breadth of an assessment and in-depth evaluation of more localised functions.

In the clinic a standard set of core tests is administered. The assessment takes approximately 1½ hours and covers the areas shown below.

## Core neuropsychological assessment

(i)     Tests of general intelligence
           Measures of premorbid or optimal level of intellectual function
(ii)    Assessment of frontal lobe function
(iii)   Tests of verbal and visual memory
(iv)    Information relating to language production and comprehension
(v)     Visuoconstructional, perceptual and spatial tasks.

## Assessment of general intelligence

The assessment of general intellectual skills gives information regarding the integrity of cortical functioning as a whole and this in itself can be of diagnostic significance. Furthermore, in many cases it is only in the context of such information that more focal syndromes can be properly identified. The concept of intelligence is a complex one. It is a hypothetical concept and many of the earlier definitions were based on what each individual theorist saw as primary to their own idea of intelligence. In practice, one tends to opt for a more operational definition such as intelligence is what is measured by intelligence tests. This has the advantage that a common concept and measuring system is used and that its limitations are known. For example, if a test has been standardized on a particular group of people of a certain age and cultural background then it is most suitable for subjects from this group and less so for those with different educational and cultural backgrounds.

## WAIS-R

The Wechsler Adult Intelligence Scale is probably the most commonly used test for the assessment of general intellectual function in adults (age range 16 to 74). It was originally developed in the USA by David Wechsler but has recently been revised (WAIS-R, Wechsler, 1981) and adapted for British use (Lea, 1981, 1986). It consists of a set of six verbal and five non-verbal tests from which a Verbal and a Performance IQ can be derived. The tests have been standardized on large samples so that the resulting IQ measures have a mean of 100 and a standard deviation of 15. This method is based on the assumption that intelligence is normally distributed in the population and the IQ scores are obtained by comparing a person's score with the scores obtained by a representative sample of the same age group. The items within each subtest are graded in difficulty and a test is discontinued after a set number of consecutive failures. When the tests are administered, raw scores are first obtained on each of the subtests. These are then converted to normalized standard scores or scaled scores which are adjusted for age. As with overall IQ, the individual subtest scores are related to the normal distribution and they are expressed on a scale with a mean of 10 and a standard deviation of 3.

Clinically, these tests are used as a means of establishing the level at which a person is functioning intellectually and not really for the purpose of assessing IQ. As one is less concerned about obtaining exact IQs, this means that all the subtests need not be administered but that a shortened form of the WAIS-R will often do. On the basis of the shortened form it is still possible to evaluate overall level of functioning and to establish whether individual subtest scores differ significantly from one another. This information can provide important pointers towards focal neurological pathology although it is not sufficient to rely exclusively on the WAIS-R for this. Four verbal and one non-verbal test from the WAIS-R are included in the memory clinic assessment and these are described in Table 6.4.

Vocabulary is a good measure of expressive verbal ability and similarities of verbal abstraction. Both are sensitive to language impairment and performance on similarities can be used to indicate frontal lobe dysfunction. Similarly, a discrepancy between forwards and backwards digit span can be a frontal sign. Low scores on arithmetic and poor forwards and backwards span may indicate an auditory verbal short-term memory deficit which often goes with impaired spelling and is associated with left parietal damage. Alternatively, in the context of impaired performance on a range of other tasks, poor performance on arithmetic and digit span would be more suggestive of attentional difficulties. Block design is used to assess constructional ability. Patients in the early stages of Alzheimer's disease often show impairment on block design which is used in combination with other more focal tests known to be sensitive to non-dominant hemisphere involvement.

**Table 6.4.** Wechsler Adult Intelligence Scale – Revised (WAIS-R)

**Verbal scale subtests**

1. *Vocabulary* is a word definition task consisting of 35 items. It starts with relatively common words such as 'winter' and 'breakfast' and concludes with 'audacious' and 'tirade'.

2. *Similarities* is a test of verbal abstraction. The subject is read pairs of words and asked to explain how they are alike. There are 14 word-pairs ranging in difficulty from 'orange-banana' to 'praise-punishment'.

3. *Arithmetic* contains 14 arithmetical questions which are time limited and range from easy questions like 'how much is £4 plus £5' to 'if 8 machines are needed to finish a job in 6 days, how many machines would be needed to finish the job in half a day'.

4. *Digit span*. In this test the subject is asked to repeat sequences of digits of increasing length (forwards span) and in reverse order (backwards span). It is a test of auditory verbal memory and concentration span.

**Performance scale subtest**

1. *Block design*. This is a visuoconstructional task where subjects are given four and later nine identical blocks, with two red sides, two white sides and two red/white sides and have to put them together to look like designs printed on cards.

## Assessment of premorbid IQ

Together with other information the WAIS-R can be used to indicate whether a patient is performing at his or her optimal level or is showing evidence of intellectual decline. Knowledge of occupational and educational background can often give a good idea of an individual's optimal or premorbid level of ability. However, this information is not always known and in some cases intellectual potential may be underestimated. There are other more objective measures of optimum performance. One commonly used is the National Adult Reading Test (NART, Nelson 1982). The NART consists exclusively of irregularly spelt words. These are words which cannot be read simply by using the familiar letter sound rules in the English language but require prior knowledge about each word for its pronunciation. The NART is graded in difficulty so that it begins with reasonably common words (chord, ache and depot) while towards the end of the test the words are much less well known (syncope, labile and campanile). Although it is influenced by educational factors to some extent, it has the advantage that there is a high correlation between measures of general intelligence and reading scores in the normal population. Another argument for using reading tests to estimate optimal ability is that

**Table 6.5.** Divisions of memory

**Short-term memory**

Limited capacity (7 plus or minus 2 items), short-term store characterized by rapid forgetting (after a few seconds).

**Long-term memory**

Unlimited capacity, long-term store where the rate of forgetting is slow.

1. *Episodic memory*: Memory for personally experienced and temporally specific events.
    (a) Retrograde memory refers to memory for past events
    (b) Anterograde memory refers to memory for new and more recent events.
2. *Semantic memory*: Permanent store of knowledge of facts, concepts, words and their meanings.

reading skills tend to remain relatively well preserved even in advanced cases of dementia.

## Memory

Since the main complaint of patients attending the clinic is poor memory, a range of memory functions needs to be assessed. Many clinicians and most patients use the term 'short-term' memory to refer to memory for events that have occurred recently over the last one or two days. Within psychology this term is used very differently which may sometimes cause confusion. In neuropsychological terms short-term memory refers to a limited capacity short-term store or working memory lasting only for a few seconds. It is assessed by the use of span tasks, i.e. digit span and letter span and it can function relatively independently from the other memory systems shown in Table 6.5.

Most of our patients' complaints of memory failure fall into the category of episodic memory loss, the part of memory which is impaired in organic amnesia and in dementia of the Alzheimer type. The main characteristic of these disorders is a severe impairment in the ability to store new information (anterograde amnesia). In this context tests of memory and learning are essential because new learning is greatly reduced even in the relatively early stages of dementia. Material specific memory deficits are not uncommon so it is necessary to assess both verbal and visual memory function. Similarly, it is advisable to use tests of recall and recognition memory as they are sensitive to different aspects of memory. Recognition tests are thought to be less vulnerable to the effects of anxiety and depression than recall tests and they have been argued to be purer measures of memory. A summary of the assessment schedule for assessing anterograde memory function is shown below. Retrograde memory is assessed informally by questioning the patient and a close relative on past personal and other salient events.

Assessment of anterograde memory

(a)  Questions of orientation in time, place and person
(b)  Information regarding topographical memory (whether the patient gets lost in familiar surroundings)
(c)  Questions about recent news and media events
(d)  Information relating to current problems and recent personal experiences
(e)  Formal assessment of recognition memory for words and faces (Warrington) and recall of passages and designs (Wechsler Memory Scale – Revised)

Recognition memory

The Warrington recognition memory test for words and faces is used to assess verbal and visual memory function, respectively (Warrington, 1984). The subject is shown 50 words (or faces). These are presented at a rate of approximately one every 3 seconds. For each item the subject is asked to judge whether they find it pleasant or not to ensure some encoding of the information to be remembered. This is followed by a two-choice recognition memory test where they are shown pairs of words. Within each pair only one word was presented earlier and the subject is asked to choose which of the two they recognize from the previous presentation.

The Warrington recognition memory test has been validated on a normal sample and a neurological group and is published with age-related norms. It does not take too long to administer and a shortened form of the test is available for those patients who for various reasons cannot perform on the more difficult version.

Recall

Recall of verbal and visual information is assessed by the logical passages and designs from the Wechsler Memory Scale – Revised (1987). Here the subject is read two short stories and immediately after each one is asked to recall as much information as they can (immediate recall). After a delay of 30 minutes, information from both stories is recalled. In the visual version of the test four relatively simple designs are shown one at a time for 10 seconds each. After each presentation the design is removed and the patient is asked to draw an exact copy. Again, memory for all four designs is tested after half an hour.

As above, these tests have the advantage of being published with normative data against which to compare a patient's scores. In addition, they allow for the assessment of memory after a delay and poor delayed recall is a good predictor of organic memory impairment. One potential disadvantage of the logical passages is that many patients from different clinical groups seem to find it difficult and often score below the normal range perhaps because of the test's sensitivity to anxiety, concentration and motivational factors. However, on the whole, the recall and recognition tests compliment each other well. This is particularly important for the identification of material specific memory problems where it is necessary to demonstrate a consistent pattern of verbal (or non-verbal) impairment across different tests. For example, a frequently observed pattern in our clinic is normal recognition memory for words and satisfactory immediate and delayed recall of designs while recognition memory for faces is poor and immediate and delayed recall of stories is impaired. This pattern is unlikely to signal material specific memory problems. However, if the tests were used in isolation there is a good chance that the wrong conclusions would be reached.

## Frontal lobe function

It is important to assess frontal lobe function for at least two reasons. First, the early behavioural and clinical signs that occur with frontal tumours can sometimes imitate depressive symptoms and be misdiagnosed at a time when other options for treatment should be considered. Secondly, it is important to assess frontal function as impairment can affect performance on a range of cognitive tasks. The changes that occur which are often misleading include slowness, loss of control of emotion, lack of responsivity to and concern for significant events and sometimes deterioration in social habits and hygiene. Memory can be influenced in various ways. Usually these patients do quite well on recognition memory tests but have greater difficulty on tasks that require more active processing and organization of the material to be remembered such as is required by more demanding recall tests. Prospective memory or the ability to remember to do something in the future may be impaired as a result of poor organisational skills rather than a memory deficit per se.

There is a host of tests available for the assessment of frontal lobe dysfunction and it has been necessary to make a small selection of those tests which, clinically, have been found to be most sensitive in the past. It should be noted that some patients with known frontal damage show very little evidence of this on testing while others may fail on relatively simple tasks. Another observation made in the clinic is that some patients with anxiety and depressive symptomatology are sometimes found to have difficulties on these tests so that failure is not necessarily always associated with organic damage. The tests adopted for our assessment are shown in Table 6.6.

In combination with the similarities and digit span subtests from the WAIS-R, they enable us to obtain information about abstract reasoning, attentional ability, strategy generation, mental flexibility/set shifting and sequencing of movement. Many frontal patients have difficulty with set shifting and the modified version of the Wisconsin card sorting test (Nelson, 1976) can provide a good measure of this. The Wisconsin is often beyond the capabilities of people with low intellectual capacity and the much simpler Weigl test will suffice. It is surprising how many patients with frontal damage fail to see the solution to this relatively easy task.

**Table 6.6.** Frontal lobe tests

1. *Verbal fluency.* This is a test of strategy generation and the subject is asked to think of as many words as they can beginning with a particular letter (F, A, and S).

2. *Alternating hand movements* is a motor sequencing test where the subject is required to use both hands, one flat and one in a fist and to reverse the hand positions by alternatively opening and closing each hand in a rhythmical sequence.

3. *Modified Wisconsin card sorting test* (Nelson, 1976). Here subjects are shown four key cards, (1 green cross, 2 yellow triangles, 3 blue circles and four red stars). They are then given one card from a pack of 48 which matches one of the key cards on the dimension of colour, shape or number. They are instructed to place each card below a key card according to certain rules. They are not told the rule but have to work it out for themselves. On each trial they are given feedback as to whether they are right or wrong and they are told when the rule is changed.

4. *Weigl colour/form sorting test* (Weigl, 1941). This is used as an alternative to the Wisconsin and consists of 12 tokens (3 shapes by 4 colours) which can be sorted into groups of either shape or colour.

## Localized cognitive functions

Due to time constraints, there is not the opportunity to assess localized function in great detail and for many of the patients seen in the clinic this would not be appropriate. However, a core assessment has to be comprehensive enough and give sufficient information to enable the identification of focal impairments.

## Language

A patient's performance on the verbal scale of the WAIS-R can often give strong pointers towards the existence of language problems and subsequently left hemisphere involvement. In combination with observations from conversational speech, the vocabulary and similarities subtests can be used to pick up speech errors and to informally assess articulation, comprehension, fluency, grammar and prosody. Impaired digit span and arithmetic may indicate problems with repetition.

One other verbal task used routinely in the clinic is the McKenna graded naming test (McKenna & Warrington, 1983). It consists of 30 line drawings of objects ranging from relatively high frequency items such as kangaroo, thimble and corkscrew to very low frequency items including cowl, centaur and retort. The items are graded in difficulty. It is well known that naming is affected by word frequency and that patients with mild to moderate word retrieval problems can name common words but are impaired in retrieving less frequent items. A graded approach is also more likely to pick up problems in patients with superior language skills and a more extended vocabulary. Performance on the McKenna has been correlated with other tests and can be compared against the vocabulary subtest of the WAIS-R such that a significant discrepancy between the two would be strongly suggestive of impairment. Similarly, even if formal tables are not available for comparison, it is useful to compare performance across tests and note unusual or unexpected discrepancies.

## Non-dominant hemisphere skills

A neuropsychological investigation is not complete without measures of posterior non-dominant hemisphere function. There is evidence for right hemisphere specialization in the processing of complex visual perceptual and spatial stimuli. Disorders at this level result from a failure to achieve a coherent perception of a stimulus. Patients with perceptual deficits often have difficulty with the interpretation of complex and degraded visual material such as incomplete letters or drawings, objects photographed from an unusual angle and overlapping pictures of different objects. In the clinic tests from the Visual Object and Space Perception Battery (VOSP, Warrington & James, 1991) are part of the core assessment. They include the following

- Fragmented letters requires the identification of incomplete letters.
- Cube analysis involves the counting of cubes arranged on top and in front of each other in a complex visual display.
- Dot counting. This test is administered when a patient has difficulty with cube analysis. The subject is asked to count different arrays of black dots.

These are relatively simple tasks which normal people with intact cognition can do with ease. Whenever there is evidence for organic impairment on these or other focal tasks, further and more detailed assessment is arranged outside the clinic.

## Interpretation of organic and functional signs

In the interpretation of neuropsychological data it is important to take advantage of the knowledge that organic brain disease conforms to anatomical specialization and that there are distinctive patterns associated with damage to specific areas of the brain. Evidence of lateralized impairment is strongly indicative of organic involvement. Right hemisphere damage is associated with impairment affecting non-verbal tasks including visual memory, face recognition, visual perception, spatial and visuoconstructional skills. Left hemisphere damage results in verbal memory impairment, language problems, dyscalculia and impaired performance on span tasks. There are signs of focal involvement even in the early stages of degenerative illness. Semantic dementia or progressive fluent aphasia is associated with deteriorating language function and disintegration of semantic knowledge. In dementia of the Alzheimer type the main characteristic is of memory impairment, while in frontal dementia memory is relatively well preserved early in the disease.

In the initial stages of dementia it can be difficult to distinguish between dementia and depression as many patients with depressive symptoms complain of memory problems and their performance on memory tests may mimic that of organic patients. In a few functional cases observed in the clinic, the patients have even shown organic patterns which have resolved with treatment for depression. However, it is probably fair to say that the performance of most patients with functional pathology does not fall into consistent organic patterns of impairment. It is worth noting that it is more difficult to evaluate patients with marked psychotic symptoms and that the following observations are most applicable to neurotically related conditions.

An important qualitative feature which can be very useful in discriminating between functional and organic disorders is the degree of consistency in a person's performance. Patients with psychiatric involvement are more likely to show variability both within and between tests while organic patients tend to be more uniform in their approach. It is not uncommon to find that the former group fail to perform satisfactorily on easy items and proceed to solve quite difficult problems within the same test. Tests from the WAIS-R are sensitive to this kind of variability. Variation between tests is also common in this group so that the results do not conform to normal neuropsychological expectations. Often this variability goes with poor performance on digit span but occurs in the absence of any other language problem and in association with motivational difficulties. Sometimes there is evidence of psychomotor slowing, although the latter could be a subcortical sign. Slowness on timed tasks such as block design results in low scores and can give a wrongful impression of impairment, even though the patient manages to solve several of the problems eventually. Patients with genuine constructional difficulties are usually unable to use the blocks to form relatively simple patterns even when given plenty of time and they often respond by putting the blocks on top of each other or on top of the pictures they are supposed to copy.

Material specific memory impairments are not uncommon in organic conditions but again, performance tends to be comparable across tests so that left hemisphere patients are consistently poorer on tests assessing verbal memory with memory for non-verbal information being relatively well preserved. Thus they do not tend to show the mixed pattern of results on recall and recognition tests described earlier.

Patients with a more global memory deficit are impaired in learning all new information and show poor incidental recall of events. They are often unable to answer questions about news or media events. They are unable to give much background information relating to their current memory problems, seem empty of content, are repetitive and often appear relieved when the interview is finished.

Conversely, it is unlikely that an individual has an organic memory impairment if they can give a lengthy and detailed history of their problems and can name several doctors or other professionals they have been in touch with. Another characteristic of the functional patient is that he or she is often more interested in talking about their problems than in focusing on the neuropsychological tests and frequently they appear reluctant to leave at the end of a session.

There is a particular group of patients where a differential diagnosis is very difficult to achieve. They show impairment on most tasks and it is unclear whether such uniformly poor performance reflects a genuine global dementia or pseudo-dementia associated with an underlying psychiatric cause. In the case of these borderline patients, one or several repeat assessments should help to clarify the picture to some extent by revealing inconsistencies or further deterioration.

Also, these patients often perform at chance level on memory tests and below the level of organic groups. One way of assessing the genuineness of their memory problem has been to give them very easy tasks which even densely amnesic patients can perform satisfactorily.

Finally, it should be noted that, in instances where patients are performing at very low levels and showing significant impairment on the standard core tests, additional and less demanding tasks are administered to assess residual cognitive capacity and to obtain scores against which to measure future change. This more flexible approach makes it possible to suit the requirements of each individual patient while still allowing comparisons to be made between different groups of patients on a set of core tests.

## REFERENCES

Hodges, J.R. (1994). *Cognitive Assessment for Clinicians*. Oxford: Oxford University Press.

Lea, M. (1981, 1986). *WAIS-R, UK. A British Supplement to the manual of the WAIS-R*. San Antonio, TS: The Psychological Corporation.

Lezak, M.D. (1995). *Neuropsychological Assessment*, 3rd edn. Oxford: Oxford University Press.

McCarthy, R.A. & Warrington, E.K. (1990). *Cognitive Neuropsychology. A Clinical Introduction*. San Diego: Academic Press.

McKenna, P. & Warrington, E.K. (1983). *The Graded Naming Test*. Windsor, Berks. UK: Nelson.

Nelson, H.E. (1976). A modified card sorting test sensitive to frontal lobe defects.*Cortex*, **12**, 313–24.

Nelson, H.E. (1982). *The National Adult Reading Test (NART)*. Windsor, Berks. UK: NFER-Nelson.

QFast (1986). *Q-Fast. The Complete Computerized Testing System*. Tusa, USA: Statsoft, Inc.

Verhey, F.R.J., Jolles, J., Ponds, R., Lugt, M. de & Vreeling, F. (1995). Psychiatric disorders in patients attending an outpatient memory clinic. *International Journal of Geriatric Psychiatry*, **10**, 899–902.

Walsh, K.W. (1987). *Neuropsychology: A Clinical Approach*, 2nd edn. Edinburgh: Churchill Livingstone.

Warrington, E.K. (1984). *Recognition Memory Test*. Windsor, Berks., UK: Nelson.

Warrington, E.K. & James, M. (1991). *The Visual Object and Space Perception Battery*. Bury St Edmunds, England: Thames Valley Test Company.

Wechsler, D. (1981). *WAIS-R Manual*. San Antonio, TS: The Psychological Corporation.

Wechsler, D.A. (1987). *Wechsler Memory Scale Revised Manual*. San Antonio, TS: The Psychological Corporation.

Weigl, E. (1941). On the psychology of so-called processes of abstraction. *Journal of Abnormal and Social Psychology*, **36**, 3–33.

Wright, N. & Lindesay, J. (1995). A survey of memory clinics in the British Isles. *International Journal of Geriatric Psychiatry*, **10**, 379–85.

# ADDENBROOKE'S COGNITIVE EXAMINATION (ACE)

| | |
|---|---|
| Name:<br><br>Date of birth:<br><br>Hospital no.:<br><br>*Addressograph* | Age at leaving education : _ _ _ _ _ _ _ _ _ _ _ _<br>*(school/college etc.)*<br><br>Date of testing : _ _ / _ _ / _ _<br><br>Tester's name : _ _ _ _ _ _ _ _ _ _ _ _ _ _ _ _ _ |

## ORIENTATION

(a) What is the Year _ _ _ _ _ _ _ _

Season _ _ _ _ _ _ _ _

Date ±2 _ _ _ _ _ _ _ _

*Record* Days _ _ _ _ _ _ _ _

*errors.* Month _ _ _ _ _ _ _ _

[*Score* 0 - 5] ▨

b) Where are we Country _ _ _ _ _ _ _ _

County _ _ _ _ _ _ _ _

Town _ _ _ _ _ _ _ _

*Record* Hospital/building _ _ _ _ _ _ _ _

*errors.* Floor *Allow if almost correct.* _ _ _ _ _ _ _ _

[*Score* 0 - 5] ▨

## REGISTRATION

Name three unrelated objects, taking one second to say each: eg. **lemon, key & ball.** Say them once only and ask the patient to repeat all three. *Give one point for each correct answer at first attempt.*
*If score <3 repeat the items until the patient learns all three*　　　　　[0 - 3] ▨

## ATTENTION / CONCENTRATION

Ask the patient to **begin with 100 and and subtract 7, and keep subtracting 7.**
Stop after five subtractions (93, 86, 79, 72, 65). *Score the total number of correct subtractions.*
*If score <5 :* Spell **WORLD backwards.** *Score is the number of letters in the correct order, eg dlorw = 3.*
*Take score of better of the two tasks. Record errors:* _ _ _ _ _ _ _ _ _ _ _ _ _ _ _ _　[0 - 5] ▨

## RECALL

Ask for the names of the three objects learned in question 3. *One point for each answer.*　[0 - 3] ▨

## MEMORY

(a) **Anterograde Memory:**

Read the name and address and ask the patient to repeat it once you have finished. Regardless of the score after the first trial, repeat the task twice in exactly the same way. *Record errors at each trial.*

| | 1st trial | 2nd | 3rd | 5 min delay | |
|---|---|---|---|---|---|
| Peter Marshall | _ _ _ _ _ _ | _ _ _ _ _ _ | _ _ _ _ _ _ | _ _ _ _ _ _ | |
| 42 Market Street | _ _ _ _ _ _ | _ _ _ _ _ _ | _ _ _ _ _ _ | _ _ _ _ _ _ | |
| Chelmsford | _ _ _ _ _ _ | _ _ _ _ _ _ | _ _ _ _ _ _ | _ _ _ _ _ _ | |
| Essex | _ _ _ _ _ _ | _ _ _ _ _ _ | _ _ _ _ _ _ | _ _ _ _ _ _ | *Trial 1–3* [0 - 21] ☐ |
| | /7 | /7 | /7 | /7 | *5 min delay* [0 - 7] ☐ |

(b) **Retrograde Memory:** Name of PM _ _ _ _ _ _ _ _ _ _ _

Last PM _ _ _ _ _ _ _ _ _ _ _

*Record* Opposition Leader _ _ _ _ _ _ _ _ _ _ _

*errors.* USA President _ _ _ _ _ _ _ _ _ _ _　[0 - 4] ☐

## VERBAL FLUENCY

(a) **Letters**   Ask the patient 'tell me as many words as you can think of beginning with the letter **P**, but not people and places. You have one minute to go'

(b) **Animals**   In the same way ask the patient to generate the names of as many **animals** as possible in one minute, beginning with **any letter of the alphabet.**
*Record all responses. Error types, perseverations and intrusions.*

|  | P |  | Animals |  |  |  |  |
|---|---|---|---|---|---|---|---|
|  | *(start here)* | *(continue)* | *(start here)* | *(continue)* | Animal | P | Score |
|  |  |  |  |  | >21 | >17 | 7 |
|  |  |  |  |  | 17–21 | 14–17 | 6 |
|  |  |  |  |  | 14–16 | 11–13 | 5 |
|  |  |  |  |  | 11–13 | 8–10 | 4 |
|  |  |  |  |  | 9–10 | 6–7 | 3 |
|  |  |  |  |  | 7–8 | 4–5 | 2 |
|  |  |  |  |  | <7 | <4 | 1 |

P:          Total _ _ _ _ _ _          No. correct _ _ _ _ _          [0 - 7] ☐

Animals:    Total _ _ _ _ _ _          No. correct _ _ _ _ _          [0 - 7] ☐

## LANGUAGE

(a) **Spontaneous speech**   • fluency (phrases >5 words)
  • paraphasic errors (phonemic or semantic)
  • word finding difficulties

(b) **Naming**          Ask the patient to name the following pictures.
           *Record errors.*          [0 - 2] ▨

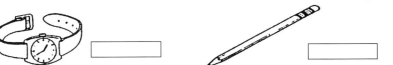

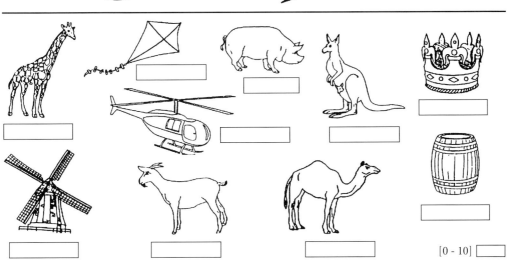

[0 - 10] ☐

(c) **Comprehension**    single-step commands
                                      • 'point to the door'
                                      • 'point to the ceiling'    [0 - 2] ▢
                                      • show written instruction:    [0 - 1] ▨

# CLOSE YOUR EYES

3-stage command
• 'Take the paper in your hand. Fold the paper
  in half. Put the paper on the floor.'
  *Score 1 for each correctly performed step.*    [0 - 3] ▨

complex grammar
• 'point to the ceiling then the door'
• 'point to the door after touching the bed/desk'
  *Score 1 for each correctly performed command.*    [0 - 2] ▢

(d) **Repetition**    single words
• 'brown'
• 'conversation'
• 'articulate'    [0 - 3] ▢

phrases
• 'No ifs, ands, or buts.'    [0 - 1] ▨
• 'The orchestra played and the
  audience applauded.'    [0 - 1] ▢

(e) **Reading**    • shed
• wipe
• board
• flame
• bridge    *Score 1 if all regular words correct.*    [0 - 1] ▢

• sew
• pint
• soot
• dough
• height    *Score 1 if all irregular words correct.*    [0 - 1] ▢

(f) **Writing**    Ask the patient to **make up a sentence and write it down** in the space below.
If stuck, suggest a topic e.g. weather, journey to hospital.
*Score 1 for a correct subject and verb in a meaningful sentence.*

------------------------------------    [0 - 1] ▨

*NOW CHECK delayed recall of name and address. Record errors on page 1 and enter result into box.*

## VISUOSPATIAL ABILITIES

(a) **Overlapping pentagons**      Ask the patient to copy this diagram:

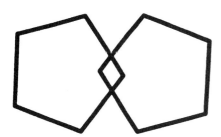

*Score 1 if both figures have 5 sides and overlap.*      [0 - 1] ▨

(b) **Wire cube**      Ask the patient to copy this drawing:

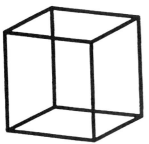

*Score 1 if correct.*      [0 - 1] ☐

(c) **Clock**      Ask the patient to draw a clockface with numbers and the hands at ten past five.

*Score 1 each for correct circle, numbers and hands.*      [0 - 3] ☐

*CHECK: Have you tested and recorded the delayed recall time of name and address (page 1)?*

OVERALL SCORES            MMSE: ▨ /30            TOTAL: ☐ /100

Normative Study based on 127 subjects aged 50 to 80
          Mean 93.9 ± 3.5          Cut off < 87 for age 50–80

# 7

# The dementias

John D.W. Greene and John R. Hodges

The concept of dementia has evolved over the past decade from one of progressive global intellectual deterioration to more modern definitions such as 'a syndrome consisting of progressive impairment in both memory and at least one of the following cognitive deficits: aphasia, apraxia, agnosia or disturbance in executive abilities, sufficient to interfere with social or occupational functioning, in the absence of delirium or major non-organic psychiatric disorders (e.g. depression, schizophrenia)' (American Psychiatric Association, 1987). This change in emphasis reflects the fact that brain diseases which cause cognitive dysfunction result in very different patterns of neuropsychological impairment, and often begin relatively focally. As will become apparent below, even this modern definition still presents problems for the diagnosis of very early cases of Alzheimer's disease who may show only memory deficits. At the other end of the spectrum, patients with frontal type dementias may not show memory deficits until very late in the course of the disease.

In this chapter, the clinical process of making a diagnosis of dementia will first be addressed, and decisions made about whether the patient appears to have a cortical or subcortical dementia. This helps narrow down the possible causes. Particular emphasis will be placed on the neuropsychology of memory, since this is central to the diagnosis of dementia.

The diagnostic process involves the following questions:
(i)     Does the patient have dementia?
(ii)    If so, does the clinical picture broadly conform to the pattern of cortical or subcortical dementia?
(iii)   Which particular disease process is giving rise to the dementia?

## Does the patient have dementia?

In patients with suspected dementia, it is first important to ensure that the patient fulfils the criteria for dementia, and that other potential causes of cognitive impairment are excluded. History taking and 'bedside' cognitive testing remain the fundamental components of diagnosis. It is vital to obtain an independent informant's account of the patient's problems and to enquire systematically about a range of cognitive, behavioural and practical abilities as described in Chapter 6 (also see Hodges, 1994a).

In the context of a memory clinic, it is important to realize the limitations of standardized brief mental test schedules such as the widely used Mini-Mental State Examination (MMSE) (Folstein et al., 1975). The MMSE is a useful instrument for grading established dementia but is insensitive for detecting the early stages of dementia of Alzheimer's type (DAT) (since orientation, immediate recall/registration and basic linguistic abilities are typically preserved – see below). Furthermore, the MMSE and other similar tests are notoriously unreliable in patients with even gross frontal executive dysfunction, as in dementia of frontal type (Gregory & Hodges, 1996a). Ideally, formal neuropsychological assessment should be performed in all cases with suspected cognitive failure, except those with clear-cut severe global impairment. Where such services are in short supply, the majority of patients can be managed on the basis of the results from bedside cognitive testing and the opinion of an experienced psychiatrist, which have been found invaluable for detecting cryptic affective illness and uncovering other important psychiatric phenomena.

## Pseudodementia

It is clearly important to ensure that the apparent dementia is not due to treatable psychiatric pathology. Up to 10% of cases presenting with presumed dementia are due to depression, which is eminently treatable (O'Connor et al., 1990). It will be discussed further in Chapter 12, while hysterical dementia is discussed in Chapters 19 and 22.

Important clues to the diagnosis are a past or family history of affective illness, a sudden or subacute onset of cognitive failure, biological features of depression (anorexia, weight loss, sleep disturbance, motor retardation, etc.), loss of interest in work, hobbies, family, etc. Overt features of depression such as pessimism, guilt or negative ruminations may be absent.

On cognitive assessment, the pattern is one of a subcortical dementia (Massman et al., 1992). On bedside cognitive testing, attentional processes are impaired, and performance on memory tests is often patchy and inconsistent. Typically, digit span is reduced and patients perform poorly on other tests of immediate (working) memory – see below. Registration of simple information, such as a name and address, is usually suboptimal but improves with repeated trials and unlike in DAT, patients with pseudodementia often do surprisingly well on tests of delayed recall. Responses on memory and other cognitive tests are frequently 'don't knows'. Language output may be slow and sparse, but paraphasic errors are not seen.

Although the above pattern may be seen in clinical practice, it should be stressed

**Table 7.1.** Differential diagnosis of delirium and dementia

| Characteristic | Delirium | Dementia |
|---|---|---|
| Onset | Acute or subacute | Insidious and chronic |
| Course | Fluctuating with lucid intervals, often worse at night | Stable over the course of the day |
| Duration | Hours to weeks | Months to years |
| Consciousness (response to environment) | Clouded | Clear |
| Attention | Impaired with marked distractability | Relatively normal |
| Orientation | Almost always impaired for time; tendency to mistakes on place and person | Impaired in later stages |
| Memory | Impaired | Impaired |
| Thinking | Disorganized, delusional | Impoverished |
| Perception | Illusions and hallucinations common, usually visual | Absent in early stages, common later |
| Speech | Incoherent, hesitant, slow or rapid | Aphasic features common |
| Sleep–wake cycle | Always disrupted | Usually normal |

that in some cases the cognitive profile may be virtually identical to that seen in organic dementias, particularly of a subcortical type. It is for this reason that all newly presenting patients with suspected dementia should ideally receive a psychiatric assessment and if doubt remains about the possible contribution of affective illness, a therapeutic trial of an alerting antidepressant is warranted.

## Delirium (acute confusional state)

This clinical syndrome is characterized by the abrupt onset of marked attentional abnormalities, disorders of perception, thinking, short- and long-term memory, psychomotor activity and the sleep–wakefulness cycle, and a marked tendency to fluctuations in cognitive performance and behaviour. The clinical differentiation between delirium and dementia is usually straightforward, and is summarized in Table 7.1. Causes of delirium are legion, including metabolic disturbance, drug or poison intoxication, drug and alcohol withdrawal, infection, head trauma, epilepsy, raised intracranial pressure, subarachnoid haemorrhage and focal brain lesions especially if right hemisphere.

## Isolated higher cerebral function disorders

Occasionally patients with focal cognitive deficits are misdiagnosed as being demented. This occurs most often in the context of the amnesic syndrome (see Chapter 8). The assessment of patients with language disorders also presents a problem since even minor deficits in either comprehension or expression will cause patients to appear fallaciously 'memory impaired'. In this situation it is vital to assess non-verbal memory by means of formal neuropsychological testing.

## Patterns of cognitive impairment: cortical versus subcortical dementia

Having established that the patient has a genuine dementia, the next step is to determine the cause. A practically useful division is between those diseases which involve the cerebral cortex (most notably Alzheimer's disease), and those which primarily affect subcortical structures (i.e. the basal ganglia, thalamus and deep white matter) such as progressive supranuclear palsy, Huntington's disease, etc. The mechanism underlying intellectual impairment in cortical disease is clear cut, but the reason why subcortical pathology results in cognitive dysfunction is perhaps less obvious: fairly recently, it has been determined that the cortex, particularly the pre-frontal area, is richly interconnected with subcortical structures via a number of feedback loops. Diseases affecting these structures will, therefore, functionally deactivate an otherwise normal cortex (Cummings & Benson, 1984), a hypothesis which has been repeatedly substantiated by the use of functional brain imaging (Perani et al., 1987). The major clinical features of cortical and subcortical dementia are summarized in Table 7.2.

It should be noted that the concept of cortical and subcortical dementias is not universally accepted (Whitehouse, 1986): DAT is associated with subcortical pathology (McDuff & Sumi, 1985), while some basal ganglia disorders, such as Huntington's disease (HD) and progressive supranuclear palsy (PSP), show some cortical pathology (Whitehouse, 1986). Moreover, not all diseases can be fitted neatly into this dichotomy. For instance, vascular dementia and cortical Lewy body disease, which are both fairly common causes of cognitive dysfunction, cause a mixed pattern (see below), while the frontal form of focal lobar atrophy (Pick's disease) presents with features which characterize subcortical dementia. Nevertheless, despite these reservations, it remains, in our opinion, a clinically useful broad classification, especially since most treatable dementias exhibit a subcortical pattern.

As memory impairment is a virtually universal feature of the dementias and is in many instances the earliest and most salient feature, a contemporary cognitive model of memory will first be reviewed briefly (for review see Brandt & Rich, 1995; Heindel et al., 1993).

**Table 7.2.** Contrasting features of cortical and subcortical dementia

| Characteristic | Cortical dementia | Subcortical dementia |
|---|---|---|
| Speed of cognitive processing | Normal | Slowed up (bradyphrenic) |
| Frontal 'executive' abilities[a] | Preserved in early stages | Disproportionately impaired from onset |
| Memory | Severe amnesia | Forgetfulness |
| | Recall and recognition affected | Recognition better |
| Language | Aphasic features | Normal except dysarthria and reduced output |
| Visuospatial and perceptual abilities | Impaired | Impaired |
| Personality | Intact until late | Typically apathetic and inert |
| Mood | Usually normal | Depression common |

*Note:*
[a] Planning, problem solving, initiation etc.

**A cognitive analysis of the memory impairment in cortical and subcortical dementias**

It is clear that memory is not a unitary cognitive ability. There is still controversy regarding the most appropriate subdivisions. The same classification has been adopted as used elsewhere in the book which has been outlined here only very briefly (also see Chapter 4).

Working (short-term or immediate) memory

The term short-term memory is a source of great confusion since, contrary to the folk (and general clinical) view, in psychology 'short-term' refers to the retention of new information for a few seconds, e.g. remembering a phone number long enough to dial it. Because of this nosological confusion, the term working memory is preferred, as defined by Baddeley (1992). Deficits in working memory can arise due to a variety of pathologies which involve either frontal attention systems or the specific slave systems. Impairment of the central executive is a consistent feature of subcortical pathology such as HD and PSP, and results in reduced digit span (especially reversed) and particularly performance on more demanding tests of dual-attention (Josiassen et al., 1983; Robbins et al., 1994). Impairment in the central executive component of working memory has been found in DAT (Baddeley et al., 1991), although recent work has suggested that this too may be spared in very early cases (Greene et al., 1995; Sahakian et al., 1990). Digit span is usually normal in the early stages of DAT (Huber et al., 1986), but deteriorates later in the disease (Kopelman, 1985).

## Episodic memory

Episodic memory refers to personally experienced and temporally specific events or episodes, which rely on temporal or contextual cues for their retrieval. It is the type of memory assessed by conventional psychometric memory tests such as the logical memory (story recall) section of the Wechsler Memory Scale – Revised (Wechsler, 1987), the Recognition Memory Test or the Doors and People Test (Baddeley et al., 1994).

A profound disruption of anterograde episodic memory is the hallmark of DAT and will be discussed in more detail below.

The episodic memory impairment seen in subcortical dementias is not only less striking than in cortical dementias, but is due to a deficit at a different stage of memory processing. Encoding is impaired (Huber et al., 1986), but less so than in cortical dementias. The rate of forgetting is relatively normal in subcortical pathology (Butters et al., 1988; Moss et al., 1986). The most striking difference is, however, the relative preservation of recognition memory in subcortical dementia (Flowers et al., 1984) which is in keeping with a deficit in retrieval (Butters et al., 1985; Pillon et al., 1993).

## Remote memory

Remote or retrograde memory refers to any memories which occurred prior to the onset of a pathological process. With a discrete insult such as trauma or a stroke, there is little difficulty in demarcating remote from anterograde memory. In a condition with an insidious onset such as DAT, it is less easy to date the onset of the pathology.

Remote memory is impaired in DAT and there is a mild temporal gradient with early-life memories being spared relative to more recent-life memories (Greene & Hodges, 1996b; Hodges et al., 1993; Kopelman, 1989). By contrast, the remote memory impairment seen in subcortical dementias shows no gradient, consistent with a retrieval deficit (Beatty et al., 1988; Sagar et al., 1988a).

## Semantic memory

Semantic memory refers to our permanent store of representational knowledge including facts, concepts, as well as words and their meaning, e.g. knowing the meaning of the word panda, that Paris is the capital of France, that the boiling point of water is 100 °C, etc. Tests of semantic memory include category fluency, naming pictures and naming from verbal description, word–picture matching, general knowledge questions, tests of vocabulary (Hodges & Patterson, 1995) and picture-picture matching tests such as the Pyramids and Palm Trees Test (Howard & Patterson, 1992).

As described below, semantic memory impairment occurs in DAT (Butters et al., 1987; Hodges et al., 1992b; Martin & Fedio, 1983), but is virtually always overshadowed by the episodic memory deficit.

A profound, yet relatively pure, loss of semantic memory is the hallmark of semantic dementia (Hodges et al., 1992a; Snowden et al., 1989; Graham & Hodges, 1997). In this syndrome, patients present with progressive anomia and show gross deficits on a range of verbal and non-verbal tests of semantic knowledge. In contrast, episodic and working memory, perception and non-verbal problem solving remain intact. As discussed elsewhere in the book (see Chapter 4) the relationship between episodic and semantic memory remains controversial.

Patients with subcortical dementias are also impaired on fluency tasks, but tend to perform less well on letter fluency than on category fluency (Rosser & Hodges, 1994). This probably reflects impaired activation and retrieval rather than true semantic breakdown (Butters et al., 1985, 1987).

## Implicit memory

Over the past decade a great deal of research has been directed to implicit memory (for review see Heindel et al., 1993). Implicit memory refers to types of learned responses not available for conscious reflection, such as conditioned reflexes, priming and motor skills, e.g. ability to drive or play a musical instrument, or the pursuit-rotor task (maintaining contact between a hand-held stylus and a rotating metallic disc). Patients with cortical and subcortical dementia perform differently on these tests of implicit memory.

While patients with subcortical dementias such as HD show impaired performance on skill-learning tasks (Heindel et al., 1989) DAT patients' motor learning is normal (Eslinger & Damasio, 1986). These results imply that the neostriatum, affected in HD but not DAT, is implicated in motor skill learning (Butters et al., 1990).

Priming refers to the temporary (and unconscious) facilitation of performance via prior exposure to stimuli (Shimamura, 1986). A wide range of priming techniques have been applied to patients with dementia but since this is still an area of research, rather than clinical neuropsychology, only two illustrative examples have been chosen. In lexical priming, subjects are initially shown words, e.g. MOTEL. They are subsequently given word stems such as MOT-, and are asked to supply the first word that comes to mind. Lexical priming causes the subject to tend to produce MOTEL, as they have been primed by the original list. In comparative studies, lexical priming has been shown to be impaired in cortical dementias but preserved in subcortical dementias such as HD (Heindel et al., 1989; Shimamura

**Table 7.3.** Recommended investigations in dementia

*Routine*
Full blood count and erythrocyte sedimentation rate (ESR)
Biochemical profile: urea or creatinine, electrolytes, calcium, liver function
Serum B12 and red blood cell (RBC) folate
Thyroid function
Serological tests for syphilis
Chest X-ray
CT scan

*Other tests which may be indicated in certain cases*
EEG (e.g. Creutzfeldt–Jakob disease and subacute sclerosing panencephalitis (SSPE))
Functional brain imaging: single photon emission computed tomography (SPECT)
CSF examination (e.g. infections, malignant meningitis, etc.)
Screening for cardiac sources of emboli
Immunological tests for vasculitides (e.g. systemic lupus erythematosus)
Slit lamp examination for Kayser–Fleischer rings and caeruloplasmin estimation (Wilson's
    disease)
Specific blood and/or urine tests for inherited metabolic disorders
Screening for HIV infection
Cerebral biopsy

et al., 1987). Lexical priming seems to require the integrity of neocortical association regions.

In semantic priming, subjects are asked to judge related word pairs (e.g. train-
station). They are later given the first word, and asked to produce the first related
word they can think of. Semantic priming refers to their tendency to produce the
second word of the original word pair. Again, DAT patients were impaired while
HD patients were not (Salmon et al., 1988).

## What is the cause of the dementia?

Having established that the patient is indeed suffering from dementia, a series of
basic investigations should be performed, as summarized in Table 7.3. The clinical
presentation will determine the choice of investigations. For example, a young
person presenting with dementia and a movement disorder who has a family
history of such a condition will require caeruloplasmin and copper studies, as well
as an ophthalmological examination for Kaiser–Fleischer rings, looking for evidence of Wilson's disease.

In those cases presenting with insidious onset of dementia, the likeliest diagnosis is Alzheimer's disease, but it is clearly important to be able to detect other potentially reversible causes of dementia. Table 7.4 illustrates the clinical pointers that may point to a diagnosis other than DAT.

## Imaging in dementia

The imaging modality widely available for clinical investigation of dementia is CT scanning. Although CT may show generalized cortical atrophy in the latter stages of degenerative dementia, scanning is done primarily to exclude other pathologies such as hydrocephalus or tumours. In one study, CT scanning elicited treatable pathology in 10% of patients presenting with dementia (Bradshaw et al., 1983), although in our experience this is almost certainly an overestimate. Since the temporal lobes are poorly visualized on conventional CT, it is a poor technique for the early diagnosis of DAT. The application of temporal lobe orientated CT scans with measurement of the medial temporal lobe width now appears to be able to detect initial perihippocampal pathology early in the course of DAT (Jobst et al., 1992).

The superior resolution of MRI allows volumetric studies of the hippocampus in early DAT, and is useful diagnostically (Jack et al., 1992; Kesslak et al., 1991; Scheltens et al., 1992).

Functional imaging in the form of PET (positron emission tomography) allows measurement of cerebral perfusion and metabolism in individual cortical areas, a reduction being suggestive of cortical pathology (Frackowiak, 1989; Frackowiak et al., 1981). Studies have shown predominantly temporoparietal hypoperfusion in DAT, with frontal changes later in the disease (Mazziotta et al., 1992). It remains, however, largely a research tool.

Although of poorer anatomical resolution, SPECT (single photon emission computed tomography) is more widely available. Alzheimer's disease tends to show a pattern of temporoparietal hypoperfusion (Montaldi et al., 1990; Waldemar et al., 1994), in contrast with the frontal or temporal changes seen in focal lobar atrophy (Neary et al., 1987) or the patchy tracer uptake seen in vascular dementia (Deutsch & Tweedy, 1987). In our own experience, however, SPECT scanning is insensitive in the early stages of DAT, and many patients with more established disease fail to show the typical pattern of temporoparietal hypoperfusion (Greene et al., 1996a).

Attempts to diagnose DAT from cerebrospinal fluid and blood have met with little success, such that neuropsychology and imaging are the principal means of investigation. Brain biopsy is very rarely carried out, as it is generally considered unethical to subject the patient to an invasive procedure when there is currently no therapeutic option.

It can be seen from Table 7.5 that many neurological diseases cause dementia. Many of these conditions cause dementia in the context of other neurological symptoms and signs, and would not present as an isolated dementia. Unfortunately, only

**Table 7.4.** Clinical features which suggest a diagnosis other than Alzheimer's disease

| | |
|---|---|
| Young age (<65) | Huntington's disease, infections (e.g. AIDS, SSPE), inherited metabolic disorders (e.g. Wilson's disease), vasculitides, neoplasia |
| Rapid progression (weeks or months) | Neoplasia, limbic encephalitis, infections, Creutzfeldt–Jakob disease |
| Personality change early in course | Pick's disease (dementia of frontal type), subcortical dementias, frontal tumours |
| Early onset incontinence | Tumours, normal pressure hydrocephalus |
| Cardiac disease, past TIA or stroke | Cerebral vascular disease (multi-infarct dementia) |
| Symptoms of raised intracranial pressure | Tumours, subdural haematoma |
| Fluctuating performance | Subdural haematoma, vascular dementia, cortical Lewy body disease |
| Immunocompromise | Infections (e.g. PML, toxoplasmosis), primary intracerebral lymphoma |
| Systemic illness | Metabolic disorders, neoplasia, infections, vasculitides |
| Family history of dementia or involuntary movements | Huntington's disease, inherited metabolic diseases |
| Anosmia | Frontal meningioma |
| Eye movement abnormalities and nystagmus | Progressive supranuclear palsy, multiple sclerosis, mitochondrial cytopathies, raised intracranial pressure, cerebellar tumours |
| Ocular signs | Syphilis, Wilson's disease, raised pressure |
| Myoclonus | Creutzfeldt–Jakob disease, SSPE, post-anoxia, myoclonic epilepsies (also DAT) |
| Alien hand sign | Cortico-basal degeneration |
| Prominent loss of vocabulary | Semantic dementia |
| Gait disturbance | Normal pressure hydrocephalus, tumours, progressive supranuclear palsy, Huntington's disease |
| Papilloedema | Hydrocephalus, tumour, subdural haematoma |
| Optic disc pallor | Multiple sclerosis |
| Visual field defect | |
| Bitemporal hemianopia | Craniopharyngioma |
| Bilateral homonymous defect | Falx meningioma, corpus callosum glioma |

**Table 7.4** (*cont.*)

| | |
|---|---|
| Kayser–Fleischer ring | Wilson's disease |
| Conjunctival ulcers | Behcet's disease |
| Diminished corneal response or unilateral deafness | Cerebellopontine angle tumour |
| Bilateral facial palsy | Sarcoidosis |
| Neck retraction | Progressive supranuclear palsy |
| Involuntary movements | Huntington's disease, Wilson's disease, Parkinson's disease |

*Notes:*
Key: SSPE  subacute sclerosing panencephalitis.
    PML  progressive multifocal leukoencephalopathy.


10–20% of hospital cases of dementias, and an even smaller proportion of community cases, are due to curable conditions.

# Cortical dementias

## Alzheimer's disease

Alzheimer's accounts for approximately two-thirds of all cases of dementia. The aetiology is currently unknown, although there are associations with increasing age, Down's syndrome, head injury and family history; in a small percentage of early-onset cases there is an autosomal dominant pattern of inheritance with the demonstration in such families of definite chromosome abnormalities (Schellenberg et al., 1992; St George-Hislop et al., 1987).

It can only be diagnosed with certainty by neuropathological confirmation of neocortical atrophy with neuronal loss, intraneuronal tangles of paired helical filaments and extraneuronal plaques containing an amyloid core. The presence of plaques and tangles correlates significantly with the presence of dementia (Wilcock & Esiri, 1982). More recently, however, it has been claimed that synaptic loss may be the primary marker of DAT, since the severity of loss correlates more closely with dementia severity (Terry et al., 1991). These neuropathological changes are found first in the medial temporal lobes, especially in the parahippocampal region, and then evolve to the posterior association cortices (Braak & Braak, 1991; Van Hoesen et al., 1991). There is also subcortical pathology present in DAT, with neuronal loss in the nucleus basalis of Meynert and the nucleus locus coeruleus, with a resultant reduction in acetylcholine and noradrenaline (Mann et al., 1984; Whitehouse et al., 1982).

**Table 7.5.** Causes of dementia

**Classification of common and treatable dementias**

Common causes

Alzheimer's disease

Multi-infarct disease

Pick's disease (focal lobar atrophy)

Parkinson's disease and diffuse cortical Lewy body disease

Huntington's disease

Treatable causes

Depressive pseudodementia

Benign tumours, expecially subfrontal meningiomas

Normal pressure hyodrcephalus

Subdural haematoma

Deficiency states – B1, B12, B6

Endocrine disease – hypothyroidism, Cushing's disease, Addison's disease

Infections – AIDS dementia complex, syphilis

Alcoholic dementia

Wilson's disease

**Classification of dementia based on aetiology**

1. Primary degenerative diseases

Alzheimer's disease

Pick's disease (focal lobar atrophy)

Huntington's disease

Parkinson's disease

Diffuse cortical Lewy body disease

Progressive supranuclear palsy (Steele–Richardson–Olszewski syndrome)

Striatonigral degeneration

Corticobasal degeneration

Olivo-ponto-cerebellar degeneration

Progressive myoclonic epilepsies

2. Vascular diseases

Multi-infarct disease secondary to atherosclerotic disease of extracranial vessels or cardiac emboli

Hypertensive encephalopathy

Binswanger's disease (subcortical arteriosclerotic encephalopathy)

Vasculitides: systemic lupus erythematosus, polyarteritis nodosa, Behcet's disease, giant cell arteritis, isolated CNS angiitis

Primary cerebral amyloid (congophilic) angiopathy

3. Infections

AIDS dementia complex

Progressive multifocal leukoencephalopathy

**Table 7.5** (*cont.*)

Cerebral toxoplasmosis
Cryptococcal meningitis
Creutzfeldt–Jakob and other prion related diseases
Syphilis
Subacute sclerosing panencephalitis and progressive rubella panencephalitis
Whipple's disease

4. Neoplastic causes
Primary intracerebral tumours: frontal gliomas crossing the corpus callosum (butterfly
glioma), posterior corpus callosal or midline (thalamic, pineal, IIIrd ventricle) tumours,
cerebral lymphoma, etc.
Extracerebral tumours: frontal meningiomas, posterior fossa tumours (acoustic neuromas)
causing hydrocephalus
Multiple cerebral metastases
Malignant meningitis
Non-metastatic (limbic) encephalitis

5. Other non-neoplastic space-occupying lesions
Chronic subdural haematoma
Normal pressure hydrocephalus

6. Chronic intoxications
Alcoholic dementia
Heavy metals: lead, mercury, manganese
Carbon monoxide poisoning
Drugs: lithium, anticholinergics, barbiturates, digitalis, neuroleptics, cimetidine,
propranolol

7. Acquired metabolic disorders and deficiency states
Cerebral anoxia
Chronic renal failure
Porto-systemic encephalopathy
Hypothyroidism
Cushing's disease
Addison's disease
Panhypopituitarism
Hypoglycaemia (chronic or recurrent)
Hypoparathyroidism
B12, B1, folic acid deficiency

8. Inherited metabolic diseases which may present with dementia in early adult life
Wilson's disease
Porphyria
Leukodystrophies: adrenoleukodystrophy, metachromatic leukodystrophy, globoid cell
leukodystrophy

**Table 7.5** (*cont.*)

Gangliosidoses
Niemann–Pick disease
Cerebro-tendinous xanthomatosis
Adult onset neuronal ceroid-lipofuscinosis (Kuf's disease)
Mitochondrial cytopathies
Subacute necrotizing encephalopathy (Leigh's disease)

9. Miscellaneous
Multiple sclerosis
Sarcoidosis
Sickle cell disease
Macroglobulinaemia
Recurrent head injury, dementia pugilistica

In the absence of a definitive in vivo diagnostic test, clinical guidelines have been constructed (e.g. NINCDS-ADRDA: McKhann et al., 1984) which incorporate inclusion and exclusion criteria. These research criteria are at least 80% accurate (Molsa et al., 1985; Wade et al., 1987).

One of the most important developments in the past decade has been the realisation that DAT does not result in 'global' cognitive impairment from the start of the illness, but progresses in a relatively predictable pattern through various stages which will be described below. The following is a guide to the most common order of deterioration (see Table 7.6).

The most pervasive feature of DAT is undoubtedly a failure of memory. When patients present in the early stages of the disease, complaints of memory difficulty are by far the commonest symptom noticed by the patient, and more particularly by their spouse. In patients who are seen for the first time at a more advanced stage of deterioration, a retrospective history of insidiously progressive memory failure can almost invariably be elicited from the carer. As will be discussed below, there are a growing number of case reports documenting atypical presentations of AD (aphasia, apraxia, visual agnosia, etc.), but our own experience suggests that these represent only a tiny minority of cases.

A decade of intensive neuropsychological research into the nature of the memory deficit has established that not all aspects of memory are affected equally in early DAT. The major impairment is in the domain of anterograde episodic memory (e.g. Grady et al., 1988; Greene et al., 1996c; Heindel et al., 1993; Hodges & Patterson, 1995; Welsh et al., 1991, 1992).

Our work has confirmed that the ability to retain new information after a period (delayed recall) is the most sensitive measure of DAT, and that memory for both

**Table 7.6.** Order of progression of symptoms in DAT

|  | Minimal | Mild | Moderate | Severe |
|---|---|---|---|---|
| Memory |  |  |  |  |
|   Working | − | + | ++ | +++ |
|   Episodic | +++ | +++ | +++ | +++ |
|   Remote | −/+ | −/+ | ++ | +++ |
|   Semantic | −/+ | + | ++ | +++ |
| Language (anomia, word-finding) | − | + | ++ | +++ |
| Visuospatial and perceptual | − | + | ++ | +++ |
| Praxis | − | −/+ | ++ | +++ |
| Thinking and problem solving | − | + | ++ | +++ |
| Social rapport and personality | − | − | −/+ | +++ |
| Incontinence | − | − | − | ++ |
| Seizures, primitive reflexes | − | − | − | ++ |

*Notes:*
− absent.
+ present.

verbal and visual material is affected in the majority of cases (Greene et al., 1996a; Hodges & Patterson, 1995). In clinical practice, this deficit can be shown on tasks such as recall of a name and address after a delay of 5 to 10 minutes. The profound deficit in episodic memory has been attributed principally to defective encoding and storage of new information, whereas an accelerated rate of forgetting appears to make only a minor contribution to the patients' memory failure (Brandt & Rich, 1994; Greene et al., 1996c; Kopelman, 1985). In other words, patients are unable to learn new information, but the little they learn is retained reasonably well.

Patients in the early amnesic prodrome of DAT cannot, according to current diagnostic criteria, be diagnosed as having probable AD, since the latter requires the presence of two or more areas of cognitive dysfunction. It is becoming increasingly evident, however, that this amnesic stage invariably proceeds to a stage of more global impairment after a period of months or years: in one recently documented case the prodomal stage persisted for 11 years (Caffarra & Venneri, 1996) and a number of such patients are being followed up in Cambridge.

It is also apparent that patients with DAT show progressive disruption of semantic memory. Patients with DAT are characteristically impaired on tests of semantic memory, including picture naming, naming from verbal descriptions, word–picture matching, general knowledge and vocabulary, and picture–picture matching tasks which rely on the ability to deduce the associative link between the items represented. Category fluency is an easily administered and sensitive measure; early in the course of DAT there is disproportionate impairment in semantic category-based, as opposed to letter-based fluency tests (for review, see Monsch et al., 1994; Rosser & Hodges, 1994). The underlying cause of the semantic deficit, at a cognitive level, has been a matter of controversy. Some researchers have claimed that the deficits found on tests of semantic memory may primarily reflect impaired access to semantic memory (for review, see Bayles et al., 1991; Nebes, 1989); but the majority of investigators support the interpretation of a breakdown in the structure of semantic memory (Chan et al., 1993; Chertkow & Bub, 1990; Hodges et al., 1992b; Martin et al., 1985). Using a battery of tests of semantic memory, all of which test knowledge about the same consistent set of 48 items, via differing modalities of sensory input and/or output, it has been established that most patients presenting with even minimal DAT (MMSE >24) show impairment on tests of semantic memory (Hodges & Patterson, 1995). This is, however, not a universal phenomenon: some patients may be severely amnesic yet perform normally on the entire semantic battery. Certainly, as the disease progresses into the moderate stages (MMSE <18) breakdown in semantic memory is a ubiquitous finding which is reflected in the increasing anomia, emptiness of language and failure on general knowledge tests.

In contrast to the deficits in these major components of longer-term memory – episodic and semantic memory – patients with DAT typically perform normally on tests of working (short-term) memory, as exemplified by their normal digit or block-tapping span. Even on dual-performance tests, designed to tap the more demanding aspects of working memory, the so-called central executive, in which subjects are required to divide their attention between two simultaneously presented streams of information, performance in the very early stages of DAT is typically unimpaired (Greene et al., 1995; Sahakian et al., 1990).

One final aspect of memory which until recently has been studied relatively little, perhaps due to the lack of quantifiable tests, is remote personal (or autobiographical) memory. Because patients often become preoccupied with, or indeed appear to 'live in', the past, it is commonly believed that such memory is spared in DAT. Recent research has shown, however, that most patients early in the course of the disease do show impaired performance on tests of autobiographical memory, although the degree of impairment is certainly less than that seen on anterograde memory tests. This loss is temporally graded with relative sparing of more distant memories; accounting, in part, for the clinical observation above. Moreover, there is no clear correlation between the degree of anterograde and retrograde memory deficit (Greene & Hodges, 1996a, b; Kopelman, 1989; Sagar et al., 1988a).

Remote memory for famous faces and events also shows impairment with a gentle temporal gradient (Greene & Hodges, 1996b; Kopelman, 1989; Sagar et al.,

1988a). This appears to be due to loss of semantic knowledge regarding people and events (Hodges et al., 1993).

The authors have concentrated on aspects of memory in DAT since this is the predominant cognitive deficit in early cases. There are, of course, other more widespread deficits which become more prominent as the disease progresses. Impairment in visuospatial and perceptual abilities are common in the middle stages of the disease, reflecting involvement of posterior higher-order visual association and parietal regions (Kaskie & Storandt, 1995; Mendez et al., 1990). The language disorder of DAT is dominated by the semantic breakdown discussed above; the phonological and syntactical components of language remain relatively intact, at least until the late stages of the disease (Hart, 1988). The ability to read aloud is also relatively preserved in DAT, although, as the disease progresses, patients have particular difficulty pronouncing irregular words that do not obey the usual rules of English orthography (e.g. pint, island, sieve, etc.) (Patterson et al., 1994a). Writing is more vulnerable than reading and patients show a range of defects in the central linguistic components, especially for irregular words, as well as the more peripheral praxis aspects of letter formation (Hughes et al., 1997; Rapcsak et al., 1989a). General ideomotor apraxia is found in patients with DAT (Rapcsak et al., 1989b) and may occasionally be severe enough to interfere with other manual tasks.

Depression is common in the early stages of DAT and often complicates the diagnosis (for review, see Wragg & Jeste, 1989). Hallucinations and delusions are commonly reported in series originating from departments of old age psychiatry (Berrios & Brook, 1985; Burns et al., 1990) but in our experience are relatively uncommon in the earlier stages of the disease. Their presence should suggest the possibility of Cortical Lewy Body disease (see below).

In marked contrast to the profile of dementia of frontal type (see below), basic aspects of personality, comportment, social interaction and behaviour are strikingly preserved in the early stages of DAT and most patients retain at least partial insight into their predicament. Many of the features of DFT such as restlessness, perseverative behaviour and echolalia may occur in the late stages of the disease but are virtually never seen at presentation, but it is notable that even in advanced cases of DAT the Kluver–Bucy syndrome is very rare.

Having stressed the amnesic presentation of DAT, it is important to point out that there have been a number of case reports of patients with pathologically verified AD presenting with atypical features including progressive aphasia (Green et al., 1990; Greene et al., 1996b; Kempler et al., 1990; Pogacar & Williams, 1984), visual apperceptual agnosia and Balint's syndrome (Berthier et al., 1991; Hof et al., 1990; Ross et al., 1990), or even progressive unilateral parietal syndrome (Crystal et al., 1982). There are, however, to the best of our knowledge, no convincing detailed case studies of patients with AD presenting with the picture of DFT, although a few such cases are included in the group studies reported by Gustafson (1987).

As the condition deteriorates, all aspects of cognition become impaired, personality disintegrates, and social misconduct and aggressive behaviour may occur. Primitive reflexes emerge, and pyramidal and extrapyramidal signs occur. There is also a greater incidence of seizures and myoclonus. Eventually incontinence and dependence lead to death.

With the fast approaching advent of disease-modifying drug therapies for DAT, it is important to confidently diagnose DAT early in its course. Neuropsychological evaluation appears to be the best discriminator of patients with early DAT from controls, in particular the delayed recall component of episodic memory (Welsh et al., 1991; 1992).

The earliest pathological changes in DAT are in the perihippocampal regions. MRI, particularly coronal sections of the medial temporal structures, is becoming increasingly able to highlight such pathology, although it is by no means infallible (Erkinjuntti et al., 1993; Jack et al., 1992; Kesslak et al., 1991). The use of SPECT in diagnosing DAT is somewhat controversial. Although some groups have found it to be very useful in discriminating patients with early DAT from elderly controls (Johnson et al., 1993), others have found it of more limited use (Greene et al., 1996b; Van Gool et al., 1995). Presently, SPECT imaging appears less sensitive than neuropsychology for diagnosing early DAT (Greene et al., 1996b; Villa et al., 1995).

### Creutzfeldt–Jakob disease

This rapidly progressive cortical dementia can be fatal within months of diagnosis (Brown et al., 1986). Given the rapidity of progression, the neuropsychological profile has been poorly characterized, although severe amnesia and aphasia are usually present, often accompanied by cortical blindness (Pietrini, 1992). Myoclonus occurs in 80% of cases, and triphasic complexes on EEG are typical, although may appear very late in the course (Chiofalo et al., 1980). Recently, there have been several cases of CJD with an earlier onset than is typical in sporadic cases (i.e. below 45) and a primarily psychiatric presentation and indolent course which may be related to consumption of beef contaminated with prion protein, termed new variant CJD (Will et al., 1996).

### Subcortical dementias

A wide range of basal ganglia and white matter diseases (see Table 7.7) may result in a pattern of so-called subcortical dementia. These disorders are characterized by mental slowing, impaired attention and frontal 'executive' function (i.e. planning,

**Table 7.7.** Major causes of subcortical dementia

Degenerative
  Progressive supranuclear palsy
  Huntington's disease
  Parkinson's disease
  Corticobasal degeneration
Vascular disorders
  Multi-infarct dementia (lacunar state)[a]
  Binswanger's disease
Metabolic
  Wilson's disease
Demyelinating disease
  Multiple sclerosis
  Leukodystrophies
  AIDS dementia complex
Miscellaneous
  Normal pressure hydrocephalus

*Note:*
[a] Cortical features often co-exist.

problem solving, self-initiated activity). Memory is moderately impaired owing to reduced attention with poor registration of new material, but severe amnesia of the type seen in DAT does not occur in the early stages. Recognition is typically much better than spontaneous recall, suggestive of a retrieval deficit (Tweedy et al., 1982). Spontaneous speech is reduced and answers to questions are slow and laconic. Features of focal cortical dysfunction such as aphasia, apraxia and agnosia are characteristically absent, but visuospatial deficits are consistently present (Josiassen et al., 1983). Change in mood, personality and social conduct are very common, resulting often in an indifferent withdrawn state (Huber & Shuttleworth, 1990).

**Progressive supranuclear palsy**

Steele–Richardson–Olszewski syndrome, or as it is more often called, progressive supranuclear palsy, was the first condition to which the term 'subcortical dementia' was applied (Albert et al., 1974). It presents with a parkinsonian syndrome, although tremor does not occur (Litvan & Agid, 1992). There is bradykinesia, extrapyramidal rigidity and a tendency to fall backwards. Axial dystonia and pseudobulbar palsy occur. A supranuclear gaze palsy – the inability to voluntarily direct the eyes or to follow a target – is the most characteristic feature of the disease.

In the early stages, vertical eye movements are affected, a feature which is easily overlooked.

Cognitive dysfunction is an early and consistent feature of the disease and, unlike PD, patients not infrequently present with mental rather than physical symptoms (Maher et al., 1985). The neuropsychological characteristics are primarily of cognitive slowing and executive dysfunction, with difficulty planning, organizing and sustaining attention (Pillon & Dubois, 1992; Pillon et al., 1986; Robbins et al., 1994). Memory is also affected (Van der Hurk & Hodges, 1995): patients show defective learning with disproportionately poor recall (vs. recognition) for new material. Subtle but consistent impairment of semantic memory has also been demonstrated, although this probably reflects a deficit in retrieval, rather than a loss of knowledge. There is also a gross reduction in verbal output reflected by impaired performance on both category and initial letter based tests of verbal fluency (Rosser & Hodges, 1994). Some patients may present with an inability to converse, and when tested show normal naming, repetition and comprehension: a pattern known as dynamic aphasia (Esmonde et al., 1996).

## Parkinson's disease

Parkinson's disease is characterized pathologically by loss of pigmented cells in the substantia nigra (Jellinger, 1987). Clinically, resting tremor, rigidity, bradykinesia and postural instability occur, and may be accompanied by bradyphrenia. Although it is rare for PD to present with dementia in the absence of a movement disorder, it is commoner for PD patients to show evidence of clinically obvious cognitive dysfunction during the course of the illness (Brown & Marsden, 1984), and up to 30% of PD patients fulfil the criteria for dementia (Mindham et al., 1982). Even more PD patients show subtle subcortical deficits on neuropsychological testing (Downes et al., 1989; Lees & Smith, 1983).

The major cognitive dysfunctions occur in the fields of executive function (Gotham et al., 1987; Mayeux et al., 1987) and memory (Sagar et al., 1988a; Sahakian et al., 1988), the latter being due to poor retrieval. The temporal ordering of newly learned information is also defective (Sagar et al., 1988b), as is visuospatial and perceptual function. In common with other subcortical disorders, language abilities are relatively spared in PD.

## Huntington's disease

This is the commonest genetic disorder to cause dementia. It is inherited in an autosomal dominant fashion, and clinical onset is usually in the fourth or fifth decade, but can be as late as the eighth. The condition is characterized neuropathologically by neostriatal degeneration (caudate nucleus and putamen) with loss of small spiny GABAergic neurones (Harper, 1991). Previous attempts to utilize neuropsychology and functional imaging to diagnose the condition preclinically have been largely superseded by confirmatory genetic testing (Huntington's Disease Collaborative Research Group, 1993): it has now been established that an abnormal expansion on chromosome 4 is the cause of HD. In apparently de novo cases, it is necessary to enquire for a family history of psychiatric illness, suicide, dementia or movement disorders.

Although characterized eventually by dementia and chorea, it is clear that cognitive and/or psychiatric changes may precede motor dysfunction by many years (Butters et al., 1978; Folstein et al., 1984). There is evidence of attentional and frontal executive dysfunction early in the disease (Lange et al., 1994; Lawrence et al., 1996). Memory impairment is seen in HD (Butters et al., 1985; Hodges et al., 1990; Moss et al., 1986): the deficit is primarily due to impaired retrieval of new information. On tests of remote memory, patients with HD show equivalent impairment over all decades which contrasts with the temporal gradient seen in DAT and Korsakoff's patients (Albert et al., 1981). Another difference is the impairment of working memory (e.g. digit span) early in the course of HD (Butters et al., 1978). Although language is preserved until late (Podoll et al., 1988), visuoperceptual deficits occur consistently (Josiassen et al., 1983).

The earliest sign of the movement disorder is a restless fidgeting of the limbs which the patient quickly learns to disguise. The choreoathetoid movements eventually affect the face and extremities. The gait becomes unsteady and reeling. On walking, characteristic finger flicking movements may be observed. A juvenile onset form with more marked extrapyramidal features and shorter life expectancy has also been described (Hayden, 1981). Dysarthria and dysphagia also develop with disease progression.

Depression is common, although a schizophreniform state with paranoid delusions may also occur (Caine & Shoulson, 1983). An insidious change in personality with the development of sociopathic behaviour is characteristic.

## Mixed cortical–subcortical dementias

### Focal lobar atrophy (Pick's disease)

Arnold Pick, after describing patients with progressive aphasia as a result of progressive temporal lobe atrophy, was the first to report the syndrome of frontal dementia (Pick, 1892, 1906). The pathological features were reported a few years later by Alzheimer (1910–1911) who described Pick cells and Pick bodies in association with focal brain atrophy. Subsequently, however, it became apparent that only a minority of cases of frontal lobe degeneration were accompanied by Pick cells and Pick bodies (Brun, 1987; Neary et al., 1986). There are essentially two major presentations which reflect the dominant locus of disease: dementia of frontal type and progressive aphasia.

## Dementia of frontal type

Dementia of frontal type (DFT) is clearly much less common than DAT, but estimates of the ratio of the two diseases range from 1 in 5 to 1 in 20 (Hodges, 1994b). Brun (1987) reported that 20 of their first 150 consecutive autopsied cases suffered from frontal or frontotemporal degeneration. On clinical grounds alone, Neary et al. (1988) estimated that 19% of 130 cases seen in the neurological unit over 5 years met criteria for DFT. In the latter two studies, however, the mean age of the total patient population was unusually young, which may well have led to an over representation of DFT patients. A definitive community-based clinicopathological study of unselected demented patients is required to answer the question of the true prevalence of DFT.

Much less controversy surrounds the age of onset. There is no doubt that DFT affects younger patients than does DAT. The peak age of onset is 45 to 65. Cases above 75 appear relatively rare (Miller et al., 1991). In our series of 15 patients, the age range was 37 to 74 with a mean of 62 years (Gregory & Hodges, 1996a). Men and women appear to be equally affected.

The presenting symptoms of DFT are quite distinct from that seen in DAT (Brun et al., 1994). In striking contrast to DAT, the majority of patients with DFT are brought along to the clinic blissfully unaware of the major changes in personality and behaviour observed by their relatives. Patients may appear apathetic and withdrawn, or alternatively become socially disinhibited with facetiousness and inappropriate jocularity. Their ability to plan and organize complex activities (work, social engagements, etc.) is almost invariably impaired, reflecting deficits in sustained attention, goal setting and attainment, mental set-shifting and flexibility. Mental rigidity and an inability to appreciate the more subtle aspects of language (irony, punning, etc.) are common. There is often indifference to domestic and occupational responsibilities, a lack of empathy for family and friends and gradual withdrawal from all social interactions. A deterioration in self-care with a reluctance to bath, groom and change clothes is frequently reported. Many patients show a change in eating habits with an escalating desire for sweet food coupled with reduced satiety; the increasing gluttony may lead to enormous weight gain. The other components of the Kluver–Bucy syndrome (hypersexuality and oral exploratory behaviour) are much less commonly observed (Cummings & Duchen, 1981).

Information regarding specific psychiatric symptoms in DFT remains scanty. Mood disturbance, obsessive–compulsive behaviour and hypochondriasis and frank psychosis have all been reported (Gregory & Hodges, 1993, 1996b; Gustafson, 1987; Mendez et al., 1993; Miller et al., 1991; Neary et al., 1988).

Memory is typically unaffected early in the course of the disease and although patients may admit, when pressed, to 'memory' difficulties, when this is explored further they usually have problems with concentration and working (immediate) memory, rather than the severe amnesia found in DAT (see above). In a recent detailed study (Hodges et al., 1999) of ten cases, who fulfilled the criteria outlined below, we found a striking lack of impairment on a battery of episodic and semantic memory tests. Likewise, tests of visuospatial function may show no significant abnormality. Tasks aimed at specific evaluation of the frontal lobes (such as the Wisconsin Card Sorting Test, Trail Making Test, Stroop Test, Shallice's Cognitive Estimates Test and verbal fluency) will often show marked impairment (see Knopman & Ryberg, 1989; Miller et al., 1991; Neary et al., 1988), but it should be stressed that in some cases with marked neurobehavioural changes, sufficient to interfere with social relations and lead to premature retirement from work, there may be very little abnormality even after rigorous neuropsychological evaluation. A number of such patients have been seen who have a 'full-house' of symptoms with eventually clear-cut frontal atrophy on MRI and a typical neuropsychological profile. With disease progression, episodic memory deteriorates but visuospatial and perceptual functions are characteristically normal even late in the disease (Gregory et al., 1999).

Language dysfunction is an early, but subtle, finding in many patients with DFT and consists of factually empty speech which is reduced in quantity. Articulation, phonology and syntax are typically preserved. Mild anomia may be present but repetition is normal. In terms of classical aphasic syndromes the picture corresponds to a dynamic aphasia. Many patients develop spontaneous echolalia (a tendency to immediately repeat the examiner's last phrase) and other reiterative speech acts such as the repetition of phrases, words, syllables or sounds. In advanced cases, comprehension may become impaired. Finally, muteness supervenes.

As mentioned above, the MMSE is insensitive in the very early amnesic phase of DAT, but falls as patients enter even the mild stages of the disease. It is, however, an even less reliable indicator of DFT; the majority of cases in our series scored above the classic cut-off of 24, while approximately a third (6/15) obtained a maximum of 30/30.

Recently clinical criteria were developed for the diagnosis of DFT which stress the neurobehavioural features of the disorder (Gregory & Hodges, 1993, 1996a; 1996b). All of the 15 patients in our prospective series had at least five of the features shown in Table 7.8.

## Progressive aphasia

In 1982 Mesulam coined the term 'slowly progressive aphasia without generalized dementia' to describe six patients with a five- to ten-year history of insidiously worsening aphasia in the absence of signs of more generalized cognitive failure. One of

**Table 7.8.** Criteria for the diagnosis of dementia of frontal type

---

1. Presentation with an insidious and progressive disorder of personality and behaviour of at least six months' duration characterized by at least five of the following features:

   loss of insight
   disinhibition
   restlessness
   distractibility
   emotional lability
   reduced empathy and unconcern for others
   lack of foresight and planning
   impulsivity
   social withdrawal
   apathy or lack of spontaneity
   poor self-care
   reduced verbal output
   verbal stereotypes or echolalia
   perseveration (verbal or motor)
   features of the Kluver–Bucy syndrome (gluttony, pica, sexual hyperactivity)

2. Historical evidence of preserved memory for day-to-day events
3. Neuropsychological evidence of disproportionate frontal dysfunction
4. Absence of history of significant head injury, stroke, score >4 on the Hachinski scale, long-term alcohol abuse, diagnosis of parkinsonism or other movement disorder
5. Psychiatric phenomena may be present

---

the six patients underwent a brain biopsy which revealed non-specific changes only. Ten years later, Mesulam and Weintraub (1992) proposed clearer diagnostic criteria for primary progressive aphasia, as follows: a progressive deterioration of language with preservation of the activities of daily living for at least two years, and evidence of relatively normal non-verbal abilities on neuropsychological testing.

There have now been over 30 papers reporting some 80 patients who fulfil the criteria for primary progressive aphasia (e.g. Caselli et al., 1992; Hodges et al., 1992a; Karbe et al., 1993; Kirshner et al., 1984; Mesulam, 1982; Poeck & Luzzatti, 1988; Scheltens et al., 1994; Snowden et al., 1992; Tyrrell et al., 1990; Weintraub et al., 1990). It seems clear that, although the language disorder in progressive aphasia is heterogeneous, two broad groups can be identified: fluent and non-fluent progressive aphasia. In both forms other, non-linguistic skills are well preserved as judged by their performance on tests of non-verbal problem solving, visuospatial and perceptual abilities. It should be noted, however, that such patients are often erroneously described as having a poor memory or being confused, as their language disorder makes it impossible for them to process verbal material. Assessment of memory in aphasic patients should be based on practical day-to-day abilities and on tests of non-verbal memory.

*Semantic dementia: progressive fluent aphasia*

Focal lobar atrophy of the temporal lobe gives rise to a form of progressive fluent aphasia which we have chosen to call semantic dementia in order to convey the concept of profound and pervasive semantic deterioration which disrupts factual memory and knowledge, language and object recognition (Hodges & Patterson, 1995, 1996; Hodges et al., 1992a, 1994; Snowden et al., 1989).

Patients typically present complaining that they have 'forgotten' the names of things and are usually unaware of the parallel decline in word comprehension. Examination reveals a fluent dysphasia with severe anomia, reduced vocabulary and prominent impairment of single-word comprehension. Category fluency is severely impaired and there is loss of general knowledge. In contrast, the sound-based (phonological) and grammatic aspects of spoken language are largely pre-served, as is comprehension of syntactically complex commands. Reading shows a pattern of surface dyslexia (i.e. a selective impairment in the ability to read words with irregular spelling to sound correspondence such as pint, island, etc. with the production of regularization errors [pint to rhyme with mint]).

In contrast to DAT, visuospatial and executive functions are preserved even late in the course of the disease. Episodic memory appears clinically to be normal in that patients recall recent events and remain well oriented, but they perform poorly on tests of verbal recall due to deficits in semantic encoding. On tests of remote memory, they show a reversal of the typical temporal gradient seen in amnesia with better performance on recent time periods than on the more distant past (Graham & Hodges, 1997; Hodges & Graham, 1998). With progression, they may develop a clinical syndrome of eating disturbance with a tendency to consume inedible things and loss of satiety, increased libido, passivity and severe associative visual agnosia. This is termed the Kluver–Bucy syndrome, and is thought to be due to bilateral amygdalar damage (Cummings & Duchen, 1981).

Radiological investigations have shown marked focal temporal neocortical atrophy involving particularly the inferior and middle temporal gyri, with relative sparing of the hippocampus. Functional imaging by SPECT appears more sensitive in early cases showing hypoperfusion of the dominant temporal lobe (Hodges et al., 1992a; Sinnatamby et al., 1996).

*Progressive non-fluent aphasia*

The most prominent clinical feature of non-fluent progressive aphasia is the dis-tortion of speech output with disturbed articulation and prosody, phonological errors, word finding pauses, and agrammatic sentence structure. The striking dysfluency results in practical communication difficulties which are obvious to the patient and observers. With disease progression, speech becomes unintelligible. Comprehension, except for syntactically complex constructions, is relatively spared in the early stages of the disease; but progressive decline in phonological processing gradually compromises speech comprehension as well as production. Eventually, patients are 'locked in' by their failure to communicate, and become socially isolated, although able to perform the activities of daily life. On formal testing, confrontational naming is impaired, but may be only mildly affected in comparison to the obvious breakdown in conversational language ability. Naming errors include many phonemic approximations (Hodges & Patterson, 1996; Patterson et al., 1994b). Repetition and short-term auditory–verbal memory are also severely disrupted.

Radiologically there is atrophy of the perisylvian language areas involving the inferior frontal and superior temporal lobe most evident on coronal MRI (Hodges & Patterson, 1996). Functional brain imaging by SPECT also implicated the left frontotemporal region and appears to be more sensitive than structural imaging.

## Vascular dementia

Cerebrovascular disease is a common cause of dementia, accounting in some studies for up to a quarter of all cases (Barclay et al., 1985; Rosen et al., 1980). Unlike DAT, there are no well-established criteria for the diagnosis, although the guidelines recently published by the NINDS–AIREN group are likely to become more widely used (Roman et al., 1993). The nature of the cognitive deficits have not been well defined (for review, see Bendixen, 1993), which almost certainly reflects the difficulty in case-definition and the heterogeneous pathologies (major infarction, lacunes, hypertensive encephalopathy, haemorrhage, etc.) which can result in vascular dementia (Hachinski & Norris, 1994).

The commonest vascular cause of dementia is the so-called multi-infarct state. In this disorder, lacunes occur usually as a result of hypertension, which leads to the development of lipohyalinosis and subsequent microaneurysms (Fisher, 1969). The clinical picture depends on the site and number of lacunes. The dementia is characterized by both cortical and subcortical features, although the latter predominate (Ishii et al., 1986; Wallin et al., 1991). It is generally unacceptable to diagnose multi-infarct dementia in the absence of a history of stroke or transient ischaemic attacks, and vascular risk factors are usually present. The progression is said to be stepwise, although this feature has probably been overemphasized, with plateaux in the course of the illness. Urinary and gait disturbances often occur early in the illness, sometimes before there is evidence of cognitive impairment (Kotsoris et al., 1987). Features of pseudobulbar palsy are characteristic. Fluctuations in cognitive performance and nocturnal confusion are very common. Emotional lability, leading to emotional incontinence, and irritability occur. There is often an accentuation of premorbid personality, with removal of inhibitions which can lead to disturbances of sexual behaviour.

Attempts have been made to differentiate vascular dementia from DAT and other dementias both clinically (Kertesz & Clydesdale, 1994) and using functional imaging (Frackowiak, 1988). Clinical pointers to vascular dementia are said to include paucity of facial expression, dysarthria, pyramidal signs and a short-stepped shuffling wide-based gait.

Cognitively, impaired attention and frontal executive features predominate (Kertesz & Clydesdale, 1994) due to a concentration of lacunes in the basal ganglia and thalamic regions, but features of cortical dysfunction are also frequently present. Although memory is also affected, the nature of the deficit has not been well characterized (Almkvist, 1994; Ricker et al., 1994). Visuospatial and perceptual deficits appear to occur less than in DAT (Gainotti et al., 1992). Multi-infarct dementia (MID) and DAT patients may be separable on the basis of speech and language impairments (Bayles & Kaszniak, 1987). Powell et al. (1988) found that DAT patients were more impaired on linguistic features of language (especially information content), while MID patients were worse on mechanical aspects of speech (especially speech melody); these aspects of speech were able to correctly classify 91% of DAT and MID patients.

So-called 'thalamic dementia' may arise from bilateral infarction of medial thalamic structures, which results in severe amnesia, marked frontal executive deficits and vertical eye movement impairment (Graff-Radford et al., 1990; Hodges & McCarthy, 1993).

## Cortical Lewy body disease

In a number of recent hospital-based pathological studies, a significant proportion (20–30%) of patients with clinically presumed DAT have been found to have cortical Lewy body disease (CLBD) (Byrne et al., 1989). Pathologically, CLBD is characterized by intraneuronal Lewy body inclusions which are widely distributed in cortical and subcortical structures (Gibb et al., 1987). In a proportion of these cases Alzheimer pathology is also present, and it remains unsettled whether CLBD represents a distinct disorder, or should more properly be regarded as a variant of Alzheimer's disease. The behavioural abnormalities are in keeping with mixed cortical–subcortical dysfunction: attentional and frontal 'executive' deficits are prominent (Galasko et al., 1994), but there are also marked visuoperceptual and memory impairments, consistent with cortical dysfunction particularly implicating posterior parieto-occipital regions (Gibb et al., 1989a; Hansen et al., 1990). Visual hallucinations, illusions and fleeting misidentification phenomena (Capgras' syndrome, etc.) appear to be particularly common. A fluctuating cognitive impairment with lucid intervals is also characteristic (McKeith et al., 1994; Perry et al., 1990). Even small doses of anti-parkinsonian drugs are liable to precipitate confusion with prominent hallucinations. Patients with CLBD have also been reported to be unusually sensitive to the side-effects of neuroleptic drugs which makes management more difficult.

## Cortico-basal degeneration

This progressive neurodegenerative disease tends to begin in late middle life, and progresses to death over 4–6 years. It presents with an asymmetric akinetic-rigid syndrome. Usually a combination of focal dystonia with myoclonus, or the alien hand sign (spontaneous coordinated hand movements outside the patient's control) develops in one upper limb (Gibb et al., 1989b). This may be accompanied by cortical sensory loss, dysarthria, ataxia, chorea and pyramidal signs. Dementia occurs in half the cases. The cognitive deficits are initially primarily parietal, with limb and constructional apraxia, severe dysgraphia, dyscalculia and spatial dysfunction (Leiguarda et al., 1994). Executive function and language impairment may supervene.

While structural imaging may show asymmetrical parietal atrophy, PET imaging shows a unique pattern of regional cortical oxygen hypometabolism and striatal fluorodopa uptake (Sawle et al., 1991). Pathologically, degeneration of the cerebral cortex and substantia nigra occurs (Gibb et al., 1989b). Swollen, achromatic neurones with Pick-like pathology have been described.

## Treatable causes of dementia

### Normal pressure hydrocephalus

In this condition, hydrocephalus develops as a result of periods of intermittent raised intracranial pressure due to raised CSF outflow resistance. Although it can be due to prior head injury, subarachnoid haemorrhage or meningitis, it is often idiopathic. The classic presentation is a clinical triad of gait apraxia, subcortical dementia and urinary dysfunction (for review, see Vanneste, 1994). In gait apraxia, the feet show the characteristic 'glued to the floor' sign when the patient tries to walk, but pyramidal or extrapyramidal signs are absent when the patient is examined lying on the bed.

The order of presentation of the clinical features helps predict whether normal pressure hydrocephalus is present: in NPH, the gait disturbance invariably precedes or accompanies dementia. If dementia occurs with no gait disorder, then it is unlikely that the patient has normal pressure hydrocephalus.

The neuropsychological profile is consistent with frontal dysfunction, both cognitively and behaviourally. This manifests as diffuse neuropsychological impairment, probably due to inertness and apathy (Stambrook et al., 1988). Impaired attention is notable. Memory shows mild impairment, but this may be secondary to poor attention. Language is preserved, while the status of visuospatial and visuoconstructional abilities is controversial.

CT shows ventricular enlargement out of proportion to the degree of cortical atrophy, sometimes with periventricular low density changes which may lead to an erroneous diagnosis of vascular dementia. Further investigation may be by intracranial pressure monitoring, or a trial of 20–50 ml CSF removal by lumbar puncture, although a negative response on the latter does not exclude the condition.

Ventricular shunting is the best treatment. Those with a short history, the typical gait disturbance, an identified cause and in whom imaging shows small sulci, respond best.

### Chronic subdural haematoma

This complication of head injury can present with subacute dementia often associated with symptoms of raised intracranial pressure. Fluctuations in conscious level or in cognitive performance are characteristic, and focal signs may be present. It occurs in those prone to head trauma (alcoholics, the elderly, patients with epilepsy) and those with coagulation defects. CT shows a peripheral mass lesion of varying signal intensity. Treatment is by surgical evacuation except if very small.

### Benign tumours

Subfrontal meningiomas may present with insidious change in personality and other frontal features. Examination may reveal anosmia or unilateral visual failure with optic atrophy. Occasionally relatively benign tumours, such as colloid cysts of the IIIrd ventricle and non-secretory pituitary tumours, may present with cognitive impairment secondary to hydrocephalus.

### Metabolic and endocrine disorders

Although cognitive impairment may occur in the context of virtually any acquired metabolic derangement, the picture is usually of delirium rather than dementia. If dementia occurs, it clinically manifests as a subcortical dementia. Chronic hypocalcaemia and recurrent hypoglycaemia may cause dementia with ataxia and involuntary movements.

Endocrine disorders more frequently cause dementia, often accompanied by psychiatric features. Hypothyroidism can present with mental slowing, apathy and poor memory. Addison's disease and hypopituitarism may manifest as a dementia of subcortical type. Cushing's disease may rarely present with dementia, but more usually results in psychiatric symptoms such as depression and paranoid delusions (Starkman & Schteingart, 1981).

It is imperative to check any young patient with dementia, especially if showing a subcortical pattern of impairment in association with a movement disorder, for Wilson's disease (Medalia et al., 1988). If left undiagnosed and untreated, the cerebral and hepatic impairment becomes resistant to therapy.

Alcohol may secondarily cause dementia by firstly producing Wernicke–Korsakoff syndrome, alcoholic pellagra, Marchiafava–Bignami disease or chronic hepatic encephalopathy. It is less clear whether alcohol may be directly neurotoxic, and cause a primary dementia (Lishman, 1981).

## Deficiency states

Although B12 deficiency can rarely cause isolated dementia, this almost always occurs without the associated subacute degeneration of the cord and peripheral neuropathy (Evans et al., 1983). Folate deficiency causes mild cognitive dysfunction, but this rarely amounts to a true dementia. B1 deficiency results in the delirium of Wernicke's encephalopathy, which if untreated will lead to the amnesic (Korsakoff's) syndrome.

## Infections

Primary CNS infection with HIV is the commonest cause of early onset dementia in some parts of the world (Forster & Pinching, 1988). The encephalopathy, termed the AIDS–dementia complex, develops early in the course of the disease and may be the sole manifestation of HIV (Navia & Price, 1987; Wilkie et al., 1990). Cognitive slowing has been reported in otherwise asymptomatic HIV-positive patients but this finding remains controversial (Grant et al., 1987). Clinically there is poor concentration, psychomotor slowing, personality change and other features of a subcortical dementia. White matter changes are seen on imaging. CSF shows increased protein, pleocytosis and oligoclonal bands. Treatment with azidothymidine (AZT) may improve cognition.

Patients with AIDS are at risk from opportunistic infections such as cerebral toxoplasmosis, cryptococcal meningitis and progressive multifocal leukoencephalopathy, all of which can present with rapidly progressive dementia.

Although now a rare cause of dementia, neurosyphilis should be considered in patients with other neurological features (seizure, dysarthria, ptosis, pupillary abnormalities, tremor, pyramidal signs, ataxia, etc.). Specific serological tests are positive and CSF shows raised protein and pleocytosis. Treatment with penicillin may result in some improvement.

Other infectious causes of dementia included subacute sclerosing panencephalitis (Jabbour et al., 1969) and progressive rubella panencephalitis (Wolinsky et al.,

1976). Whipple's disease may give rise to a dementia in association with ocular palsies, ataxia or a hypothalamic syndrome, and may be reversible with antibiotics (Ryser et al., 1984).

## REFERENCES

Albert, M.L., Feldman, R.G. & Willis, A.L. (1974). The 'subcortical dementia' of progressive supranuclear palsy. *Journal of Neurology, Neurosurgery and Psychiatry*, **37**, 121–30.

Albert, M.S., Butters, N. & Brandt, J. (1981). Development of remote memory loss in Huntington's disease. *Journal of Clinical Neuropsychology*, **3**, 1–12.

Almkvist, O. (1994). Neuropsychological deficits in vascular dementia in relation to Alzheimer's disease: reviewing evidence for functional similarity or divergence. *Dementia*, **5**, 203–9.

Alzheimer, A. (1910–1911). Uber eigenartige Krankheitsfalle des spateren Alters. *Gesellschaft Neurologische Psychiatrik*, **4**, 356–85.

American Psychiatric Association (1987). *Diagnostic and Statistical Manual of Mental Disorders*, Volume IV. Washington, DC: American Psychiatric Association.

Baddeley, A. (1992). Working memory. *Science*, **255**, 556–9.

Baddeley, A.D., Bressi, S., Della Sala, S., Logie, R. & Spinnler, H. (1991). The decline of working memory in Alzheimer's disease: a longitudinal study. *Brain*, **114**, 2521–42.

Baddeley, A.D., Emslie, H. & Nimmo-Smith, I. (1994). *The Doors and People Test: A Test of Visual and Verbal Recall and Recognition*. Bury St Edmunds: Thames Valley Test Company.

Barclay, L.L., Zemcov, A., Blass, J.P. & Sansone, J. (1985). Survival in Alzheimer's disease and vascular dementias. *Neurology*, **35**, 834–40.

Bayles, K.A. & Kaszniak, A.W. (1987). *Communication and Cognition in Normal Aging and Dementia*. Boston, MA: Little Brown & Co.

Bayles, K.A., Tomoeda, C.K., Kasniak, A.W. & Trosset, M.W. (1991). Alzheimer's disease effects on semantic memory: loss of structure or impaired processing. *Journal of Cognitive Neuroscience*, **3**, 166–82.

Beatty, W.W., Salmon, D.P., Butters, N., Heindel, W.C. & Granholm, E.L. (1988). Retrograde amnesia in patients with Alzheimer's disease or Huntington's disease. *Neurobiology of Ageing*, **9**, 181–6.

Bendixen, B. (1993). Vascular dementia: a concept in flux. *Current Opinions in Neurology and Neurosurgery*, **6**, 107–12.

Berrios, G.E. & Brook, P. (1985). Delusions and psychopathology of the elderly with dementia. *Acta Psychiatrica Scandinavica*, **72**, 296–301.

Berthier, M.L., Leiguarda, R., Starkstein, S.E., Sevlever, G. & Taratuto, A.L. (1991). Alzheimer's disease in a patient with posterior cortical atrophy. *Journal of Neurology, Neurosurgery and Psychiatry*, **54**, 1110–11.

Braak, H. & Braak, E. (1991). Neuropathological staging of Alzheimer-related changes. *Acta Neuropathology*, **82**, 239–59.

Bradshaw, J.R., Thomson, J.L.G. & Campbell, M.J. (1983). Computed tomography in the investigation of dementia. *British Medical Journal*, **1**, 277–80.

Brandt, J. & Rich, J.B. (1994). Memory disorders in the dementias. In *Handbook of Memory Disorders*, ed. A.D. Baddeley, B.A. Wilson & F. Watts, pp. 243–71. Chichester, UK: John Wiley.

Brown, P., Cathala, F., Castaigne, P. & Gajdusek, D. (1986). Creutzfeldt–Jakob disease: clinical analysis of a consecutive series of 230 neuropathologically verified cases. *Archives of Neurology*, 20, 597–602.

Brown, R.G. & Marsden, C.D. (1984). How common is dementia in Parkinson's disease? *Lancet*, i, 1262–5.

Brun, A. (1987). Frontal lobe degeneration of non-Alzheimer's type. I. Neuropathology. *Archives of Gerontology and Geriatrics*, 6, 209–33.

Brun, A., Englund, B., Gustafson, L., Passant, U., Mann, D.M.A. & Neary, D. (1994). Clinical and neuropathological criteria for frontotemporal dementia. *Journal of Neurology, Neurosurgery and Psychiatry*, 57, 416–18.

Butters, N., Sax, D. & Montgomery, K. (1978). Comparison of the neuropsychological deficits associated with early and advanced Huntington's disease. *Archives of Neurology*, 35, 585–9.

Butters, N., Wolfe, J., Martone, M., Granholm, E. & Cermak, L.S. (1985). Memory disorders associated with Huntington's disease: verbal recall, verbal recognition and procedural memory. *Neuropsychologia*, 23, 729–43.

Butters, N., Granholm, E., Salmon, D.P., Grant, I. & Wolfe, J. (1987). Episodic and semantic memory: a comparison of amnesic and demented patients. *Journal of Clinical and Experimental Neuropsychology*, 9, 479–97.

Butters, N., Salmon, D.P., Cullum, M.C., Cairns, P., Troster, A.I., Jacobs, D., Moss, M. & Cermak, L.S. (1988). Differentiation of amnesic and demented patients with the Wechsler Memory Scale-Revised. *Clinical Neuropsychology*, 2, 133–48.

Butters, N., Heindel, W.C. & Salmon, D.P. (1990). Dissociation of implicit memory in dementia: neurological implications. *Bulletin of the Psychonomic Society*, 28, 359–66.

Byrne, E.J., Lennox, G., Lowe, J. & Godwin-Austen, R.B. (1989). Diffuse Lewy body disease: clinical features in 15 cases. *Journal of Neurology, Neurosurgery and Psychiatry*, 52, 709–17.

Caffarra, P. & Venneri, A. (1996). Isolated degenerative amnesia without dementia: an 8-year longitudinal study. *Neurocase*, 2, 99–106.

Caine, E.D. & Shoulson, I. (1983). Psychiatric syndromes in Huntington's disease. *American Journal of Psychiatry*, 140, 728–33.

Caselli, R.J., Jack, C.R., Petersen, R.C., Wahner, H.W. & Yanagihara, T. (1992). Asymmetric cortical degenerative syndrome – clinical and radiologic correlations. *Neurology*, 42, 1462–8.

Chan, A.S., Butters, N., Paulson, J.S., Salmon, D.P., Swenson, M. & Maloney, L. (1993). An assessment of the semantic network in patients with Alzheimer's disease. *Journal of Cognitive Neuroscience*, 5, 254–61.

Chertkow, H. & Bub, D. (1990). Semantic memory loss in dementia of Alzheimer's type. *Brain*, 113, 397–417.

Chiofalo, N., Fuentes, A. & Galvez, S. (1980). Serial EEG findings in 27 cases of Creutzfeldt–Jakob disease. *Archives of Neurology*, 37, 143–5.

Crystal, H.A., Horoupian, D.S., Katzman, R. & Jotkowitz, S. (1982). Biopsy-proved Alzheimer disease presenting as a right parietal lobe syndrome. *Annals of Neurology*, 12, 186–8.

Cummings, J.L. & Duchen, L.W. (1981). Kluver–Bucy syndrome in Pick's disease: clinical and pathological correlations. *Neurology*, **31**, 1415–22.

Cummings, J.L. & Benson, D.F. (1984). Subcortical dementia. Review of an emerging concept. *Archives of Neurology*, **41**, 874–9.

Deutsch, G. & Tweedy, J.R. (1987). Cerebral blood flow in severity-matched Alzheimer and multi-infarct patients. *Neurology*, **37**, 431–8.

Downes, J.J., Roberts, A.C., Sahakian, B.J., Evenden, J.L., Morris, R.E. & Robbins, T.W. (1989). Impaired extra-dimensional shift performance in medicated and unmedicated Parkinson's disease. Evidence for specific attentional dysfunction. *Neuropsychologia*, **27**, 1329–43.

Erkinjuntti, T., Lee, D.H., Gao, F., Steenhuis, R., Eliasziw, M., Fry, R., Merskey, H. & Hachinski, V.C. (1993). Temporal lobe atrophy on magnetic resonance imaging in the diagnosis of early Alzheimer's disease. *Archives of Neurology*, **50**, 305–10.

Eslinger, P. & Damasio, A. (1986). Preserved motor learning in Alzheimer's disease: implications for anatomy and behaviour. *Journal of Neuroscience*, **6**, 3006–9.

Esmonde, T., Giles, E., Xuereb, J. & Hodges, J. (1996). Progressive supranuclear palsy presenting with dynamic aphasia. *Journal of Neurology, Neurosurgery and Psychiatry*, **60**, 403–10.

Evans, D.L., Edelsohn, G.A. & Golden, R.N. (1983). Organic psychosis without anaemia or spinal cord symptoms in patients with vitamin B12 deficiency. *American Journal of Psychiatry*, **140**, 218–21.

Fisher, A.M. (1969). The arterial lesions underlying lacunes. *Acta Neuropathologica (Berlin)*, **12**, 1–15.

Flowers, K.A., Pearce, I. & Pearce, J.M.S. (1984). Recognition memory in Parkinson's disease. *Journal of Neurology, Neurosurgery and Psychiatry*, **47**, 1174–81.

Folstein, M.F., Folstein, S.E. & McHugh, P.R. (1975). 'Mini-mental state'. A practical method for grading the mental state of patients for the clinician. *Journal of Psychiatric Reseearch*, **12**, 189–98.

Folstein, S.E., Abbott, M.H., Franz, M.L., Huang, S., Chase, G.A. & Folstein, M.F. (1984). Phenotypic heterogeneity in Huntington's disease. *Journal of Neurogenetics*, **1**, 175–84.

Forster, S.M. & Pinching, A.J. (1988). Acquired immune deficiency syndrome (AIDS) and its neurological complications. In *Recent Advances in Clinical Neurology*, ed. C. Kennard, vol. 5, pp. 27–46. Edinburgh: Churchill Livingstone.

Frackowiak, R.S.J. (1988). PET scanning and the pathophysiology of vascular and multi-infarct dementia. In *Vascular and Multi-infarct Dementia*, ed. J.S. Meyer, H. Lechner, J. Marshall & J. F. Toole. Mount Kisco, NY: Future Publishing Co.

Frackowiak, R.S.J. (1989). PET: studies in dementia. *Psychiatry Research*, **29**, 353–5.

Frackowiak, R.S.J., Pozzillic, C., Legg, N.J., Duboulay, G., Marshall, J., Lenzi, G. & Jojnes, T. (1981). Regional cerebral oxygen supply and utilisation in dementia. A clinical and physiological study with oxygen 15 and Positron Emission Tomography. *Brain*, **104**, 753–78.

Gainotti, G., Parlato, V., Monteleone, D. & Carlomagno, S. (1992). Neuropsychological markers of dementia on visual-spatial tasks: a comparison between Alzheimer's type and vascular forms of dementia. *Journal of Clinical and Experimental Neuropsychology*, **14**, 239–52.

Galasko, D., Hansen, L.A., Katzmann, R., Wiederholt, W., Masliah, E. & Terry, R. et al. (1994). Clinical-neuropathological correlations in Alzheimer's disease and related dementias. *Archives of Neurology*, **51**, 888–95.

Gibb, W.R.G., Esiri, M.M. & Lees, A.J. (1987). Clinical and pathological features of diffuse cortical Lewy body disease (Lewy body dementia). *Brain*, **110**, 1131–53.

Gibb, W.R.G., Luthert, P.J., Janota, I. & Lantos, P.L. (1989a). Cortical Lewy body dementia, clinical features and classification. *Journal of Neurology, Neurosurgery and Psychiatry*, **52**, 185–192.

Gibb, W.R.G., Luthert, P.J. & Marsden, C.D. (1989b). Corticobasal degeneration. *Brain*, **112**, 1171–92.

Gotham, A.M., Brown, R.G. & Marsden, C.D. (1987). 'Frontal' cognitive function in patients with Parkinson's disease. *Brain*, **111**, 299–321.

Grady, C.L., Haxby, J.V., Horwitz, B., Sundaram, M., Berg, G., Schapiro, M., Friedland, R.P. & Rapoport, S.I. (1988). Longitudinal study of the early neuropsychological and cerebral metabolic changes in dementia of the Alzheimer type. *Journal of Clinical and Experimental Neuropsychology*, **10**, 576–96.

Graff-Radford, N.R., Tranel, D., Van Hoesen, G.W. & Brandt, J.P. (1990). Diencephalic amnesia. *Brain*, **113**, 1–26.

Graham, K.S. & Hodges, J.R. (1997). Differentiating the roles of the hippocampal complex and the neocortex in long-term memory storage; evidence from the study of semantic dementia and Alzheimer's disease. *Neuropsychology*, **11**, 77–89.

Grant, I., Atkinson, J.H., Hesselink, J.R., Kennedy, C.J., Richman, D.D., Spector, S.A. & McCutchan, J.A. (1987). Evidence for early cerebral nervous system involvement in the acquired immunodeficiency syndrome (AIDS) and other human immunodeficiency virus (HIV) infections. *Annals of Internal Medicine*, **107**, 828–36.

Green, J., Morris, J.C., Sandson, J., McKeel, D.W. & Miller, J.W. (1990). Progressive aphasia: a precursor of global dementia? *Neurology*, **40**, 423–9.

Greene, J.D.W. & Hodges, J.R. (1996a). Fractionation of remote memory: evidence from a longitudinal study in dementia of Alzheimer type. *Brain*, **119**, 129–142.

Greene, J.D.W. & Hodges, J.R. (1996b). Identification of Famous Faces and Famous Names in early Alzheimer's disease: relationship to anterograde episodic and general semantic memory. *Brain*, **119**, 111–28.

Greene, J.D.W., Hodges, J.R. & Baddeley, A.D. (1995). Autobiographical memory and executive function in early dementia of Alzheimer type. *Neuropsychologia*, **33**, 1647–70.

Greene, J.D.W., Miles, K. & Hodges, J.R. (1996a). Neuropsychology of memory and SPECT in the diagnosis and staging of dementia of Alzheimer type. *Journal of Neurology*, **243**, 175–90.

Greene, J.D.W., Patterson, K., Xuereb, J. & Hodges, J.R. (1996b). Alzheimer's disease presenting with nonfluent progressive aphasia. *Archives of Neurology*, **53**, 1072–8.

Greene, J.D.W., Baddeley, A.D. & Hodges, J.R. (1996c). Recall and recognition of verbal and nonverbal material in early Alzheimer's disease: applications of the Doors and People Test. *Neuropsychologia*, **34**, 537–51.

Gregory, C.A. & Hodges, J.R. (1993). Dementia of frontal type and the focal lobar atrophies. *International Review of Psychiatry*, **5**, 397–406.

Gregory, C.A. & Hodges, J.R. (1996a). Clinical features of frontal lobe dementia in comparison to Alzheimer's disease. *Journal of Neural Transmission*, **47**, 103–23.

Gregory, C.A. & Hodges, J.R. (1996b). Dementia of frontal type: use of consensus criteria and prevalence of psychiatric features. *Neuropsychiatry, Neuropsychology and Behavioural Neurology*.

Gregory, C.A., Serra-Mestres, J. & Hodges, J.R. (1999). The early diagnosis of the frontal variant of frontotemporal dementia: how sensitive are standard neuroimaging and neuropsychological tests. *Neuropsychiatry, Neuropsychology and Behavioural Neurology*, **12**, 128–35.

Gustafson, L. (1987). Frontal lobe degeneration of non-Alzheimer type. II. Clinical picture and differential diagnosis. *Archives of Gerontology and Geriatrics*, **6**, 209–33.

Hachinski, V. & Norris, J.W. (1994). Vascular dementia: an obsolete concept. *Current Opinion in Neurology*, **7**, 3–4.

Hansen, L., Salmon, D.P., Galasko, D., Masliah, E., Katzman, R., DeTeresa, R., Thal, L., Pay, M.M., Hofstetter, R., Klauber, M., Rice, V., Butters, N. & Alford, M. (1990). The Lewy body variant of Alzheimer's disease: a clinical and pathological entity. *Neurology*, **40**, 1–8.

Harper, P.S. (1991). Huntington's disease. In *Major Problems in Neurology*, ed. L. Walton & C.P. Warlow. London: W.B. Saunders Co. Ltd.

Hart, S. (1988). Language and dementia: a review. *Psychological Medicine*, **18**, 99–112.

Hayden, M.R. (1981). *Huntington's chorea*. Berlin: Springer-Verlag.

Heindel, W.C., Salmon, D.P., Shults, C.W., Walicke, P.A. & Butters, N. (1989). Neuropsychological evidence for multiple implicit memory systems: a comparison of Alzheimer's, Huntington's and Parkinson's disease patients. *Journal of Neuroscience*, **9**, 582–7.

Heindel, W.C., Salmon, D.P. & Butters, N. (1993). Cognitive approaches to the memory disorders of demented patients. In *Comprehensive Handbook of Psychopathology*, ed. P.B. Sutker & H.E. Adams, pp. 735–61. New York: Plenum Press.

Hodges, J.R. (1994a). *Cognitive Assessment for Clinicians: A Practical Guide*. Oxford: Oxford University Press.

Hodges, J.R. (1994b). Pick's disease. In *Dementia*, ed. A. Burns & R. Levy, pp. 739–53. London: Chapman and Hall.

Hodges, J.R. & McCarthy, R.A. (1993). Autobiographical amnesia resulting from bilateral paramedian thalamic infarction: a case study in cognitive neurobiology. *Brain*, **116**, 921–40.

Hodges, J.R. & Patterson, K. (1995). Is semantic memory consistently impaired early in the course of Alzheimer's disease? Neuroanatomical and diagnostic implications. *Neuropsychologia*, **33**, 441–59.

Hodges, J.R. & Patterson, K. (1996). Non-fluent progressive aphasia and semantic dementia: a comparative neuropsychological study. *Journal of the International Neuropsychological Society*, **2**, 511–24

Hodges, J.R. & Graham, K.S. (1998). A reversal of the temporal gradient for person knowledge in semantic dementia: implications for the neural organisation of long-term memory. *Neuropsychologia*, **36**, 803–25.

Hodges, J.R., Salmon, D.P. & Butters, N. (1990). Differential impairment of semantic and episodic memory in Alzheimer's and Huntington's diseases: a controlled prospective study. *Journal of Neurology, Neurosurgery and Psychiatry*, **53**, 1089–95.

Hodges, J.R., Patterson, K., Oxbury, S. & Funnell, E. (1992a). Semantic dementia: progressive fluent aphasia with temporal lobe atrophy. *Brain*, **115**, 1783–806.

Hodges, J.R., Salmon, D.P. & Butters, N. (1992b). Semantic memory impairment in Alzheimer's disease: failure of access or degraded knowledge? *Neuropsychologia*, **30**, 310–14.

Hodges, J.R., Salmon, D.P. & Butters, N. (1993). Recognition and naming of famous faces in Alzheimer's disease: a cognitive analysis. *Neuropsychologia*, **31**, 775–88.

Hodges, J.R., Patterson, K. & Tyler, L.K. (1994). Loss of semantic memory: implications for the modularity of mind. *Cognitive Neuropsychology*, **11**, 505–42.

Hodges, J.R., Patterson, K., Garrard, P., Bak, T., Perry, R. & Gregory, C. (1999). The differentiation of semantic dementia and frontal lobe dementia (temporal and frontal variants of frontotemporal dementia) from early Alzheimer's disease: a comparative neuropsychological study. *Neuropsychology*, **13**, 31–40.

Hof, P.R., Bouras, C., Constantinidis, J. & Morrison, J.H. (1990). Selective disconnection of specific visual association pathways in cases of Alzheimer's disease presenting with Balint's syndrome. *Journal of Neuropathology and Experimental Neurology*, **49**, 168–84.

Howard, D. & Patterson, K. (1992). *Pyramids and Palm Trees: A Test of Semantic Access from Pictures and Words*. Bury St Edmunds, Suffolk: Thames Valley Publishing Company.

Huber, S.J. & Shuttleworth, E.C. (1990). Neuropsychological assessment of subcortical dementia. In *Subcortical Dementia*, ed. J.L. Cummings, pp. 71–86. Oxford: Oxford University Press.

Huber, S.J., Shuttleworth, E.C., Paulson, G.W., Bellchambers, M.J. & Clapp, L.E. (1986). Cortical vs. subcortical dementia: neuropsychological differences. *Archives of Neurology*, **43**, 392–4.

Hughes, J.C., Graham, N., Patterson, K. & Hodges, J.R. (1997). Dysgraphia in mild dementia of Alzheimer type. *Neuropsychologia*, **35**, 533–45.

Huntington's Disease Collaborative Research Group. (1993). A novel gene containing a trinucleotide repeat that is expanded and unstable on Huntington's disease chromosomes. *Cell*, **72**, 971–83.

Ishii, N., Nishahara, Y. & Imamura, T. (1986). Why do frontal lobe symptoms predominate in vascular dementia with lacunes. *Neurology*, **36**, 340–5.

Jabbour, J.T., Garcia, J.M., Lemmi, H., Ragland, J., Duenas, D.A. & Sever, J.L. (1969). Subacute sclerosing panencephalitis. *Journal of the American Medical Association*, **207**, 2248–54.

Jack, C.R., Petersen, R.C., O'Brien, P.C. & Tangalos, E.G. (1992). MR-based hippocampal volumetry in the diagnosis of Alzheimer's disease. *Neurology*, **42**, 183–8.

Jellinger, K. (1987). The pathology of parkinsonism. In *Movement Disorders 2: Neurology*, vol. 7, ed. C.D. Marsden & S. Fahn, pp. 124–65. London: Butterworth.

Jobst, K.A., Smith, A.D., Szatmari, M., Molyneux, A., Esiri, M.E. & King, E. (1992). Detection in life of confirmed Alzheimer's disease using a simple measurement of medial temporal lobe atrophy by computed tomography. *Lancet*, **340**, 1179–83.

Johnson, K.A., Kijewski, M.F., Becker, J.A., Garada, B., Satlin, A. & Holman, B.L. (1993). Quantitative Brain SPECT in Alzheimer's disease and normal ageing. *Journal of Nuclear Medicine*, **34**, 2044–8.

Josiassen, R.C., Curry, L.M. & Mancall, E.L. (1983). Development of neuropsychological deficits in Huntington's disease. *Archives of Neurology*, **40**, 791–6.

Karbe, H., Kertesz, A. & Polk, M. (1993). Profiles of language impairment in primary progressive aphasia. *Archives of Neurology*, **50**, 193–201.

Kaskie, B. & Storandt, B. (1995). Visuospatial deficit in dementia of Alzheimer type. *Archives of Neurology*, **52**, 422–5.

Kempler, D., Metter, E.J., Riege, W.H., Jackson, C.A., Benson, D.F. & Hanson, W.R. (1990). Slowly progressive aphasia: three cases with language, memory, CT and PET data. *Journal of Neurology, Neurosurgery and Psychiatry*, **53**, 987–93.

Kertesz, A. & Clydesdale, S. (1994). Neuropsychological deficits in vascular dementia vs Alzheimer's disease: frontal lobe deficits prominent in vascular dementia. *Archives of Neurology*, **51**, 1226–31.

Kesslak, J.P., Nalcioglu, O. & Cotman, C.W. (1991). Quantification of magnetic resonance scans for hippocampal and parahippocampal atrophy in Alzheimer's disease. *Neurology*, **41**, 51–4.

Kirshner, H.J., Webb, W.G., Kelly, M.P. & Wells, C.E. (1984). Language disturbance: an initial symptom of cortical degenerations and dementia. *Archives of Neurology*, **41**, 491–6.

Knopman, D.S. & Ryberg, S. (1989). A verbal memory test with high predictive accuracy for dementia of the Alzheimer type. *Archives of Neurology*, **46**, 141–5.

Kopelman, M.D. (1985). Rates of forgetting in Alzheimer-type dementia and Korsakoff's syndrome. *Neuropsychologia*, **23**, 623–38.

Kopelman, M.D. (1989). Remote and autobiographical memory, temporal context memory and frontal atrophy in Korsakoff and Alzheimer patients. *Neuropsychologia*, **27**, 437–60.

Kotsoris, H., Barclay, L.L., Kheyfets, S., Hulyalkar, A. & Dougherty, J. (1987). Urinary and gait disturbances as markers for early multi-infarct dementia. *Stroke*, **18**, 138–41.

Lange, K.W., Sahakian, B.J., Quinn, N.P., Marsden, C.D. & Robbins, T.W. (1994). Comparison of executive and visuospatial memory function in Huntington's disease and dementia of Alzheimer-type matched for degree of dementia. *Journal of Neurology, Neurosurgery and Psychiatry*, **58**, 598–606.

Lawrence, A.D., Sahakian, B.J., Hodges, J.R., Rosser, A.E., Lange, K.W. & Robbins, T.W. (1996). Executive and mnemonic functions in early Huntington's disease. *Brain*, **119**, 1633–45.

Lees, A.J. & Smith, E. (1983). Cognitive deficits in the early stages of Parkinson's disease. *Brain*, **106**, 257–70.

Leiguarda, R., Lees, A.J., Merello, M., Starkstein, S. & Marsden, C.D. (1994). The nature of apraxia in corticobasal degeneration. *Journal of Neurology, Neurosurgery and Psychiatry*, **57**, 455–9.

Lishman, W.A. (1981). Cerebral disorder in alcoholism, syndromes of impairment. *Brain*, **104**, 1–20.

Litvan, I. & Agid, Y. (1992). *Progressive Supranuclear Palsy: Clinical and Research Approaches*. Oxford: Oxford University Press.

Maher, E.R., Smith, E.M. & Lees, A.J. (1985). Cognitive deficits in the Steele-Richardson-Olszewski syndrome (progressive supranuclear palsy). *Journal of Neurology, Neurosurgery and Psychiatry*, **48**, 1234–9.

Mann, D.M.A., Yates, P.O. & Marcyniuk, B. (1984). A comparison of changes in the nucleus basalis and locus coeruleus in Alzheimer's disease. *Journal of Neurology, Neurosurgery and Psychiatry*, **47**, 201–3.

Martin, A. & Fedio, P. (1983). Word production and comprehension in Alzheimer's disease: the breakdown of semantic knowledge. *Brain and Language*, **19**, 124–41.

Martin, A., Brouwers, P., Cox, C. & Fedio, P. (1985). On the nature of the verbal memory deficit in Alzheimer's disease. *Brain and Language*, **25**, 323–41.

Massman, P.J., Delis, D.C., Butters, N., Dupont, R.M. & Gillin, J.C. (1992). The subcortical dysfunction hypothesis of memory deficits in depression: neuropsychological validation in a subgroup of patients. *Journal of Clinical and Experimental Neuropsychology*, **14**, 687–706.

Mayeux, R., Stern, Y., Sano, M.C., Cote, L. & Williams, D.S.W. (1987). Clinical and biochemical correlates of bradyphrenia in Parkinson's disease. *Neurology*, **37**, 1130–4.

Mazziotta, J.C., Frackowiak, R.S.J. & Phelps, M.E. (1992). The use of positron emission tomography in the clinical assessment of dementia. *Seminars in Nuclear Medicine*, **22**, 233–46.

McDuff, T. & Sumi, S.M. (1985). Subcortical degeneration in Alzheimer's disease. *Neurology*, **35**, 123–6.

McKeith, I.G., Fairbairn, A.F., Perry, R.H. & Thompson, P. (1994). The clinical diagnosis and misdiagnosis of senile dementia of Lewy body type (SDLT). *British Journal of Psychiatry*, **165**, 324–32.

McKhann, G., Drachman, D., Folstein, M., Katzman, R., Price, D. & Stradlan, E.M. (1984). Clinical diagnosis of Alzheimer's disease. *Neurology*, **34**, 939–44.

Medalia, A., Isaacs-Glaberman, K. & Scheinberg, I.H. (1988). Neuropsychological impairment in Wilson's disease. *Archives of Neurology*, **45**, 502–4.

Mendez, M.F., Mendez, M.A., Martin, R., Smyth, K.A. & Whitehouse, P.J. (1990). Complex visual disturbances in Alzheimer's disease. *Neurology*, **40**, 439–43.

Mendez, M.F., Selwood, A., Mastri, A.R. & Frey, W.H. (1993). Pick's disease versus Alzheimer's disease: a comparison of clinical characteristics. *Neurology*, **43**, 289–92.

Mesulam, M.M. (1982). Slowly progressive aphasia without generalized dementia. *Annals of Neurology*, **11**, 592–8.

Mesulam, M.M. & Weintraub, S. (1992). Primary progressive aphasia. In *Heterogeneity of Alzheimer's Disease*, ed. F. Boller, pp. 43–66. Berlin: Springer-Verlag.

Miller, B.L., Cummings, J.L., Villanueva-Meyer, J., Boone, K., Mehringer, C.M., Lesser, I.M.& Mena, I. (1991). Frontal lobe degeneration: clinical, neuropsychological and SPECT characteristics. *Neurology*, **41**, 1374–82.

Mindham, R.H.S., Ahmed, S.W.A. & Clough, C.G. (1982). A controlled study of dementia in Parkinson's disease. *Journal of Neurology, Neurosurgery and Psychiatry*, **45**, 969–74.

Molsa, P.K., Paljvari, L., Rinne, J.O., Rinne, U.K. & Sako, E. (1985). Validity of clinical diagnosis in dementia: a prospective clinicopathological study. *Journal of Neurology, Neurosurgery and Psychiatry*, **48**, 1085–90.

Monsch, A.U., Bondi, M.W., Butters, N., Pauslen, J.S., Salmon, D.P., Brugger, P. & Swenson, M.R. (1994). A comparison of category and letter fluency in Alzheimer's disease and Huntington's disease. *Neuropsychology*, **8**, 25–30.

Montaldi, D., Brooks, D.N., McColl, J.H., Wyper, D., Patterson, J., Barron, E. & McCulloch, J. (1990). Measurements of regional cerebral blood flow and cognitive performance in Alzheimer's disease. *Journal of Neurology, Neurosurgery and Psychiatry*, **53**, 33–8.

Moss, M.B., Albert, M.S., Butters, N. & Payne, M. (1986). Differential patterns of memory loss among patients with Alzheimer's disease, Huntington's disease, and alcoholic Korsakoff's syndrome. *Archives of Neurology*, **43**, 239–46.

Navia, B.A. & Price, R.W. (1987). The acquired immunodeficiency syndrome: dementia as the presenting sole manifestation of human immunodeficiency virus infection. *Archives of Neurology*, **44**, 65–9.

Neary, D., Snowden, J.S., Bowen, D.M., Sims, N.R., Mann, D.M.A., Benton, J.S., Northen, B., Yates, P.O. & Davison, A.N. (1986). Neuropsychological syndromes in presenile dementia due to cerebral atrophy. *Journal of Neurology, Neurosurgery and Psychiatry*, **49**, 163–74.

Neary, D., Snowden, J.S., Shields, R.A., Burjan, A.W.I., Northen, B., MacDermott, N., Prescott, M.C. & Testa, H.J. (1987). Single photon emission tomography using 99mTc-HM-PAO in the investigation of dementia. *Journal of Neurology, Neurosurgery and Psychiatry*, **50**, 1101–9.

Neary, D., Snowden, J.S., Northen, B. & Goulding, P. (1988). Dementia of frontal lobe type. *Journal of Neurology, Neurosurgery and Psychiatry*, **51**, 353–61.

Nebes, R.B. (1989). Semantic memory in Alzheimer's disease. *Psychological Bulletin*, **106**, 377–94.

O'Connor, D.W., Pollitt, P.A., Roth, M., Brook, P.B. & Reiss, B.B. (1990). Memory complaints and impairment in normal, depressed and demented elderly persons identified in a community survey. *Archives of General Psychiatry*, **47**, 224–7.

Patterson, K., Graham, N. & Hodges, J.R. (1994a). Reading in Alzheimer's type dementia: a pre-served ability? *Neuropsychology*, **8**, 395–407.

Patterson, K.E., Graham, N. & Hodges, J.R. (1994b). The impact of semantic memory loss on phonological representations. *Journal of Cognitive Neuroscience*, **6**, 57–69.

Perani, D., Vallar, G., Cappa, S., Messa, C. & Fazio, F. (1987). Aphasia and neglect after subcortical stroke. *Brain*, **110**, 1211–29.

Perry, R.H., Irving, D., Blessed, G., Fairbairn, A. & Perry, E.K. (1990). Senile dementia of Lewy body type. A clinically and neuropathologically distinct form of Lewy body dementia in the elderly. *Journal of Neurological Science*, **95**, 119–39.

Pick, A. (1892). Uber die Beziehungen der senilen Hirnatrophie zur Aphasie. *Prager Medicinische Wochenschrift*, **17**, 165–7.

Pick, A. (1906). Uber einen weiteren symptomenkomplex im Rahmen der Dementia senilis, bedingt durch umschriebene starkere Hirnatrophie (gemische Apraxie). *Monatschrift für Psychiatrie und Neurologie*, **19**, 97–108.

Pietrini, V. (1992). Creutzfeldt-Jakob disease presenting as Wernicke–Korsakoff syndrome. *Journal of Neurological Science*, **108**, 149–53.

Pillon, B. & Dubois, B. (1992). Cognitive and behavioral impairments. In *Progressive Supranuclear Palsy: Clinical and Research Approaches*, ed. I. Litvan & Y. Agid, pp. 223–39. Oxford: Oxford University Press.

Pillon, B., Dubois, B., Lhermitte, F. & Agid, Y. (1986). Heterogeneity of cognitive impairment in progressive supranuclear palsy, Parkinson's disease, and Alzheimer's disease. *Neurology*, **36**, 1179–85.

Pillon, B., Deweer, B., Agid, Y. & Dubois, B. (1993). Explicit memory in Alzheimer's, Huntington's, and Parkinson's diseases. *Archives of Neurology*, **50**, 374–9.

Podoll, K., Caspary, P., Lange, H.W. & Noth, J. (1988). Language functions in Huntington's disease. *Brain*, **111**, 1475–503.

Poeck, K. & Luzzatti, C. (1988). Slowly progressive aphasia in three patients: the problem of accompanying neuropsychological deficit. *Brain*, **111**, 151–68.

Pogacar, S. & Williams, R.S. (1984). Alzheimer's disease presenting as slowly progressive aphasia. *Rhode Island Medical Journal*, **67**, 181–5.

Powell, A.L., Cummings, J.L., Hill, M.A. & Benson, D.F. (1988). Speech and language alterations in multi-infarct dementia. *Neurology*, **38**, 717–19.

Rapcsak, S.Z., Arthur, S.A., Bliklen, D.A. & Rubens, A.B. (1989a). Lexical agraphia in Alzheimer's disease. *Archives of Neurology*, **46**, 65–8.

Rapcsak, S.Z., Croswell, S.C. & Rubens, A. (1989b). Apraxia in Alzheimer's disease. *Neurology*, **39**, 664–8.

Ricker, J.H., Keenan, P.A. & Jacobson, M.W. (1994). Visuoperceptual–spatial ability and visual memory in vascular dementia and dementia of the Alzheimer type. *Neuropsychologia*, **32**, 1287–96.

Robbins, T.W., James, M., Owen, A.M., Lange, K.W., Lees, A.J., Leigh, P.N., Marsden, C.D., Quinn, N.P. & Summers, B.A. (1994). Cognitive deficits in progressive supranuclear palsy, Parkinson's disease, and multiple system atrophy in tests sensitive to frontal lobe dysfunction. *Journal of Neurology, Neurosurgery and Psychiatry*, **57**, 79–88.

Roman, G.C., Tatemichi, T.K., Erkinjuntti, T., Cummings, J.L., Masdeu, J.C., Garcia, J.H., Amaducci, L., Orgogozo, J.M., Brun, A., Hofman, A. et al. (1993). Vascular dementia: diagnostic criteria for research studies. Report of the NINDS-AIREN International Workshop. *Neurology*, **43**, 250–60.

Rosen, W.G., Terry, R.D., Fuld, P.A., Katzman, R. & Peck, A. (1980). Pathological verification of ischaemic score in differentiation of the dementias. *Annals of Neurology*, **7**, 486–8.

Ross, G.W., Benson, D.F., Verity, A.M. & Victoroff, J.I. (1990). Posterior cortical atrophy: neuropathological correlations. *Neurology*, **40**, 200.

Rosser, A. & Hodges, J.R. (1994). Initial letter and semantic category fluency in Alzheimer's disease, Huntington's disease and progressive supranuclear palsy. *Journal of Neurology, Neurosurgery and Psychiatry*, **57**, 1389–94.

Ryser, R.J., Locksley, R.M., Eng, S.C., Dobbins, W.O., Schoenknecht, F.D. & Rubin, C.E. (1984). Reversal of dementia associated with Whipple's disease by trimethoprim-sulfamethoxazole, drugs that penetrate the blood–brain barrier. *Gastroenterology*, **86**, 745–52.

Sagar, H.A., Cohen, N.J., Sullivan, E.V., Corkin, S. & Growdon, J.H. (1988a). Remote memory function in Alzheimer's disease and Parkinson's disease. *Brain*, **111**, 185–206.

Sagar, H.J., Sullivan, E.V., Gabrieli, J.D.E., Corkin, S. & Growdon, J.H. (1988b). Temporal ordering deficits and bradyphrenia in Parkinson's disease. *Brain*, **111**, 525–39.

Sahakian, B.J., Morris, R.G., Evenden, J.L., Heald, A., Levy, R., Philpot, M. & Robbins, T.W. (1988). A comparative study of visuospatial memory and learning in Alzheimer-type dementia and Parkinson's disease. *Brain*, **111**, 695–718.

Sahakian, B.J., Downes, J.J., Eagger, S., Evenden, J.L., Levy, R., Philpot, M.P., Roberts, A.C. & Robbins, T.W. (1990). Sparing of attentional relative to mnemonic function in a subgroup of patients with dementia of the Alzheimer type. *Neuropsychologia*, **28**, 1197–213.

Salmon, D.P., Shimamura, A.P., Butters, N. & Smith, S. (1988). Lexical and semantic priming deficits in patients with Alzheimer's disease. *Journal of Clinical and Experimental Neuropsychology*, **10**, 477–94.

Sawle, G.V., Brooks, D.J., Marsden, C.D. & Frackowiak, R.S.J. (1991). Corticobasal degeneration. *Brain*, **114**, 541–56.

Schellenberg, G.D., Bird, T.D., Wijsman, E.M., Orr, H.T., Anderson, L., Nemense, White, J.A., Bonnycastle, L., Weber, J.L., Alonso, M.E., Potter, H., Heston, L.L. & Martin, G.M. (1992). Genetic linkage evidence for a familial Alzheimer's disease locus on chromosome 14. *Science*, **258**, 68–671.

Scheltens, P., Leys, D., Barkhof, F., Huglo, D., Weinstein, H.C., Vermersch, P., Kuiper, M.,

Steinling, M., Wolters, E.Ch. & Valk, J. (1992). Atrophy of medial temporal lobes on MRI in 'probable' Alzheimer's disease and normal ageing: diagnostic value and neuropsychological correlates. *Journal of Neurology, Neurosurgery and Psychiatry*, 55, 967–72.

Scheltens, P., Ravid, R. & Kamphorst, W. (1994). Pathologic findings in a case of primary progressive aphasia. *Neurology*, 44, 279–82.

Shimamura, A. (1986). Priming effects in amnesia: evidence for a dissociable memory function. *Quarterly Journal of Experimental Psychology*, 38, 619–44.

Shimamura, A.P., Salmon, D.P., Squire, L.R. & Butters, N. (1987). Memory dysfunction and word priming in dementia and amnesia. *Behavioural Neuroscience*, 101, 347–51.

Sinnatamby, R., Antoun, N.A., Freer, C.E.L., Miles, K.A. & Hodges, J.R. (1996). The neuroradiological findings in primary progressive aphasia: a comparison of CT, MRI and cerebral perfusion SPECT. *Neuroradiology*, 38, 232–8.

Snowden, J.S., Goulding, P.J. & Neary, D. (1989). Semantic dementia: a form of circumscribed cerebral atrophy. *Behavioural Neurology*, 2, 167–82.

Snowden, J.S., Neary, D., Mann, D.M.A., Goulding, P.J. & Testa, H.J. (1992). Progressive language disorder due to lobar atrophy. *Annals of Neurology*, 31, 174–83.

St George-Hislop, P., Tanzi, R., Polinsky, R., Haines, J.L., Nee, L., Watkins, P.C., Myers, R.H., Feldman, R.G., Pollen, D., Drachman, D., Growdon, J., Bruni, A., Foncin, J.F., Salmon, D., Frommelt, P., Amaducci, L., Sorbi, S., Piacentini, S., Stewart, G.D., Hobbs, W.J., Conneally, P.M. & Gusella, J.F. (1987). The genetic defect causing familial Alzheimer's disease maps on chromosome 21. *Science*, 235, 885–90.

Stambrook, M., Cardoso, E.R., Hawryluk, G.A., Erikson, P., Piatek, D. & Sicz, G. (1988). Neuropsychological changes following the neurosurgical treatment of normal pressure hydrocephalus. *Archives of Clinical Neuropsychology*, 3, 323–30.

Starkman, M.N. & Schteingart, D.E. (1981). Neuropsychiatric manifestations of patients with Cushing's syndrome: relationship to cortical and adrenocorticotropic hormone levels. *Archives of Internal Medicine*, 141, 215–19.

Terry, R.D., Masliah, E., Salmon, D.P., Butters, N., DeTeresa, R., Hill, R., Hansen, L.A. & Katzman, R. (1991). Physical basis of cognitive alterations in Alzheimer's disease: synapse loss is the major correlate of cognitive impairment. *Annals of Neurology*, 30, 572–80.

Tweedy, J.R., Langer, K.G. & McDowell, F.H. (1982). The effect of semantic relations on the memory deficit associated with Parkinson's disease. *Journal of Clinical Neuropsychology*, 4, 235–47.

Tyrrell, P.J., Warrington, E.K., Frackowiak, R.S.J. & Rossor, M.N. (1990). Heterogeneity in progressive aphasia due to focal cortical atrophy. A clinical and PET study. *Brain*, 113, 1321–36.

Van der Hurk, P. & Hodges, J.R. (1995). Episodic and semantic memory in Alzheimer's disease and progressive supranuclear palsy. *Journal of Clinical and Experimental Neuropsychology*, 17, 459–71.

Van Gool, W.A., Walstra, G.J.M., Teunisse, S., Van der Zant, F.M., Weinstein, H.C. & Van Royen, E.A. (1995). Diagnosing Alzheimer's disease in elderly, mildly demented patients: the impact of routine single photon emission computed tomography. *Journal of Neurology*, 242, 401–5.

Van Hoesen, G.W., Hyman, B.T. & Damasio, A.R. (1991). Entorhinal cortex pathology in Alzheimer's disease. *Hippocampus*, 1, 1–8.

Vanneste, J.A.L. (1994). Three decades of normal pressure hydrocephalus: are we wiser now? *Journal of Neurology, Neurosurgery and Psychiatry*, **57**, 1021–5.

Villa, G., Cappa, A., Tavolozza, M., Gainotti, G., Giordano, A., Calcagni, M.L. & De Rossi, G. (1995). Neuropsychological tests and [99mTc]-HMPAO SPECT in the diagnosis of Alzheimer's dementia. *Journal of Neurology*, **242**, 359–66.

Wade, J.P.H., Mirsen, T.R., Hachinski, V.C., Fishman, M., Lau, C. & Merskey, H. (1987). The clinical diagnosis of Alzheimer's disease. *Archives of Neurology*, **44**, 24–9.

Waldemar, G., Bruhn, P., Kristensen, M., Johnsen, A., Paulson, O.B. & Lassen, N.A. (1994). Heterogeneity of neocortical cerebral blood flow deficits in dementia of the Alzheimer type: a [$^{99m}$Tc]-d,l-HMPAO SPECT study. *Journal of Neurology, Neurosurgery and Psychiatry*, **57**, 285–95.

Wallin, A., Blennow, K.A.J. & Goffries, C.G. (1991). Subcortical symptoms predominate in vascular dementia. *International Journal of Geriatric Psychiatry*, **6**, 137–45.

Wechsler, D.A. (1987). *Wechsler Memory Scale – Revised*. San Antonio: Psychological Corporation.

Weintraub, S., Rubin, N.P. & Mesulam, M.-M. (1990). Primary progressive aphasia: longitudinal course, neuropsychological profile, and language features. *Archives of Neurology*, **47**, 1329–35.

Welsh, K., Butters, N., Hughes, J., Mohs, R. & Heyman, A. (1991). Detection of abnormal memory decline in mild cases of Alzheimer's disease using CERAD neuropsychological measures. *Archives of Neurology*, **48**, 278–81.

Welsh, K.A., Butters, N., Hughes, J.P. & Mohs, R.C. (1992). Detection and staging of dementia in Alzheimer's disease: use of the neuropsychological measures developed for the Consortium to Establish a Registry for Alzheimer's disease. *Archives of Neurology*, **49**, 448–52.

Whitehouse, P.J. (1986). The concept of subcortical and cortical dementia: another look. *Annals of Neurology*, **19**, 1–6.

Whitehouse, P.J., Price, D.L., Struble, R.G., Clark, A.W., Coyle, J.T. & DeLong, M.R. (1982). Alzheimer's disease and senile dementia: loss of neurons in the basal forebrain. *Science*, **215**, 1237–9.

Wilcock, G.K. & Esiri, M.M. (1982). Plaques, tangles and dementia: a quantitative study. *Journal of Neurological Science*, **56**, 343–56.

Wilkie, F.L., Eisdorfer, C., Morgan, R., Loewenstein, D.A. & Szapocznik, J. (1990). Cognition in early human immunodeficiency virus infection. *Archives of Neurology*, **47**, 433–40.

Will, R.G., Ironside, J.W., Zeidler, M., Cousens, S.N., Estibeiro, K., Alperovitch, A., Poser, S., Pocchiari, M., Hofman, A. & Smith, P.G. (1996). A new variant of Creutzfeldt–Jakob disease in the UK. *Lancet*, **347**, 921–5.

Wolinsky, J.S., Berg, B.O. & Maitland, C.J. (1976). Progressive rubella panencephalitis. *Archives of Neurology*, **33**, 722–3.

Wragg, R.E. & Jeste, D.V. (1989). Overview of depression and psychosis in Alzheimer's disease. *American Journal of Psychiatry*, **146**, 577–87.

## 8

# The amnesic syndrome

Ennio De Renzi

Patients with complaints of poor memory are frequently encountered in clinical practice, but not all of them prove to be truly amnesic when assessed clinically and with objective criteria. Anxiety, hypochondrial worries and depression may hinder the focusing of attention on the event, or task, which the patient is trying to register, and can cause memory gaps that are overemphasized and become the subject of worries. Lapses of attention are also common in patients with organic brain syndromes and may be responsible, along with inadequate encoding strategy, for their poor memory performance. These patients aside, a number of cases remain in which the inability to remember ongoing and past events is the main manifestation of disease and points to the damage of specific anatomical structures. From a clinical perspective, it is important to classify these patients into two groups, depending on whether amnesia appears either in isolation and reflects a focal lesion, or is a component of a more complex pattern of cognitive deficits, consequent to diffuse cortical damage, such as in Alzheimer's disease (see Chapter 7). Although the patients of the latter group are by far the more frequent in clinical practice, it is the former group that has provided the main source of information for delineating the amnesic syndrome and for understanding its anatomico-functional underpinnings.

## The amnesic syndrome

### Clinical features

Patients with the amnesic syndrome have an unclouded sensorium and appear alert, able to concentrate and are cooperative. Perceptual and intellectual skills are preserved. Speech is fluent and appropriate and patients easily understand the examiner's questions and test instructions, although it may be necessary to repeat them in the course of the session, because they have been forgotten. Patients are aware of their predicament, but are usually not particularly concerned about it.

The amnesic deficit does not affect all the types of information the patient has acquired, to the same degree. Assessment of memory must therefore, be carried out, keeping in mind the factors that have been found to play a role in the patient's performance. They are the interval between the processing of information and its retrieval, the nature of the memoranda, and their chronological relation with respect to the onset of disease. For a discussion of these distinctions see Chapter 4.

### Short- and long-term memory

Amnesic patients do not score differently from normals on tasks that require the immediate reproduction of a sequence of stimuli not exceeding the capacity of the short-term (working) memory store (memory span). Thus performance on tests like digits forward and Corsi block-tapping test, which assess verbal and spatial short-term memory respectively, is within the normal range. On the other hand, the deficit becomes immediately apparent as soon as the memoranda exceed the memory span or a distractor activity intervenes between the presentation and recall of stimuli, namely, when the information must be recovered from the long-term store. Thus three items given by the examiner are repeated correctly, but if they are requested after a filled delay of a few seconds, the patient may ask 'What names?', having completely forgotten the episode.

### Anterograde and retrograde amnesia

Amnesia does not affect equally memories acquired after and before the onset of disease (anterograde and retrograde amnesia, respectively). Anterograde amnesia is a constant feature of the amnesic syndrome and results in the inability to retain new experiences, even when they are repeated or are emotionally laden. The most severe patients do not remember the date and the name of the hospital, do not recognize the examiner and the testing room and cannot remember any recent event, even those that have occurred a few minutes before, as soon as the focus of their attention shifts.

An exhaustive examination of the scope and severity of the anterograde deficit calls for the administration of a variety of tests, differing in the type of stimuli (meaningless, meaningful, requiring a logical reconstruction), the modality through which they are conveyed (verbal, visual and spatial) and the retrieval procedure (free recall, cued recall, recognition). Popular verbal tests are the following: (i) *Story recall*: a short story is read out and its recall is assessed immediately and after a filled delay. (ii) *Paired associate learning*: a list of word pairs is presented for the patient to retrieve the second member of the pair when the first is given. Pairs may differ in difficulty, depending on the strength of semantic association between the two words (e.g. east–west vs. grass–shoe) and amnesics usually fail to learn any difficult association. (iii) *Word list learning*: a list of unrelated words is repeatedly read to the patient, who, after each presentation, tries to retrieve them in whatever order he/she prefers. Recall is again requested after a filled delay of 10 to 15 minutes. Normal subjects remember better the words that occupy the early and last positions in the list (primary position effect and recency effect, respectively), the former because they are not affected by proactive interference, the latter because they can be retrieved from the short-term (working) memory store. Only the recency effect is preserved in amnesics, due to the integrity of their short-term (working) memory. Proper testing of visual memory should avoid meaningful stimuli, since they lend themselves to be verbally coded. The Rey figure, a complex abstract drawing that the patient must first copy and then reproduce from memory after a filled delay, represents a suitable stimulus for testing visual memory. Spatial memory is assessed with tasks that require the patient to memorize a sequence of visual stimuli that have the same shape and are only identifiable by their position in space, such as Corsi blocks and stepping stone mazes (Milner, 1972).

Contrary to anterograde amnesia, retrograde amnesia (RA) shows a considerable variability in its extent and severity. In the past its study has been relatively neglected because, while the conditions in which new stimuli are presented for learning can be strictly controlled and made equal across subjects, it is impossible to ascertain what the patient actually knew before the onset of amnesia. Some progress has been made recently in developing procedures that permit a standardized assessment of retrograde memory for general facts and autobiographic events. Memory for facts is tested with chronologically organized questionnaires, which investigate the knowledge of events and persons whose fame has been associated with a specific period of time and since then have only rarely been rehearsed (e.g. who is Uri Gagarin?). They permit the evaluation of the extent of RA and whether it shows a temporal gradient, namely, an impairment limited to more recent periods. The performance on these tasks must be compared with that on questions which refer to facts generally known in our culture and whose acquisition is not chronologically defined (e.g. what is the Eiffel Tower, which is the capital of France, what is a root square ?). Autobiographical memory can be assessed in individual cases by constructing, with the assistance of the patient's relatives, an inventory of the main personal events or episodes that have marked his/her life. However, this procedure does not permit a comparison between patients and is, therefore, usefully complemented by semi-structured interviews (Borrini et al., 1989; Kopelman et al., 1989), which call for the retrieval of episodes of the patient's life across a number of time bands (primary school, first job, etc.). The distinction between episodes (specific events, whose recall makes reference to the temporal and spatial circumstances of their acquisition) and facts (knowledge that is independent of where and when it was acquired) also applies to autobiographic memory. These semi-structured interviews probe episodic and factual memory with separate lists of questions, e.g. tell me about a quarrel with a school mate vs. tell me the name of your elementary teacher.

Explicit and implicit memory

The term 'memory' is usually reserved for the conscious recollection of events or facts acquired in the past and stored as individual units of knowledge in our mind. There is, however, another way past experiences affect our present behaviour, i.e. through the improvement of our motor, perceptual and even cognitive skills. We learn to ski, to read, to develop strategies in solving certain types of mental tasks and in all of these performance proficiency is dependent on the modification undergone by our nervous system, thanks to previous experiences. Yet when we ski, read or solve a new problem, we have no feeling of remembering the past, which is incorporated in the performance, but not consciously retrieved. Let us take the example of a subject first trying to learn to ski. There are two ways in which the subject can memorize this experience, either by remembering it as an episode that has definite temporospatial coordinates (explicit memory) or by showing an improvement in the ability to keep his/her balance on a snow-covered slope (memory for procedures, or implicit memory). Amnesia honours this distinction, in that it disrupts explicit memory and does not affect implicit memory, both in its retrograde and anterograde components (Corkin, 1968; Milner, 1972).

Another area where amnesics show preservation of past knowledge is language. Its integrity attests that not only their phonetic and grammatical competence but also their lexicon is spared and this very fact has been taken as evidence that word knowledge represents a separate type of memory (semantic memory) from knowledge of single events (Tulving, 1983). This claim is, however, open to question, since it confounds the nature of stimuli with the time of their acquisition. The verbal thesaurus a human being owns is mostly acquired in the early period of life and its sparing might therefore, reflect the integrity of very remote memory and not the existence of a discrete memory domain. When amnesics have been tested for their ability to learn words that entered the lexicon post-morbidly, they were found to be as severely impaired as in the learning of other material (Gabrieli et al. 1988; Verfaellie et al., 1995a). Moreover, Korsakoff patients and a severe postencephalitic amnesic have been found impaired even in the knowledge of words whose entry in the vocabulary ante-dated the onset of disease, particularly if they were acquired during more recent time periods. Only very old words were preserved (Verfaellie et al., 1995a, b).

Confabulations

A phenomenon that occurs in a minority of amnesics is the tendency to generate false memories, in spite of clear consciousness. It can take two forms, provoked and spontaneous confabulations. Provoked confabulations are given in response to questions that the patient is unable to answer, apparently as an attempt to fill memory gaps. They tend to be plausible and circumscribed and are transient and

easily abandoned (momentary or embarassment confabulations, according to
Berlyne, 1972). They have been reported in Korsakoff and Alzheimer patients and
even in normal subjects, when recall is tested after a long delay (Kopelman, 1987).
Spontaneous confabulations are clinically more relevant. They are fantastic fabrica-
tions, often grandiose and bizarre, which may be elicited by the misinterpretation of
an external stimulus. Apparently, patients believe they have experienced the fabricated events. When their implausibility or inconsistency is pointed out, they usually
remain perplexed and accept the correction, but after a while invent a new confabulation. This behaviour is observed in the acute stage of Korsakoff disease and in a
few patients with head injury or with rupture of an anterior communicating artery
aneurysm, while it has never been reported in temporal lobe amnesics. Although the
presence of a memory defect is a consistent feature of spontaneous confabulations,
its severity is not necessarily related to their flourishing and the two phenomena are
to a certain degree independent, as shown by the fact that confabulations generally
clear in the chronic stage of Korsakoff syndrome, while amnesia persists.

Confabulations can be investigated in a structured setting by asking questions
that address different issues, remote and recent autobiographic memory, famous
facts and people, tales and also 'I don't know' questions (i.e. questions to which
most normal people would answer 'I don't know'), such as, 'Who was the winner
of the fencing world championship in 1983?' (Mercer et al., 1977; Dalla Barba et al.,
1990). Only a minority of confabulators produce false responses to the last type of
questions. Dalla Barba et al. (1990) have reported a Korsakoff patient who showed
amnesia and confabulations confined to autobiographic memory.

Most authors are inclined to attribute spontaneous confabulations to the concomitant damage to the frontal lobes that would deprive the patient of the monitoring function this region exerts on behaviour. Frontal damage has been
demonstrated both pathologically and radiologically in Korsakoff patients (Stuss et
al., 1978) and in patients with rupture of anterior communicating artery aneurysms (Alexander & Freedman, 1984; Damasio et al., 1985; Vilkki, 1985), in which
the lesion encroaches upon the orbitofrontal and septal areas. In agreement with
this view, Benson et al. (1996) reported a Korsakoff patient with florid confabulations, whose SPECT showed hypoperfusion in the orbital frontal region and medial
diencephalic region. Four months later, the confabulations and the frontal hypometabolism had disappeared, while amnesia and a certain degree of diencephalic
hypometabolism persisted.

## Is the amnesic profile related to the locus of lesion and its aetiology?

As will be discussed below, the amnesic syndrome can result from a variety of
lesions, affecting the discrete anatomical structures that compose the circuit of

memory. It is therefore, logical to raise the question of whether there are features distinguishing the amnesic profile, depending on the locus and nature of damage. The answer is uncertain. Amnesia linked to medial temporal damage has been claimed to be marked by the absence of confabulations and the presence of a temporal gradient in RA, which would be, at most, limited to the few years preceding the onset of disease and even less when the lesion is confined to the hippocampus. This pattern has been contrasted with that of Korsakoff patients, who often confabulate in the acute stage and manifest a RA extending over several decades, though being more severe in the recent pre-morbid period. However, it is open to question whether these features reflect the differential contribution made by the temporal and diencephalic structures to memory functions or are consequent to the concomitant damage to frontal areas, frequently found in the alcoholic Korsakoff syndrome. Extensive RA is not consistently observed in patients with other types of diencephalic pathology. Mamillary body damage (Dusoir et al., 1990; Squire et al., 1989; Kapur et al., 1996) is not accompanied by RA, while the retrograde component of amnesia in thalamic damage varies from mild (Michel et al., 1982; Speedie & Heilman, 1982) to severe (Gentilini et al., 1987; Hodges & McCarthy, 1993; Markowitsch et al., 1993a,b). As to confabulations, they have only rarely been reported after unilateral thalamic damage, but were present in five patients with an infarct involving both the thalamus and the occipito-temporal cortex (Servan et al., 1994) and in three out of eight consecutive patients with bilateral paramedian thalamic artery infarcts, and in one of them they were very florid (Gentilini et al., 1987). It is possible that, in these cases, the confabulation is contingent on frontal lobe deafferentation. More data are needed before a firm position can be taken, but on the whole it would appear that there is no compelling evidence that the components of the Papez circuit play a different role in subserving memory functions.

Amnesia consequent to hypoxia has been claimed (Volpe & Hirst, 1983; Volpe et al., 1986) to show a peculiar dissociation between the poor performance on recall tasks and the relatively preserved performance on recognition tests. There are, however, methodological pitfalls inherent in this kind of comparison (Haist et al., 1992), which invite caution in accepting the conclusions based on a few cases.

## Other types of amnesia

The literature has reported patterns of memory deficit that differ from that of the classical amnesic syndrome, because they affect a selective area of knowledge or are extended to domains spared by global amnesia, or are confined to the retrograde compartment of memory. Transient global amnesia and other forms of temporary memory loss are dealt with in Chapter 9.

## Prosopamnesia (amnesia for faces and people)

There are patients who manifest the inability to recognize familiar faces, in spite of having no visuoperceptual disorder and retaining full verbal knowledge of the biography and the context in which the target person is encountered. The deficit is confined to the visual modality (familiar voices are normally recognized) and is therefore, conceptualized as a particular form of visual agnosia, associative prosopagnosia, a condition in which the subsector of semantic memory storing information about familiar people is no longer accessible from the output of the visual system. Although the term mnestic prosopagnosia or loss of person-specific semantics is applied to patients, who, though not being amnesic in other domains, have lost the ability to identify a person, whatever the modality through which it is assessed (Hècaen, 1981; Ellis, 1989), it must be admitted that none of the so far reported cases shows a deficit strictly confined to people. Hanley et al. (1989) reported a post-encephalitic patient who, in the context of a semantic impairment for living things, showed a prominent difficulty in recognizing famous people from their face, voice and name. There was, however, evidence from learning tasks that he could gain covert access to information that he was unable to retrieve consciously. The same pattern of deficit was reported in a patient who had undergone a right temporal lobectomy (Ellis et al., 1989), but again it was not isolated, in that it extended to the semantic knowledge of other single entities, such as the names of famous animals (e.g. Moby Dick or Lassie), buildings (the Kremlin) and old products. More specific was the amnesia for faces and voices (but not names) of people that had first become famous after the onset of disease in the patient of Hanley et al. (1990) who had a right frontotemporal lesion. Yet he was also impaired in learning unknown faces and objects. A transition from pure prosopagnosia to amnesia for all information concerning a person was reported (Evans et al., 1995) in a patient, who had no other recognition disorders and was affected by a progressive atrophy of the anterior part of the right temporal lobe.

These cases add to the available evidence from associative prosopagnosia (De Renzi et al., 1994) and point to a key role for the right inferomedial temporal lobe in retrieving knowledge about familiar faces.

## Topographical amnesia

This term designates patients who lose their bearings in familiar surroundings, in the absence of confusion, general memory deficit and severe visuospatial disorders. Following Paterson and Zangwill (1945), the inability to find one's way has been traced back to two basic disorders, topographical agnosia, i.e. the failure to recognize buildings, streets and landmarks that assist the subject in localizing a place within a spatial context and topographical amnesia, i.e. the loss of the ability to map the routes and turns into a mental representation that recapitulates the scheme of a pathway (De Renzi, 1982). In such a case, even the identification of landmarks may be of little help, because the patient no longer remembers what spatial information they convey and does not know therefore, whether they mean that he/she must go straightforward, turn left, come back, etc. Topographical disorientation is frequently, but not necessarily, associated with amnesia for famous faces and is mostly associated with a right occipitotemporal lesion (McCarthy et al., 1996). It can occur transiently, either as a selective form of transient amnesic attacks (Stracciari et al., 1994b), or as the early manifestation of a disorder that subsequently evolves towards an Alzheimer disease.

## Semantic amnesia

Contrary to global amnesics, who have an intact verbal and visual lexicon, semantic amnesics have lost knowledge of the meaning of words and their pictorial referents. They differ from aphasics, because their impairment does not extend to non-lexical aspects of language, such as prosody, phonology, grammar and syntax and also involves non-verbal stimuli, and they differ from agnosics, because the deficit is not confined to a single sensory modality. The impairment shows up in naming and verbal comprehension tasks, but it is also apparent in non-verbally based tasks that demand semantic processing of the stimulus (e.g. association and categorization tasks requiring sorting pictures having a semantic relation or belonging to the same category) as in the Hodges and Patterson (1995) semantic battery. When presented with stimulus names, the patient is unable to retrieve the physical and functional features of their reference and to make comparisons between them.

A number of these patients present a surprising dissociation between the severe impairment of certain categories of stimuli and the relative, or even complete, integrity of others. The most frequently reported pattern, first pointed out by Warrington and Shallice (1984), is the living–non-living dissociation, with loss of knowledge of stimuli from natural or biological categories (animals, fruit, vegetables and flowers) and intact knowledge of artefacts. The opposite dissociation – impairment confined to non-living categories – is more rare (Warrington & McCarthy, 1983, 1987). It must be stressed, however, that the living–non-living contrast does not capture the complexity of clinical findings and should be considered a convenient shorthand rather than a rigid boundary. First, in a number of cases the impairment only concerned the animal class. Other living categories were spared or not studied. Secondly, even when the deficit seems to cover the full range of animate things (De Renzi & Lucchelli, 1994), a thorough investigation brings out a pattern of dissociation that does not comply with the living–non-living dichotomy: e.g. body parts (a living category) are frequently preserved and food, which strictly speaking is not a living category, is impaired. Thirdly, in a patient who showed a disruption selective for artificial objects (Warrington & McCarthy, 1987), the deficit mainly concerned manipulable objects and spared non-manipulable objects.

The nature of the dissociation remains a matter of debate. A few authors have claimed that it is an artefact of testing, depending on the lower frequency and familiarity (Funnell & Sheridan, 1992; Stewart et al., 1992) or the greater visual complexity and similarity (Humphreys & Riddoch, 1987) of natural items in comparison with artificial items. However, even when these factors were taken into account, and their influence on the performance partialled out, the animal category remained more impaired (Farah et al., 1991; Laiacona et al., 1993; Sartori et al., 1993). If it is accepted that the difference is genuine, does it point to the anatomical segregation of semantic categories in the brain, or is it secondary to the type of information that plays a crucial role in the identification of living and non-living things, respectively? Most authors have followed Warrington and Shallice (1984) in positing that there are classes of things, like animals, that are mainly discriminated by their perceptual features and others, like artificial objects, whose identification is mainly based on their function. The basic deficit underlying the living category impairment would be the inability to retrieve the perceptual features of stimuli, but while this deficit has devastating consequences for the entities that are defined by their physical properties, it does not substantially affect those that are defined by their function. In agreement with this assumption, there is evidence from the literature (Basso et al., 1988; Silveri & Gainotti, 1988; Farah et al., 1989; De Renzi & Lucchelli, 1994) that patients with living category impairment are unable to retrieve the perceptual features of living things, while they retain knowledge of their functional–contextual attributes. One may ask, however, why a general impairment, such as the failure to retrieve perceptual features, is only apparent with living things and does not emerge for artificial things, even when expressly probed. De Renzi and Lucchelli (1994) speculated that a crucial difference between non-living and living things is that, only in the former, is there congruency between form and function. The shape of artificial objects is strictly determined by the aim they are meant to fulfil, while that of animals (and other living things) has been modelled by nature. The close relation existing in artefacts between these two aspects means that it is possible to rely on the knowledge of an object's functional properties to recover its perceptual features. No comparable compensation is possible for living things and there is, therefore, no means to circumvent the failure of perceptual information to access the semantic store. This hypothesis also accounts for the discrepancies within the living–non-living dichotomy: body parts, which are mainly defined by their function, usually escape the disruption affecting biological entities, while food, which is mainly defined by its physical properties, tends to follow the fate of living things.

Patients showing the reverse dissociation – a more marked impairment for non-living things – are generally affected by severe aphasia and do not lend themselves to exhaustive testing. The nature of their deficit is, consequently, less clearly understood. The syndrome of semantic dementia in which there is a slowly progressive loss of semantic memory in association with focal atrophy of the temporal lobes is discussed elsewhere (see Chapter 7, this volume).

## Focal retrograde amnesia

Global amnesia is characterized by a prevailing deficit in the acquisition of new memories and by a variable degree of impairment of memories that had been stored before the disease. The opposite pattern – dense retrograde amnesia and preserved learning skills – has come to the attention of neuropsychologists in recent years and it still represents a matter of debate. Leaving aside the ancient literature, which is of difficult evaluation, the first modern case has been reported by Roman Campos in 1980. Thirteen years later, Kapur (1993a) could find eight cases and in the following three years at least 13 new cases were published (Yoneda et al., 1992; De Renzi & Lucchelli, 1993; Markowitsch et al., 1993a; Ogden, 1993; Stracciari et al., 1994a; De Renzi et al., 1995; Hunkin et al., 1995; Lucchelli et al., 1995; Maravita et al., 1995; Mattioli et al., 1996; Barbarotto et al., 1996; Evans et al., 1996). The feature common to all these patients is the persistent dissociation between the loss of past memories and the integrity, or at least the much less severe impairment, of learning abilities. Thanks to the latter, patients are able to relearn what they have forgotten, autobiographic episodes included, capitalizing on information acquired from relatives, friends, the media, etc, but they never recover the feeling of familiarity and intimacy associated with personal experiences, and are never able to elaborate on them, beyond what they have been told. In all other respects, patients appear normal.

The extent of retrograde amnesia varies, with respect to both the quality of memories and the life span involved. In a few patients only autobiographic memories were impaired, in others (Kapur et al., 1989) the deficit was more marked for famous facts, while in the majority, both kinds of memories were lost. There are even patients in whom the deficit extends to the recognition of word and object meaning. A temporal gradient of variable length (from 1 to 40 years) has been observed in some patients, while in others amnesia covers their entire life.

A number of factors have been found to be associated with the appearence of the syndrome. In some patients it follows a definite organic disease with documented brain damage: severe head injury with coma, encephalitis, cerebral vasculitis, infarct. There are, however, patients who manifest the sudden loss of retrograde memories, in the absence of a proportionate organic cause. In many of them amnesia was triggered by a mild head trauma, not accompanied by loss of consciousness or any other sign of brain pathology, which was, therefore, unlikely to have caused a lasting damage of brain structures. One would expect the features of the retrograde deficit and its long-term outcome to be different in the two groups, but this is not the case. In the majority of patients, RA appears to be a persistent phenomenon that does not recover with passage of time. There are, however, a few cases of either group, in which a complete recovery occurred within a year after the onset (Lucchelli et al., 1995).

While the clinical profile of the syndrome is known, its interpretation is a conundrum. The main issue of contention is whether it is legitimate to cover under the same label of focal retrograde amnesia patients who show definite evidence of brain damage and patients in whom no apparent organic aetiology can be invoked and for whom a radically different mechanism should be entertained. When confronted with patients who exhibit a dramatic disruption of nervous functions, in the absence of any detectable organic sign, clinicians are prone to invoke the action of psychological mechanisms, either voluntary (malingering), or involuntary (hysteria). It is, therefore, not surprising that some authors were inclined to dispose of the cases of focal retrograde amnesia that occur without a proportionate organic aetiology, by labelling them as psychogenic. However, a psychogenic interpretation rests on weak grounds if it is simply based on the absence of demonstrable organic factors and cannot marshal in its support positive findings, showing that emotional events or life stress were associated with the onset of amnesia and that there were, in the patient's history, clues pointing to a psychological maladjustment. The search for this evidence has been pursued by the authors who have reported these patients, but it has always been negative. In no case was it possible to uncover elements suggestive of primary or secondary gains that the patients could derive from forgetting their past, and no precedent of psychiatric disorders or psychological difficulties could be brought out. It is always possible to argue that probing for the intricacies of human psychology is such a hard task that one can never be confident of having carried it out exhaustively, but it is also true that even if we were successful in bringing out a psychological event or stress preceding amnesia, this would not, of its own, represent unequivocal evidence that the cause of the memory deficit is psychological, since the association might be accidental as it occurs in some organic cases (Kopelman et al., 1994). It is of note that a patient with focal retrograde amnesia who recovered after amytal injection (Stuss & Guzman, 1988) had lost his memories following an episode of encephalitis. The nature of RA without organic damage will probably long remain a subject of different interpretations. The author believes that labelling it as psychogenic is hazardous and proposes to define it with the more neutral term of 'functional'. Although it is often used as tantamount to psychogenic, in its proper sense it means that the lesion affects the function and not the substrate and, as such, it does not claim to have provided an answer to a question that is still unsettled and that would not benefit from a dogmatic definition.

It must be added that even the cases with documented brain damage are not easy to frame in current theories on memory and its anatomical correlates. First, it is hard to understand how a patient can retrieve post-morbid information and fail to retrieve that stored before the disease. The hypothesis of discrete mechanisms underlying old and more recent memories is untenable, because the critical variable determining the fate of memories is not the age of their acquisition, but the chronological position they occupy with respect to the disease, namely, a factor that simply does not exist in normals. Secondly, the location of lesion differs from patient to patient and in most cases it does not involve the structures that are known to constitute the circuit of memory. Markowitsch (1995) advocated a crucial role of the right temporal pole and the anterolateral frontal cortex for the recall of episodic information from long-term memory, but the evidence is flimsy and contradictory.

In conclusion, we are faced with a new clinical picture that can be triggered by different mechanisms and which defies any straightforward interpretation. It can be surmised that the trauma causes a widespread inhibition of the keys of access to the neuronal networks embodying the engrams that had already been stored at the time of amnesia onset, leaving the retrieval mechanism itself undamaged.

## The anatomical correlates of amnesia

The study of amnesia has been of paramount importance to the identification of the cerebral structures that mediate memory. They are located in discrete areas of the brain, which are interconnected and constitute the so called Papez circuit, where information must circulate before it can be permanently stored in the cortex. The elements of this loop are: (i) the hippocampus, which receives and sends information to the associative cortex and whose main subcortical outflow is the fornix; (ii) the fornix, whose anterior pillars end at the mamillary bodies, though some of the hippocampal fibres leave the body of the fornix to project directly to the anterior nucleus of the thalamus and the septal nuclei; (iii) the mamillary bodies, which are connected with the anterior thalamic nuclei, via the mamillothalamic tract; (iv) an alternative route linking the medial temporal lobe with the thalamus is represented by the amygdalofugal fibres that run to the dorsomedial nuclei of the thalamus, which in turn project to the frontal lobe; (v) the anterior thalamic nuclei are interconnected with the retrosplenial cortex, which is linked with the hippocampal region (subiculum and presubiculum).

### Hippocampal amnesia

Probably no single case (including Tan-Tan, whose report by Broca opened a new era in the study of aphasia) has played a role in the history of neuropsychology comparable to that of H.M., a patient who was found by Scoville and Milner (1957) to have become severely amnesic, following a bilateral temporal lobectomy, carried out to relieve his epilepsy. The resection involved the uncus, the amygdala, the anterior two-thirds of the hippocampus and the parahyppocampal gyrus for a distance from the temporal pole of approximately 8 cm, while it spared the temporal neocortex. Subsequent studies of patients with different aetiologies (infarcts, encephalitis, etc.) have fully confirmed the crucial contribution of this region to memory function, although the role of its different structures is still open to question. In humans, the role of the amygdala is probably subsidary (Andersen, 1978; Zola-Morgan & Squire, 1989), and limited to non-verbal memory (Tranel & Hyman, 1990), or to the reactivation of emotionally laden events (Sarter & Markowitsch, 1985), while that of the hippocampus seems to be crucial for learning new memories. This has been confirmed by the study of a few privileged cases with restricted lesions. Anterograde amnesia was severe in a patient with disappearence of the pyramidal cells of both hippocampi, following an anoxic accident (Cummings et al., 1984) and in a patient, affected by Hodgkin's disease, who showed an almost complete bilateral neuronal loss of the amygdala and the hippocampus (Duychaerts et al., 1985). Retrograde memory was remarkably less impaired. In the case of R.B. (Zola-Morgan et al., 1986), the lesion was confined to the entire rostrocaudal extent of the CA1 sector of the hippocampus and caused a clinically disabling anterograde amnesia, which was, however, less marked than in patient H.M., whose damage involved other hippocampal structures.

## Diencephalic amnesia

The medial temporal region has strong connections, via the fornix, with the mamillary bodies, which in turn project to the anterior nuclei of the thalamus, via the mamillothalamic tract. Another thalamic region that has been held responsible for amnesia is the mediodorsal thalamic nuclei regions, which receive a pathway from the ventral amygdala, running adjacent to the mamillothalamic tract (Graff-Radford et al., 1990) and project to the frontal lobes. Which of these structures is mainly responsible for diencephalic amnesia has not been definitely settled, because the lesion often involves more than one. Damage to the mamillary bodies was originally thought to represent the anatomical basis of the alcoholic Korsakoff syndrome, but this notion was subsequently disputed (Victor et al., 1971), since in a few patients with damage confined to these structures there was no memory loss and the main role in Korsakoff amnesia was attributed to the concomitant lesion of the mediodorsal thalamic nuclei. However, in another series of 11 patients, in whom autopsy data were available, mamillary body damage was present in all, while only seven had damage to the dorsomedial nuclei (Brion & Mikol, 1978). Evidence that the thalamic lesion per se can give rise to amnesia is also provided by patients with dorsomedial thalamic infarcts, who often show anterograde amnesia as a prominent symptom (Von Cramon et al., 1985; Gentilini et al., 1987; Graff-Radford et al., 1990; Hodges & McCarthy, 1993). It must be stressed, however, that the lesion also involves the mamillothalamic tract and sometimes extends to the anterior thalamic nuclei, making it difficult to disentangle the role played by damage to these different structures.

The role of the fornix in mnestic process is a matter of controversy. Fornicotomy, carried out in epileptics to control seizure activity, was not followed by marked memory defects (Garcia-Begonchea & Friedman, 1987) and a review of the literature on lesional patients was negative, if the damage did not encroach upon neighbouring structures (Squire & Moore, 1979). However, more recently a few cases showing anterograde amnesia associated with fornix involvement have been reported (Grafman et al., 1985; Gaffan et al., 1991; Calabrese et al., 1995).

### Posterior cingulate and retrosplenial area

A severe amnesic syndrome is thought to be a constant feature of callosal tumours involving the splenium. This association, which was already known to neurologists (Ironside & Guttmacher, 1929), has been confirmed by recent case reports (Valenstein et al., 1987; Rudge & Warrington, 1991). Anterograde amnesia is profound, while retrograde amnesia shows a distinct temporal gradient, dating back to a few years and leaving undamaged more remote memories. It is unlikely that the memory deficit is contingent upon the hemisphere disconnection (except when the left hippocampus is damaged), since the section of the splenial fibres, in the absence of complicating factors and of extracallosal damage, is not followed by a persistent amnesia (Clark & Geffen, 1989). Retrosplenial amnesia has been attributed to the encroachment of the lesion upon the hippocampal–thalamic connections running in the fornix (Rudge & Warrington, 1991), but since fornix damage does not consistently result in memory deficit, Valenstein et al. (1987) surmised that the crucial role was played by damage to the retrosplenial cortex and the posterior cingulate cortex, which would interrupt the fibres linking the anterior thalamus with the hippocampus.

### Basal forebrain and septal nuclei

The participation in memory processes of the basal forebrain, a region comprising a set of structures located in the medial and ventral cortex of the hemispheres, is suggested by the frequent occurrence of memory disorders following the rupture of anterior communicating artery aneurysms, when they are associated with postoperative spasm or an infarction in the distribution of anterior communicating artery perforators (Alexander & Freedman, 1984; Vilkki, 1985). There is increasing consensus that the crucial area is the region of the septum, which contains lateral and medial septal nuclei, the nucleus of the diagonal band of Broca and the nucleus basalis of Meynert. The neurons of these nuclei are cholinergic and project to the

**Table 8.1.** Causes of relatively pure amnesia

Neurodegenerative
  Early Alzheimer's disease
  Subcortical diseases (Huntington's chorea, progressive supranuclear palsy)
  Slowly progressive amnesia

Vascular
  Posterior cerebral artery infarction
  Bilateral thalamic infarction
  Anterior communicating artery aneurysms
  Anoxic encephalopathy

Infective and inflammatory
  Herpes simplex virus encephalitis
  Paraneoplastic limbic encephalitis

Trauma
  Closed head injury
  Following fornix damage usually in association with surgery on the IIIrd ventricle
    (colloid cysts, etc.)

Alcohol and deficiency states
  Korsakoff's syndrome

hippocampus, the amygdala and the neocortex. The connections with the hippo-campus have their main origin in the nucleus of Broca, are reciprocal and travel through the precommissural fornix. Those with the amygdala and the cortex arise from the nucleus of Meynert, whose degeneration has been held partly responsible for the memory deficits of Alzheimer's disease (Whitehouse et al., 1981). It is con-ceivable that the reduction of the cholinergic output from the damaged septal nuclei to the medial temporal structures and the neocortex results in the dysfunction of the latter structures (see Chapter 5, this volume for further discussion of this topic).

**Aetiology of amnesia** (see Table 8.1)

Amnesia is the symptom that most commonly brings a patient affected by Alzheimer's disease (AD) to medical consultation and the doctor should always suspect this aetiology, in the presence of a patient presenting a slowly progressive forgetfulness, especially if the deficit also extends to memory for words. A thorough neuropsychological assessment usually points out that the impairment also involves other cognitive domains, intelligence, language, visuospatial and con-structive skills, etc. The substitution of neurons by neurofibrillary tangles and neu-ritic plaques that represent the bulk of AD pathology affects the hippocampal region (particularly layer II and IV of the entorhinal cortex and the subiculum), the nucleus basalis of Meynert and the higher order association cortex at an early stage of disease.

Memory disorders are a frequent component of the symptomatology of other neurodegenerative diseases (Huntington's chorea, progressive supranuclear palsy, etc.), but they are less marked in those mainly affecting the subcortical structures and always appear in the context of a syndrome involving several cognitive and non-cognitive systems. Quite recently a form of slowly developing amnesia that at a certain point stops its progression and remains unchanged for years has been pointed out (Kritchevsky & Squire, 1993; Lucchelli et al., 1994; Tanabe et al., 1994; Miceli et al., 1996). Other cognitive abilities are intact. This clinical pattern has parallels to the other forms of so-called 'focal dementia' syndromes including slowly progressive aphasia (Mesulam, 1982), apraxia, or agnosia (De Renzi, 1986), all characterized by impairment confined to one cognitive domain, but differs in that the deficit appears to stabilize. MRI and PET studies have shown atrophy and/or hypometabolism of the hippocampal region. New case reports, more prolonged follow-up and pathological data are necessary, before attempting a classification of this form. Vascular lesions affecting areas that subserve memory functions give rise to pretty pure amnesic syndromes. A memory deficit is a frequent component of the syndrome ensuing the left posterior cerebral artery infarct (De Renzi et al., 1987b; Servan et al., 1994), which may involve the dorsomedial nucleus of the thalamus or the hippocampus or both. When the infarct is bilateral, not a rare event, given the common origin of the posterior cerebral arteries from the basilar artery, the memory deficit is particularly severe. Also the infarcts of the septal area, which commonly accompany the rupture of anterior communicating artery aneurysms, give rise to an amnesic syndrome. Anoxic encephalopathy, following a cardiac arrest, or strangulation, causes a selective damage to the hippocampus (Zola-Morgan et al., 1986), producing a classical amnesic syndrome.

Herpes simplex encephalitis typically produces necrosis of the inferomedial areas of the temporal and frontal lobes. The hippocampus, the amygdala, the parahippocampal gyrus and the posterior orbital cortices are damaged bilaterally, though sometimes asymmetrically. Damage may extend to the cingulate gyri and the anterolateral and anteroinferior temporal neocortex. The disease used to be fatal, but, since effective antiviral therapy has been introduced, a remarkable number of patients survive, some with complete recovery and others with cognitive deficits that predominantly impair memory. The amnesic impairment is variable, depending on the location and extension of brain damage, but basically two profiles can be identified: one corresponds to the typical amnesic syndrome with severe learning defect and retrograde amnesia for facts and autobiographic episodes, but preservation of the lexicon and perceptuomotor skills. The other is featured by a profound deficit of semantic knowledge that covers the lexicon and object recognition and, as has been mentioned above, may preferentially affect living things. Memory impairment for facts and events is often associated, but in at least one case autobiographic memory was completely preserved (De Renzi et al., 1987a). Closed head injury, accompanied by loss of consciousness, is commonly followed by a period of post-traumatic amnesia and often by residual memory deficit, whose intensity is related to the severity of trauma and the locus of lesion (Levin, 1989). Retrograde amnesia covering a brief period preceding the trauma (usually not longer than 30 minutes) is frequent. More rarely it dates back to years and even decades, but shows a tendency to shrink (Benson & Geschwind, 1967).

Chronic alcohol abuse represents the main aetiology of Korsakoff syndrome, but rarely is the memory deficit as pure as that observed in hippocampal lesion.

## Conclusion

The amnesic syndrome, although rare in clinical practice, remains extremely important theoretically for understanding the organisation and neural basis of memory. There is still debate as to whether the amnesic syndrome represents a unitary entity, but there is clear variability in the extent of remote memory loss depending upon the site of pathology.

A number of variants of the classic amnesic syndrome have been described in the recent past, including prosopamnesia (inability to recognize previously familiar faces), topographical amnesia and semantic amnesia. Recently, much interest has been directed to the entity of focal retrograde amnesia which is now clearly established as a manifestation of brain disease. Despite a century of research, much remains to be learnt about human memory disorders.

## REFERENCES

Alexander, M.P. & Freedman, M. (1984). Amnesia after anterior communicating artery aneurysm rupture. *Neurology*, **34**, 752–7.

Andersen, R. (1978). Cognitive changes after amigdalotomy. *Neuropsychologia*, **16**, 439–51.

Barbarotto, R., Laiacona, M. & Cocchini, G. (1996). A case of simulated, psychogenic or focal pure retrograde amnesia: did an entire life become unconscious ? *Neuropsychologia*, **34**, 575–85.

Basso, A., Capitani, E. & Laiacona, M. (1988). Progressive language impairment without dementia: a case with isolated category specific semantic defect. *Journal of Neurology, Neurosurgery and Psychiatry*, **51**, 1201–7.

Benson, D.F. & Geschwind, N. (1967). Shrinking retrograde amnesia. *Journal of Neurology, Neurosurgery and Psychiatry*, **30**, 539–44.

Benson, D.F., Djenderedjian, A., Miller, B.L., Pachana, L.A., Chang, L., Itti, L. & Mena, I. (1996). Neural basis of confabulation. *Neurology*, **46**, 1239–43.

Berlyne, N. (1972). Confabulation. *British Journal of Psychiatry*, **120**, 31–9.

Borrini, G., Dall' Ora, P., Della Sala, S., Marinelli, R. & Spinnler, H. (1989). Autobiographic memory. Sensitivity to age and education of a standardized enquiry. *Psychological Medicine*, **19**, 215–24.

Brion, S. & Mikol, J. (1978). Atteinte du noyau laterale dorsale du thalamus et syndrome de Korsakoff alcoholique. *Journal of Neurological Science*, **38**, 249–61.

Calabrese, P., Markowitsch, H.J., Harders, A.G., Scholz, M. & Gehlen, W. (1995). Fornix damage and memory. A case report. *Cortex*, **31**, 555–64.

Clark, C.R. & Geffen, G.M. (1989). Corpus callosum surgery and recent memory. A review. *Brain*, **12**, 165–75.

Corkin, S. (1968). Acquisition of motor skill after bilateral medial temporal-lobe excision. *Neuropsychologia*, **6**, 255–65.

Cummings, J.L., Tomiyasu, U., Read, S. & Benson, F. (1984). Amnesia with hippocampal lesions after cardiopulmonary arrest. *Neurology*, **34**, 679–81.

Dalla Barba, G., Cipolotti, L. & Denes, F. (1990). Autobiographic memory loss and confabulation in Korsakoff' s syndrome. *Cortex*, **26**, 525–34.

Damasio, A., Graf-Radford, N., Eslinger, P., Damasio, H. & Kassel, N. (1985). Amnesia following basal forebrain lesion. *Archives of Neuro*logy, **42**, 263–71.

De Renzi, E. (1982). *Disorders of Space Exploration and Cognition*. Chichester, UK: John Wiley.

De Renzi, E. (1986). Slowly progressive visual agnosia or apraxia without dementia. *Cortex*, **22**, 171–80.

De Renzi, E. & Lucchelli, F. (1993). Dense retrograde amnesia, intact learning capability and abnormal forgetting rate: a consolidation deficit ? *Cortex*, **29**, 449–66.

De Renzi, E. & Lucchelli, F. (1994). Are semantic systems separately represented in the brain? The case of living category impairment. *Cortex*, **30**, 3–25.

De Renzi, E., Liotti, M. & Nichelli, P. (1987a). Semantic amnesia with preservation of autobiographic memory. A case report. *Cortex*, **23**, 575–97.

De Renzi, E., Zambolin, A. & Crisi, G. (1987b). The pattern of neuropsychological impairment associated with left posterior cerebral artery infarcts. *Brain*, 110, 1099–116.

De Renzi, E., Perani, D., Carlesimo, G.A., Silveri, M.C. & Fazio, F. (1994). Prosopagnosia can be associated with damage confined to the right hemisphere. An MRI and PET study and a review of the literature. *Neuropsychologia*, **32**, 893–902.

De Renzi, E., Lucchelli, F., Muggia, S. & Spinnler, H. (1995). Persistent retrograde amnesia following a minor trauma. *Cortex*, **31**, 531–42.

Dusoir, H., Kapur, N., Bymes, D., McKinstry, S. & Hoare, R.D. (1990). The role of diencephalic pathology in human memory disorder: evidence from a penetrating paranasal brain injury. *Brain*, **113**, 1695–706.

Duychaerts, C., Derouesné, C., Signoret, J.L., Gray, F., Escourolle, R. & Castaigne, P. (1985). Bilateral and limited amygdalohippocampal lesions causing a pure amnesic syndrome. *Annals of Neuro*logy, **18**, 314–19.

Ellis, H.D. (1989). Past and recent studies of prosopagnosia. In *Developments in Clinical and Experimental Neuropsychology*, ed. J.R. Crawford & D.M. Parker, pp.51–165. New York: Plenum Press.

Ellis, A.W., Young, A.W. & Critchley, E.M.R. (1989). Loss of memory for people following temporal lobe damage. *Brain*, **112**, 1469– 83.

Evans, J.J., Heggs, A.J., Antoun, N. & Hodges, J.R. (1995). Progressive prosopagnosia associated with selective right temporal lobe atrophy. A new syndrome ? *Brain*, **118**, 1–13.

Evans, J.J., Breen, E.K., Antoun, N. & Hodges, J.R. (1996). Focal retrograde amnesia for autobiographical events following cerebral vasculitis: a connectionist account. *Neurocase*, **2**, 1–11.

Farah, M.J., Hammond, K.M., Metha, Z. & Ratcliff, G. (1989). Category-specificity and modality-specificity in semantic memory. *Neuropsychologia*, **27**, 193–200.

Farah, M.J., McMullen, P. & Meyer, M.M. (1991). Can recognition of living things be selectively impaired ? *Neuropsychologia*, **29**, 185–91.

Fisher, C.M. & Adams, R.D. (1964). Transient global amnesia. *Acta Neurologica Scandinavica*, **40**, 7–83.

Funnell, E. & Sheridan, J. (1992). Categories of knowledge ? Unfamiliar aspects of living and non-living things. *Cognitive Neuropsychology*, **9**, 135–53.

Gabrieli, J.D.E., Cohen, N.J. & Corkin, S. (1988). The impaired learning of semantic knowledge following bilateral medialtemporal-lobe resection. *Brain Cognition*, **7**, 525–39.

Gaffan, E.A., Gaffan, D. & Hodges, J.R. (1991). Amnesia following damage to the fornix and other sites. *Brain*, **114**, 1297–313.

Garcia-Begonchea, F. & Friedman, W.A. (1987). Persistent memory loss following section of the anterior fornix in humans: a historical review. *Surgical Neurology*, **27**, 361–4.

Gentilini, M., De Renzi, E. & Crisi, G. (1987). Bilateral paramedian thalamic artery infarcts: report of eight cases. *Journal of Neurology, Neurosurgery and Psychiatry*, **50**, 900–9.

Graff-Radford, N. R., Tranel, D., Van Hoesen, G.W. & Brandt, J.P. (1990). Diencephalic amnesia. *Brain*, **113**, 1–25.

Grafman, J., Salazar, A.M., Weingartner, H., Vance, S.C. & Ludlow, C. (1985). Isolated impairment of memory following a penetrating lesion of the fornix cerebri. *Archives of Neurology*, **42**, 1162–8.

Haist, F., Shimamura, A.P. & Squire, L.R. (1992). On the relationship between recall and recognition memory. *Journal of Experimental Psychology: Learning, Memory and Cognition*, **18**, 691–702.

Hanley, J.R., Young, A.W. & Pearson, N.A. (1989). Defective recognition of familiar people. *Cognitive Neuropsychology*, **6**, 179–210.

Hanley, J.R., Pearson, N.A. & Young, A.W. (1990). Impaired memory for new visual forms. *Brain*, **113**, 1131–48.

Hécaen, H. (1981). The neuropsychology of face recognition. In *Perceiving and Remembering Faces*, ed. G. Davies, H. Ellis & G. Shepherd. London: Academic Press.

Hodges, J.R. & McCarthy, R.A. (1993). Autobiographic amnesia resulting from paramedian thalamic infarction. *Brain*, **116**, 921–40.

Hodges, J.R. & Patterson, K.E. (1995). Is semantic memory consistently impaired early in the course of Alzheimer's disease? Neuroanatomical and diagnostic implications. *Neuropsychologia*, 33, 441–59.

Humphreys, G.W. & Riddoch, M.J. (1987). On telling your fruit from your vegetables: a consideration of category-specific deficits after brain damage. *Trends in Neuroscience*, **10**, 145–8.

Hunkin, N.M., Parkin, A.Q.J., Bradley, V.A., Burrows, E.H., Aldrich, F.K., Jansari, A. & Burdon-Cooper, C. (1995). Focal retrograde amnesia following closed head injury: a case study and theoretical account. *Neuropsychologia*, **33**, 509–23.

Ironside, R. & Guttmacher, M. (1929). The corpus callosum and its tumours. *Brain*, **52**, 442–83.

Kapur, N. (1993a). Focal retrograde amnesia in neurological disease: a critical review. *Cortex*, **29**, 217–34.

Kapur, N. (1993b). Transient epileptic amnesia. A clinical update and a reformulation. *Journal of Neurology, Neurosurgery and Psychiatry*, **56**, 1184–90.

Kapur, N., Young, A., Bateman, D. & Kennedy, F. (1989). Focal retrograde amnesia: a long-term clinical and neuropsychological follow-up. *Cortex*, **25**, 387–402.

Kapur, N., Thompson, S., Cook, P., Lang, L. & Brice, J. (1996). Anterograde but not retrograde memory loss following combined mammillary body and medial thalamic lesions. *Neuropsychologia*, **34**, 1–8.

Kopelman, M.D. (1987). Two types of confabulations. *Journal of Neurology, Neurosurgery and Psychiatry*, **50**, 1482–7.

Kopelman, M.D., Wilson, B.A. & Baddeley, A.D. (1989). The autobiographical memory interview: a new assessment of autobiographical and personal semantic memory in amnesic patients. *Journal of Clinical and Experimental Neuropsychology*, **11**, 724–44.

Kopelman, M.D., Panayotopoulos, C.P. & Lewis, P. (1994). Transient epileptic amnesia differentiated from psychogenic 'fugues': neuropsychological, EEG and PET findings. *Journal of Neurology, Neurosurgery and Psychiatry*, **57**, 1002–4.

Kritchevsky, M. & Squire, L.S. (1993). Permanent global amnesia with unknown etiology. *Neurology*, **43**, 326–32.

Laiacona, M., Barbarotto, R. & Capitani, E. (1993). Perceptual and associative knowledge in category specific impairment of semantic memory: a study of two cases. *Cortex*, **29**, 727–40.

Levin, H.S. (1989). Memory deficit after closed head injury. In *Handbook of Neuropsychology*, ed. F. Boller & J. Grafman, vol. 3, pp. 183–207. Amsterdam: Elsevier.

Lucchelli, F., De Renzi, E., Perani, D. & Fazio, F. (1994). Primary amnesia of insidious onset with subsequent stabilization. *Journal of Neurology, Neurosurgery and Psychiatry*, **57**, 1366–70.

Lucchelli, F., Muggia, S. & Spinnler, H. (1995). The 'Petites Madeleines' phenomenon in two amnesic patients. Sudden recovery of forgotten memories. *Brain*, **113**, 1673–94.

McCarthy, R.A., Evans, J.J. & Hodges, J.R. (1996). Topographical amnesia: spatial memory disorder, building agnosia or category specific semantic memory impairment. *Journal of Neurology, Neurosurgery and Psychiatry*, **60**, 318–25.

Maravita, A., Spadoni, M., Mazzucchi, A. & Parma, M. (1995). A new case of retrograde amnesia with abnormal forgetting rate. *Cortex*, **31**, 653–68.

Markowitsch, H.J. (1995). Which brain regions are critically involved in the retrieval of old episodic memory ? *Brain Research Review*, **21**, 117–27.

Markowitsch, H.J., Calabrese, P., Liess, J., Haupts, M., Durwen, H.F. & Gehlen, W. (1993a). Retrograde amnesia after traumatic injury of the fronto-temporal cortex. *Journal of Neurology, Neurosurgery and Psychiatry*, **56**, 988–92.

Markowitsch, H.J., Von Cramon, D.Y. & Schuri,U. (1993b). Mnestic performance profile of a bilateral diencephalic infarct patient with preserved intelligence and severe amnesic disturbances. *Journal of Clinical and Experimental Neuropsychology*, **15**, 627–52.

Mattioli, F., Grassi, F., Perani, D., Cappa, S.F., Miozzo, A. & Fazio, F. (1996). Persistent post-traumatic retrograde amnesia. A neuropsychological and (18F) FDG PET study. *Cortex*, **32**, 121–9.

Mercer, B., Wapner, W., Gardner, H. & Benson, D.F. (1977). A study of confabulation. *Archives of Neurology*, 34: 429–33.

Mesulam, M.M. (1982). Slowly progressive aphasia without generalized dementia. *Annals of Neurology*, **11**, 592–8.

Miceli, G., Colosimo, C., Daniele, A., Perani, D. & Fazio, F. (1996). Isolated amnesia with slow onset and stable course, without ensuing dementia: MRI and PET data and six-year neuropsychological follow-up. *Dementia*, **7**, 104–10.

Michel, D., Laurent, B., Foyatier, N., Blanc, A. & Portafaix, M. (1982) Infarctus thalamique gauche. Etude de la mémoire et du langage. *Revue Neurologique*, **138**, 533–50.

Milner, B. (1972). Disorders of learning and memory after temporal lobe lesions in man. *Clinical Neurosurgery*, **19**, 421–46.

Ogden, J.A. (1993). Visual object agnosia, prosopagnosia, achromatopsia-loss of visual imagery and autobiographic amnesia following recovery from cortical blindness: case M.H. *Neuropsychologia*, **31**, 571–89.

Paterson, A. & Zangwill, O.L. (1945). A case of topographical disorientation associated with a unilateral cerebral lesion. *Brain*, **68**, 188–211.

Roman Campos, G., Poser, C.M. & Wood, F.B. (1980). Persistent retrograde memory deficit after transient global amnesia. *Cortex*, **16**, 509–18.

Rudge, P. & Warrington, E.K. (1991). Selective impairment of memory and visual perception in splenial tumours. *Brain*, **114**, 349–60.

Sarter, M. & Markowitsch, H.J. (1985). The amygdala' s role in human mnemonic processing. *Cortex*, **21**, 7–24.

Sartori, G., Miozzo, M. & Job, R. (1993). Category-specific naming impairment ? Yes. *Quarterly Journal of Experimental Psychology*, **46A**, 489–504.

Scoville, W.B. & Milner, B. (1957). Loss of recent memory after bilateral hippocampal lesions. *Journal of Neurology, Neurosurgery and Psychiatry*, **20**, 11–21.

Servan, J., Verstichel, P., Catala, M. & Rancurel, G. (1994). Syndrome amnésiques et fabulations au cours d' infarctus du territoire de l' artére cérébrale postérieure. *Revue Neurologique*, **150**, 201–8.

Silveri, M.C. & Gainotti, G. (1988). Interaction between vision and language in category-specific semantic impairment. *Cognitive Neuropsychology*, **5**, 677–709.

Speedie, L.J. & Heilman, K.M. (1982). Amnesic disturbance following infarction of the left dorsomedial nucleus of the thalamus. *Neuropsychologia*, **20**, 597–604.

Squire, L.R. & Moore, R.Y. (1979). Dorsal thalamic lesion in a noted case of human memory dysfunction. *Annals of Neurology*, **6**, 503–6.

Squire, L.R., Amaral, D.G, Zola-Morgan, S., Kritchevsky, M. & Press, G. (1989). Description of brain injury in the amnesic patient N.A. based on magnetic resonance imaging. *Experimental Neurology*, **105**, 23–35.

Stewart, F., Parkin, A.J. & Hunkin, N.M. (1992). Naming impairments following recovery from herpes simplex encephalitis: category-specific? *Quarterly Journal of Psychology*, **44A**, 261–84.

Stracciari, A., Ghidoni, E., Guarino, M., Poletti, M. & Pazzaglia, P. (1994a). Post-traumatic retrograde amnesia with selective impairment of autobiographic memory. *Cortex*, **30**, 459–68.

Stracciari, A., Lorusso, S. & Pazzaglia, P. (1994b). Transient topographical amnesia. *Journal of Neurology, Neurosurgery and Psychiatry*, **57**, 1423–5.

Stuss, D.T. & Guzman, D.A. (1988). Severe remote memory loss with minimal anterograde amnesia: a clinical note. *Brain and Cognition*, **8**, 21–30.

Stuss, D.T., Alexander, M.P., Lieberman, A. & Levine, H. (1978). An extraordinary form of confabulation. *Neurology*, **28**, 1166–72.

Tanabe, H., Kazui, H., Ikeda, M., Hashikawa, K., Hashimoto, M., Yamada, N. & Eguchi, Y. (1994). Slowly progressive amnesia without dementia. *Neuropathology*, **14**, 105–14.

Tranel, D. & Hyman, B.T. (1990). Neuropsychological correlates of bilateral amygdala damage. *Archives of Neurology*, **47**, 349–55.

Tulving, E. (1983). *Elements of Episodic Memory*. Oxford: Oxford University Press.

Valenstein, E., Bowers, D., Verfaellie, M., Heilman, K.M., Day, A. & Watson, R.T. (1987). Retrosplenial amnesia. *Brain*, **110**, 1631–46.

Verfaellie, M., Croce, P. & Millberg, W.P. (1995a). The role of episodic memory in semantic learning: an examination of vocabulary acquisition in a patient with amnesia due to encephalitis. *Neurocase*, **1**, 291–304.

Verfaellie, M., Reiss, L. & Roth, H.D. (1995b). Knowledge of new English vocabulary in amnesia: an examination of premorbidly acquired semantic memory. *Journal of International Neuropsychological Society*, **1**, 443–53.

Victor, M., Adams, R.D. & Collins, G.H. (1971). *The Wernicke–Korsakoff Syndrome: A Clinical and Pathological Study of 245 Patients, 82 with Post-Mortem Examination*. Oxford: Blackwell.

Vilkki, J. (1985). Amnesic syndromes after surgery of anterior communicating artery aneurysms. *Cortex*, **21**, 431–44.

Volpe, B.T. & Hirst, W. (1983). The characterization of an amnesic syndrome following hypoxic ischemic injury. *Archives of Neurology*, **40**, 436–40.

Volpe, B.T., Holtzman, J.D. & Hirst, W. (1986). Further characterization of patients with amnesia after cardiac arrest: preserved recognition memory. *Neurology*, **36**, 408–11.

Von Cramon, D.Y., Hebel, N. & Schuri, U. (1985). A contribution to the anatomical basis of thalamic amnesia. *Brain*, **108**, 993–1008.

Warrington, E.K. & McCarthy, R.A. (1983). Category specific access dysphasia. *Brain*, **106**, 859–78.

Warrington, E.K. & Shallice, T. (1984). Category specific semantic impairments. *Brain*, **107**, 829–54.

Warrington, E.K. & McCarthy, R.A. (1987). Categories of knowledge: further fractionations and an attempted integration. *Brain*, **110**, 1273–96.

Whitehouse, P.J., Price, D.L., Clark, A.W., Coyle, J.T. & De Long, M.R. (1981). Alzheimer disease: evidence for selective loss of cholinergic neurons in the nucleus basalis. *Annals of Neurology*, **10**, 122–6.

Yoneda, Y., Yamadori, A., Mori, E. & Yamashima, H. (1992). Isolated prolonged retrograde amnesia. *European Neurology*, **32**, 340–2.

Zola Morgan, S., Squire, L.R. & Amaral, D.G. (1986). Human amnesia and the temporal medial lesion: enduring memory impairment following a bilateral lesion limited to field CA1 of the hippocampus. *Journal of Neuroscience*, **6**, 2950–67.

Zola-Morgan, S., Squire, L.R. & Amaral, D.G. (1989). Lesions of the amygdala that spare adjacent cortical regions do not impair memory or exacerbate the impairment following lesions of the hippocampal formation. *Journal of Neuroscience*, **9**, 1922–36.

# 9

# Transient global amnesia and transient epileptic amnesia

Adam Zeman and John R. Hodges

## Historical introduction

Fisher and Adams (1964) coined the term 'transient global amnesia' (TGA) to describe a syndrome which was reported independently by several authors in the 1950s (Bender, 1956; Guyotat & Courjon, 1956). This profound but temporary 'defect of memory, involving the events of the recent past and the present', had probably been classified previously as a manifestation of hysteria (Hodges, 1991). Once recognized, the syndrome proved highly distinctive and over 1500 cases have been described (Frederiks, 1993).

Many years before the delineation of TGA, Hughling-Jackson's classical description of the case of a physician with epilepsy, Dr Z., suggested that amnesia for episodes of complex and well-integrated behaviour can be a manifestation of temporal lobe epilepsy (TLE, Hughlings-Jackson, 1889). Fisher and Adams speculated that TGA might result from seizure activity disrupting 'the recording and recall of recent events'. Subsequent research, outlined below, has shown that true TGA does not have an epileptic basis, but has also confirmed that epilepsy can cause a distinctive variety of transient amnesia. Numerous terms have been applied to episodes of epileptic amnesia including pure amnestic seizures (Palmini et al., 1992), ictal amnesia (Rowan, 1991), epileptic amnesic attacks (Pritchard et al., 1985; Galassi et al., 1986) and epileptic transient amnesia (Stracciari et al., 1990). The term suggested recently by Kapur, transient epileptic amnesia (TEA, Kapur, 1993), has been adopted, which highlights the similarity of this syndrome to, but also its distinction from, TGA.

In this chapter the clinical and neuropsychological features of TGA and TEA are reviewed and contrasted, their pathophysiology discussed and an approach to the management of patients with transient amnesia is outlined.

## Transient global amnesia

### Definition

TGA is a distinctive syndrome of profound but transient amnesia lasting for some hours. During the attack sufferers are unable to acquire new lasting memories,

**Table 9.1.** Diagnositc criteria for TGA

1. Attacks must be witnessed.
2. There must be clear-cut anterograde amnesia during the attack.
3. There must be no clouding of consciousness or loss of personal identity, and the cognitive impairment must be limited to amnesia.
4. There should be no associated focal neurological symptoms or signs.
5. Epileptic features must be absent.
6. Attacks must resolve within 24 hours.
7. Patients with recent head injury or known active epilepsy are excluded.

although immediate or 'working' memory is intact. This anterograde amnesia leads to a permanent memory gap for the period of the attack. The amnesia is global in the sense that memory for both new verbal and new non-verbal material is severely impaired. Sufferers also lose access to past memories: this retrograde amnesia later resolves almost completely. Awareness of personal identity is always preserved. The criteria used to define TGA have varied from series to series, helping to explain some differences of opinion about the syndrome described below. Table 9.1 lists the strict diagnostic criteria used in the Oxford study for cases of 'pure' TGA (Hodges, 1991).

**Epidemiology and clinical features**

TGA is a condition of later life, with a mean age of around 60 years (Hodges, 1991). Attacks below the age of 40 are very rare. Men and women are equally affected. Estimates of incidence range from three to ten cases/100 000/year (Frederiks, 1993). Familial cases of TGA have been described but the vast majority are sporadic. Most patients experience a single attack but there is an annual risk of recurrence of around 3% (Hodges, 1991; Frederiks, 1993). Risk factors for TGA are discussed below.

Attacks begin abruptly, and sufferers may be aware at the outset that something is amiss with their memory. They may appear perplexed and are invariably disoriented, in time, and often in place, but never in person. They typically question their companions repetitively about their immediate circumstances, rapidly forgetting the answers they are given. Their remarks also reveal some impairment of recall for events preceding the attack: in contrast to the anterograde amnesia which is invariably severe, this retrograde amnesia may vary in extent from a few hours to many years. Although sufferers remain able to perform complex manoeuvres, such as driving, bell ringing and ballroom dancing, several authors have noted a 'flattening' of affect. Working memory, required, for example, for immediate repetition of a sentence is unimpaired. Overt distress and agitation occasionally develop. A minority of patients complain of headache, nausea, sleepiness and non-specific dizziness. After some hours, typically 4–6 and almost always less than 12, the symptomatic impairment of memory gradually resolves, the retrograde component shrinking along a temporal gradient from the remote to the recent past. There is a permanent dense memory gap for the period of the attack, and, as a rule, for a few hours preceding the attack. There is evidence from neuropsychological testing, discussed below, that a subclinical impairment of memory may persist after the attack.

Attacks of TGA can follow a wide variety of stresses, including strenuous exertion, sexual intercourse, immersion in water, pain and emotive events. A recent case control study (Inzitari et al., 1997) has confirmed this observation, and supplied some evidence that phobic personality traits may predispose to attacks of TGA.

## Neuropsychology

Neuropsychological testing during attacks has confirmed that amnesia is much the most striking deficit in TGA, and is often the only impairment (Kritchevsky et al., 1988; Kritchevsky & Squire, 1989; Hodges, 1991, 1994; Evans et al., 1993). Some authors have reported mild impairments of naming, of the reproduction of complex geometric figures and of performance on tests of frontal lobe function, such as verbal fluency for words beginning with certain letters. These additional deficits are relatively minor, inconsistent and unlikely to be causally related to the primary disorder of memory; they do, however, hint that the process which gives rise to TGA is not always confined to structures subserving memory.

Unlike anterograde amnesia, which is invariably dense, the extent of retrograde amnesia varies widely from case to case, from a few hours to 40 years in six personally studied cases (Hodges, 1991). Recall for more recent events is more severely affected than recall for remote events. The retrograde amnesia resolves almost entirely after the attack. Taken together, these findings have the theoretical implication that retrograde amnesia with a temporal gradient can be caused by temporary failure of memory retrieval. It is of interest that patients have particular difficulty in assigning a temporal order to public events which they are able recognize, and in recalling episodic details about personal events which they can describe in bare outline (Evans et al., 1993). Cueing appears to facilitate the retrieval of personal memories during attacks of TGA. The permanent 'memory gap' which often remains for events occurring during the few hours before the onset of TGA suggests that the memory for such events is peculiarly vulnerable to the underlying dysfunction.

While a profound temporary impairment of declarative anterograde memory is the neuropsychological hallmark of TGA, there is evidence that several other aspects of memory are unaffected. It has already been noted that immediate or working memory remains intact. Recent reports suggest that it is possible to acquire new implicit or procedural memories during episodes of TGA (Goldenberg et al., 1991; Kazui et al., 1995). Semantic memory in TGA has received little detailed attention but is not overtly impaired (Hodges, 1991, 1994; Goldenberg, 1995).

Serial testing has shown that recovery from an episode of TGA takes at least 24 hours and sometimes continues over days or months. There is also evidence for a subtle, subclinical but permanent impairment of anterograde verbal memory and of remote memory in some patients following TGA (Hodges & Oxbury, 1990). Whether this results from, or predisposes to, TGA is uncertain: serial study of patients with successive attacks could resolve this issue, but such patients are rare.

## Pathophysiology and aetiology

The amnesia which occurs transiently in TGA strikingly resembles the permanent 'amnesic syndrome' described in, for example, H.M., the intensively studied Canadian patient who underwent bilateral medial temporal lobectomy for epilepsy, in 'Clive', the post-encephalitic patient featured on British TV, and in individuals with Korsakoff's amnesia. The classical amnesic syndrome can follow either bilateral damage to medial temporal structures, in particular the hippocampal formation and parahippocampal gyrus, or bilateral damage to the mamillary bodies, thalamus or basal forebrain nuclei which are linked with the medial temporal structures, in part via the 'circle of Papez' (see Chapters 4 and 8, this volume). It is generally supposed therefore, that TGA results from temporary bilateral inactivation of some part of this system. The pathophysiology and aetiology of TGA remain uncertain, but three main hypotheses have been advanced.

### Epilepsy

Fisher and Adams (1964) initially suspected that TGA was a type of epilepsy. This now appears very unlikely. Epilepsy causes recurent episodes of neurological dysfunction while most patients have only a single episode of TGA (Hodges, 1991). The EEG is normal or shows only non-specific abnormalities in the great majority of patients with TGA both during and after their attacks (Miller et al., 1987). Finally, the clinical phenomena which are now associated with transient epileptic amnesia differ from those of transient global amnesia. It seems reasonable therefore, to conclude that TGA is not a variety of epilepsy. If an EEG performed during or after an episode of transient amnesia reveals an epileptiform focus in one or both temporal lobes, the diagnosis is likely instead to be TEA, which we describe in detail below.

### Transient thrombo-embolic ischaemia

Permanent amnesia sometimes results from cerebral infarction in the territory of the posterior cerebral arteries, which provide the predominant blood supply to the limbic structures mediating memory described above (Graff-Radford et al., 1990; Hodges & McCarthy, 1993). The observation that transient ischaemia in this vascular territory can give rise to transient amnesia naturally suggested the possibility that TGA might be a form of thromboembolic transient ischaemic attack (TIA). Observations in some early series of patients with TGA supported this hypothesis, but in retrospect this was probably due to the inclusion of patients who had neurological symptoms and signs suggestive of brainstem or diencephalic ischaemia as well as transient amnesia. More recent case-control studies, using stricter diagnostic criteria, like those stated in Table 9.1, have shown clear-cut epidemiological differences between patients with strictly defined TGA and TIAs: (i) risk factors for stroke, such as ischaemic heart disease and a history of smoking, are strongly associated with TIAs but are no more common among patients with TGA than in the general population; (ii) TGA has a benign prognosis, while patients with TIAs are at a considerably elevated risk of major vascular events and death from vascular causes. Thus while there is no doubt that 'transient ischaemic amnesia' can occur in conjunction with other features of transient ischaemia in the posterior cerebral circulation, it is not the cause of TGA.

### Migraine

Case-control studies have indicated that migraine is more common among patients with TGA than among healthy matched controls. For example, in Hodges' series 30% of patients gave a history suggestive of common or classical migraine in the past, and 25% of patients satisfied strict research criteria for the diagnosis of migraine. The corresponding frequencies in matched healthy controls were 17% and 12% (Hodges, 1991). Headache and nausea occasionally accompany TGA. Their absence does not exclude a migrainous cause for neurological disturbance: focal neurological symptoms in migraineurs can occur independently of headache and this is not uncommon in the elderly (Fisher, 1980). However, TGA most commonly occurs as a solitary event in patients without headache at the time or a history of migraine in the past. It would, therefore, be premature to conclude that TGA is, in general, a form of 'isolated migraine accompaniment'.

The epidemiological link between migraine and TGA has given rise to a 'unifying hypothesis' for the pathophysiology of TGA. This is best considered in the light of the limited evidence available about TGA from functional neuroimaging (Table 9.2).

### Functional imaging in TGA

Prior to 1998 there were 11 reports of functional imaging performed in 14 patients during or in the few hours immediately after attacks of TGA, eight using SPECT, two using PET and one using a non-tomographic xenon inhalation technique

**Table 9.2.** Functional neuroimaging during transient global amnesia

| Author | Age, sex, hand | Timing | Technique | Findings | Comments |
|---|---|---|---|---|---|
| Volpe & Hirst, 1983 | 71, F, ? | 'during', 1/7 later | PET | global reduction $O_2$ metab, reduced mesial temporal $O_2$ extraction: during attack only | control group not described |
| Trillet et al., 1987 | (i) 52, F, R | 7 h, 3 d later | Xenon inhln. | global decrease CBF, esp. R temporal at 7 h; decreased R hem CBF at 3 d | migraineur; IV naloxone given between scans; |
| | (ii) 74, F, R | 3 h, 5 h (recovered at 5h) | Xenon inhln. | global decrease CBF, esp L temporofrontal at 3 h; decreased CBF at 5 h | hypertensive; controls younger than patients (i) and (ii) |
| Stillhard et al., 1990 | 71, F, R | 7 h, 3 d, 1 y | SPECT | bitemporal and ?bifrontal hypoperfusion at 7 h compared to later scans | migraineur, previous TGA; 'frontal'; enlarged R T horn on MRI |
| Tanabe et al., 1991 | 63, F, R | 6 h, 1 w, 5 m (6 h = early recovery) | SPECT | bilateral mesial temporal hypoperfusion at 6 h compared to later scans | hypertensive; small L hippocampal lesion on MRI |
| Goldenberg et al., 1991 | 55, F, ? | 6 h, 12 d, 40 d | SPECT | decreased global and L thalamic CBF at 6 h; decreased L frontal perfusion at 12 and 40 d. | 'frontal'; episode of visual disturbance 2 w later; control group younger |
| Lin et al., 1993 | 37, F, R | 6 h, 3 d (6 h = early recovery) | SPECT | multiple perfusion defects in occipital and medial temporal lobes and L thalamus at 6 h; occipital defects only at 3 d | headache |

| Study | Patient (age, sex, hand) | Timing | Modality | Findings | Comments |
|---|---|---|---|---|---|
| Evans et al., 1993 | 55, F, R | 'during', 7 w | SPECT | bilateral hypoperfusion posteromedial temporal lobes in attack only | |
| Sakashita et al., 1993 | (i) 45, M, R | 15 h, 15 d (15 h = 3 h post-recovery) | SPECT | L inferior temporal hypoperfusion at 15 h only | aged-matched controls in this study |
| | (ii) 54, F, R | 20 h, 9 d (20 h = 1 h post-recovery) | | R hippocampal and bi-thalamic hypoperfusion at 20 h; bi-hippocampal and bi-thalamic at 9 d. | |
| Baron et al., 1994 | 56, F, R | 5 h, 3 m (5 h = early recovery) | PET | CBF and $CMRO_2$ reduced in R prefrontal cortex in comparison to L (absolute values normal); $CMRO_2$ reduced in R thalamus and lentiform nucleus | hypertensive, hyperlipidaemic |
| Goldenberg, 1995 | 75, F, ? | 'during', 2 w (during = early recovery) | SPECT | hypoperfusion of both thalami, L frontal and temporal lobes including medial temporal region during attack only | migraineur, headache in attack, 'frontal', possible previous episode |
| Kazui et al., 1995 | [a](iii) 57, M,R | 'during', 1 w | SPECT | medial temporal hypoperfusion, especially L, during episode only | migraineur |
| | (iv) 63, M, R | 'during', 1 d | | symmetrical medial temporal hypoperfusion during episode only | |

Notes:

Key: hand = handedness; h = hours, d = days, w = weeks, m = months, y = years; PET = positron emission tomography, SPECT = single photon emission computed tomography; metab = metabolism, CBF = cerebral blood flow, $CMRO_2$ = rate of cerebral oxygen metabolism, L = left, R = right, 'frontal' = impaired performance on tests of executive function.

[a] Case (i) in this paper is described in Tanabe et al., 1991, no SPECT was performed in case (ii).

**Table 9.3.** Diagnostic criteria for TEA

1. There must be a history of recurrent episodes of transient amnesia, which may affect anterograde or retrograde memory or both.
2. Cognitive functions other than memory must be judged intact during typical episodes by a reliable witness.
3. There must be evidence for underlying partial epilepsy from all or any of:
   (a) reproducible epileptiform discharges on EEG;
   (b) co-occurrence of other seizure types (if concurrent onset and/or close association with episodes of transient amnesia suggests a connection);
   (c) a clear-cut response to anticonvulsant therapy (with abolition or definite reduction in frequency of amnesic episodes).

(Table 9.3). The studies differ widely in the details of their methodology, and most are single case reports. Temporal lobe hypoperfusion was detected in 12/14 patients studied during attacks, specifically involving medial temporal structures in 7/12; the abnormalities were bilateral in nine. Thalamic hypoperfusion was detected in five patients, and frontal cortex was involved in four. These results broadly support the view that TGA is caused by a disturbance of the function of limbic structures in the temporal lobe and thalamus. They also suggest some variablity from case to case and indicate that attacks of TGA are accompanied by local hypoperfusion. It is uncertain whether the hypoperfusion is primary or the result of diminished metabolism. Further studies of larger numbers of patients using both PET and functional MRI are likely to clarify these issues of localization and mechanism. The first such study (Strupp et al., 1998) has recently reported left medial temporal lobe high signal abnormalities on diffusion weighted MRI in seven out of eight patients studied within 40 hours of attack onset. In three patients, including the only patient studied during an attack, these abnormalities were bilateral.

## A unifying hypothesis?

The 'unifying hypothesis' proposed by Olesen (Olesen & Jorgensen, 1986) suggests that depression of hippocampal metabolism underlies TGA and the associated abnormalities on functional imaging. These authors propose that the 'spreading depression of Leao' (SD), is the underlying mechanism both of the focal neurological symptoms occuring in migraine and of the hippocampal dysfunction taken to cause TGA. 'Spreading depression' is a phenomenon observed in experimental animals, involving the gradual spread of a wave of depolarization, followed by neuronal depression, across the cortex, in response to a wide variety of insults. According to this hypothesis a single final common pathway is utilized by the numerous triggers of TGA: this involves the release of glutamate by volleys of sensory stimuli arriving in the hippocampus, provoking an episode of SD.

Glutamate, an excitatory neurotransmitter, is a potent cause of SD in experimental animals, and SD is known to occur in the human hippocampus. While this account accommodates the evidence from epidemiology, neuropsychology and functional imaging better than the alternatives outlined above, it remains a speculative theory of the pathophysiology of TGA.

## Transient epileptic amnesia

### Definition

Although there are no grounds for supposing that typical cases of TGA are caused by epilepsy, there is growing evidence that temporal lobe epilepsy (TLE) can manifest itself in amnesic episodes somewhat resembling attacks of TGA. This syndrome has been less well characterized than TGA. However, at least 21 cases have now been documented in the literature, in 15 publications (Lou, 1968; Shuping, 1980; Deisenhammer, 1981; Dugan et al., 1981; Meador et al., 1985; Pritchard et al., 1985; Galassi et al., 1986, 1988; Miller et al., 1987; Kapur, 1989, 1993; Stracciari et al., 1990; Tassinari et al., 1991; Kopelman et al., 1994; Vuilleumier et al., 1996). A further ten cases have recently been studied prospectively, adopting the term proposed by Kapur, 'transient epileptic amnesia' (TEA) (Kapur, 1993), to refer to this disorder (Zeman et al., 1998). Suggested criteria for the diagnosis of TEA are stated in Table 9.3. A number of clinical pointers help to suggest an epileptic aetiology for episodes of transient amnesia: these are outlined below.

### Epidemiology and clinical features

Patients with TEA are usually middle-aged or elderly. Only two of the 31 patients described in the literature, including our series, were under 40. The mean age overall was 60, with a range from 22–82. Men predominate, with a ratio of 2.25:1. The cause of the epilepsy is usually obscure, but half of our patients gave a history of ischaemic (4) or valvular (1) heart disease, suggesting a possible thromboembolic aetiology, perhaps by way of ischaemic injury to medial temporal structures in which lesions are known to be potentially epileptogenic. Attacks are recurrent, with a range from 3–20 and a mean of nine in our series: these attacks occurred at a mean rate of three per year. This is in sharp contrast to TGA, which has a low recurrence rate.

The attacks themselves typically involve a combination of anterograde and retrograde amnesia, with perplexity and repetitive questioning. In these respects they resemble episodes of TGA, but there are several distinctive features which should raise suspicion of underlying epilepsy. (i) Attacks are relatively brief: over 80% of patients have at least some attacks lasting less than 1 hour. Such brief attacks of TGA are exceptional. (ii) Attacks on waking are characteristic. Every patient in our series reported at least one such attack, and they were a typical feature in many. In contrast, episodes of TGA probably occur on waking no more often than would be expected by chance (Fisher, 1982). (iii) The anterograde amnesia is often incomplete. Patients may recall some details about their episodes of amnesia, 'remembering not being able to remember' recent events during attacks.

While episodes of TEA generally involve elements of both anterograde and retrograde amnesia there are reports of anterograde amnesia, unnoticed by the patient, occurrring in isolation in some attacks (Palmini et al., 1992); occasionally retrograde amnesia may predominate (Kapur, 1989).

Although the majority of patients with episodes of TEA exhibit other seizure types, usually simple or complex partial seizures with symptomatology pointing to an origin in the temporal lobe, transient amnesia is the sole manifestation of epilepsy in about one-third of cases.

There is growing evidence that patients with episodes of TEA are prone to a characteristic and persistent impairment of retrograde memory. This has been highlighted by both Kapur (1989) and Kopelman (Kopelman et al., 1994); seven of our ten patients likewise complained of a patchy loss of recall for salient episodes from their personal past. The impairment tends to be more severe for episodes from recent years, but in half of our cases it affected recall for events predating the clinical onset of TEA. In addition to their amnesia for salient episodes, six of our patients complained of difficulty in recognizing familiar landmarks and in recalling familiar routes, three of problems in recognizing familiar faces, and two had lost their recall for some professional skills. Despite their complaints of retrograde memory impairment, only one of the seven complained of a comparable disturbance of day-to-day memory, and the group performed normally on a number of standard tests of anterograde memory.

Anti-convulsant therapy is usually highly effective in controlling episodes of TEA. Its effect on the associated retrograde amnesia requires further study but appears to be less clear cut.

Thus TEA is distinguished from TGA by the relatively high frequency and brief duration of attacks and by their common occurrence on waking. The predominance of retrograde amnesia in some attacks, and the emergence of a persisting symptomatic retrograde amnesia are also helpful pointers to an epileptic aetiology in patients with amnesic episodes which might otherwise be mistaken for TGA.

## Pathophysiology

While the evidence for the existence of TEA is now strong, its pathophysiology remains uncertain. The evidence bearing on four key questions is briefly considered. (i) Does the epileptic activity associated with TEA arise in the mesial temporal lobes? (ii) Is bilateral temporal lobe dysfunction required? (iii) Is TEA an ictal or post-ictal state? (iv) What is the explanation for the interictal disturbance of retrograde memory which sometimes accompanies TEA?

### Is the focus in the medial temporal lobe

There is no doubt that the temporal lobes, which are particularly vulnerable to epilepsy, are the usual location of the electrical foci responsible for TEA. Surface EEG does not permit precise localization of a focus within the temporal lobe, but the limited data available from studies using intracranial electrodes indicate that medial temporal structures may be involved (Palmini et al., 1992; Morrell, 1980; Bridgman et al., 1989; Lee et al., 1992). Neuroimaging is generally normal in this disorder, and therefore unhelpful in pinpointing the focus of pathology.

### Is bilateral dysfunction required?

Permanent amnesia is only seen after bilateral damage to the limbic structures mentioned above. It is therefore a reasonable hypothesis that TEA only occurs in patients with bilateral temporal lobe dysfunction. Of the 18 cases of TEA with epileptiform abnormalities on surface EEG, 12 had bilateral abnormalities. Bilateral neuropsychological or EEG abnormalities were noted in six out of the eight patients reported by Palmini with episodes of pure anterograde amnesia in the context of established temporal lobe epilepsy (Palmini et al., 1992). Thus more than half of these patients show signs of bilateral disturbance of temporal lobe function, providing some support for the view that this is the basis of episodes of epileptic amnesia.

### Is TEA an ictal or post-ictal state?

EEG studies using electrodes implanted in the mesial temporal lobes have shown that brief bilateral mesial temporal discharges can disrupt anterograde or retrograde memory, and that this disruption may go unnoticed by the subject (Bridgman et al., 1989; Palmini et al., 1992). Lee et al. (1992) report the remarkable case of a woman who entered a 12-day period of continuous anterograde amnesia with additional retrograde amnesia for events of the last 4 months, as a result of semi-continuous epileptic activity in both medial temporal lobes. Such evidence shows that both short-lived and prolonged amnesia, affecting anterograde or retrograde memory, can occur as isolated ictal phenomena. On the other hand, prolonged amnesic states can also occur in the aftermath of ictal activity, as a form of 'Todd's paralysis' of memory (Morrell, 1980). Detailed EEG studies during episodes of TEA are required to clarify the relative importance of ictal activity and post-ictal dysfunction of TL structures in this disorder.

What is the basis of the interictal retrograde amnesia?

In principle, the patchy impairment of remote memory which affects a high pro-portion of patients with TEA must have one of three explanations: failure to encode episodes into long-term memory, failure to consolidate and maintain such memo-ries or failure to retrieve memories which have been successfully stored. Further work is required to resolve this issue, but there is some suggestive evidence that the main underlying deficit is failure of consolidation.

A number of the patients in the authors' series have told them that their memo-ries for recent personal events appear to be intact initially but may then disappear without trace, suggesting that acquisition is normal but consolidation impaired. This is in keeping with their normal performance on standard tests of anterograde memory. Current computational neural network models of long-term memory processing, based upon human neuropsychological and animal data (Alvarez & Squire, 1995; McLelland et al., 1995; Murre, 1996) suggest that the medial tempo-ral lobe complex plays a critical, but temporally limited, role in the encoding and storage of new episodic memories. Over time, a process of consolidation occurs whereby memories become independent of the hippocampus. Ictal activity in the mesial temporal lobes might be capable of disrupting recent memories during this vulnerable stage of consolidation. In this context, it is of interest that TEA often occurs in relation to sleep, as there is accumulating evidence that processes of memory consolidation may be particularly active in sleep (Karni, 1994; Wilson, 1994).

While this hypothesis merits further study, it is likely that the extensive persis-tent retrograde amnesia we have observed in some patients, affecting recall for events over 30 years, cannot be accounted for by a defect in consolidation alone. Disruption of such well established memories may point to pathology affecting the infero-temporal neocortex, which is implicated in the storage of well-established semantic knowledge, including knowledge about people (Evans et al., 1995; Patterson & Hodges, 1995). It is an open question whether the pathology underly-ing retrograde amnesia for remote events in these patients caused by or the cause of the episodes of TEA.

## Management of transient amnesia

The differential diagnosis of episodes of transient amnesia is summarized in Table 9.4. The management of such episodes turns on selecting the correct diag-nosis from among the possibilities listed in Table 9.4.

It is vital to obtain as full a history of the episodes as possible. A description from a witness is invaluable: in the absence of an eye-witness description it is not pos-sible to make a firm diagnosis. A full background medical and psychiatric history should be taken, with specific enquiry about risk factors for epilepsy (birth

**Table 9.4.** Differential diagnosis of transient amnesia

| Diagnosis | Pointers |
| --- | --- |
| Transient global amnesia | 4–6 hours, isolated, profound AGA, variable RGA; few/no vasc RFs |
| Transient epileptic amnesia | Brief, recurrent, occur on waking, partial recall, other seizures, interictal amnesia |
| Migraine | Headache, nausea in attack, past history |
| Thromboembolic transient ischaemic amnesia | Post. circ. symptoms or signs, prominent vasc RFs |
| Psychogenic amnesia | Young, past psychiatric history, current stressors, loss of personal identity, profound RGA but little AGA |
| Head injury | History, examination |
| Drugs: alcohol | History |
|     benzodiazepines | History |
|     anticholinergics | History |
| Miscellaneous: symptomatic transient amnesia | History, examination, brain imaging |

*Notes:*
Key: AGA = anterograde amnesia, RGA = retrograde amnesia, vasc RFs = risk factors for vascular disease, post circ = posterior circulation.

trauma, febrile convulsions, head injury, CNS infections, alcohol use and family history) and for vascular disease (such as hypertension, diabetes and smoking). History of drug use may be relevant. The patient and a witness should be asked if there is any persistent disturbance of anterograde or remote memory. A general medical examination should be performed with particular attention to evidence of vascular disease, and a neurological examination particularly seeking signs of vertebrobasilar ischaemia, such as abnormalities of eye movement or long tract signs.

Psychogenic amnesia is discussed in detail in Chapter 19, this volume. Helpful pointers to this diagnosis include younger age than is usual in patients with TGA, TEA or TIAs, a past psychiatric history and/or major current life stress, loss of personal identity during the episode and profound retrograde amnesia in the face of normal anterograde memory. Occasional reports of transient amnesia in association with a variety of systemic and neurological disorders, and following angiography, require the inclusion of the 'miscellaneous' category in Table 9.4 (Hodges, 1991). With the exception of transient amnesia following angiography, which is extremely rare, such cases seldom if ever conform to the criteria for pure TGA stated in Table 9.1.

Where the history is typical of TGA, without any evidence of epilepsy or cerebrovascular disease from clinical assessment, there is probably no need for further investigation. If there are features of TEA (see Table 9.3), the patient should be investigated further with routine wake EEG and neuroimaging, CT or, if possible, MRI, with specific views of the temporal lobes. If wake EEG is unhelpful, it is worthwhile to record a sleep EEG. If there are prominent vascular risk factors, or symptoms or signs pointing to vertebrobasilar ischaemia, patients should be screened for causes of vascular disease, with investigations including full blood count, ESR, blood glucose, and lipids, syphilis serology, renal and liver function tests, electrocardiograph and chest radiograph. A CT scan of the head is helpful and further vascular imaging may be indicated by the clinical context (echocardiogram, carotid ultrasound or formal cerebral angiography). If migraine is thought to be the underlying disorder, no further investigation is usually required, although it is worth bearing in mind the possibilty of symptomatic migraine, due, for example, to the presence of anticardiolipin antibodies.

Once the diagnosis has been identified, treatment can follow standard lines. TGA requires no more than explanation and reassurance. TEA is usually managed effectively with anti-convulsants. Carbamazepine and sodium valproate are currently first-line drugs for temporal lobe seizures. Transient ischaemic attacks demand control of risk factors, exclusion of treatable cardiac pathology and aspirin if platelet emboli are suspected; ischaemia arising in the posterior cerebral circulation is rarely amenable to vascular surgery. A range of symptomatic and prophylactic therapies is available for migraine. Psychogenic amnesia requires psychiatric assessment and advice.

## Conclusions

Transient Global Amnesia (TGA) is a fairly common and clearly defined clinical syndrome the aetiology of which remains obscure. It has been established that conventional thromboembolic cerebrovascular disease and epilepsy are not the cause and there is a strong link with migraine. The most plausible unifying hypothesis is that various physical and emotional stressors may provoke spreading depression via the release of glutamate or other excitotoxic neurotransmitters (see Hodges, 1998). Neuropsychologically, TGA produces profound anterograde but variable retrograde amnesia. The more recently defined disorder, Transient Epileptic Amnesia (TEA) occurs in the same age group as TGA. It is characterized by brief recurrent episodes of amnesia, sometimes with partial recall of the attack. Attacks on waking are characteristic and there is often a progressive impairment of remote memory with recurring attacks. The most helpful diagnostic procedure is a sleep EEG. Patients with TEA often benefit from anti-convulsant medication.

## REFERENCES

Alvarez, P. & L.R. Squire (1995). Memory consolidation and the medial temporal lobe: a simple network model. *Proceedings of the National Academy of Sciences, USA*, **91**, 7041–5.

Baron, J.C., Petittaboue, M.C., Ledoze, F., Desgranges, B., Ravebel, N. & Marchal, G. (1994). Right frontal-cortex hypometabolism in transient global amnesia – a pet study. *Brain*, **117**, 545–52.

Bender, M.B. (1956). Syndrome of isolated episode of confusion with amnesia. *Journal of Hillside Hospital*, **5**, 212–15.

Bridgman, P.A., Malamut, B.L., Sperling, M.R., Saykin, A.J. & O'Connor, M.J. (1989). Memory during subclinical hippocampal seizures. *Neurology*, **39**, 853–6.

Deisenhammer, E. (1981). Transient global amnesia as an epileptic manifestation. *Journal of Neurology*, **225**, 289–92.

Dugan, T.M., Nordgren, R.E. & O'Leary, P. (1981). Transient global amnesia associated with bradycardia and temporal lobe spikes. *Cortex*, **17**, 633–8.

Evans, J.J., Wilson, B., Wraight, E.P. & Hodges, J.R. (1993). Neuropsychological and SPECT scan findings during and after transient global amnesia: evidence for the differential impairment of remote episodic memory. *Journal of Neurology, Neurosurgery and Psychiatry*, **56**, 1227–30.

Evans, J.J., Heggs, A.J., Antoun, N. & Hodges, J.R. (1995). Progressive prosopagnosia associated with selective right temporal lobe atrophy: a new syndrome? *Brain*, **118**, 1–13.

Fisher, C.M. (1980). Late-life migraine accompaniments as a cause of unexplained transient ischaemic atttacks. *The Canadian Journal of Neurological Sciences*, **7**, 9–17.

Fisher, C.M. (1982). Transient global amnesia: precipitating activities and other observations. *Archives of Neurology*, **39**, 605–8.

Fisher, C.M. & Adams, R.D. (1964). Transient global amnesia. *Acta Neurologica Scandanavica*, **40**, 1–81.

Frederiks, J.A.M. (1993). Transient global amnesia. *Clinical Neurology and Neurosurgery*, **95**, 265–83.

Galassi, R., Pazzaglia, P., Lorusso, S. & Morreale, A. (1986). Neuropsychological findings in epi-leptic amnesic attacks. **25**, 299–303.

Galassi, R., Morreale, A., Lorusso, S., Pazzaglia, P. & Lugaresi, E. (1988). Epilepsy presenting as memory disturbances. *Epilepsia*, **29**(5), 624–9.

Goldenberg, G. (1995). Transient global amnesia. *Handbook of Memory Disorders*, ed. A.D. Baddeley, B.A. Wilson & F.N. Watts, pp. 109–33. Chichester, UK: John Wiley.

Goldenberg, G., Podreka, I., Pfafflmeyer, N., Wessely, P. & Deecke, L. (1991). Thalamic ischaemia in transient global amnesia. *Neurology*, **41**, 1748–52.

Graff-Radford, N.R., Tranel, D., Van Hoesen, G.W. & Brandt, J.P. (1990). Diencephalic amnesia. *Brain*, **113**, 1–25.

Guyotat, J. & Courjon, J. (1956). Les ictus amnesiques. *Journal de Medicine de Lyon*, 37, 697–701.

Hodges, J.R. (1991). *Transient Global Amnesia*. London: W.B. Saunders Co. Ltd.

Hodges, J.R. (1994). Semantic memory and frontal executive function during transient global amnesia. *Journal of Neurology, Neurosurgery and Psychiatry*, 57, 605–8.

Hodges, J.R. (1998). Unraveling the enigma of transient global amnesia. *Annals of Neurology*, 43, 151–153

Hodges, J.R. & Oxbury, S.M. (1990). Persistent memory inpairment following transient global amnesia. *Journal of Clinical and Experimental Neuropsychology*, 12(6), 904–20.

Hodges, J.R. & McCarthy, R. (1993). Autobiographical amnesia resulting from bilateral parame-dian thalamic infarction. *Brain*, 116, 921–40.

Hughlings-Jackson, J. (1889). On a particular variety of epilepsy ('intellectual aura'), one case with symptoms of organic brain disease. *Brain*, XI, 179–207.

Inzitari, D., Pantoni, L., Lamassa, M., Pallanti, S., Pracucci, G. & Marini, P. (1997). Emotional arousal and phobia in transient global amnesia. *Archives of Neurology*, 54, 866–73.

Kapur, N. (1989). Focal retrograde amnesia: a long term clinical and neuropsychological follow-up. *Cortex*, 25, 387–402.

Kapur, N. (1993). Transient epileptic amnesia – a clinical update and a reformulation. *Journal of Neurology, Neurosurgery and Psychiatry*, 56, 1184–90.

Karni, A. (1994). Dependence on REM sleep of overnight improvement of a perceptual skill. *Science*, 265, 679–82.

Kazui, H., Tanabe, H., Ikeda, M., Nakagawa, Y., Shiraishi, J. & Hashikawa, K. (1995). Memory and cerebral blood flow in cases of transient global amnesia during and after the attack. *Behvioural Neurology*, 8, 93–101.

Kopelman, M.D., Panayiotopoulos, C.P. & Lewis, P. (1994). Transient epileptic amnesia differentiated from psychogenic 'fugue': neuropsychological, EEG and PET findings. *Journal of Neurology, Neurosurgery and Psychiatry*, 57, 1002–4.

Kritchevsky, M. & Squire, L.R. (1989). Transient global amnesia: evidence for extensive, tempo-rally graded retrograde amnesia. *Neurology*, 39, 213–18.

Kritchevsky, M., Squire, L.R. & Zouzounis, J.A. (1988). Transient global amnesia: characterisa-tion of anterograde and retrograde amnesia. *Neurology*, 38, 213–19.

Lee, B.I., Lee, B.C., Hwang, Y.M., Sohn, Y.H., Jung, J.W., Park, S.C & Han, M.H. (1992). Prolonged ictal amnesia with transient focal abnormalities on magnetic resonance imaging. *Epilepsia*, 33, 1042–6.

Lin, K.N., Liu, R.S., Yeh, T.P., Wang, S.J. & Liu, H.C. (1993). Posterior ishcemia during an attack of transient global amnesia. *Stroke*, 24, 1093–5.

Lou, H. (1968). Repeated episodes of transient global amnesia. *Acta Neurological Scandanavica*, 44, 612–18.

McClelland, J.L., McNaughton, B.L. & O'Reilly, R.C. (1995). Why are there complementary learning systems in the hippocampus and neocortex: insights from the successes and failures of connectionist models of learning and memory. *Psychological Review*, 102, 419–57.

Meador, K.J., Adams, R.J. & Flanigin, H.F. (1985). Transient global amnesia and meningioma. *Neurology*, 35, 769–71.

Miller, J.W., Yanagihara, T., Petersen, R.C. & Klass, D.W. (1987). Transient global amnesia and epilepsy: electroencephalographic distinction. *Archives of Neurology*, 44, 629–63.

Morrell, F. (1980). Memory loss as a Todds paralysis. *Epilepsia*, 21, 185.

Murre, J. M. J. (1996). Implicit and explicit memory in amnesia: some explanations and predictions by the TraceLink model. *Memory*, 5, 213–32.

Olesen, J. & Jorgensen, M.B. (1986). Leao's spreading depression in the hippocampus explains transient global amnesia. *Acta Neurological Scandinavica*, 73, 219–20.

Palmini, A.L., Gloor, P. & Jones-Gotman, M. (1992). Pure amnestic seizures in temporal lobe epilepsy. *Brain*, 115, 749–69.

Patterson, K. & Hodges, J.R. (1995). Disorders of semantic memory. *Handbook of Memory Disorders*, ed. A.D. Baddeley, B.A. Wilson & F.N. Watts, pp. 167–86. Chichester, UK: John Wiley.

Pritchard, P.B., Holmstrom, V.L., Roitzsch, J.C. & Giacinto, J. (1985). Epileptic amnesic attacks: benefit from antiepileptic drugs. *Neurology*, 35, 1188–9.

Rowan, A.J. (1991). Ictal amnesia and fugue states. *Neurobehavioural Problems in Epilepsy*, ed. D. Smith, D. Treiman & M. Trimble, pp. 357–67. New York: Raven Press.

Sakashitsa, Y., Sugimoto, T., Taki, S. & Matsuda, H. (1993). Abnormal cerebral blood flow following transient global amnesia. *Journal of Neurology, Neurosurgery and Psychiatry*, 56, 1327.

Shuping, J. R. (1980). Transient global amnesia due to glioma in the dominant hemisphere. *Neurology*, 30, 88–90.

Stillhard, G., Landis, T., Schiess, R., Regard, M. & Sialer, G. (1990). Bitemporal hypoperfusion in transient global amnesia: a 99m-Tc-HM-PAO SPECT and neuropsychological findings during and after an attack. *Journal of Neurology, Neurosurgery and Psychiatry*, 53, 339–42.

Stracciari, A., Ciucci, G., Bianchedi, G. & Rebucci, G.G. (1990). Epileptic transient amnesia. *European Neurology*, 30, 176–9.

Strupp, M., Brüning, R., Wu, R.H., Deimling, M., Reiser, M. & Brandt, T. (1998). Diffusion-weighted MRI in transient global amnesia: elevated signal intensity in the left mesial temporal lobe in 7 of 10 patients. *Annals of Neurology*, 43, 164–70.

Tanabe, H., Hashikawa, K., Nakagawa, Y., Ikeda, M., Yamamoto, H., Harada, K., Tsunoto, T., Nishimura, T., Shiraishi, J. & Kimura, K. (1991). Memory loss due to transient hypoperfusion in the medial temporal lobes including hippocampus. *Acta Neurologica Scandinavica*, 81, 22–7.

Tassinari, C.A., Ciarmatori, C., Alesi, C., Cardinaletti, L., Salvi, F., Rubboli, G., Plasmati, R., Forti, A. & Michelucci, R. (1991). Transient global amnesia as a postictal state from recurrent partial seizures. *Epilepsia*, 32, 882–5.

Trillet, M., Croisile, B., Philippon, B., Vial, C., Laurent, B. & Guillot, M. (1987). Transient global amnesia and cerebral blood-flow. *Revue Neurologique*, 143, 536-9.

Volpe, B.T. & Hirst, W. (1983). The characterization of an amnesic syndrome following hypoxic ischaemic injury. *Archives of Neurology*, 40, 436–40.

Vuilleumier, P., Despland, P.A. & Regii, F. (1996). Failure to recall (but not to remember). *Neurology*, 46, 1036–9.

Wilson, M. A. (1994). Reactivation of hippocampal ensemble memories during sleep. *Science*, 265, 676–9.

Zeman, A.Z.J., Boniface, S.J. & Hodges, J.R. (1998) Transient epileptic amnesia: a description of the clinical and neuropsychological features in 10 cases and a review of the literature. *Journal of Neurology, Neurosurgery and Psychiatry*, 64, 435–43.

# 10

# Insight into memory deficits

Ivana S. Marková and German E. Berrios

In recent years increasing interest has been shown in the empirical study of insight and related notions in psychiatric and neurological/neuropsychological disciplines. In clinical psychiatry, insight has been explored predominantly in patients with psychotic illnesses, particularly schizophrenia (McEvoy et al., 1989; Amador et al., 1991, 1993; David et al., 1992). Insight in patients with affective disorders has received much less attention (Michalakeas et al., 1994; Ghaemi et al., 1996). The focus of these studies has been on the relationship between levels of insight and severity of psychopathology, compliance with treatment, prognosis, neuropsychological impairment, etc. The inconsistent results achieved so far are likely to result from differences in the methods of evaluation, these in turn reflecting diverse conceptualizations of insight (Marková & Berrios, 1995a). In general, recent views conceive of insight as a multidimensional concept including not only the patient's *awareness* of the symptoms/disease, but also elaboration of the said experience, variously conceptualized as, e.g. a correct attribution (Amador et al., 1991), a relabelling of symptoms as pathological (David, 1990), or a deeper knowledge of the effects of the symptoms/disease on the individual in the context of his/her environment (Marková & Berrios, 1992, 1995b).

In contrast to this broad conceptualization of insight in psychiatry, the neurological and neuropsychological disciplines have tended to conceive insight in the much narrower sense of awareness of specific deficits. Since the late nineteenth century, there have been reports of patients seemingly oblivious to major neurological deficit, maintaining their 'unawareness' and/or explicitly denying any disability in the face of confrontative evidence to the contrary (Anton, 1899). 'Anosognosia', the term coined by Babinski in 1914 to refer to the unawareness of hemiplegia seen in patients following stroke, has since then also been used to refer to the unawareness displayed in patients in relation to other neurological/neuropsychological syndromes, e.g. cortical blindness (Anton's syndrome), aphasia (Rubens & Garrett, 1991), hemiballismus (Roth, 1944), amnesic syndromes (McGlynn & Schacter, 1989), dementia (Reed et al., 1993; Starkstein et al., 1995), head injury (Prigatano, 1991), tardive dyskinesia (Myslobodsky, 1986), to mention but a few. The 'impaired insight' of anosognosia has been conceptualized as a dysfunction in an 'awareness system' which in turn is envisaged as general or module-specific (Schacter, 1990, 1991, 1992). Structured studies of anosognosia have tried to evaluate degrees of anosognosia and focus on localization of unawareness in specific structural/functional brain systems. Results have also been mixed (see below).

Attempts have been made to link neurological and psychiatric models of anosognosia/insight but their success is unclear. For example, studies have concentrated on searching for correlations between neuropsychological variables specific to frontal lobe and right hemispheric dysfunction and impaired insight in patients with schizophrenia (McEvoy et al., 1993; Young et al., 1993; Cuesta & Peralta, 1994) or with bipolar affective disorders (Ghaemi et al., 1996). Such studies appear to be based on the finding that anosognosia has been linked with frontal lobe dysfunction and right hemisphere damage (e.g. Bisiach et al., 1986; Starkstein et al., 1992). In other words, it is assumed that anosognosia as assessed in neurological conditions and impaired insight as assessed in schizophrenia, are both referring to the same phenomenon. Young et al. (1993), for example, whilst acknowledging difficulties in determining a clear definition of 'unawareness' in relation to schizophrenia, nevertheless base their study on a possible association between such unawareness and anosognosia in neurological states. They define 'unawareness' in schizophrenia as 'the phenomena in which individuals with long standing schizophrenic symptomatology state upon intensive questioning that they are not ill, do not have symptoms or have no difficulties or abnormalities which they attribute to a psychiatric illness' (Young et al., 1993, p. 118). They consider this an analogous phenomenon to the anosognosia seen in neurological disorders. Mullen et al. (1996) are even more explicit in equating these phenomena. They state that 'the ability to relabel certain mental events as pathological <u>corresponds closely</u> to the concept of anosognosia . . . the recognition by a patient of neurological symptoms is <u>conceptually identical</u> with the recognition of psychiatric symptoms' (p. 645, our emphases). In consequence, common explanatory hypotheses and underlying mechanisms are sought for the impaired insight and unawareness present in schizophrenia and neurological states.

This assumption, however, that the same phenomenon is being studied, whether this is termed 'insightlessness' in mental illness or 'anosognosia' in neurological states, has neither a theoretical nor empirical basis (Marková, 1998a). Yet, the issue is an important one, not only because of the implications this carries for possible explanatory mechanisms sought to underlie insight, but because, in addition, the nature of insight itself, as a clinical phenomenon and theoretical construct, is under question. It is therefore from this perspective, i.e. from the questioning of the phenomenon under investigation, that insight into memory function will be examined. Perforce this chapter must be selective and will concentrate on the issue of insight and memory function.

Research in this area has focused primarily on insight in relation to memory deficits. Both awareness of memory dysfunction and awareness of memory function (implicit memory) have been studied in relation to focal brain disease (amnestic syndromes) and generalized brain disease (dementias) and this line will be followed here. With respect to 'normal' or non-ill subjects, self-reports of memory function have been treated mainly in experimental psychology where, rather than 'insight' or 'awareness', somewhat different frameworks are used. Hermann (1982), for example, reviewing the current self-report questionnaires on everyday memory function found only a moderate correlation between self-assessments and performance on clinical tests of memory. These results were then discussed in terms of people's beliefs about their memory and factors that might influence such beliefs. Similarly, in functional psychiatric disorders, whilst memory function/dysfunction has not in itself been the subject of insight research, there is indirect reference to this issue, e.g. in the recognition of the syndrome of 'pseudodementia' (Gelder et al., 1996). Likewise, studies examining subjective memory complaints in depressed patients have noted discrepancies between such complaints and actual memory performance (Grut et al., 1993), thereby implying some disturbance in awareness or insight.

## Insight into memory function in focal brain disease

Interest and research in issues of awareness into memory function in relation to focal brain disease, such as amnestic syndrome, brain injury, strokes, etc. has been directed to two specific areas, namely, (a) awareness of memory knowledge and (b) awareness of memory deficit.

(a) Korsakoff (1889) in his original description of the amnestic syndrome, was more interested in this former aspect of insight. Thus, whilst commenting on the lack of concern (rather than lack of awareness) shown by patients about their memory impairment, he was struck by the level of their unconscious knowledge. For example, patients, whilst not recognizing Korsakoff on repeated daily contact, nevertheless recognized that he was a doctor. Moreover, months or even years after their illness, patients could recollect conversations or events occurring during their illness of which they seemed to have no awareness at the time. In addition, Korsakoff observed that unconscious awareness was evident to differing extents in relation to different aspects of memory. For example, pleasant, sympathetic behaviour towards certain individuals/events and hostile or unsympathetic behaviour towards others, suggested that patients preserved unconsciously affective responses in the face of a lack of conscious recollection of the situations evoking such responses. Since the early observations by Korsakoff and others (for review, also see Schacter, 1991), such unconscious knowledge, later termed 'memory without awareness' (Jacoby & Witherspoon, 1982) or 'implicit memory' (Schacter, 1995), has only been developed as an area of systematic research since the 1970s. Implicit memory has been demonstrated in patients with the amnesic syndrome, who are able, for example, to show effects of priming on memory tests without recalling the priming itself (Warrington & Weiskrantz, 1968, 1974, 1982; Cermak et al., 1985; Shimamura, 1986; McAndrews et al., 1987; Schacter, 1991). Assessment of this type of awareness has tended to be restricted to demonstrating its presence in amnesic patients, either by such priming tasks or by skill-learning tasks. In these latter studies, patients are taught to learn and retain new skills such as computer training and yet they remain 'unaware' of having such training or skills (Glisky et al., 1986).

(b) Lack of awareness of memory deficit has been commonly noted in relation to amnesic syndromes, particularly where there is also evidence of frontal lobe dysfunction. Talland (1965), for example, refers to 'lack of insight' for memory deficit as a characteristic feature of Korsakoff syndrome. Unawareness of memory impairment is also prominent in Luria's (1976) case descriptions of patients with frontal lobe tumours and patients with ruptured aneurysms of the anterior communicating artery (ACAA). In contrast, he describes patients whose memory impairment is secondary to IIIrd ventricle lesions or pituitary tumours, as being 'adequately aware of their [memory] defect' (p. 342). Because such studies are concerned predominantly with the delineation of the memory dysfunction itself, together with associated cognitive features in relation to the different brain lesions, the issue of subjective knowledge or insight into the memory problems is restricted to either direct comments on its absence or indirect inferences from the accounts by the patients. There have been relatively few studies focusing specifically on the notion of awareness of memory deficits and its assessment in relation to these disorders. Some studies appear to address this issue indirectly. For example, Sunderland et al. (1983) designed a study examining the relationship between subjects' perceived everyday memory and their memory function as assessed by performance on clinical tests. They administered a questionnaire rating the frequency with which some memory-dependent tasks were experienced as difficult to patients with severe head injury, their relatives and a group of controls. Results showed that the responses of the relatives (about patients' everyday memory) correlated much better with the objective memory test results than did the responses of the patients or controls. Rather than viewing the results in terms of disturbed awareness/insight on the part of patients, the authors explained the subjective–objective discrepancies on the basis of a mismatch between the sort of information being captured by standard memory tests and the sort of memory problems experienced by patients in everyday tasks. A subsequent study using a refined version of the questionnaire

(Sunderland et al., 1984) yielded similar results but, again without invoking disturbed awareness, the authors suggested that the memory defect itself was in part responsible for the subjective–objective discrepancy (i.e. patients were inaccurate in their assessments of memory failures because of their inability to remember their mistakes). Arguments against this view have since been put forward on the grounds that patients with certain amnesic syndromes, performing equally badly on memory tests, nevertheless do have awareness into their deficits (Schacter, 1991).

Foremost amongst studies that do, however, focus specifically on unawareness of memory deficits in amnesic syndromes has been the work by Schacter and colleagues (e.g. McGlynn & Schacter, 1989; Schacter 1991, 1992). A detailed assessment measure of awareness of memory deficits comprising three main components is described by Schacter (1991). The first part consists of a General Self-Assessment Questionnaire in which patients rate on a seven-point scale the degree to which they experience difficulty with various aspects of memory compared to before their illness. Relatives also complete this scale. The second part consists of an Everyday Memory Questionnaire in which a number of hypothetical situations are described and patients are asked to rate the probability that they would remember information in these situations (currently and before their illness) after delays of a minute, an hour, a day and a week. In addition, patients are asked to make similar ratings of their relatives' abilities to remember the same situations. Similarly, the relatives also complete this for themselves and the patients. The last part consists of an Item Recall Questionnaire in which patients have to predict how many items they would remember (currently and prior to illness) if they were shown lists of ten items (further subdivided into 'easy' and 'difficult' items) and are subsequently tested at each of the delays. Using this assessment in two densely amnesic patients, Schacter (1991) describes different patterns of results. One patient whose amnesia was secondary to ACAA rupture showed poor awareness of memory deficits and overestimated his ability to recall items on the questionnaire, compared with his wife who made more accurate predictions. In contrast, the other patient whose amnesia was secondary to herpes simplex encephalitis showed much greater awareness of her memory problems, with ratings on the questionnaires consistent with her spouse's ratings and with her performance on testing. The severity of memory deficits as measured by the tests was equivalent in both patients and the IQ of the second patient was much lower than that of the first, suggesting that the difference in awareness was unlikely to be due to generalized intellectual impairment.

This type of detailed assessment of awareness of memory deficit illustrates well the neuropsychological approach in the conceptualization of awareness in general. Thus, similar methods have been applied in the assessment of awareness of various impairments including social, behavioural and emotional in relation to head injury (Prigatano, 1991), cognitive and motor deficits in Huntington's disease (McGlynn

& Kaszniak, 1991b) and similar deficits in Alzheimer's disease (McGlynn & Kaszniak, 1991a; Green et al., 1993; see below). This approach is characterized by a relatively narrow underlying concept of awareness as a unitary function. Patients either know or do not know they have a memory problem and/or are rated according to the perceived frequency with which they make 'mistakes' on account of this problem, and on the perceived severity with which such mistakes affect them. This does not mean to say that the concept of awareness is thus regarded as an all-or-none phenomenon and Schacter (1992) explicitly argues against this, but that the qualitative differences in awareness are dependent on the types of memory tasks used to elicit them.

Mechanisms proposed to underlie anosognosia in relation to focal memory pathology (as well as other neuropsychological deficits), in the main, reflect this view of awareness as a unitary function. Such mechanisms have been comprehensively reviewed by McGlynn and Schacter (1989) and fall broadly into three main groups, namely: (i) neuroanatomical, (ii) neuropsychological and (iii) motivational.

## Neuroanatomical theories

In brief, amongst the many neuroanatomical theories proposed to underlie anosognosia in general, such as thalamic damage (Roth, 1944; Watson & Heilman, 1979), striatal damage (Healton et al., 1982), right hemisphere, particularly right parietal involvement (Price & Mesulam, 1985; Bisiach et al., 1986; Starkstein et al., 1992; Heilman et al., 1993), the most consistent finding, as far as anosognosia of memory deficit in relation to amnesic syndromes is concerned, has been the association with frontal lobe dysfunction. Evidence here has come from a variety of sources. For example, it has been observed that patients with amnesic syndromes involving frontal lobe impairment tend to be unaware of their memory deficit, in contrast to patients whose amnesic syndromes are due to temporal lobe damage and who tend to show some awareness of their memory difficulties (McGlynn & Schacter, 1989; Schacter, 1991). Frontal lobe dysfunction has similarly been implicated in the pathogenesis of anosognosia in relation to other neuropsychological deficits (Mesulam, 1986; Stuss & Benson, 1986; Stuss, 1991; Prigatano, 1991). However, there have also been reports of patients with frontal lobe dysfunction with preserved awareness of memory deficits (Luria, 1976; Vilkki, 1985; Schacter, 1991). Most studies reporting these associations have not assessed awareness in a systematic way and simply state it as present or absent. Where there has been a structured assessment of awareness, this tends to be in single case studies and hence it is difficult on empirical grounds to conclude much about the relationship between unawareness and frontal lobe dysfunction. Of theoretical interest, Stuss and Benson (1986) have suggested a model of brain functioning in which the frontal lobes are viewed as serving an executive or control function, monitoring, exploring, selecting and judging all nervous system activities. Interestingly, they make a distinction between self-awareness and awareness of deficits in behavioural disorders such as neglect and aphasia (Stuss, 1991). The former is seen as the highest psychological attribute of the frontal lobes, interacting closely with organized function systems subserving various psychological processes, e.g. attention, language and memory. Thus, damage to the frontal lobes would result in a general disturbance of self-awareness, which, because of the varied nature of the 'self', in turn would lead to 'fractionation' of disordered self-awareness (Stuss, 1991). Awareness of deficits, on the other hand, is related to the specific functional systems themselves, e.g. language, and hence impaired awareness of deficit involves impaired knowledge associated with the specific system and would relate to dysfunction in posterior or basal brain regions. Similar views, concentrating on the interaction between frontal and parietal regions and emphasizing to different extents the functional role of each in relation to general and specific awareness, have been put forward by Prigatano (1991), Mesulam (1986) and Bisiach et al. (1986). The latter authors state that anosognosia for a specific deficit 'betrays a disorder at the highest levels of organization of that function. This implies that monitoring of the internal working is not secured in the nervous system by a general, superordinate organ, but is decentralized and apportioned to the different functional blocks to which it refers' (Bisiach et al., 1986, p. 480).

## Neuropsychological theories

With the advances in development of cognitive neuropsychology (Shallice, 1988; McCarthy & Warrington, 1990), interest has focused on applying cognitive neuropsychological theories to both normal brain function and to explaining specific deficits in brain dysfunction. In particular, models are being developed which seek to link neuroanatomical approaches with cognitive psychological approaches, aiming to integrate these into both a structural and functional level of explanation. Unawareness of neurological deficits, in the context of the concept of awareness or consciousness in general, has thus been important in this regard and subject to a variety of related theories (Marcel & Bisiach, 1988; Heilman, 1991).

An interesting model attempting to account for the different types of awareness levels in relation to neurological deficits, primarily memory, has been proposed by Schacter (1990). This model, termed DICE (dissociable interactions and conscious experience), postulates the existence of a 'conscious awareness system' (CAS) which has direct links to individual 'knowledge modules' such as lexical, conceptual, spatial, etc., as well as to an episodic memory information system. Whilst such modules/systems are in constant/ongoing operation to affect behaviour normally, it is only when the CAS is activated and when it interacts with such systems, that a conscious experience of the particular information is obtained. Concentrating on memory deficits, Schacter goes on to discuss how damage at different levels in such a model can explain both global and specific impairments of awareness. He then proposes different levels of explanation within his model to account for these various types of unawareness, including not only unawareness of deficits but also unawareness of knowledge or 'implicit memory'. A first-order level of explanation would involve damage or impairment within the CAS or with its individual connections. He himself favours a second-order level of explanation which would involve dysfunction at the level of the knowledge modules themselves. Sharing similarities with the various models proposed by Stuss and Benson (1986), Bisiach et al. (1986), Mesulam (1986), and Prigatano (1991), Schacter further links his model with neuroanatomical theories. He postulates that the CAS is a posterior system involving the inferoparietal lobes, with connections to the 'executive system' situated in the frontal lobes (McGlynn & Schacter, 1989; Schacter, 1990, 1991). In this way, the model is an attempt to provide both a structural and a functional explanation of impairment in awareness and the dissociations in awareness found in relation to different 'modules' or functions. In line with cognitive theory, it assumes modularity of mental processes, and hence the level of functional explanation is directed at the connections and at the result of damaged connections between individual 'psychological' systems.

## Motivational theories

In contrast to the preceding 'organic' approaches, others have argued that the pathogenesis of 'anosognosia' can be explained on the basis of psychological processes or motivational factors within the patient. The main proponents of these theories were Weinstein and Kahn (1955), who suggested that people are motivated to varying extents to deny the presence of illness or disability in order to protect themselves from the consequent distress of recognition of dysfunction. Using the term 'denial of illness' preferentially, though interchangeably with 'anosognosia', they brought the level of explanation underlying unawareness of deficits to that of psychoanalytical theory. In other words, they invoked the action of defence mechanisms as the unconscious mental processes involved in the protection against overt distress. Whilst proposing psychological mechanisms, the authors stressed, none the less, the necessity of the presence of brain dysfunction itself, in contributing to the presence and expression of the multiple forms of denial/anosognosia. Thus, as Weinstein (1991, p. 254) later stated, '. . . The existence and form of denial/anosognosia are determined by the location and rate of development of the brain lesion, the situation in which the denial is elicited, the type of disability, and the way the patient perceives its meaning on the basis of his past experience.'

Furthermore, following clinical observation, Weinstein and Kahn (1955) suggested that a particular personality type predisposed to the development of denial. Such patients premorbidly considered illness as a weakness/failure and were strongly concerned about the opinions of others and had strong drives to do well and succeed. Subsequently, Weinstein et al. (1994) assessed such traits in the form of Denial Personality Ratings in their research on denial/anosognosia in dementia.

As McGlynn and Schacter (1989) point out, there are a number of problems with viewing anosognosia/unawareness of deficits predominantly in terms of motivational/psychological processes. For example, such theories don't account for the specificity of anosognosia seen frequently in relation to neurological states. Nor, if unconscious psychological mechanisms are postulated should the site of the lesion make much difference. Likewise, the time course of anosognosia is often inconsistent with the views on onset and course of motivated denial. Lewis (1991) also emphasized these difficulties and, consequently, she distinguishes between psychogenic and neurogenic denial. However, she stresses the importance of interaction of both psychological and neurological factors in the overall picture presented.

## Insight into memory function in generalized brain disease (dementias)

In the last decade, there has been growing interest in the concept of insight in relation to dementia. In particular, there have been increasing numbers of systematic studies focusing on the development of specific measures to assess insight as well as investigating the possible neurological and neuropsychological mechanisms underlying impaired insight. In contrast to the relatively consistent approach to awareness/insight in the neurological states (as reviewed above), studies examining insight in the dementias are striking in the range of different approaches used (Kaszniak & Christenson, 1996). This suggests that, as in functional psychiatric disorders, a variety of different conceptual frameworks underlying the notion of insight are being applied in such research. This makes comparisons between studies problematic and may contribute in part to the reported mixed outcomes.

One of the reasons for the different approaches to the concept of insight in the dementias may lie in the clinical status of the dementias themselves. Dementias, or chronic organic brain syndromes, occupy both neurological and psychiatric domains, and hence are subject to the differing influences of physiological/neuropsychological vs. psychiatric/psychological methods characteristic of each discipline. Another reason may lie in the nature of the clinical features of the dementias. Thus, rather than involving single/several specific neurological deficits, dementias may be characterized by various cognitive (including memory) deficits, motor abnormalities, affective and personality changes, psychotic symptoms and behavioural disturbances. Consequently, studies exploring insight in dementias include, to different extents, insight not only into memory function, but also insight into the other impairments.

Evidence for the different approaches to conceptualization of insight into memory deficits in dementias comes from two main sources: (a) terminology used, (b) assessments of insight.

## Terminology

A number of related terms are used in the research on insight in dementias including, 'loss of insight' (De Bettignies et al., 1990), 'lack of awareness' (Ott & Fogel, 1992; Green et al., 1993; Auchus et al., 1994), 'anosognosia' (Reed et al., 1993; Starkstein et al., 1995), 'denial' (Sevush & Leve, 1993; Weinstein et al., 1994) and more recently, 'impaired self-awareness' (Kaszniak & Christenson, 1996). This raises questions concerning first, whether these terms are referring to the same concept and, secondly, whether they are used in the same way by the different researchers. At a very basic level, the terms do of course imply differences. Thus, 'anosognosia' as stated earlier, refers to unawareness of a specific neuropsychological deficit, the latter being 'objectively' ascertainable. 'Lack of awareness' is a less specific term in that it carries no implication concerning the 'object' of awareness whether this be a neurological, physical or 'psychological' phenomenon. As mentioned earlier, 'awareness' in relation to neurological states appears to be used in a more specific sense of a function, differentiated from judgment. 'Insight' on the other hand, following lexical definition and the 'psychiatric' approach, seems to refer to more than awareness. It includes also an understanding of what the object of awareness (memory deficit, paralysis, hallucination, etc.) actually means for the individual. In this sense, awareness can be deemed necessary but not sufficient for insight. The more recently used term 'self-awareness' (recent, that is, in neurological usage) is suggestive of a closer relationship with insight. The term suggests an awareness of something as it relates to the individual and hence, implies some form of additional judgment. In common with general usage of these terms in dementia research, insight assessed as 'self-awareness' rather than 'awareness', does not, however, necessarily reflect this difference in meaning (Loebel et al., 1990). 'Denial' tends to have both a general and specific meaning with problems arising when these are not differentiated. In a general sense, 'denial' is often used descriptively to refer to the refusal made by a patient to admit to an overt dysfunction. However, the term is also frequently used in the sense of defensive denial or 'motivated denial' (McGlynn & Schacter, 1989) where the implication lies in an underlying psychological process operating to inhibit overt acknowledgement of the dysfunction. In this sense, the term has a two-fold meaning in that not only does it refer to 'unawareness' (though implying awareness at an unconscious level), but it also suggests a psychological mechanism underlying this unawareness (i.e.

defence mechanisms, etc.). The term 'denial' in the specific sense, has generally been applied to functional psychiatric illnesses and particularly to the 'neurotic' disorders where lack of awareness or denial of symptoms has been explained as 'a mental mechanism without conscious awareness and employed to resolve emotional conflict and allay anxiety by denying a problem' (Goodwin, 1989). Denial has also been used in this latter sense in dementia (Weinstein & Kahn, 1955).

Problems arise when such terms are not defined and/or are used interchangeably without reference to possible distinctions. As a result, it becomes difficult to identify the particular sense or underlying concept (Feher et al., 1991). McGlynn and Schacter (1989), acknowledge such difficulties and they use the terms 'anosognosia', 'unawareness of deficit' and 'loss of insight' interchangeably. They make it clear, however, that they are using these terms to refer to an underlying concept of unawareness in the neuropsychological sense, maintaining the same meaning as used in relation to amnesic syndromes. On the other hand, they distinguish this concept from motivated denial which they view as a distinct and separate phenomenon. In contrast, however, Weinstein et al. (1994) use the terms 'anosognosia' and 'denial' interchangeably and differentiate these from 'loss of insight' which they consider as a distinct and unitary phenomenon. Unfortunately, they do not actually define their concept of 'loss of insight' and it is consequently difficult to understand the grounds for their distinction. It is not clear, for example, why 'loss of insight implies a unitary defect, which should become more marked as the disease [Alzheimer's disease] progresses' (Weinstein et al., 1994, p. 182). Using the term 'anosognosia', Starkstein et al. (1995) accept a definition of 'loss of insight, misinterpretation and explicit denial', thus broadening the concept in another direction. Along different lines, Mangone et al. (1991) consider impaired insight following frontal lobe dysfunction as equivalent to 'confabulation'. In contrast, they equate impaired insight following right hemisphere dysfunction, with 'anosognosia'. They do not examine the concepts themselves but define them by putative underlying brain mechanisms.

## Assessments of insight in dementias

The number and variety of assessment methods used in exploring insight in dementia likewise suggest differences in approaches to the concept of insight. These are reflected in both the range of methods developed by which insight is inferred and the different types of content deemed relevant to the determination of insight and hence sought by the various assessment measures. First, in terms of methods, most earlier studies do not define their assessment criteria and on the basis of subjective evaluation, subjects are categorized into those having and those not having insight/awareness (e.g. Gustafson & Nilsson, 1982). More recently, however, attempts have been made to use qualitative and quantitative methods. For example, structured or semistructured interviews have been administered in order to categorize degrees of insight in Alzheimer's disease (AD) (Sevush & Leve, 1993; Weinstein et al., 1994). In these cases patients are rated, on the basis of responses to specific questions, as having either no insight, i.e. no acknowledgement of memory impairment, or full insight, i.e. acknowledgement of both the presence and the severity of memory impairment, or partial insight, i.e. showing some awareness of the presence of memory impairment but not its full extent. Similar categorical divisions have been used to evaluate insight in patients with Huntington's Disease (HD) (Caine et al., 1978) and Parkinson's disease (Danielczyk, 1983). Others have complemented information by interviewing relatives/caregivers before making such distinctions (Ott & Fogel, 1992). These methods thus seek to grade patients' insight or awareness on the basis of a fairly general and non-specific concept of insight but without attempting to identify or qualitatively discriminate between different types or aspects of awareness.

More specific notions of insight or awareness appear to underlie the insight assessments based on discrepancy measures. These methods determine levels of insight on the basis of discrepancies between the patient's assessment of self-functioning and either: (i) 'objective' measures of impairment such as a battery of neuropsychological tests (Anderson & Tranel, 1989) and/or, (ii) the carer's assessment of patient functioning (De Bettignies et al., 1990; Mangone et al., 1991; Michon et al., 1992, 1994; Verhey et al., 1993; Vasterling et al., 1995). The greater the discrepancy obtained on these measures, indicates a greater degree of unawareness or insightlessness shown by the patient. In other words, these methods assume that the 'objective' assessments of functioning (either clinical tests or carers' views) provide the standard, or relatively accurate representation of the level of functioning (memory or other) in the patient. Lack of concordance is thus attributed to disturbed awareness on the part of the patient. The concept of insight underlying such methods is thus fairly specific in that it is conceived as a ('correct') evaluation of function in a particular area. In the sense that they focus on the differences between subjective and 'objective' evaluations, these methods stress quantitative differences in awareness, but again tend not to explore the actual nature of awareness itself. Instead, qualitative differences, following the neuropsychological models of awareness, relate more to differential scores in discrepancy/awareness in relation to different tasks or functions (Green et al., 1993; Vasterling et al., 1995). Such ratings also cannot discriminate between impaired awareness and denial in the 'motivated' or 'defensive' sense. Furthermore, some of the assumptions behind these methods can be questioned. It can be argued for example, that even if clinical tests of memory/cognitive function provide valid and accurate measures of ability, they may not necessarily correspond to the sort of subjective experiences of memory impairment that are asked in questionnaires/interviews (Sunderland et al., 1983; Kaszniak & Christenson, 1996). Similarly, some carers may not provide 'objective' assessments of functioning in patients but may, for various reasons, both overestimate and underestimate levels of impairment in the patient. De Bettignies et al. (1990), for example, used discrepancy measures between patients (with AD and multi-infarct dementia) and informants as a measure of patients' insight into their living skills. They found that, whilst insight was not correlated with age, mental status, education or level of depression in the patients, it was significantly related to the degree of caregiver concern or burden. In other words, the higher the degree of the burden perceived by the caregiver, the higher the discrepancy between patient and informant report. The authors suggested that the elicited impaired insight in this situation was not only due to the overestimation of capacity by the patients, but that caregivers with a greater perceived burden were underestimating the capacity of the patients. Most studies, however, seem to indicate that carers' assessments of patients' memory function have a good correlation with patients' performances on 'objective' (psychometric) tests (Freidenberg et al., 1990; McGlone et al., 1990; Feher et al., 1991; Koss et al., 1993; Jorm et al., 1994).

Reisberg et al. (1985) (for review, see McGlynn & Kaszniak (1991b)) compared ratings made by patients with AD of their own and their caregivers' cognitive (memory) function with equivalent ratings made by the caregivers of their's and the patients' memory function. This assessment of insight was thus based on the difference between patients' self-judgment and their judgment of others' function. A similar method has also been used by McGlynn and Kaszniak (1991a, see below), who suggest that in dementia, the cognitive breakdown results in patients being unable to monitor their own cognitive performance whilst still being able to make accurate judgments of their relatives' abilities.

One interesting and comprehensive method of assessing quantitatively patients' insight into deficits was devised by McGlynn and Kaszniak in relation to AD (1991a) and HD (1991b). This was developed using a similar approach to that described by Schacter (1991, as above) in the assessment of awareness of memory deficit in amnesic syndromes. Similarly, involving comparisons between patients and their caregivers, with respect to HD, three aspects of 'insight' were explored. First, a structured questionnaire (Daily Difficulties Questionnaire) was administered to both patients and caregivers to assess their own and their relatives' present functioning as compared to 5 years previously. Then, the two other aspects of insight were assessed as the differences between patients' (and caregivers') predictions of performance on various motor and cognitive tasks and their actual subsequent performance. In other words, 'insight' was evaluated as a predictive judgment on tasks which could then be directly verified. A similar approach was used by Green et al. (1993) who likewise used the difference between patients' prediction of their performance on a word recall test with their actual subsequent performance, as one aspect of insight assessment in dementia.

Apart from such differences in the methods used in assessing insight, the content of the information sought in such assessments also varies considerably, reflecting further the different notions underlying insight in these measures. This variation in content of insight assessment measures can, for the purposes here, be roughly divided into two main areas.

First, the object itself of the insight assessment is not always the memory function. Indeed, many studies do not directly specify the object of awareness and the general implication is that the insight refers to the disease as a whole (e.g. Danielczyk, 1983; Schneck et al., 1982). Some studies specify memory impairment as the sole object of the insight assessment (Feher et al., 1991; McGlynn & Kaszniak, 1991a; Michon et al., 1992; Reed et al., 1993). In other studies the object of insight is defined as 'independent living skills' and awareness into memory impairment is not part of the assessment (De Bettignies et al., 1990). Still others assess insight into memory function alongside insight into other cognitive, behavioural, affective and personality functions. For example, McGlynn and Kaszniak (1991b) looked at insight in *motor* as well as cognitive performance. Ott and Fogel (1992), in turn, examined insight in relation to the patient's situation, memory impairment, impairment in activities of daily living (ADL) and progression of deficits. The assessment devised by Anderson and Tranel (1989), explored awareness in eight specific areas. These included the following: reasons for hospitalization, motor impairments, general thinking and intellect, orientation, memory, speech and language, visual perception and lastly, abilities on tests and future activities. Green et al. (1993) focused on recent memory, remote memory, attention and everyday activities. On the other hand, Vasterling et al. (1995), assessed memory, general health, self-care ability and mood disturbance.

Secondly, even when the 'object' of the insight assessment is memory, differences still occur in the insight assessments according to the type of memory function/dysfunction that is being examined. For example, some assessments focus on awareness of a general memory impairment (Mangone et al., 1991; Sevush & Leve, 1993; Verhey et al., 1993), whilst others examine awareness of memory impairment in relation to numerous specific memory-dependent tasks (Feher et al., 1991; Green et al., 1993 ). Some researchers also explore patients' awareness of the effects of memory impairment in different aspects of their lives (Sevush & Leve, 1993; Starkstein et al., 1995, 1997). In a different vein, some insight assessments concentrate on awareness of current memory function (Mangone et al., 1991; Verhey et al., 1993) whilst others focus also on awareness of change in memory functioning (McGlynn & Kaszniak, 1991a,b; Vasterling et al., 1995). Further disparities between studies are evident, e.g. in the ratings of anosognosia/unawareness made by Reed et al. (1993) and Weinstein et al. (1994). The ratings in these studies are in part determined by views on patients' affective responses and level of concern about deficits. Other researchers (Anderson & Tranel, 1989; Verhey et al., 1993), on the other hand, limit their evaluations to awareness or knowledge of the deficits themselves.

## Outcome studies

Not surprisingly, results of empirical studies are inconclusive. Variability in terms, definitions, assessment methods, and 'object of insight' all contribute to this, as well as the fact that different outcome measures have been used. In addition, most of this work has been carried out in relation to AD, where loss of insight is recognized as an important feature of the disease (American Psychiatric Association, 1994). There has been little systematic work on other types of dementia. In general, it is claimed that patients with cortical dementias (e.g. AD, Pick's disease) show greater loss of insight (Lishman, 1987; McGlynn & Kaszniak, 1991b). Some studies also suggest that there is an earlier loss of insight in Pick's disease (Gustafson & Nilsson, 1982). It has also been claimed that 'subcortical' dementias are not associated with a great degree of insightlessness (e.g. Caine & Shoulson, 1983; Danielczyk, 1983). Patients with multi-infarct dementia (MID) are said to have preserved insight as compared with AD patients (Lishman, 1987; De Bettignies et al., 1990), although more recent work has found no significant difference (Sultzer et al., 1993). Most of these findings, however, are based on work where insight is not assessed in a structured way or where the criteria for assessing its presence/absence (most studies assume a unitary conceptualization) are not defined (Danielczyk, 1983). In addition, difficulties arise in the assessment of the stage of the disease, the rate of progression and the severity of dementia, all of which may influence the level and type of insight. In general, there has been less work on traumatic, radiation, space-occupying, myxoedematous, B12 deficiency, normal-pressure hydrocephalus, etc. types of dementia, perhaps reflecting the lesser prevalence of these clinical groups as compared with AD. A summary of the results from recent studies on insight in dementias is given in Table 10.1.

## Stage of dementia

With respect to *stage* of the dementia, most studies suggest that insight is preserved early on in the disease (Schneck et al., 1982; Seltzer et al., 1993) and diminishes with progression of the disease (Freidenberg et al., 1990; Starkstein et al., 1997), though others point at a more complicated relationship. Thus, Reisberg et al. (1985), for review, see McGlynn and Kaszniak (1991b), found that patients showed less insight at the earliest stage of the illness, becoming more insightful during the 'confusional' phase, before losing this insight in the later stages. Neary et al. (1986) suggest that there is considerable variation in the amount of insight held by patients with AD,

**Table 10.1.** Summary of studies examining insight in dementias

| Study | Patient sample | Terminology: (a)<br>'Object' of insight: (b) | Assessment of 'insight' | Outcome variables | Main findings |
|---|---|---|---|---|---|
| Anderson & Tranel (1989) | n = 100 dementia: 49 CVA: 32 head trauma: 19 | (a) unawareness = anosognosia (b) cognitive and motor deficits | awareness index (AI): discrepancy between patients' description of ability and performance on neurophsychology tests | neuropsychology tests: 1–8 CT and/or MRI | – three groups no different on AI. – unawareness associated with: right-hemisphere damage, IQ, temporal disorientation |
| De Bettignies et al. (1990) | AD: 12 MID: 12 elderly control: 12 | (a) level of insight (b) independent living skills | discrepancy between scores on questions rated by patient and rated by caregivers | physical self-maintenance scale instrumental activities of daily living HDRS | – AD greater loss of insight than MID and controls. – loss of insight not related to level of depression – loss of insight significantly related to degree of caregivers' burden |
| Feher et al. (1991) | AD: 38 | (a) anosognosia, unawareness of symptoms, denial of memory deficits (b) memory deficits | 'denial score' – discrepancy between scores on questions rated by patient and rated by caregivers | MMSE, GDS, HDRS, memory tests: 4, 9, 10 | – degree of denial correlated weakly with severity of dementia and severity of memory impairment – degree of denial correlated negatively with depression |
| McGlynn & Kaszniak (1991a) | AD: 8 | (a) unawareness of deficits, loss of insight (b) memory deficits | discrepancy between scores on DDQ and CTPP as rated by patients and caregivers | MMSE neuropsychology tests: 11–22 | – degree of unawareness correlated with severity of dementia – patients had little insight into own memory deficits but better insight into carers' performances |

**Table 10.1** (*cont.*)

| Study | Patient sample | Terminology: (a)<br>'Object' of insight: (b) | Assessment of 'insight' | Outcome variables | Main findings |
|---|---|---|---|---|---|
| McGlynn &<br>Kaszniak<br>(1991b) | HD: 8 | (a) unawareness of<br>deficits<br>(b) memory deficits<br>and motor disturbance | discrepancy between scores<br>on DDQ, CTPP and MTPP<br>as rated by patients and<br>caregivers | MMSE, neuropsychology<br>tests: 10, 22<br>motor tasks: a–e | – discrepancy between HD and<br>caregivers on ratings<br>– HD showed accuracy at<br>predicting own performance on<br>some memory tests |
| Mangone<br>et al. (1991) | AD: 41 | (a) insight – 2<br>components-<br>confabulation,<br>anosognosia<br>(b) physical self<br>maintenance activities<br>and ADL | 'impaired insight score (IIS)'<br>– discrepancy between scores<br>on items rated by patients<br>and caregivers | MMSE, GDS, BDRS,<br>BPRS<br>neuropsychology tests:<br>9, 23–33 | – lower insight correlated with<br>increased severity of dementia<br>– lower insight in AD with<br>delusions<br>– significant correlation between<br>IIS and GDS, BDRS, MMSE<br>– no correlation with duration of<br>memory loss<br>– negative correlation between IIS<br>and all neuropsychology tests<br>– best predictors of IIS = GDS, 23,<br>30. |
| Michon et al.<br>(1992) | AD: 15 | (a) anosognosia<br>(b) memory | 'nosognosic score' –<br>discrepancy between patient<br>and family ratings | MMSE<br>neuropsychology tests:<br>22, 34–37 | – no correlation between<br>anosognosia and 34<br>– marginal correlation with MMSE<br>– high (negative) correlation with<br>'frontal' tests score |

| Study | Sample | Awareness measure | Method | Instruments | Findings |
|---|---|---|---|---|---|
| Ott & Fogel (1992) | $n = 50$ (AD: 37, rest: vascular, frontal lobe, etc.) | (a) insight, awareness of dementia (b) situation, memory impairment, impairment in ADL, progression of deficits | 'insight rating scale' – score based on information from both patient and caregiver, scoring in each domain | MMSE, HDRS, COR, GDS, CDRS | – significant correlation between impaired insight and severity of dementia<br>– poor correlation with depression |
| Reed et al. (1993) | AD: 57 (47-probable, 10-possible) | (a) anosognosia, lack of awareness of symptoms (b) memory impairment | ratings by two psychologists from notes of interviews made by neurologist and psychiatrist – four categories identified | MMSE, DSM III neuropsychology tests: 38–41 SPECT – ($n = 20$) | – no relationship between level of awareness and dementia severity<br>– no relationship between level of awareness and presence of depression<br>– association between anosognosia and right dorsolateral frontal perfusion |
| Sevush & Leve (1993) | AD: 128 | (a) denial of deficits, anosognosia (b) memory | structured clinical interview – three categories identified | cognitive abilities: 42, 3-item depression scale | – correlation between denial and severity of cognitive deficit<br>– negative correlation between denial and depression |
| Verhey et al. (1993) | AD: 103 VD: 43 other: 24 (HD, PD, etc.) | (a) insight, awareness, anosognosia – 'absence of knowledge/ recognition' (b) cognitive deficits (mainly memory) | semistructured interview of patient and caregiver – four categories identified | GerDS, HDRS, DSM IIIR | – level of awareness related to severity of dementia<br>– no relationship to depression (presence or severity)<br>– modest correlation between awareness and item 'psychic anxiety' on HDRS |

**Table 10.1** (*cont.*)

| Study | Patient sample | TermTerminology: (a) 'Object' of insight: (b) | Assessment of 'insight' | Outcome variables | Main findings |
|---|---|---|---|---|---|
| Green et al. (1993) | AD: 20 | (a) awareness of deficits (b) recent memory, remote memory, attention, everyday activities | – questionnaire discrepancy = discrepancy between patient and family judgment in the four areas – recall discrepancy = discrepancy between patient prediction on recall performance and actual performance | Dementia Rating Scale (n = 9) neuropsychology tests: 2 (n = 11), 38 (n = 20) | – patients show variable awareness in relation to the four domains – greatest unawareness in relation to recent memory and everyday activities – no correlation between unawareness and severity of dementia |
| Auchus et al. (1994) | AD: 28 | (a) unawareness, anosognosia, anosodiaphoria (b) cognitive impairment | retrospective review – patients judged aware (13) and unaware (15) on basis of self-report and responses to direct questions on memory | neuropsychology tests: 2, 9, 30, 39, 40, 41, 43 | – no correlation between unawareness and severity of dementia or memory function tests – only significant correlation between unawareness and visuoconstructive ability (41,43) |
| Michon et al. (1994) | AD: 24 | (a) anosognosia (b) memory deficits | 'anosognosia score' – discrepancy between patient's self-rating score and rating by family member on 20-item questionnaire | MMSE neuropsychology tests: 9, 10, 22, 30, 34, 35, 39 behavioural abnormalities: 'frontal score' | – no correlation between anosognosia score and MMSE, Wechsler Memory Scale or linguistic abilities – significant correlation (negative) with frontal score, particularly Wisconsin Card Sorting Test |

| Study | Sample | Measures | Method | Tests | Findings |
|---|---|---|---|---|---|
| Weinstein et al. (1994) | AD: 41 (30-probable, 11-possible) | (a) anosognosia, lack of knowledge of disease, denial, unawareness of impairment, etc – not loss of insight (b) memory, ADL | specific questions as part of structured interview – three categories identified | MMSE, neuropsychology tests: 43–45 presence of psychotic features denial personality rating (carers) | – no correlation between denial and severity of dementia – denial associated with confabulation, delusions and misidentifications – denial more frequent when initial presentation was memory loss, behavioural disturbance |
| Vasterling et al. (1995) | AD: 43 | (a) awareness of deficits, degree of agreement between patients and carers (b) memory, general health, self-care ability, mood disturbance | discrepancy between ratings made by patients and carers on five-point scale in each domain | MMSE, CDR, COR, PEAS, EMQ | – greatest unawareness in memory and self-care – moderate unawareness in anxiety and irritability – minimal unawareness in health and depression – unawareness associated with advanced disease – unawareness associated with cognitive impairment |
| Starkstein et al. (1995) | AD: 24 12-anosognosia 12-without anosognosia | (a) anosognosia, unawareness, denial, misinterpretation (b) illness – intellectual function, interests, personality | anosognosia questionnaire for dementia (AQ-D) – 30 questions given to patients and carers. Final score is discrepancy between the two scores. | MMSE, HDRS, FIM, STC, neuropsychology tests: 19, 35, 39, 40, 41, 46–49 SPECT | – no correlations between anosognosia and depression, functional level, social ties, neuropsychology – significant relationship between anosognosia and blood flow continues. |

**Table 10.1** (*cont.*)

| Study | Patient sample | Terminology: (a) 'Object' of insight: (b) | Assessment of 'insight' | Outcome variables | Main findings |
|---|---|---|---|---|---|
| | | | | | deficits in frontal inferior and superior areas of right hemisphere |

*Notes:*

*Abbreviations:* AD – Alzheimer's disease; MID – Multi-infarct dementia; HD – Huntington's disease; ADL – Activities of Daily Living; MMSE – Mini-Mental State Examination; HDRS – Hamilton Depression Rating Scale; GDS – Global Deterioration Scale; BDRS – Blessed Dementia Rating Scale; BPRS – Behavioral Pathology Rating Scale; CDRS – Clinical Dementia Rating Scale; GerDS – Geriatric Depression Scale; COR – Cornell Depression Scale; DDQ – Daily Difficulties Questionnaire; CTPP – Cognitive Tasks Performance Predictions; MTPP – Motor Tasks Performance Predictions; EMQ – Everyday Memory Questionnaire; PEAS – Performance of Everyday Activities Scale; FIM – Functional Independence Measure; STC – Social Ties Checklist

*Motor tasks:* (a) write word list, (b) grooved pegboard, (c) walk on line, (d) catch ball, (e) finger tapping, (f) pronounce words

*Neuropsychology tests:* 1 – Benton Orientation Questionnaire, 2 – Wechsler Adult Intelligence Scale-Revised, 3 – Rey Auditory-Verbal Learning Test, 4 – Benton Visual Retention Test, 5 – Rey-Osterrith Complex Figure Recall Test, 6 – Multilingual Aphasia Examination, 7 – Test of Facial Recognition, 8 – Judgment of Line Orientation, 9 – Logical Memory [from Wechsler Memory Scale], 10 – Paired Associates [from Wechsler Memory Scale], 11 – Word Recall-immediate, 12 – Word Recall-delayed, 13 – Picture Recall-immediate, 14 – Picture Recall-delayed, 15 – Picture Recognition-immediate, 16 – Picture Recognition-delayed, 17 – Word Recognition-immediate, 18 – Word Recognition-delayed, 19 – Digit Span, 20 – Verbal Span, 21 – Spatial Span, 22 – Verbal Fluency, 23 – Continuous Performance Test, 24 – Alternating Sequences Test, 25 – Go-No-Go Paradigm, 26 – Alzheimer's Disease Assessment Scale, 27 – Ideomotor Praxis Test, 28 – Ideational Praxis Test, 29 – Constructional Praxis Test, 30 – Visual Reproduction [from Wechsler Memory Scale], 31 – Right-Left Differentiation Test, 32 – Spatial Relationship Test, 33 – Word List Generation, 34 – Wechsler Memory Scale, 35 – Wisconsin Card Sorting Test, 36 – Graphic Series, 37 – Frontal Behaviours, 38 – California Verbal Learning Test, 39 – Boston Naming Test, 40 – Controlled Oral Word Association Test, 41 – Block Design [from WAIS-R], 42 – Assessment of Cognitive Abilities in Dementia, 43 – Clock Drawing, 44 – Face-Hand Test, 45 – Immediate Recall of Test Story, 46 – Token Test, 47 – Raven's Progressive Matrices, 48 – Apraxia Subtest of Western Aphasia Battery, 49 – Selective Reminding Test of Buschke and Fuld.

some patients with more global impairment showing greater insight into their illness than patients at an earlier stage.

## Severity of dementia

Examination of the relationship between severity of the dementing illness and loss of insight has yielded mixed results, with some workers reporting a strong positive correlation (Mangone et al., 1991; Ott & Fogel, 1992; Sevush & Leve, 1993; Verhey et al., 1993; Vasterling et al., 1995). Others find a weaker association (Feher et al., 1991; Michon et al., 1992) and yet others claim that there is no relationship between the severity of dementia and loss of insight (Green et al., 1993; Reed et al., 1993; Auchus et al., 1994; Weinstein et al., 1994). Results in this area are particularly variable (see Table 10.1) and are likely to reflect not just the different methods used in assessing insight but the difficulty and variability in determining the severity of the dementia itself. For example, many studies use the severity of cognitive impairments as a measure of severity of the dementia, whereas others rely to different extents also on measures of functional abilities, behavioural disturbance and personality change.

## Depression

In their attempt to 'explain' depression in dementia, some studies have examined the relationship between depressive symptoms and level of insight in dementia. Results are conflicting as, for example, Reed et al. (1993), found no relationship between 'anosognosia' in AD patients and a diagnosis of major depression (according to DSM III criteria). De Bettignies et al. (1990) and Verhey et al. (1993) found no relationship between loss of insight in dementia (mixed groups of AD, vascular dementia and others) and degree of depression (as assessed by the Hamilton Depression Rating Scale [HDRS]). On the other hand, Feher et al. (1991) have described a weak relationship between loss of insight and HDRS scores, and Sevush and Leve (1993) claimed a significant relationship between loss of insight and severity of depression (depression in this study was rated on a three-item scale). In other words, the more insightful patients were found to be more depressed, and both studies suggested that the depression present in the patients with dementia might, in part, have developed as a reaction to the awareness patients had concerning their disease. In a large study, involving 235 patients with AD, Seltzer et al. (1993) also found that preserved insight was significantly related to the presence of depression, but in this study, neither insight nor depression (or other symptoms) were assessed in a structured or systematic way. Instead, together with ten other psychiatric symptoms, they were rated simply as being present or absent. Interestingly, in direct contrast to the previous studies, Freidenberg et al. (1990) found a significant relationship between diminished insight in patients with

Alzheimer's disease and both depressive and psychotic symptoms. On the other hand, Kaszniak et al. (1993) found no correlation between impaired awareness in Alzheimer's disease patients and ratings of depression or delusions. The 'type' of depression in AD was found to be differentially related to anosognosia in the recent study by Starkstein et al. (1997). In this longitudinal study, the authors found that in their AD patients with dysthymia, there was a significant worsening of anosognosia over a 16 month follow-up period which significantly correlated with lower depression rating scores at the follow-up evaluation. This was in contrast to the AD patients with major depression for whom no significant correlation with anosognosia scores was obtained. The authors explained this on the basis that dysthymia may be an emotional reaction to the AD whereas major depression represents a more severe biological dysfunction specific to the neuronal loss of AD.

## Brain mechanisms

In line with 'neurological' research, where associations have been described between 'anosognosia' and frontal lobe pathology (McGlynn & Schacter, 1989; Prigatano, 1991; Starkstein et al., 1993), attempts have also been made to examine the role of the frontal lobe in the relationship between loss of insight and dementia. Weinstein et al. (1994) showed that AD patients presenting with memory loss and behavioural disturbances indicative of frontal lobe involvement, had less awareness of deficits than patients presenting with features suggestive of posterior brain involvement such as writing/reading difficulties or visuospatial problems. Similarly, Mangone et al. (1991) and Michon et al. (1992, 1994) found a strong correlation between anosognosia and scores on frontal lobe dysfunction tests. Reed et al. (1993) carried out SPECT studies in 20 patients with AD and found a significant correlation between 'anosognosia' and right dorsolateral frontal lobe perfusion. Anosognosia in this particular study was determined on the basis of ratings made from case notes on the patients, who were categorized as having 'full awareness', 'shallow awareness' or 'no awareness'. Starkstein et al. (1995), found that patients with anosognosia in AD had significantly lower regional cerebral blood flow in the right frontal lobe on SPECT studies than did patients without anosognosia, although there were no differences on neuropsychological testing. The authors in this study used the discrepancies between patients' answers and caregivers' answers on a structured questionnaire as a measure of anosognosia. They conceptualized anosognosia broadly, examining awareness of intellectual functioning, changes in interests and personality changes. However, they then categorized the patients into those with and those without anosognosia on the basis of a cut-off point on their questionnaire score. It is not clear, therefore, whether the two groups differed simply in degree of awareness into deficits or in the *types* of deficits towards which they were unaware. Auchus et al. (1994) have reported that patients with AD showed a significant correlation between unawareness of deficits and visuocon-structional dysfunction (as assessed by clock drawing and block designing) suggest-ing that right hemisphere dysfunction might also be important as an underlying mechanism of unawareness. Unawareness of deficits (rated as present or absent) in this retrospective study, however, was elicited on the basis of clinical judgment and no criteria were given to explain how this was determined.

For the sake of completion, a brief mention should be made concerning one of the other aspects of awareness or insight that has been studied in relation to dementia, namely, implicit or unconscious memory. Work in this area has fol-lowed the neuropsychological approach to awareness as already described in amnesic syndromes. Using priming tasks, patients with AD have been shown to display implicit memory in a similar manner to other patients with amnesic syn-dromes (McGlynn & Schacter, 1989; Schacter, 1995). In addition, dissociations have been found between not only implicit and explicit memory, but also between the types of implicit memory preserved. For example, the commonest finding with respect to AD has been a dissociation between priming deficits in word-related priming tasks, visual tasks and motor tasks (Burke et al., 1994; Russo & Spinnler, 1994; Schacter, 1995). The converse, i.e. deficits in procedural, motor-related tasks and sparing of verbal-related tasks, has been found in Huntington's disease (Butters et al., 1994). In a detailed study, Keane et al. (1991) have been able to dem-onstrate a dissociation between perceptual priming (spared) and verbal priming (involved) in AD, which is in keeping with the view that these functions are served by the occipital and temporo-parietal lobe, respectively. More recently, Gallie et al. (1993) compared 20 patients with AD (mild, moderate and severe) with 40 con-trols on four different priming tasks (i.e. using spoken and written words, pictures and objects). They found that the patients with AD and controls showed similar levels of priming on spoken and written word category completion tests (thus showing a dissociation between implicit and explicit memory in AD). However, the patients with AD showed lower priming effects on pictures (i.e. priming deficits) and greater priming effects on tactile identification (i.e. priming pre-served) than did the control subjects. Differences were also observed at different stages of the disease.

Studies, examining this aspect of awareness in dementia, have generally been limited to demonstrating the presence (sparing) or absence (deficit) of implicit memory with respect to different modality-specific tests. In this sense, implicit memory is viewed very much as a distinct and separate neuropsychological phe-nomenon, with theories concerning its mechanism following the neuropsycholog-ical lines as described earlier. There has been little attempt to conceptualize this notion either theoretically or empirically within the framework of insight as a whole. Future work might, for example, explore the relationship between this sort of unawareness of function and the impaired insight in relation to deficits in patients with dementia.

## Conclusions

This chapter has emphasized the diversity of approaches to the study of insight into memory function which, in turn, reflects different conceptualizations of insight. The latter are likely to influence the way in which the 'clinical' phenomena of insight/awareness and anosognosia are perceived and measured. Consequently, the issue of whether the same or different phenomena are being examined needs to be addressed, as this, in turn, carries implications for the validity of explanatory mechanisms across different studies and patient groups.

## REFERENCES

Amador, X.F., Strauss, D.H., Yale, S.A. & Gorman, J.M. (1991). Awareness of illness in schizophrenia. *Schizophrenia Bulletin*, 17, 113–32.

Amador, X.F., Strauss, D.H., Yale, S.A., Flaum, M.M., Endicott, J. & Gorman, J.M. (1993). Assessment of insight in psychosis. *American Journal of Psychiatry*, 150, 873–9.

American Psychiatric Association (1994). *Diagnostic and Statistical Manual of Mental Disorders*, 4th edn (DSM-IV). Washington, DC: APA.

Anderson, S.W. & Tranel, D. (1989). Awareness of disease states following cerebral infarction, dementia and head trauma: standardized assessment. *The Clinical Neuropsychologist*, 3, 327–39.

Anton, G (1899). Ueber die Selbstwahrnehmung der Herderkrankungen des Gehirns durch den Kranken bei Rindenblindheit und Rindentaubheit. *Archiv für Psychiatrie und Nervenkrankheiten*, 32, 86–127.

Auchus, A.P., Goldstein, F.C., Green, J. & Green, R.C. (1994). Unawareness of cognitive impairments in Alzheimer's disease. *Neuropsychiatry Neuropsychology and Behavioral Neurology*, 7, 25–9.

Babinski, M.J. (1914). Contribution à l'Étude des Troubles Mentaux dans l'Hémiplégie organique cérébrale (Anosognosie). *Revue Neurologique*, 27, 845–8.

Bisiach, E., Vallar, G., Perani, D., Papagno, C. & Berti, A. (1986). Unawareness of disease following lesions of the right hemisphere: anosognosia for hemiplegia and anosognosia for hemianopia. *Neuropsychologia*, 24, 471–82.

Burke, J., Knight, R.G. & Partridge, F.M. (1994). Priming deficits in patients with dementia of the Alzheimer type. *Psychological Medicine*, 24, 987–93.

Butters, N., Salmon, D. & Heindel, W.C. (1994). Specificity of the memory deficits associated with basal ganglia dysfunction. *Revue Neurologique*, 150, 580–7.

Caine, E.D. & Shoulson, I. (1983). Psychiatric syndromes in Huntington's disease. *American Journal of Psychiatry*, 140, 728–33.

Caine, E.D., Hunt, R.D., Weingartner, H. & Ebert, M.H. (1978). Huntington's dementia, clinical and neuropsychological features. *Archives of General Psychiatry*, **35**, 377–84.

Cermak, L.S., Talbot, N., Chandler, K. & Wolbarst, L.R. (1985). The perceptual priming phenomena in amnesia. *Neuropsychologia*, **23**, 615–22.

Cuesta, M.J. & Peralta, V. (1994). Lack of insight in schizophrenia. *Schizophrenia Bulletin*, **20**, 359–66.

Danielczyk, W. (1983). Various mental behavioral disorders in Parkinson's disease, primary degenerative senile dementia and multiple infarction dementia. *Journal of Neural Transmission*, **56**, 161–76.

David, A.S. (1990). Insight and psychosis. *British Journal of Psychiatry*, **156**, 798–808.

David, A.S., Buchanan, A., Reed, A. & Almeida, O. (1992). The assessment of insight in psychosis. *British Journal of Psychiatry*, **161**, 599–602.

De Bettignies, B.H., Mahurin, R.K. & Pirozzolo, F.J. (1990). Insight for impairment in independent living skills in Alzheimer's disease and multi-infarct dementia. *Journal of Clinical and Experimental Neuropsychology*, **12**, 355–63.

Feher, E.P., Mahurin, R.K., Inbody, S.B., Crook, T.H. & Pirozzolo, F.J. (1991). Anosognosia in Alzheimer's disease. *Neuropsychiatry, Neuropsychology and Behavioral Neurology*, **4**, 136–46.

Freidenberg, D.L., Huber, S.J. & Dreskin, M. (1990). Loss of insight in Alzheimer's disease. *Neurology*, **40**, 240 (abstract).

Gallie, K.A., Graf, P. & Tuokko, H. (1993). Implicit memory in Alzheimer's disease: performance on different tests. *Journal of Clinical and Experimental Neuropsychology*, **15**, 30 (abstract).

Gelder, M., Gath, D., Mayou, R. & Cowen, P. (1996). *Oxford Textbook of Psychiatry*, 3rd edn. Oxford: Oxford University Press.

Ghaemi, S.N., Hebben, N., Stoll, A.L. & Pope, H.G. (1996). Neuropsychological aspects of lack of insight in bipolar disorder: a preliminary report. *Psychiatry Research*, **65**, 113–20.

Glisky, E.L., Schacter, D.L. & Tulving, E. (1986). Computer learning by memory-impaired patients: acquisition and retention of complex knowledge. *Neuropsychologia*, **24**, 313–28.

Goodwin, D.M. (1989). *A Dictionary of Neuropsychology*. Heidelberg: Springer.

Green, J., Goldstein, F.C., Sirockman, B.E. & Green, R.C. (1993). Variable awareness of deficits in Alzheimer's disease. *Neuropsychiatry, Neuropsychology and Behavioral Neurology*, **6**, 159–65.

Grut, M., Jorm, A.F., Fratiglioni, L., Forsell, Y., Viitanen, M. & Winblad, B. (1993). Memory complaints of elderly people in a population survey: variation according to dementia stage and depression. *Journal of the American Geriatrics Society*, **41**, 1295–300.

Gustafson, L. & Nilsson, L. (1982). Differential diagnosis of presenile dementia on clinical grounds. *Acta Psychiatrica Scandinavica*, **65**, 194–209.

Healton, E.B., Navarro, C., Bressman, S. & Brust, J.C.M. (1982). Subcortical neglect. *Neurology*, **32**, 776–8.

Heilman, K.M. (1991). Anosognosia: possible neuropsychological mechanisms. In *Awareness of Deficit After Brain Injury*, ed. G.P. Prigatano & D.L. Schacter. Oxford: Oxford University Press.

Heilman, K.M., Watson, R.T. & Valenstein, E. (1993). Neglect and related disorders. In *Clinical Neuropsychology*, ed. K.M. Heilman & E. Valenstein, pp. 279–336. Oxford: Oxford University Press.

Hermann, D.J. (1982). Know the memory: the use of questionnaires to assess and study memory. *Psychological Bulletin*, **92**, 434–52.

Jacoby, L.L. & Witherspoon, D. (1982). Remembering without awareness. *Canadian Journal of Psychology*, **36**, 300–24.

Jorm, A.F., Christensen, H., Henderson, A.S., Korten, A.E., Mackinnon, A.J. & Scott, R. (1994). Complaints of cognitive decline in the elderly: a comparison of reports by subjects and informants in a community survey. *Psychological Medicine*, **24**, 365–74.

Kaszniak, A.W., Ditraglia, G. & Trosset, M.W. (1993). Self-Awareness of cognitive deficit in patients with probable Alzheimer's disease. *Journal of Clinical and Experimental Neuropsychology*, **15**, (abstract), 30.

Kaszniak, A.W. & Christenson, G.D. (1996). Self-awareness of deficit in patients with Alzheimer's disease. In *Toward a Science of Consciousness. The First Tucson Discussions and Debates*, ed. S.R. Hameroff, A.W. Kaszniak & A.C. Scott, pp. 227–42. Cambridge, MA: MIT Press.

Keane, M.M., Gabrieli, J.D.E., Fennema, A.C., Growden, J.H. & Corkin, S. (1991). Evidence for a dissociation between perceptual and conceptual priming in Alzheimer's disease. *Behavioral Neurosciences*, **105**, 326–42.

Korsakoff, S.S. (1889). Étude médico-psychologique sur une forme des maladies de la mémoire. *Revue Philosophique*, **28**, 501–30.

Koss, E., Patterson, M.B., Ownby, R., Stuckey, J.C. & Whitehouse, P.J. (1993). Memory evaluation in Alzheimer's disease, caregivers' appraisals and objective testing. *Archives of Neurology*, **50**, 92–7.

Lewis, A. (1934). The psychopathology of insight. *Journal of Medical Psychology*, **14**, 332–48.

Lewis, L. (1991). Role of psychological factors in disordered awareness. In *Awareness of Deficit After Brain Injury*, ed. G.P. Prigatano & D.L. Schacter. Oxford: Oxford University Press.

Lishman, W.A. (1987). *Organic Psychiatry*, 2nd edn. Oxford: Blackwell.

Loebel, J.P., Dager, S.R., Berg, G. & Hyde, T.S. (1990). Fluency of speech and self-awareness of memory deficit in Alzheimer's disease. *International Journal of Geriatric Psychiatry*, **5**, 41–5.

Luria, A.R. (1976). *The Neuropsychology of Memory*. New York: John Wiley.

McAndrews, M.P., Glisky, E.L. & Schacter, D.L. (1987). When priming persists: Long-lasting implicit memory for a single episode in amnesic patients. *Neuropsychologia*, **25**, 497–506.

McCarthy, R.A. & Warrington, E.K. (1990). *Cognitive Neuropsychology*. London: Academic Press.

McEvoy, J.P., Apperson, L.J., Appelbaum, P.S., Ortlip, P., Brecosky, J., Hammill, K., Geller, J.L. & Roth, L. (1989). Insight in schizophrenia. Its relationship to acute psychopathology. *Journal of Nervous and Mental Disease*, **177**, 43–7.

McEvoy, J.P., Freter, S., Merritt, M. & Apperson, L.J. (1993). Insight about psychosis among outpatients with schizophrenia. *Hospital and Community Psychiatry*, **44**, 883–4.

McGlone, J., Gupta, S., Humphrey, D. & Oppenheimer, T. (1990). Screening for early dementia using memory complaints from patients and relatives. *Archives of Neurology*, **47**, 1189–93.

McGlynn, S.M. & Schacter, D.L. (1989). Unawareness of deficits in neuropsychological syndromes. *Journal of Clinical and Experimental Neuropsychology*, **11**, 143–205.

McGlynn, S.M. & Kaszniak, A.W. (1991a). When metacognition fails: impaired awareness of deficit in Alzheimer's disease. *Journal of Cognitive Neuroscience*, **3**, 183–9.

McGlynn, S.M. & Kaszniak, A.W. (1991b). Unawareness of deficits in dementia and schizophrenia. In *Awareness of Deficit After Brain Injury*, ed. G.P. Prigatano & D.L. Schacter. Oxford: Oxford University Press.

Mangone, C.A., Hier, D.B., Gorelick, P.B., Ganellen, R.J., Langenberg, P., Boarman, R. & Dollear, W.C. (1991). Impaired Insight in Alzheimer's Disease. *Journal of Geriatric Psychiatry and Neurology*, 4, 189–93.

Marcel, A.J. & Bisiach, E. (eds.) (1988). *Consciousness in Contemporary Science.* Oxford: Oxford University Press.

Marková, I.S. (1998). Towards a structure of insight: a clinical and conceptual analysis. *MD thesis.* Glasgow: Glasgow University Library.

Marková, I.S. & Berrios, G.E. (1992). The meaning of insight in clinical psychiatry. *British Journal of Psychiatry*, **160**, 850–60.

Marková, I.S. & Berrios, G.E. (1995a). Insight in clinical psychiatry revisited. *Comprehensive Psychiatry*, **36**, 367–76.

Marková, I.S. & Berrios, G.E. (1995b). Insight in clinical psychiatry: a new model. *Journal of Nervous and Mental Disease*, **183**, 743–51.

Mesulam, M-M. (1986). Frontal cortex and behavior. *Annals of Neurology*, **19**, 320–5.

Michalakeas, A., Skoutas, C., Charatambous, A., Peristeris, A., Marinos, V., Keramari, E. & Theologou, A. (1994). Insight in schizophrenia and mood disorders and its relation to psychopathology. *Acta Psychiatrica Scandinavica*, **90**, 46–9.

Michon, A., Deweer, B., Pillon, B., Agid, Y. & Dubois, B. (1992). Anosognosia and frontal dysfunction in SDAT. *Neurology*, **42**, 221.

Michon, A., Deweer, B., Pillon, B., Agid, Y. & Dubois, B. (1994). Relation of anosognosia to frontal lobe dysfunction in Alzheimer's disease. *Journal of Neurology, Neurosurgery and Psychiatry*, **57**, 805–9.

Mullen, R., Howard, R., David, A. & Levy, R. (1996). Insight in Alzheimer's disease. *International Journal of Geriatric Psychiatry*, **11**, 645–51.

Myslobodsky, M.S. (1986). Anosognosia in tardive dyskinesia: 'tardive dysmentia' or 'tardive dementia'? *Schizophrenia Bulletin*, **12**, 1–6.

Neary, D., Snowden, J.S., Bowen, D.M., Sims, N.R., Mann, D.M.A., Benton, J.S., Northen, B., Yates, P.O. & Davison, A.N. (1986). Neuropsychological syndromes in presenile dementia due to cerebral atrophy. *Journal of Neurology, Neurosurgery and Psychiatry*, **49**, 163–74.

Ott, B.R. & Fogel, B.S. (1992). Measurement of depression in dementia: self vs. clinician rating. *International Journal of Geriatric Psychiatry*, 7, 899–904.

Price, B.H. & Mesulam, M. (1985). Psychiatric manifestation of right hemisphere infarctions. *Journal of Nervous and Mental Disease*, **173**, 610–14.

Prigatano, G.P. (1991). Disturbances of self-awareness of deficit after traumatic brain injury. In *Awareness of Deficit After Brain Injury*, ed. G.P. Prigatano & D.L. Schacter. Oxford: Oxford University Press.

Reed, B.R., Jagust, W.J. & Coulter, L. (1993). Anosognosia in Alzheimer's disease: relationships to depression, cognitive function, and cerebral perfusion. *Journal of Clinical and Experimental Neuropsychology*, **15**, 231–44.

Roth, N. (1944). Unusual types of anosognosia and their relation to the body image. *Journal of Nervous and Mental Disease*, **100**, 35–43.

Rubens, A.R. & Garrett, M.F. (1991). Anosognosia of Linguistic Deficits in Patients with Neurological Deficits. In *Awareness of Deficit After Brain Injury*, ed. G.P. Prigatano & D.L. Schacter. Oxford: Oxford University Press.

Russo, R. & Spinnler, H. (1994). Implicit verbal memory in Alzheimer's disease. *Cortex*, **30**, 359–75.

Schacter, D.L. (1990). Toward a cognitive neuropsychology of awareness: implicit knowledge and anosognosia. *Journal of Clinical and Experimental Neuropsychology*, **12**, 155–78.

Schacter, D.L. (1991). Unawareness of deficit and unawareness of knowledge in patients with memory disorders. In *Awareness of Deficit After Brain Injury*, ed. G.P. Prigatano & D.L. Schacter. Oxford: Oxford University Press.

Schacter, D.L. (1992). Consciousness and awareness in memory and amnesia: critical issues. In *The Neuropsychology of Consciousness*, ed. A.D. Milner & M.D. Rugg, pp. 179–200. London: Academic Press.

Schacter D.L. (1995). Implicit memory: a new frontier for cognitive neuroscience. In *The Cognitive Neurosciences*, ed. M.S. Gazzaniga, pp. 815–24. Cambridge, MA: MIT Press.

Schneck, M.K., Reisberg, B. & Ferris, S.H. (1982). An overview of current concepts in Alzheimer's disease. *American Journal of Psychiatry*, **139**, 165–73.

Seltzer, B., Buswell, A. & Vasterling, J. (1993). Awareness of deficit in Alzheimer's disease (AD): association with psychiatric symptoms and other disease variables. *Journal of Clinical and Experimental Neuropsychology*, **15**, (abstract), 30.

Sevush, S. & Leve, N. (1993). Denial of memory deficit in Alzheimer's disease. *American Journal of Psychiatry*, **150**, 748–51.

Shallice, T. (1988). *From Neuropsychology to Mental Structure*. Cambridge, UK: Cambridge University Press.

Shimamura, A.P. (1986). Priming effects in amnesia: evidence for a dissociable memory function. *Quarterly Journal of Experimental Psychology*, **38A**, 619–44

Starkstein, S.E., Fedoroff, J.P., Price, T.R., Leiguarda, R. & Robinson, R.G. (1992). Anosognosia in patients with cerebrovascular lesions. A study of causative factors. *Stroke*, **23**, 1446–53.

Starkstein, S.E., Fedoroff, J.P., Price, T.R., Leiguarda, R. & Robinson, R.G. (1993). Neuropsychological deficits in patients with anosognosia. *Neuropsychiatry, Neuropsychology and Behavioral Neurology*, **6**, 43–8.

Starkstein, S.E., Vázquez, S., Migliorelli, R., Tesón, A., Sabe, L. & Leiguarda, R. (1995). A single-photon emission computed tomographic study of anosognosia in Alzheimer's disease. *Archives of Neurology*, **52**, 415–20.

Starkstein, S.E., Chemerinski, E., Sabe, L., Kuzis, G., Petracca, G., Tesón, A. & Leiguarda, R. (1997). Prospective longitudinal study of depression and anosognosia in Alzheimer's disease. *British Journal of Psychiatry*, **171**, 47–52.

Stuss, D.T. (1991). Disturbance of self-awareness after frontal system damage. In *Awareness of Deficit After Brain Injury*, ed. G.P. Prigatano & D.L. Schacter., Oxford: Oxford University Press.

Stuss, D.T. & Benson, D.F. (1986). *The Frontal Lobes*. New York: Raven Press.

Sultzer, D.L., Levin, H.S., Mahler, M.E., High, W.M. & Cummings, J.L. (1993). A comparison of psychiatric symptoms in vascular dementia and Alzheimer's disease. *American Journal of Psychiatry*, **150**, 1806–12.

Sunderland, A., Harris, J.E. & Baddeley, A.D. (1983). Do laboratory tests predict everyday memory? A neuropsychological study. *Journal of Verbal Learning and Verbal Behavior*, **22**, 341–57.

Sunderland, A., Harris, J.E. & Gleave, J. (1984). Memory failures in everyday life following severe head injury. *Journal of Clinical Neuropsychology*, **6**, 127–42.

Talland, G.A. (1965). *Deranged Memory*. New York: Academic Press.

Vasterling, J.J., Seltzer, B., Foss, J.W. & Vanderbrook, V. (1995). Unawareness of deficit in Alzheimer's disease. Domain-specific differences and disease correlates. *Neuropsychiatry, Neuropsychology and Behavioral Neurology*, **8**, 26–32.

Verhey, F.R.J., Rozendaal, N., Ponds, R.W.H.M. & Jolles, J. (1993). Dementia, awareness and depression. *International Journal of Geriatric Psychiatry*, **8**, 851–6.

Vilkki, J. (1985). Amnesic syndromes after surgery of anterior communicating artery aneurysms. *Cortex*, **21**, 431–44.

Warrington, E.K. & Weiskrantz, L. (1968). New method of testing long-term retention with special reference to amnesic patients. *Nature*, **217**, 972–4.

Warrington, E.K. & Weiskrantz, L. (1974). The effect of prior learning on subsequent retention in amnesic patients. *Neuropsychologia*, **12**, 419–28.

Warrington, E.K. & Weiskrantz, L. (1982). Amnesia: a disconnection syndrome? *Neuropsychologia*, **20**, 233–48.

Watson, R.T. & Heilman, K.M. (1979). Thalamic neglect. *Neurology*, **29**, 690–4.

Weinstein, E.A. (1991). Anosognosia and denial of illness. In *Awareness of Deficit After Brain Injury*, ed. G.P. Prigatano & D.L. Schacter. Oxford: Oxford University Press.

Weinstein, E.A. & Kahn, R.L. (1955). *Denial of Illness: Symbolic and Physiological Aspects*. Springfield: Thomas.

Weinstein, E.A., Friedland, R.P. & Wagner, E.E. (1994). Denial/unawareness of impairment and symbolic behavior in Alzheimer's disease. *Neuropsychiatry, Neuropsychology and Behavioral Neurology*, **7**, 176–84.

Young, D.A., Davila, R. & Scher, H. (1993). Unawareness of illness and neuropsychological performance in chronic schizophrenia. *Schizophrenia Research*, **10**, 117–24.

# 11

# Memory in functional psychosis

Peter J. McKenna, A. Paula McKay and Keith Laws

The term psychosis refers to mental disorders which affect widespread areas of mental functioning and which are often, but not necessarily always, accompanied by the hallmark symptoms of delusions, hallucinations, and incoherence of speech. The qualification of functional serves to distinguish two such states, schizophrenia and manic–depressive psychosis, from the so-called organic psychoses of delirium and dementia – which also affect mental functioning in a global way and which can themselves be accompanied by delusions, hallucinations as well as many other psychiatric symptoms. The distinction turns on the presence or absence of a single clinical feature, cognitive impairment. This is always present, if sometimes subtle, in delirium and dementia, but the absence of memory impairment, disorientation and other evidence of disturbed intellectual function is invariably held to be a prerequisite for the diagnosis of schizophrenia or manic–depressive psychosis.

Why, then, is there a chapter on functional psychosis in a book about memory disorders? The answer to this question lies in the history of psychosis and the uneasy nosological position occupied by functional psychosis, in particular, over the course of the twentieth century. Established in the nineteenth century (see Berrios, 1987, 1996; Beer, 1996), the concept of psychosis underwent various modifications and subdivisions in accordance with the currents of thought of the period. One important distinction that appeared was between exogenous and endogenous psychoses: the former were due to toxic and infectious agents whereas in the latter the cause lay principally in the individual, often in an apparent hereditary predisposition. Another distinction was borrowed from the neurological tradition of organic vs. functional, which in its original sense separated diseases where there was structural nervous system abnormality from those where there was none and in which a purely physiological disturbance of function had to be assumed. Already similar, by the beginning of the twentieth century these distinctions had begun to overlap. By this time, however, the organic–functional distinction had undergone a radical transformation: principally at the hands of Charcot it had come to refer, on the one hand, to organically determined nervous system disease, and on the other to hysterical, psychogenic, or psychologically determined disability. These influences led ultimately to a firm differentiation being established between organic psychoses – somatic illnessess with psychic disturbances including all the known forms of dementia, plus illnesses associated with cerebral trauma, tumour, infections and endocrine disorders – and functional psychoses – a category which always included schizophrenia and affective psychosis, plus at various times other disorders such as paranoia and epilepsy.

Although one of the earliest references to functional psychosis (Mendel, 1907 cited by Berrios, 1987) used it merely to refer to mental diseases in which no anatomical findings could as yet be demonstrated, by the end of the 1920s, the prevailing view was that in organic psychoses the examination had to be made in the brain, whereas for functional psychoses it was the mind that had to be studied (Bumke, cited by Beer, 1996). For the next half century the psychological approach to functional psychosis held sway. At a theoretical level psychodynamic theories flourished and psychoanalysis, at least in America, became the basic science of psychiatry. In day-to-day clinical terms, absence of cognitive impairment became the cornerstone of diagnosis of functional psychosis, to the extent that, if a patient presenting with schizophrenia, mania or depression showed any evidence of this, investigations would normally be undertaken to exclude neurological or other underlying physical disease.

Then, in the 1960s, a sea change in thinking took place. Psychoanalysis, whose influence had previously been ever-widening, began to undergo an inexorable loss of prestige (D. Rogers, unpublished MD thesis); at the same time a range of newly discovered drug treatments for schizophrenia and depression were being developed and were proving to be disconcertingly successful (e.g. Healy, 1996). The biological approach to functional psychosis began to gain ground and went on to become the dominant explanatory paradigm. As part of this, the neuropsychology of functional psychosis went from being a topic of little serious interest to a legitimate field of study. In schizophrenia, studies of memory now rival, and may even have overtaken, the other main area of neuropsychological investigation, frontal or executive function. In affective psychosis, the long-standing observation that memory may be affected in depression has gone from being automatically considered secondary to motivational or other factors, to a phenomenon deserving recognition and investigation in its own right. Nevertheless, as will be seen, the chequered career of functional psychosis has left a legacy of ambivalence about the nature of memory impairment in both conditions.

## Schizophrenia

### General intellectual impairment

The original descriptions of schizophrenia were characterized by equivocation and ambivalence on the question of whether cognitive function was affected. Kraepelin

(1913a) considered that the disorder he named dementia praecox led in the great majority of cases to a state that exhibited many features in common with other forms of dementia; but he then went on to comment that the injury predominated in the emotional and volitional spheres and that memory and orientation were not usually and comparatively little affected. Part of Bleuler's (1911) stated reason for renaming dementia praecox as schizophrenia was that he believed the connotation of intellectual decline to be misleading. However, he dwelt at length on what he variously referred to as schizophrenic dementia, schizophrenic intellectual deterioration and the schizophrenic disorder of intelligence – all the while arguing that it was fundamentally different from 'dementia, in the sense of the organic psychoses'.

Over succeeding decades this uncertainty hardened into the dogma that there could be no compromise of intellectual function in schizophrenia. To some extent this reflected the rise of psychoanalysis and psychodynamic psychiatry, especially in the USA; any hint of organicity, of brain disease in schizophrenia was, and is, anathema to this school of thought. But, to some extent also, it was a consequence of simple clinical observation: the vast majority of schizophrenic patients encountered in everyday clinical practice do not show disorientation or any of the other forms of cognitive failure that are seen in brain damage or dementia. It is only among the most severely and chronically ill patients, i.e. those residing on the long-stay wards of mental hospitals, that such impairments begin to be found, and even then they are unobtrusive.

Nevertheless, as psychological studies began to be carried out over the first half of the century, they uniformly found that patients with schizophrenia tended to perform more poorly than normals on virtually all cognitive tasks (see Chapman & Chapman, 1973). Somewhat later, when intelligence testing became popular, schizophrenic patients were found to have lower IQs than the rest of the population, markedly so in the most severe cases, with some of the impairment appearing to represent decline after the onset of illness (Payne, 1973). At first, these findings were attributed to factors such as poor co-operation, lack of motivation, or the interfering effects of mental state abnormalities such as distractibility and incoherence of speech. For example, Slater (1936), criticizing an early study of memory in psychotic patients, argued that it would be surprising if anyone at all in an asylum consisting 'to a large extent of stuporose catatonics, self-absorbed and hallucinating hebephrenics, suspicious paranoiacs, scatter-brained and distractible manics and worried and retarded depressives' reached a standard of normality. Similarly, in Chapman and Chapman's (1973) account referred to above, they considered that 'to a large extent, lowered IQ test performance by schizophrenics reflects severity of pathology . . . schizophrenics earn low IQ scores because they are disturbed, rather than because they are dull.' Later, it became a widely held view that the sedative effects of neuroleptic drugs were responsible for poor performance on cognitive tests. This was despite the unanimous conclusion of many studies that drug treatment had little or no effect on most or all aspects of cognitive function in normal individuals – and if anything, tended to improve this in schizophrenic patients (e.g. King, 1990; Goldberg & Weinberger, 1996).

In the 1970s, the climate of opinion began to change (see Goldberg & Gold, 1995; Rogers, 1996). After administering neuropsychological tests to 66 chronic schizophrenic patients, Klonoff et al. (1970) suggested 'with the utmost caution' that the poor performance found might reflect brain damage. In 1978 three reviews were published (Goldstein, 1978; Heaton et al., 1978; Malec, 1978), which all came to the conclusion that it was impossible to distinguish chronic schizophrenic patients from patients with organic brain disease on the basis of their performance on a variety of neuropsychological tests. At around the same time Crow and coworkers (Stevens et al., 1978; Owens & Johnstone, 1980; see also Liddle & Crow, 1984; Buhrich et al., 1988) embarked on a series of studies documenting the phenomenon of age-disorientation in schizophrenia. They found that up to 25% of chronically hospitalized schizophrenic patients were unable to give their correct age, that this was invariably part of a wider pattern of poor intellectual test performance, and that it was not attributable to a variety of confounding factors including physical treatments and low premorbid intelligence. The obvious interpretation was that something essentially indistinguishable from dementia supervenes in a minority of patients with the disorder.

Perhaps the best evidence of general intellectual impairment in schizophrenia comes from a number of studies which have applied batteries of neuropsychological tests to patients and normal controls. Those using modern diagnostic criteria, and which have employed explicit matching for age and education (or parental education, which has been argued to be a better index of educational achievement in schizophrenic patients), are summarized in Table 11.1. It can be seen that every study found some evidence of impairment. In most of the studies significantly poorer performance was found in most or all of the areas of function examined. However, one study (Kolb & Whishaw, 1983) only found significant impairment on tests of memory and executive function, and another (Goldberg et al., 1990) found that impairment was restricted to memory, executive function and a vigilance task. These studies also reinforce the view that drug treatment is not an important confounding factor: two of the studies were carried out on drug-free patients (Saykin et al., 1991; Blanchard & Neale,1994), and one on never-treated patients (Saykin et al; 1994).

## Memory impairment

Given a general tendency to poor cognitive performance in schizophrenia, it would be surprising if impairment were not found on memory tests. Cutting (1985)

**Table 11.1.** Studies applying neuropsychological test batteries to schizophrenic patients

| Study | Numbers | Diagnostic criteria | Patient type | Matching | Tests | Findings | Comment |
|---|---|---|---|---|---|---|---|
| Kolb & Whishaw (1983) | 30 patients 30 normals | DSM III | Acute | Age Education | IQ Memory Visual/visuospatial function Face processing Executive function Other | Patients sig. worse on performance but not verbal IQ, memory tests and executive function | Deficits found mainly in memory and executive function |
| Goldberg et al. (1990) | 16 patients 16 normals | DSM IIIR | Chronic | Controls were unaffected MZ co-twins | IQ Memory Vigilance Executive function | Patients sig. worse on IQ, memory tests, some executive tests, and vigilance | Affected co-twins performed more poorly than unaffected, on all tests but not always significantly so |
| Braff et al. (1991) | 40 patients 40 normals | DSM IIIR | Chronic | Age Education | IQ Executive function Memory Language Visuospatial function Auditory perception Tactile perception Motor skill | Patients sig. worse on all tests except motor skill, visuospatial and language | — |
| Saykin et al. (1991) | 36 patients 36 normals | DSM IIIR | Chronic | Age Parental education | IQ Executive function Memory Language | Patients sig. worse on all tests except language | All patients drug-free Disproportionately poor performance on memory tests |

| Study | Sample | Criteria | Course | Matching | Tests | Results | Notes |
|---|---|---|---|---|---|---|---|
| | | | | | Auditory perception Motor skill | | |
| Saykin et al. (1994) | 37 patients 131 normals | DSM-IIIR | Acute | Age Parental education | IQ Executive function Memory Language Auditory perception Motor skill | Patients sig. worse on all tests except motor skill tests | All patients first episode and drug-naive |
| Blanchard & Neale (1994) | 28 patients 15 normals | DSM IIIR | Chronic | Age Education | Executive function Memory Language Visual perception Tactile perception Motor function | Patients sig. worse on almost all tests | All patients drug-free |

reviewed approximately 30 studies of memory carried out mainly in the 1960s and 1970s. He concluded that memory remained superficially intact in acute schizophrenic patients, although there was evidence of subtle deficits in some areas. In chronic schizophrenia, however, poor memory performance was commonly found and could amount to what he called 'marked amnesia'.

Studies of memory carried out since Cutting's (1985) review are summarized in Table 11.2. Only studies of non-elderly patients, which employed diagnostic criteria and which compared patients with well-matched normal controls are included. The emphasis is on studies using general memory measures or batteries of memory tests such as the Wechsler Memory Scale; studies directed principally to particular aspects of memory are reviewed later. It can be seen that eight of the ten studies found evidence of impairment on some or all of the measures used, and only two of them failed to find significant differences between patients and controls on any measure (Shoqeirat & Mayes, 1988; Morrison-Stewart et al., 1992).

An idea of the prevalence and degree of memory impairment in schizophrenia can be gained from a study carried out by McKenna et al. (1990) using the Rivermead Behavioural Memory Test (RBMT) (Wilson et al., 1985). This is a clinically oriented, relatively undemanding test made up of 12 subtests covering recall, recognition, orientation and memory for a simple route, together with three measures of prospective memory, the capacity to remember to do things. An overall 'screening' score is derived from the sum of pass/fail scores for each of the 12 subtests. The patient group consisted of 60 patients meeting Research Diagnostic Criteria for schizophrenia (which exclude co-existing neurological disease and drug or alchohol abuse) aged 18–68, and included approximately equal numbers of outpatients in fair or good remission, inpatients on acute wards, rehabilitation patients, and patients on long stay wards. Their performance was compared with that of two groups on which the RBMT was originally validated: 118 normal individuals aged 19–69 and 176 patients with moderate or severe brain injury, aged 14–69. Figure 11.1 shows the performance of the three groups, expressed as cumulative percentages. It can be seen that, whereas less than 5% of the normal individuals scored 7 or fewer, over half the schizophrenic patients were below this level, and some patients fell into the severely impaired range. It is also evident that the performance of the schizophrenic patients was essentially indistinguishable from that of the head-injured patients. As expected, memory impairment was found to be significantly correlated with severity and chronicity of illness, and also with overall intellectual impairment. Impairment was not, however, restricted to chronically hospitalized patients, and was found in some acutely ill or remitted patients. Closely similar findings were obtained by Duffy and O'Carroll (1994) in a replication of this study.

None of the above studies of memory was carried out on drug-free patients.

**Table 11.2.** Recent studies of memory performance in schizophrenic patients

| Study | Numbers | Matching | Significant test differences | Non-significant test differences | Comments |
|---|---|---|---|---|---|
| Calev et al. (1987b) | 20 patients All treated 20 controls | Age Education Estimated current IQ | Word list recall Design recall | – | No sig. differences between pts taking and not taking anti-cholinergics |
| Shoqeirat & Mayes (1988) | 16 patients All treated 16 controls | Age Education | – | Recognition memory Object recall Spatial recall | Diagnostic criteria uncertain |
| Gruzelier et al. (1988) | 36 patients Some treated 29 controls | Age Education (see comments) | Digit span Block span Recurring digit span Associate learning | Recurring block span | Educational matching not perfect |
| Morrison-Stewart et al. (1992) | 30 patients Some treated 30 controls | Age Estimated current IQ | – | WMS Benton visual retention test | – |
| Gold et al. (1992a) | 36 patients All treated 18 controls | Age Education Estimated IQ (vocabulary) | Word list recall Word recognition | – | – |
| Landro et al. (1993) | 30 patients Some treated 18 controls | Age Education | Word recall Trigram recall (Peterson task) | – | Chronic patients worse than non-chronic on some but not all measures |

**Table 11.2** (*cont.*)

| Study | Numbers | Matching | Significant test differences | Non-significant test differences | Comments |
|---|---|---|---|---|---|
| Goldberg et al. (1993) | 24 patients All treated 24 controls | Controls were unaffected MZ Co-twins | WMS immediate logical memory, immediate Design reproduction, paired associates | WMS delayed logical memory, delayed design Reproduction. RMT (faces and words) Digit span (forward and backward) | Two patients had delusional disorder, not schizophrenia |
| Elliott et al. (1995) | 32 patients All treated 24 controls | Age Estimated premorbid IQ | Recognition memory for patterns and spatial position | – | – |
| Paulsen et al. (1995) | 175 patients All treated 229 controls | None (See comments) | CVLT recall measures and recognition measures | A few miscellaneous CVLT measures | Similar results for age and education matched subgroups  Impairment correlated with anti-cholinergic dose, chronicity and negative symptoms |
| Rushe et al. (1999) | 34 patients All treated 53 controls | Age Estimated premorbid IQ | WMS logical memory, visual reproduction, paired associates | Digit span Block span Memory for temporal order | No sig. differences between patients on and off anti-cholingergic medication on most tests. |

*Notes:*
Key: WMS – Weschler Memory Scale; CVLT – California Verbal Learning Test; RMT – Warrington Recognition Memory Test.

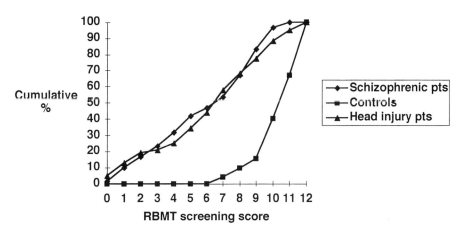

Fig. 11.1    Memory test scores in 60 schizophrenic patients, 176 head-injured patients and 118 normal individuals (from McKenna et al., 1990).

However, three of the studies of general cognitive function in schizophrenia (Saykin et al., 1991, 1994; Blanchard & Neale, 1994) examined only drug-free, or drug-naive patients, and all of these found evidence of memory impairment. There is little to support a link between memory impairment and anti-cholinergic drug treatment: memory impairment has been documented in patients who were not taking anti-cholinergic drugs (Calev, 1987a; Goldberg et al., 1993), and the degree of impairment has been found not to differ between patients who were on and off such medication at the time of testing (Calev et al., 1987b; McKenna et al., 1990; Duffy & O'Carroll, 1994; Rushe et al., 1999). One study (Paulsen et al., 1995) did find significant inverse correlations between an overall measure of recall and anti-cholinergic dose ($r = -0.44$, $P = 0.005$) in 175 schizophrenic patients, but a subsequent multiple regression analysis indicated that this accounted for a non-significant proportion of the variance compared to negative symptoms, age of onset and inpatient vs. outpatient status.

The question of whether memory impairment in schizophrenia can be attributed to the confounding factors of motivation, co-operation and distraction by psychotic experiences has also been considered. McKenna et al. (1990) found that excluding 16 of their 60 patients in whom poor co-operation was evident at the time of testing made little difference to the mean RBMT screening score (there was an improvement of less than one point). In their replication of this study, Duffy and O'Carroll (1994) rated motivation and co-operation on a five-point scale and found no correlation between this and the patients' memory performance. Finally, Gold et al. (1992b) assessed the possible role of attentional factors by comparing performance on the 'attention' subscale of the Wechsler Memory Scale between schizophrenic patients with large and small intelligence–memory quotient discrepancies.

Although the two groups differed markedly on the four memory-based subscales of the WMS-R, they did not differ on the attention subscale.

## The pattern of memory impairment

### Short-term vs. long-term memory

All of the ten studies listed in Table 11.2 employed long-term memory measures. Five found significant impairment on most such measures (Calev et al., 1987b; Landro et al., 1993; Elliott et al., 1995; Paulsen et al., 1995; Rushe et al., 1999); two found impairment on some but not all such measures (Gruzelier et al., 1988; Goldberg et al., 1993); and two found no impairment (Shoqeirat & Mayes, 1988; Morrison-Stewart et al., 1992).

There has been much less investigation of short-term memory in schizophrenia. A number of early studies (for review, see Cutting, 1985) reported significant differences between schizophrenic patients and controls in a variety of span tasks. This finding has also been reported in three recent studies (Gruzelier et al.,1988; Park & Holzman, 1992; Gold et al., 1997); in these studies, though, the differences were small, of the order of a single digit. Two further studies failed to find significant differences (Goldberg et al.,1993; Morice & Delahunty, 1996). Rushe et al. (1999) initially found modest but significant differences between schizophrenic patients and controls on digit span and block-tapping span, but these disappeared when subgroups matched for estimated IQ were compared.

Some authors have gone further and argued that schizophrenic memory impairment shows a dissociation between short-term and long-term memory. Thus Tamlyn et al. (1992) found that only 14% of the 60 patients of McKenna et al. (1990) had digit spans that were outside the normal range, in contrast to 80% who were in the impaired range on a long-term memory test, prose recall. Similarly, Duffy and O'Carroll (1994) found that all of their patients scored within the normal range on forward digit span but that there was substantial impairment on a long-term memory task, the Benton Visual Retention Test. Some other group studies have had findings that can be interpreted in the same direction (Goldberg et al., 1993; Rushe et al., 1999).

In recent years, the concept of short-term memory has been elaborated into that of working memory (Baddeley, 1986), conceived of as a set of interacting systems for the temporary holding and manipulation of information necessary for comprehension, learning and reasoning. As an area of high level integration of cognitive activity, working memory is currently a focus of interest in schizophrenia (e.g. Goldman-Rakic, 1991; Fleming et al., 1994). Three studies (Park & Holzman, 1992; Fleming et al., 1995; Gold et al., 1997) have found evidence of working memory impairment in schizophrenic patients. Two further studies (Goldberg et al., 1993;

Morice & Delahunty, 1996) had equivocal results, respectively finding a trend towards impairment and impairment on two out of four tests.

## Semantic memory

One major subdivision within long-term memory is that between episodic and semantic memory (Tulving, 1983; Baddeley, 1990). Episodic memory is memory for personally experienced events (e.g. what one had for breakfast, who one met on holiday last year), whereas semantic memory refers to the storage of information in pure, impersonal form, or, in other words, knowledge. This encompasses knowledge for use in language (for example, knowing the meaning of the word generous), through general knowledge (for example, knowing the capital of France), to abstract concepts (for example, understanding what is meant by justice) and the rules governing social behaviour (for example, knowing not to order the dessert course along with the starter and main course in a restaurant).

There are many indications that semantic memory is affected along with episodic memory in schizophrenia. Using a test in which subjects have to state whether simple sentences such as 'pliers are found in tool chests' and 'vans grow in gardens' are true or false, Tamlyn et al. (1992) and Duffy and O'Carroll (1994) found that schizophrenic patients were slower than normal and also commonly made multiple errors – normal individuals typically make no more than one or two errors on this test. Other studies have found impaired performance on tests directed to knowledge about words (Clare et al., 1993; Chen et al., 1994; McKay et al., 1996), and on tests of social and practical knowledge about the world (Cutting & Murphy,1988).

## Procedural and implicit memory

A final distinction within long-term memory is between declarative memory, which includes both episodic and semantic memory, and procedural memory: memory for skills, including motor, perceptual and some intellectual skills. A number of lines of evidence suggest that another form of memory, implicit memory, is closely related to procedural memory (see Baddeley, 1990). Implicit memory refers to the phenomenon of memory without conscious recollection, and is usually tested by means of priming effects. A typical example involves first giving subjects a list of words and asking them to remember them. Later, a list of three-letter word stems, some of which can be completed using words from the original list, is presented and the subjects are requested to complete them with any words that come to mind. Priming is measured by the number of stems that are completed with words from the previously presented list.

There has been little study of procedural memory in schizophrenia. Studies using an archetypal motor skill task, the pursuit rotor, have demonstrated slower (Schwartz et al., 1996) or normal rates of learning (Goldberg et al., 1993; Kern et al., 1997). Clare et al. (1993) investigated procedural memory in schizophrenic patients who showed substantial general memory impairment. They compared performance on the pursuit rotor and two other procedural memory tests, jigsaw learning and mirror reading, in 12 patients who scored in the moderately or severely impaired range on the RBMT, with that of 12 normal controls individually matched for age and estimated IQ. The pattern was found to be similar on all three tasks: while the patients' level of performance was poorer than controls at the beginning and end of testing, their rate of improvement, i.e. their procedural learning, was similar. The authors argued that procedural learning and memory remains intact even when memory is generally impaired in schizophrenia, and even though the level of performance on such tasks is affected by the general schizophrenic tendency to poor cognitive task performance.

Studies of implicit memory in schizophrenia have had mixed findings. Using word stem completion tasks, Randolph et al. (1990) found significant impairment, but Gras-Vincendon et al. (1994) found this to be normal whereas explicit recall of the same words was impaired. Schwartz et al. (1993) found normal implicit memory for degraded words coupled with impaired explicit memory for paired associate learning. In the study of Clare et al. (1993), implicit memory, like procedural memory, was found to be normal in the presence of moderate or severe general memory impairment, using a procedure involving priming of homophone spelling.

### Intact recognition and impaired recall: a pathognomonic feature of schizophrenic memory impairment?

A number of early studies of memory in schizophrenia found that patients showed impairment on tests of recall but not of recognition (e.g. Bauman & Murray, 1968; Nachmani & Cohen, 1969; Koh, 1978). The finding of such a discrepancy was accorded considerable significance, and has been used to support various arguments about the nature of schizophrenic memory impairment: for example, that there is a selective deficit at the stage of retrieval as opposed to encoding, that there is a failure to take advantage of organization, or that the impairment affects effortful as opposed to automatic information processing (for a review, see Landro, 1994). All of these interpretations carry the implication that schizophrenic memory impairment is not a primary abnormality but instead is a secondary consequence of abnormality in other areas of function, such as attention, executive function, or even motivation.

A number of more recent studies, however, have documented recognition memory impairments in schizophrenic patients (Gold et al., 1992a; Tamlyn et al., 1992; Clare et al., 1993; Elliott et al., 1995; Paulsen et al., 1995), and impaired recall coupled with normal recognition has been found in only two further studies

(Goldberg et al., 1989, 1993). Recognition tasks are typically much easier than recall tasks and so it is quite possible that some of the earlier positive findings reflected differences in task difficulty rather than a true neuropsychological dissociation. Two studies by Calev and coworkers (Calev et al., 1984a, b) used recall and recognition tests which were matched for difficulty and found that, though relatively worse at recall, schizophrenics also had significantly poorer recognition than controls.

In summary, poor memory performance in schizophrenia is a robust finding, with the few negative findings probably reflecting the fact that it is a function of severity and chronicity of illness and can be minor in acute or remitted patients. Schizophrenic memory impairment forms part of a wider pattern of cognitive impairment seen in the disorder and, like this, can become marked in some patients with chronic, severe illness. There are prominent deficits in both episodic and semantic long-term memory, but short-term memory, procedural memory and implicit memory appear, on balance, to be spared or relatively spared. Working memory function is probably compromised in schizophrenia but, with some negative and trend-level findings, the indications so far are that the deficit is not of the same order of magnitude as that seen in long-term memory.

## Affective psychosis

### General intellectual impairment

Manic–depressive psychosis was separated from schizophrenia at the beginning of the century on a number of grounds (see Berrios, 1996), one of the most important of which was that full recovery took place between episodes and there was no progression to a state of permanent deterioration. Kraepelin (1913b), for example, stated that '. . . attacks of manic–depressive insanity never lead to profound dementia, not even when they continue throughout life almost without interruption. Usually all morbid manifestations completely disappear; but where that is exceptionally not the case only a rather slight peculiar psychic weakness develops. . . .' Leaving aside the ambiguity about what Kraepelin meant by dementia, this and other similar pronouncements seemed to preclude the occurrence of cognitive impairment in affective psychosis.

Such a view, however, ignored certain aspects of the clinical picture. In the first place, as was well recognized by the beginning of the twentieth century (see Berrios, 1996), patients with depression frequently complain of poor memory and other subjective cognitive symptoms. Also well described by the end of the nineteenth century was the phenomenon of reversible dementia associated with melancholia (see Berrios, 1985); this referred to an uncommon clinical presentation in which patients become depressed and at the same time develop objective evidence of cognitive impairment – sometimes to a degree suggesting a diagnosis of dementia – but then go on to recover fully.

Nevertheless, for the first half of the twentieth century, the idea of cognitive impairment in affective psychosis was paid little, if any, attention. Then in the 1950s reversible dementia associated with depression was rediscovered by Madden et al. (1952) and others, and was given its modern name, depressive pseudodementia (see also Chapter 12, this volume). Subsequently it has become widely accepted that all degrees of poor cognitive performance can accompany depression, with pseudodementia merely representing the most severe expression of this. Thus in frequently cited reviews, Miller (1975) and McAllister (1981) concluded that severely depressed patients often demonstrate mild to moderate impairment in cognitive function, and Cassens et al. (1990) concluded that 'some depressed patients present with few cognitive deficits, some with rather focal or discrete neuropsychological deficits, and some with moderate or severe global deficits.' The question of cognitive impairment in mania, however, has remained little investigated: McAllister (1981) was able to find only two studies devoted to this issue, and there have only been a handful since then (e.g. Gruzelier et al., 1988; Morice, 1990; Bulbena & Berrios, 1993).

Studies applying neuropsychological test batteries to patients with affective psychosis are shown in Table 11.3. Because of their small number, three studies (Friedman, 1964; Raskin et al., 1982; Robertson & Taylor, 1985) which did not employ diagnostic criteria are included; however, as in the section on schizophrenia, studies which did not match patients for age and educational level are excluded. Also excluded are studies carried out on elderly depressed patients: although cognitive deficits are regularly found in this population, the interpretation of these is complicated by factors like the decline in cognitive performance seen in the normal elderly, the possibility of co-existing early dementia, and the increased susceptibility of the elderly to cognitive side effects of drugs (see Jorm, 1986).

Three of the studies were carried out on depressed patients. One of these (Miller et al., 1991) found no evidence of impairment and another (Friedman, 1964) only found impairment on 9 out of 82 test scores (which could have been due to chance given the large number of statistical comparisons). The remaining study (Raskin et al., 1982) found evidence of impairment on most measures, across all areas of function. Two studies were carried out on a combination of manic and depressed patients. One of these (Robertson & Taylor, 1985), carried out on patients who were depressed, manic or euthymic at the time of examination, found impairment affecting intelligence, memory and executive function (the only areas examined). The other (Coffman et al., 1990), which was carried out on bipolar patients not further specified, found significant impairment on approximately half the tests

**Table 11.3.** Studies applying neuropsychological test batteries to patients with affective psychosis

| Study | Numbers | Diagnostic criteria | Patient type | Matching | Tests | Findings | Comments |
|-------|---------|---------------------|--------------|----------|-------|----------|----------|
| Friedman (1964) | 55 patients<br>Not stated if treated<br>65 controls | Clinical (rigorous, conforming closely to major depression) | Unipolar and bipolar depressed | Age<br>Education<br>Estimated current IQ | Memory<br>Executive function<br>Motor skill<br>Various perceptual tests<br>Vigilance | Sig. impairment on 9 of 82 test scores (memory, psychomotor speed) | Controlling for multiple comparison would have abolished all differences |
| Raskin et al. (1982) | 277 patients<br>Most drug free<br>112 controls | None | Depressed, not otherwise specified | Age<br>Education<br>Estimated current IQ | Memory<br>Executive function<br>Psychomotor tests<br>visual/visuospatial function | Sig. impairment on 11 of 13 tests, affecting all areas of function | 11 patients were 'schizoaffective'<br>Some of differences would not have survived controlling for multiple comparisons |
| Robertson & Taylor (1985) | 30 patients<br>Not stated if treated<br>41 controls | None | Mixed unipolar and bipolar depressed, elated, euthymic | Age<br>Education | IQ<br>Memory<br>Executive function | Sig. impairment on on all tests | Both patients and controls were prisoners on remand<br>6 patients had diagnosis of 'reactive depression' |
| Miller et al. (1991) | 28 patients<br>All drug free<br>28 controls | RDC | Depressed, not otherwise specified | Age<br>Education | General intellectual function<br>Visual and tactile perception<br>Language<br>Memory | No significant impairment on any of the tests | – |

**Table 11.3** (*cont.*)

| Study | Numbers | Diagnostic criteria | Patient type | Matching | Tests | Findings | Comment |
|-------|---------|---------------------|--------------|----------|-------|----------|---------|
| Coffman et al. (1990) | 30 patients All treated 52 controls | DSM IIIR | Bipolar | Education (age corrected for in analysis) | IQ Memory Executive function Tactile perception Language Motor skill | Significant impairment on 14 of 25 tests Especially executive function, tactile performance, motor skill Also non-verbal but not verbal memory | Controlling for neuroleptic dose did not affect findings |

used, but spanning almost all areas of function. Most of the studies which found impairment were carried out on patients who were receiving drug treatment, but one (Raskin et al., 1982) found impairment in mainly drug-free patients. It should also be noted that anti-depressant drugs and lithium have generally been found to exert only minimal effects on cognitive function (e.g. Judd et al., 1977; Lader & Bhanji, 1980; Thompson, 1991).

In contrast to the corresponding studies in schizophrenia, the findings are very mixed in these studies. One inference that can be drawn is that depressed patients on the whole show only minor degrees of general cognitive impairment. Another is that impairment is more prevalent in patients with bipolar as opposed to uni-polar illnesses: two of the three studies which explicitly included such patients found evidence of impairment. On the basis that bipolar patients generally have more severe illnesses than unipolar depressives, a tentative conclusion might therefore be that neuropsychological impairment is a function of severity of illness.

Adding support to such a view are two further studies which suggest that, as in schizophrenia, cognitive impairment may become pronounced and clinically evident in some patients with most severe and chronic forms of affective psycho-sis. Johnstone et al. (1985) examined a sample of 26 institutionalized patients meeting strict criteria for affective illness (either unipolar or bipolar) using a clin-ical dementia screening test. They found that 40% scored more than two standard deviations below the mean for a control group of patients institutionalized because of physical illness. Waddington and Youssef (1988) also found that impairment was frequent on a clinical dementia scale in a similar group of institutionalized affective patients.

## Memory impairment in depression

Memory has always been a particular focus of interest in studies of cognitive func-tion in depression. McAllister (1981) reviewed ten studies and noted that significant memory impairment was found in seven. Johnson and Magaro (1987), reviewing these and several more studies, concurred that most demonstrated some memory impairment in depressed patients, although they noted that a minority continued to find no significant differences.

More recent studies are summarized in Table 11.4. As in the previous section on schizophrenia, only studies using diagnostic criteria and matching for age and education and/or IQ are included; once again the emphasis is on studies which are directed to memory in general rather than one or another subdivision of this. Studies carried out on elderly depressed patients are also excluded, for the reasons given above. All the studies found significant impairment on some of the tests used, and most found impairment on a majority. Two studies, however,

**Table 11.4.** Recent studies of memory performance in depressed patients

| Study | Numbers | Matching | Significant test differences | Non-significant test differences | Comments |
|---|---|---|---|---|---|
| Calev et al. (1986) | 10 patients All drug free 10 controls | Age Education | Verbal recall Design recall | – | Tests matched for difficutly |
| Roy-Byrne et al. (1986) | 10 patients Some treated 10 controls | Age Education | Verbal recall | Verbal recognition | – |
| Wolfe et al. (1987) | 20 unipolar patients 12 bipolar patients All drug free 20 controls | Age Education | Verbal recall Verbal recognition | – | Bipolar patients sig. worse than unipolar on both tests |
| Golinkoff & Sweeney (1989) | 18 patients Not stated if treated 18 controls | Age Estimated current IQ | Paired associate recall Paired associate recognition | – | Patients did not differ significantly from a group of patients with personality disorder |
| Richards & Ruff (1989) | 30 patients All drug free 30 controls | Age Education Estimated current IQ | Visuospatial learning and recall | Digit span Block span WMS logical memory Rey figure recall Selective reminding test | – |

| Study | Subjects | Matching | Impaired tasks | Unimpaired tasks | Notes |
|---|---|---|---|---|---|
| Danion et al. (1991) | 36 patients, Some drug free, 18 controls | Age, Education | WMS memory quotient, logical memory, paired associates, visual reproduction, digit span | WMS personal and current information, orientation, mental control | No sig. difference; between treated and untreated patients |
| Austin et al. (1992a) | 40 patients, Some drug free, 20 controls | Age, Education, Estimated premorbid IQ | Word list recall/learning, AVLT learning, recall and recognition | Digit span forward and backward | – |
| Brand et al. (1992) | 24 patients, All drug free, 24 controls | Age, Education | Word recall and learning, Word recognition (hard task) | Delayed word recall, Word recognition (easy task) | – |
| Ilsley et al. (1995) | 15 patients, All treated, 15 controls | Age, Estimated premorbid IQ | Prose recall | RBMT profile score, Digit span, Recognition | – |
| Elliott et al. (1996) | 28 patients, All treated, 22 controls | Age, Estimated premorbid IQ | Pattern recognition, Spatial recognition, Spatial span | – | – |

*Notes:*

Key: WMS – Weschler Memory Scale; AVLT – Rey Auditory Verbal Learning Test; RBMT – Rivermead Behavioural Memory Test.

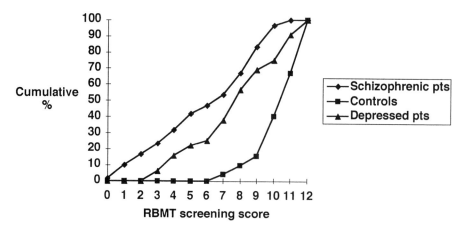

Fig. 11.2     Memory test scores in 33 depressed patients, 60 schizophrenic patients and 118 normal individuals (data from Tarbuck & Paykel, 1995; McKenna et al., 1990).

found predominantly intact memory: Richards and Ruff (1989) found impairment on only 4 of 13 measures, and Ilsley et al. (1995) found no overall differences between 15 patients and 15 controls on a general measure, the RBMT, although there was significant impairment on two of the subtests, prose recall and recall of a route.

An idea of the extent and severity of memory impairment in depression can be gained from a study by Tarbuck and Paykel (1995), which applied the RBMT to 37 young and elderly patients meeting DSM IIIR criteria for major depression. The scores, expressed as cumulative percentages, for 33 patients in the age range 23–73 are shown in Fig. 11.2, where they are compared with the 60 schizophrenic and 118 normal individuals with a similar age range described earlier. It can be seen that the depressed patients showed a range of performance which was intermediate between that of the other two groups.

Drug effects seem unlikely to account for memory impairment in depression. In the above studies significant impairment was found in three studies carried out on drug-free patients (Calev et al., 1986; Wolfe et al., 1987; Brand et al., 1992). Status as medicated or unmedicated also failed to emerge as a significant determinant of memory impairment in a meta-analysis of 147 studies of recall and recognition memory carried out by Burt et al. (1995).

The potential confounding factor of poor motivation has been addressed in the study of Richards and Ruff (1989) (although it should be noted that this study only found impairment on a minority of tests). As part of this study these authors randomly assigned their 30 depressed patients to 'motivated' or 'non-motivated' conditions; in the former, but not the latter, they received encouragement, assurances that they were doing well, and were informed that they would receive payment if they tried hard (a $10 bill remained in full view throughout testing). No difference between the conditions was found on any of the 13 memory measures used. The role of motivational factors is discussed further in the section on effortful vs. automatic processing, below.

### Memory between episodes in affective psychosis

Clinical impression, aided and abetted by the dogma of no compromise of intellectual function in functional psychosis, has favoured the view that any cognitive impairment accompanying depression returns to normal with clinical recovery. In support of this, McAllister (1981) found that four out of five studies which retested patients after treatment and/or following clinical improvement found corresponding improvement in memory performance, although typically this did not amount to complete reversal of the deficit.

Two more recent studies have tended to uphold the orthodox view. Bulbena and Berrios (1993) retested 33 affectively ill patients (the majority of whom were depressed at initial evaluation) and found significant improvement in measures of immediate and delayed recall. Tarbuck and Paykel (1995), in the study cited above, found that the RBMT scores of both their young and elderly depressed patients improved signicantly when they were retested (using a parallel form of the test) after recovery: when depressed, 9 of the 37 patients fell into the moderately or severely impaired memory range, but after recovery none of the 34 available for follow-up did so. One study, however, goes against the grain: Marcos et al. (1994) examined 28 patients previously meeting DSM-IIIR criteria for major depression, who had been euthymic for at least three months. Compared to 19 age and educationally matched normal controls, the patients showed significantly poorer performance on four out of five memory tests.

Reversibility of memory impairment may be even less of a general rule in certain types of depressed patient. One such group may be patients presenting with pseudodementia: Bulbena and Berrios (1986) found that 6 of a series of 15 patients who received a diagnosis of depressive pseudodementia were found to be demented (not further specified) at follow-up 15–47 months later. Another group may be elderly patients: Abas et al. (1990) and Altshuler (1993) noted that a number of studies of elderly depressed patients found that some degree of cognitive impairment could still be detected in some patients after resolution of depression. In their own study, Abas et al. (1990) found persistent cognitive deficits in 35% of a sample of 20 elderly depressed patients. Yet another group may be patients with severe, chronic illness: McKay et al. (1995) assessed memory, using the RBMT, in ten such patients who met DSM IIIR criteria for major depression, or bipolar disorder when they were (sometimes only briefly) euthymic. Four of the ten patients' scores were found to fall in the moderately or severely impaired memory range.

## The pattern of memory impairment in depression

### Short-term versus long-term memory

It is evident from Table 11.4 that memory impairment in depression is found on tests which explicitly tap long-term memory, such as word list recall, prose recall, paired associate learning and verbal recognition. Accordingly, there can be no doubt that, as in schizophrenia, this memory store is affected.

Studies of short-term memory in depression have almost always found it to be normal. Thus in the review of Cassens et al. (1990) only 1 of 11 studies found a significant reduction of forward digit span. Four more recent studies which were well controlled and used diagnostic criteria (Richards & Ruff, 1989; Austin et al., 1992a; Channon et al., 1993; Ilsley et al., 1995) failed to find any evidence of impairment. One contemporary study (Gruzelier et al., 1988) did find a significant reduction in digit span and block-tapping span in 12 depressed patients; however, in this study the patients were significantly older than the controls. Other studies have found normal performance on a task requiring recognition over a 1-second interval (Glass et al., 1981) and on a recall task with a delay of only a few seconds (Cohen et al., 1982).

The only study to date examining working memory in depression is that of Channon et al. (1993). They compared 24 depressed patients with 21 age and sex matched controls on four tasks tapping working memory function, backward digit span, backward block-tapping span and serial addition (in which subjects were required to add continuously the last two of a series of digits). The patients were found to show significant impairment on backward digit span, but not on any of the other tests.

### Semantic memory

This has only been investigated in one study. Ilsley et al. (1995), in the study summarized in Table 11.4, used the same sentence verification test as Tamlyn et al. (1992) and Duffy and O'Carroll (1994) and found no differences in either speed of verification or number of errors.

### Procedural and implicit memory

Procedural memory has not been formally studied in depression, a perhaps surprising omission, given the many reports of slowing on psychomotor tasks. Studies of implicit memory have been reviewed by Ilsley et al. (1995) and Watts (1995), who noted that four studies (Danion et al., 1991; Denny & Hunt, 1992; Watkins et al., 1992; Bazin et al., 1994) found this to be intact despite significant impairment of explicit memory. One further study (Elliott & Greene, 1992) found both implicit and explicit memory to be impaired. In their own study, Ilsley et al. (1995) found that implicit memory, measured by priming in word stem completion, was normal; however, in this study the patients also showed normal performance on the corresponding explicit recall task.

## Intact automatic vs. impaired effortful processing: a pathognomonic feature of depressive memory impairment?

As in schizophrenia, some early studies of memory in depression found evidence of impaired recall coupled with intact recognition (Stömgren, 1977; Cohen et al., 1982; Weingartner & Silberman, 1982). In others, effects such as poorer performance on later as opposed to earlier items in a word list, impairments on delayed but not immediate recall and failure to organize to-be-remembered material were noted (see Willner, 1984). This seemed to fit well with a distinction made in information processing theory between effortful and automatic processing, and led to an influential proposal that the cognitive deficit of depression was not in memory per se, but in the ability to apply mental effort.

However, this hypothesis, which is similar to the selective recall deficit hypothesis of schizophrenia but goes further in its imputation of motivational factors, faces difficulties. In the first place, the original finding of a dissociation between recall and recognition performance has not been consistently replicated and a number of more recent studies have documented poor recognition memory performance in depression (Calev & Erwin, 1985; Wolfe et al., 1987; Golinkoff & Sweeney, 1989; Austin et al., 1992a; see also the meta-analysis of Burt et al., 1995). Secondly, two studies which deliberately varied the amount of effort associated with memory tasks have failed to find that this affects performance in depressed patients. Golinkoff and Sweeney (1989) found that increasing task difficulty affected memory performance no more in depressed patients than in controls. In a procedure which experimentally manipulated the effort associated with recall, Hertel and Rude (1991) also found that depressed patients showed the same degree of better recall in high-effort compared to low-effort conditions as controls.

In summary, the findings on memory in affective psychosis form a less coherent picture than in schizophrenia. There is good evidence for memory impairment in depression, but it is unclear whether a similar deficit is seen in mania – although the limited findings to date (e.g. Gruzelier et al., 1988; Bulbena & Berrios, 1993) are suggestive of this. Memory impairment in depression may sometimes form part of a wider pattern of cognitive impairment, but it remains uncertain whether this is invariably, sometimes, or even only uncommonly the case. As in schizophrenia, memory and other cognitive deficits in affective psychosis appear to be a function of severity and chronicity of illness – at least in as much as the evidence suggests that they are more evident in bipolar than unipolar patients and they become most pronounced in chronically hospitalized patients. Unlike schizophrenia, memory and other neuropsychological deficits in depression seem to be reversible, remitting or at least improving with resolution of the affective episode. This reversibility may, however, not be absolute and there are strong hints that elderly patients, patients with pseudodementia, and patients with severe illness may sometimes develop persistent impairment. Findings concerning the pattern of memory impairment in depression are limited, but they support the view that long-term memory is affected but short-term memory remains intact. Semantic memory and implicit memory may also remain intact, but the studies are probably too few in the former and too inconsistent in the latter for any strong conclusions to be drawn.

## Discussion

The occurrence of memory deficits in schizophrenia and manic-depressive psychosis appears to be established beyond reasonable doubt. This impairment cannot easily be attributed to confounding factors like poor motivation and drug treatment, and so it follows that the disease process of functional psychosis sometimes affects memory. As well as overturning long-held views, such a conclusion has implications for the understanding of the nature of functional psychosis and its relationship to organic neurological disease.

A notable feature of the memory impairment of functional psychosis is that it shows dissociations. In schizophrenia an obvious impairment in long-term memory is coupled with preserved or relatively preserved short-term memory, and the balance of evidence also favours a sparing of procedural and implicit memory. The same seems to be true of affective psychosis, at least from the studies of depressive memory impairment. This pattern is similar to a well-known form of neurological memory impairment, the so-called amnesic syndrome. This is classically seen in the Wernicke–Korsakoff syndrome and following bilateral medial temporal lobectomy (e.g. Baddeley, 1990), but other neurological disorders such as transient global amnesia (Hodges, 1991) and closed head injury (Baddeley et al., 1987) also show some or all of the same features. There is, however, to be at least one difference: semantic memory remains normal in the amnesic syndrome, at least for information acquired before the onset of amnesia (e.g. Squire, 1987), whereas in schizophrenia there is now a considerable body of evidence for widespread deficits affecting the most basic aspects of knowledge.

That the pattern of memory impairment in schizophrenia shows similarities to some forms of neurological disease is perhaps not surprising. Based on incontrovertible evidence for a genetic factor in its aetiology (Gottesman, 1991), equally strong evidence for the effectiveness of neuroleptic drug treatment (Davis, 1985), and rather weaker direct evidence of structural and functional brain abnormality (see Chua & McKenna, 1995), schizophrenia is regarded by contemporary mainstream psychiatry as a biological brain disease. This being the case, the simplest hypothesis to explain schizophrenic memory impairment is that it due to to the damaging effects of schizophrenia on the brain.

At first sight the same argument can be applied to affective psychosis. There is the same evidence for a genetic factor in this disorder as schizoprenia, and also much the same response to biological rather than psychological treatments (e.g. see Paykel, 1992). There is even a roughly similar amount of evidence for underlying brain abnormality (see below). Some authorities believe that the two forms of functional psychosis lie on a continuum with one another, and there is certainly no dispute that significant numbers of patients with intermediate, 'schizoaffective' presentations exist (for a review, see McKenna, 1994). Here, though, there is a serious obstacle to attributing the memory impairment of depression to brain damage – this is the fact that it is reversible. Memory impairment which appears and disappears over weeks or months, sometimes repeatedly, may not be entirely without precedent in neurology but seems to point to an underlying mechanism, which is very different from the relatively crude processes of tissue destruction, cell loss and ischaemia.

If it is biological, the memory impairment of functional psychosis might be expected to have correlates in abnormal brain structure or function. Schizophrenia is associated with only one unequivocally established structural abnormality, lateral ventricular enlargment (for a review, see Chua & McKenna, 1995). This, however, is minor, and based on studies which have found it to present early in the course of the illness and not to be progressive, it is widely believed to be a neurodevelopmental 'trait marker' for schizophrenia rather than the manifestation of a degenerative process (e.g. Lewis, 1990; Jones et al., 1994). Neither lateral ventricular enlargement nor any other, less well-established structural abnormalities have been consistently found to be associated with memory or general intellectual impairment (Lewis, 1990; Chua & McKenna, 1995).

Affective disorder is probably also associated with significant lateral ventricular enlargement (Elkis et al., 1995). Here, one study (Abas et al., 1990) has found that this abnormality is associated with poor cognitive performance (not specifically poor memory performance), and another has found correlations between various aspects of neuropsychological performance and indices of structural abnormality (Coffman et al., 1990). However, given the inconsistency of the corresponding findings in schizophrenia, it is probably premature to draw any strong conclusions from these studies.

Functional imaging is currently in a certain amount of disarray in schizophrenia, with the leading candidate for abnormality, hypofrontality, now being seriously questioned as a general finding (see Chua & McKenna, 1995; Gur & Gur, 1995). There are, however, indications that hypofrontality is associated with certain 'deficit' aspects of the clinical picture, especially chronicity and negative symptoms (see Chua & McKenna, 1995). Whether this extends to an association with cognitive impairment is unclear: two studies have found this (Paulman et al., 1990; Sagawa et al.,1990), but a third (Cohen et al., 1987) did not. Depression may also be associated with abnormal findings on functional imaging (see Austin & Mitchell, 1996; Dolan & Goodwin, 1996), although no clear or consistent pattern has yet been described. There are some preliminary indications that particular abnormalities are associated with cognitive impairment (Austin et al., 1992b; Bench et al., 1993; Dolan et al., 1994). As in schizophrenia, however, the findings are not consistent.

## Conclusion

To sum up, both schizophrenia and manic–depressive psychosis are associated with memory deficits as part of a wider pattern of cognitive impairments, which can occasionally become severe. The features of the impairment in both disorders, plus other circumstantial evdence, suggest that it is 'biological' in nature, but not 'neurological', i.e. that it has different underlying causes than those normally encountered in neurology. Clear evidence for a basis in structural and/or functional brain abnormality is so far lacking.

## REFERENCES

Abas, M.A., Sahakian, B.J. & Levy, R. (1990). Neuropsychological deficits and CT scan changes in elderly depressives. *Psychological Medicine*, **20**, 507–20.

Altshuler, L. (1993). Bipolar disorder: are repeated episodes associated with neuroanatomic and cognitive changes? *Biological Psychiatry*, **33**, 563–65.

Austin, M.-P. & Mitchell, P. (1996). Functional neuroimaging in affective disorders. In *Melancholia: a Disorder of Movement and Mood*, ed. G. Parker & D. Hadzi-Pavlovic. Cambridge: Cambridge University Press.

Austin, M.-P., Ross, M., Murray, C., O'Carroll, R.E., Ebmeier, K.P. & Goodwin, G.M. (1992a). Cognitive function in major depression. *Journal of Affective Disorders*, **25**, 21–30.

Austin, M.-P., Dougall, N., Ross, M., Murray, C., O'Carroll, R.E., Moffoot, A., Ebmeier, K.P. & Goodwin, G. (1992b). Single photon emission tomography with $^{99m}$Tc-exametrazine and the pattern of brain activity underlying the psychotic/neurotic continuum. *Journal of Affective Disorders*, **26**, 31–44.

Baddeley, A.D. (1986). *Working Memory*. Oxford: Clarendon Press.

Baddeley, A.D. (1990). *Human Memory: Theory and Practice*. Hove: Erlbaum.

Baddeley, A.D., Harris, J., Sunderland, A., Watts, K.P. & Wilson, B.A. (1987). Closed head injury and memory. In *Neurobehavioral Recovery from Head Injury*, ed. H.S. Levin, J. Grafman & H.M. Eisenberg. New York: Oxford University Press.

Bauman, E. & Murray, D.J. (1968). Recognition versus recall in schizophrenia. *Canadian Journal of Psychology*, **22**, 18–25.

Bazin, N., Perruchet, P., De Bonis, M. & Féline, A. (1994). The dissociation of explicit and implicit memory. *Psychological Medicine*, **24**, 239–45.

Beer, M.D. (1996). Psychosis: a history of the concept. *Comprehensive Psychiatry*, **37**, 273–91.

Bench, C.J., Friston, K.J., Brown, R.G., Frackowiak, R.S.J. & Dolan, R.J. (1993). Regional cerebral blood flow in depression measured by positron emission tomography: the relationship with clinical dimensions. *Psychological Medicine*, **23**, 579–90.

Berrios, G.E. (1985). 'Depressive pseudodementia' or 'melancholic dementia': a 19th century view. *Journal of Neurology, Neurosurgery and Psychiatry*, **48**, 393–400.

Berrios, G.E. (1987). Historical aspects of the psychoses: 19th century issues. *British Medical Bulletin*, **43**, 484–98.

Berrios, G.E. (1996). *The History of Mental Symptoms: Descriptive Psychopathology Since the Nineteenth Century*. Cambridge: Cambridge University Press.

Blanchard, J.J. & Neale, J.M. (1994). The neuropsychological signature of schizophrenia – generalized or differential deficit. *American Journal of Psychiatry*, **151**, 40–8.

Bleuler, E. (1911). *Dementia Praecox, or the Group of Schizophrenias* (translated 1950 by J. Zinkin). New York: International Universities Press.

Braff, D.L., Heaton, R., Kuck, J., Cullum, M., Moranville, J., Grant, I. & Zisook, S. (1991). The generalized pattern of neuropsychological deficits in outpatients with chronic schizophrenia with heterogeneous Wisconsin Card Sorting Test results. *Archives of General Psychiatry*, **48**, 891–8.

Brand, A.N., Jolles, J. & Gispen-de-Weid, C. (1992). Recall and recognition memory deficits in depression. *Journal of Affective Disorders*, **25**, 77–86.

Bulbena, A. & Berrios, G.E. (1986). Pseudodementia: facts and figures. *British Journal of Psychiatry*, **148**, 87–94.

Bulbena, A. and Berrios G.E. (1993). Cognitive function in the affective disorders: a prospective study. *Psychopathology*, **26**, 6–12.

Buhrich, N., Crow, T.J., Johnstone, E.C. & Owens, D.G.C. (1988). Age disorientation in chronic schizophrenia is not associated with pre-morbid intellectual impairment or past physical treatments. *British Journal of Psychiatry*, **152**, 466–9.

Burt, D.B., Zembar, M.J. & Niederehe, G. (1995). Depression and memory impairment: a meta-analysis of the association, its pattern and specificity. *Psychological Bulletin*, **117**, 285–305.

Calev A. (1984a). Recall and recognition in chronic nondemented schizophrenics: the use of matched tasks. *Journal of Abnormal Psychology*, **93**, 172–7.

Calev, A. (1984b). Recall and recognition in mildly disturbed schizophrenics: the use of matched tasks. *Psychological Medicine*, **14**, 425–9.

Calev, A. & Erwin, P.G. (1985). Recall and recognition in depressives. *British Journal of Clinical Psychology*, **24**, 127–8.

Calev, A., Korin, Y., Shapira, B., Kugelmass, S. & Lerer, B. (1986). Verbal and non-verbal recall by depressed and euthymic affective patients. *Psychological Medicine*, **16**, 789–94.

Calev, A. Berlin, H. & Lerer, B. (1987a). Remote and recent memory in long-hospitalized chronic schizophrenics. *Biological Psychiatry*, **22**, 79–85.

Calev, A., Korin, Y., Kugelmass, S. and Lerer, B. (1987b). Performance of chronic schizophrenics on matched word and design recall tasks. *Biological Psychiatry*, **22**, 699–709.

Cassens, G. Wolfe, L. & Zola, M. (1990). The neuropsychology of depressions. *Journal of Neuropsychiatry*, **2**, 202–13.

Channon, S., Baker, J.E. & Robertson, M.M. (1993). Working memory in clinical depression: an experimental study. *Psychological Medicine*, **23**, 87–91.

Chapman, L.J. & Chapman, J.P. (1973). *Disordered Thought in Schizophrenia*. New York: Appleton-Century-Crofts.

Chen, E.Y.H, Wilkins, A.J. & McKenna, P.J. (1994). Semantic memory is both impaired and anomalous in schizophrenia. *Psychological Medicine*, **24**, 193–202.

Chua,S.E. & McKenna, P.J. (1995). Schizophrenia – a brain disease? A critical review of structural and functional cerebral abnormality in the disorder. *British Journal of Psychiatry*, **166**, 563–82.

Clare, L., McKenna, P.J., Mortimer, A.M. & Baddeley, A.D. (1993). Memory in schizophrenia: what is impaired and what is preserved? *Neuropsychologia*, **31**, 1225–41.

Coffman, J.A., Bornstein, R.A., Olson, S.C., Schwartzkopf, S.B. & Nasrallah, H.A. (1990). Cognitive impairment and cerebral structure by MRI in bipolar disorder. *Biological Psychiatry*, **27**, 1188–96.

Cohen, R.M., Weingartner, H., Smallberg, S.A., Pickar, D. & Murphy, D.L. (1982). Effort and cognition in depression. *Archives of General Psychiatry*, **39**, 593–8.

Cohen, R.M., Semple, W.E., Gross, M., Nordahl, T.E., DeLisi, L.E., Holcomb, H.H., King, A.C., Morihisa, J.M. & Pickar, D. (1987) Dysfunction in a prefrontal substrate of sustained attention in schizophrenia. *Life Sciences*, **40**, 2031–9.

Cutting, J. (1985). *The Psychology of Schizophrenia*. Edinburgh: Churchill Livingstone.

Cutting, J. and Murphy, D. (1988). Schizophrenic thought disorder: a psychological and organic interpretation. *British Journal of Psychiatry*, **152**, 310–19.

Danion, J.-M., Willard-Schroeder, D., Zimmerman, M.-A., Grange, D., Schlienger, J.-L. & Singer, L. (1991). Explicit memory and repetition priming in depression: preliminary findings. *Archives of General Psychiatry*, **48**, 707–11.

Davis, J.M. (1985). Antipsychotic drugs. In *Comprehensive Textbook of Psychiatry*, ed. H.I. Kaplan & B.J. Sadock. Baltimore: Williams and Wilkins.

Denny, E.B. & Hunt, R.R. (1992). Affective valence and memory in depression: dissociation of recall and fragment completion. *Journal of Abnormal Psychology*, **101**, 575–80.

Dolan, R.J. & Goodwin, G.M. (1996). Brain imaging in affective disorders. In *Brain Imaging in Psychiatry*, ed. S. Lewis & N. Higgins. Oxford: Blackwell.

Dolan, R.J., Bench, C.J., Brown, R.G., Scott, L.C. & Frackowiak, R.S.J. (1994). Neuropsychological dysfunction in depression: the relationship to regional cerebral blood flow. *Psychological Medicine*, **24**, 849–57.

Duffy, L. & O'Carroll, R. (1994). Memory impairment in schizophrenia – a comparison with that observed in the alcoholic Korsakoff syndrome. *Psychological Medicine*, **24**, 155–66.

Elkis, H., Friedman, L., Wise, A. & Meltzer, H.Y. (1995). Meta-analysis of studies of ventricular enlargement and cortical sulcal prominence in mood disorders. *Archives of General Psychiatry*, **52**, 735–46.

Elliott, C.L. & Greene, R.L. (1992). Clinical depression and implicit memory. *Journal of Abnormal Psychology*, **101**, 572–4.

Elliott, R., McKenna, P.J., Robbins, T.W. & Sahakian, B.J. (1995). Neuropsychological evidence for fronto-striatal dysfunction in schizophrenia. *Psychological Medicine*, **25**, 619–30.

Elliott, R., Sahakian, B.J., McKay, A.P., Herrod, J.J., Robbins, T.W. & Paykel, E.S. (1996). Neuropsychological impairments in unipolar depression: the influence of perceived failure on subsequent performance. *Psychological Medicine*, **26**, 975–89.

Fleming, K., Goldberg, T.E. & Gold, J.M. (1994). Applying working memory constructs to schizophrenic cognitive impairment. In *The Neuropsychology of Schizophrenia*, ed. A.S. David & J.C. Cutting. Hove: Erlbaum.

Fleming, K., Goldberg, T.E., Gold, J.M. & Weinberger, D.R. (1995). Verbal working memory dysfunction in schizophrenia: use of a Brown-Peterson paradigm. *Psychiatry Research*, **56**, 155–61.

Friedman, A. (1964). Minimal effects of severe depression on cognitive functioning. *Journal of Abnormal and Social Psychology*, **69**, 237–43.

Glass, R.M., Uhlenhuth, E.H., Hartel, F.W., Matuzas, W. & Fischman, M.W. (1981). Cognitive dysfunction and imipramine in outpatient depressives. *Archives of General Psychiatry*, **38**, 1048–51.

Gold, J.M., Randolph, C., Carpenter, C.J., Goldberg, T.E. & Weinberger, D.R. (1992a). Forms of memory failure in schizophrenia. *Journal of Abnormal Psychology*, **101**, 487–94.

Gold, J.M., Randolph, C. & Carpenter, C.J. (1992b). The performance of patients with schizophrenia on the Wechsler Memory Scale-Revised. *Clinical Neuropsychologist*, **6**, 367–70.

Gold, J.M., Carpenter, C., Randolph, C., Goldberg, T.E. & Weinberger, D.R. (1997). Auditory working memory and Wisconsin Card Sorting Test performance in schizophrenia. *Archives of General Psychiatry*, **54**, 159–65.

Goldberg, T.E. & Gold, J.M (1995). Neurocognitive deficits in schizophrenia. In *Schizophrenia*, ed S.R. Hirsch & D.R. Weinberger. Oxford: Blackwell.

Goldberg, T.E. & Weinberger, D.R. (1996). Effects of neuroleptics on the cognition of patients with schizophrenia: a review of recent studies. *Journal of Clinical Psychiatry*, **57**, 62–5.

Goldberg, T.E., Weinberger, D.R., Pliskin, N.H., Berman, K.F. & Podd, M.H. (1989). Recall memory deficit in schizophrenia: a possible manifestation of prefrontal dysfunction. *Schizophrenia Research*, **2**, 251–7.

Goldberg, T.E., Ragland, J.D., Gold, J.M., Bigelow, L.B., Torrey, E.F. & Weinberger, D.R. (1990). Neuropsychological assessment of monozygotic twins discordant for schizophrenia. *Archives of General Psychiatry*, **47**, 1066–72.

Goldberg, T.E., Torrey, E.F., Gold, J.M., Ragland, J.D., Bigelow, L.B. & Weinberger, D.R. (1993). Learning and memory in monozygotic twins discordant for schizophrenia. *Psychological Medicine*, **23**, 71–85.

Goldman-Rakic, P.S. (1991). Prefrontal cortical dysfunction in schizophrenia: the relevance of working memory. In *Psychopathology and the Brain*, ed. B.J. Carroll & J.E. Barrett. New York: Raven Press.

Goldstein, G. (1978). Cognitive and perceptual differences between schizophrenics and organics. *Schizophrenia Bulletin*, **4**, 160–85.

Golinkoff, M. & Sweeney, J.A. (1989). Cognitive impairments in depression. *Journal of Affective Disorders*, **17**, 105–12.

Gottesman, I.I. (1991). *Schizophrenia Genesis: the Origins of Madness.* New York: Freeman.

Gras -Vincendon, A., Danion, J.-M., Grange, D., Bilik, M., Willard-Schroeder, D., Sichel, J.-P. & Singer, L. (1994). Explicit memory, repetition priming and cognitive skill learning in schizophrenia. *Schizophrenia Research,* **13**, 117-26.

Gruzelier, J., Seymour, K., Wilson, L., Jolley, A. & Hirsch, S. (1988). Impairments on neuropsychological tests of temporohippocampal and frontohippocampal function in remitting schizophrenia and affective disorders. *Archives of General Psychiatry,* **45**, 623–9.

Gur, R.C. & Gur, R.E. (1995). Hypofrontality in schizophrenia: RIP. *Lancet,* **i**, 1383–4.

Healy, D. (1996.) *The Psychopharmacologists.* London: Altman/Chapman & Hall.

Heaton, R.K., Baade, L.E. & Johnson, K.L. (1978). Neuropsychological test results associated with psychiatric disorders in adults. *Psychological Bulletin,* **85**, 141–62.

Hertel, P.T. & Rude, S.S. (1991). Depressive deficits in memory: focusing attention improves subsequent recall. *Journal of Experimental Psychology: General,* **120**, 301–9.

Hodges, J.R. (1991). *Transient Amnesia: Clinical and Neuropsychological Aspects.* London: W.B. Saunders Co. Ltd.

Ilsley, J.E., Moffoot, A.P.R. & O'Carroll, R.E. (1995). An analysis of memory dysfunction in major depression. *Journal of Affective Disorders,* **35**, 1–9.

Johnson, M.H. & Magaro, P.A. (1987). Effects of mood and severity on memory processes in depression and mania. *Psychological Bulletin,* **101**, 28–40.

Johnstone, E.C., Owens, D.G.C., Frith, C.D. & Calvert, L.M. (1985). Institutionalisation and the outcome of functional psychoses. *British Journal of Psychiatry,* **146**, 36–44.

Jones, P.B., Harvey, I., Lewis, S.W. & Murray, R.M. (1994). Cerebral ventricle dimensions as risk factors for schizophrenia and affective psychosis. *Psychological Medicine,* **24**, 995–1011.

Jorm, A.F. (1986). Cognitive deficit in the depressed elderly: a review of some basic unresolved issues. *Australian and New Zealand Journal of Psychiatry,* **20**, 11–22.

Judd, L.L., Hubbard, B., Janowsky, D.S., Huey, L.Y. & Takahashi, K.I. (1977). The effect of lithium carbonate on the cognitive functions of normal subjects. *Archives of General Psychiatry,* **34**, 355–7.

Kern, R.S., Green, M.S. & Wallace, C.J. (1997). Declarative and procedural learning in schizophrenia: a test of the integrity of divergent memory systems. *Cognitive Neuropsychiatry,* **2**, 39–50.

King, D.J. (1990). The effect of neuroleptics on cognitive and psychomotor function. *British Journal of Psychiatry,* **157**, 799–811.

Klonoff, H., Fibiger, C.H. & Hutton, C.H. (1970). Neuropsychological patterns in chronic schizophrenia. *Journal of Nervous and Mental Disease,* **150**, 291–300.

Koh, S.D. (1978). Remembering of verbal materials by schizophrenic young adults. In *Language and Cognition in Schizophrenia,* ed. S. Schwartz. Hillsdale, NJ: Erlbaum.

Kolb, B. & Whishaw, I.Q. (1983). Performance of schizophrenic patients on tests sensitive to left or right temporal or parietal function in neurological patients. *Journal of Nervous and Mental Disease,* **171**, 435–43.

Kraepelin, E. (1913a). *Dementia Praecox and Paraphrenia* (translated by. R.M. Barclay, 1919). Edinburgh: Livingstone.

Kraepelin, E. (1913b). *Manic-Depressive Insanity and Paranoia* (translated by R.M. Barclay, 1921). Edinburgh: Livingstone.

Lader, M. & Bhanji, S. (1980). Physiological and psychological effects of antidepressants in man. In *Psychotropic Agents, Part I (Handbook of Experimental Pharmacology, Vol. 55)*, ed. F. Hoffmeister & G. Stille. New York: Springer Verlag.

Landro, N.I. (1994). Memory function in schizophrenia. *Acta Psychiatrica Scandinavica*, **90**, 87–94.

Landro, N.I., Orbeck, A.L. & Rund, B.R. (1993). Memory functioning in chronic and non-chronic schizophrenics, affectively disturbed patients and normal controls. *Schizophrenia Research*, **10**, 85–92.

Lewis, S.W. (1990). Computerised tomography in schizophrenia 15 years on. *British Journal of Psychiatry*, **157**, 16–24.

Liddle, P.F. & Crow, T.J. (1984). Age disorientation in chronic schizophrenia is associated with global intellectual impairment. *British Journal of Psychiatry*, **144**, 193–9.

McAllister, T.W. (1981). Cognitive functioning in the affective disorders. *Comprehensive Psychiatry*, **22**, 572–86.

McKay, A.P., Tarbuck, A.F., Shapleske, J. & McKenna, P.J. (1995). Neuropsychological impairment in manic-depressive psychosis: evidence for persistent deficits in patients with chronic, severe illness. *British Journal of Psychiatry*, **167**, 51–7.

McKay, A.P., McKenna, P.J., Mortimer, A.M., Bentham, P. & Hodges, J.R. (1996). Semantic memory is impaired in schizophrenia. *Biological Psychiatry*, **39**, 929–37.

McKenna, P.J. (1994). *Schizophrenia and Related Syndromes*. Oxford: Oxford University Press.

McKenna, P.J., Tamlyn, D., Lund, C.E., Mortimer, A.M., Hammond, S. & Baddeley, A.D. (1990). Amnesic syndrome in schizophrenia. *Psychological Medicine*, **20**, 967–72.

Madden, J.J., Luban, J.A., Kaplan, L.A. & Manfredi, H.M. (1952). Non-dementing psychoses in older persons. *Journal of the American Medical Association*, **150**, 1567–72.

Malec, J. (1978). Neuropsychological assessment of of schizophrenia versus brain damage: a review. *Journal of Nervous and Mental Disease*, **166**, 507–16.

Marcos, T., Salamero, M., Gutiérrez, F., Catalán, R., Gasto, C. & Lázarro, L. (1994). Cognitive dysfunctions in recovered melancholic patients. *Journal of Affective Disorders*, **32**, 133–7.

Miller, I.S., Faustman, W.O., Moses, J.A. & Csernansky, J.G. (1991). Evaluating cognitive impairment in depression with the Luria-Nebraska neuropsychological battery. *Psychiatry Research*, **37**, 219–27.

Miller, W.R. (1975). Psychological deficits in depression. *Psychological Bulletin*, **82**, 238–60.

Morice, R. (1990). Cognitive inflexibility and and pre-frontal dysfunction in schizophrenia and mania. *British Journal of Psychiatry*, **157**, 50–4.

Morice, R. & Delahunty, A. (1996). Frontal/executive impairments in schizophrenia. *Schizophrenia Bulletin*, **22**, 125–37.

Morrison-Stewart,S.L., Williamson, P.C., Corning, W.C., Kutcher, S.P., Snow, W.G. & Merskey, H. (1992). Frontal and non-frontal lobe neuropsychological test performance and clinical symptomatology in schizophrenia. *Psychological Medicine*, **22**, 353–9.

Nachmani, G. & Cohen, B.D. (1969). Recall and recognition free learning in schizophrenics. *Journal of Abnormal Psychology*, **74**, 511–16.

Owens, D.G.C. & Johnstone, E.C. (1980). The disabilities of chronic schizophrenia – their nature and the factors contributing to their development. *British Journal of Psychiatry*, **136**, 384–93.

Park, S. & Holzman, P.S. (1992). Schizophrenics show spatial working memory deficits. *Archives of General Psychiatry*, **49**, 975–82.

Paulman, R.G., Devous, M.D., Gregory, R.R., Herman, J.H., Jennings, L., Bonte, F.J., Nasrallah, H.A. & Raese, J.D. (1990). Hypofrontality and cognitive impairment in schizophrenia: dynamic single-photon tomography and neuropsychological assessment of schizophrenic brain function. *Biological Psychiatry*, **27**, 377–99.

Paulsen, J.S., Heaton, R.K., Sadek, J.R., Perry, W., Delis, D.C., Braff, D., Kuck, J., Zisook, S. & Jeste, D.V. (1995). The nature of learning and memory impairments in schizophrenia. *Journal of the International Neuropsychological Society*, **1**, 88–99.

Paykel, E.S. (ed.) (1992). *Handbook of Affective Disorders*. Edinburgh: Churchill Livingstone.

Payne, R.W. (1973). Cognitive abnormalities. In *Handbook of Abnormal Psychology*, ed. H.J. Eysenck. London: Pitman.

Randolph, C., Gold, J.M, Carpenter, C.J., Goldberg, T.E. & Weinberger, D.R. (1990). Implicit memory in patients with schizophrenia and normal controls: effects of task demands and susceptibility to priming. *Journal of Clinical and Experimental Neuropsychology*, **15**, 853–66.

Raskin, A., Friedman, A.S. & DiMascio, A. (1982). Cognitive and performance deficits in depression. *Psychopharmacology Bulletin*, **18**, 196–202.

Richards, P.M. and Ruff, R.M. (1989). Motivational effects on neuropsychological functioning: comparison of depressed versus nondepressed individuals. *Journal of Consulting and Clinical Psychology*, **57**, 396–402.

Robertson, G. & Taylor, P.J. (1985). Some cognitive correlates of affective disorders. *Psychological Medicine*, **15**, 297–309.

Rogers, D.G.C. (1996). The cognitive disorders of psychiatric illness: a historical perspective. In *Schizophrenia: A Neuropsychological Perspective*, ed. C. Pantelis, H.E. Nelson & T.R.E. Barnes. Chichester, UK: Wiley.

Roy-Byrne, P.P., Weingartner, H., Bierer, L.M. & Post, R.M. (1986). Effortful and automatic cognitive processes in depression. *Archives of General Psychiatry*, **43**, 265–7.

Rushe, T.M., Woodruff, P.W.R., Murray, R.M. & Morris, R.G. (1999). Episodic memory and learning in patients with chronic schizophrenia. *Schizophrenia Research*, **35**, 85–6.

Sagawa, K., Kawakatsua, S., Shibuya, I., Oiji, A., Morinobu, S., Komatani, A. Yazaki, M. & Totsuka, S. (1990). Correlation of regional cerebral blood flow with performance of neuropsychological tests in schizophrenic patients. *Schizophrenia Research*, **3**, 241–6.

Saykin, A.J., Gur, R.C., Gur, R.E., Mozley, P.D., Mozley, L.H., Resnick, S.M., Kester, D.B. & Stafiniak, P. (1991). Neuropsychological function in schizophrenia: selective impairment in memory and learning. *Archives of General Psychiatry*, **48**, 618–24.

Saykin, A.J., Shtasel, D.L., Gur, R.E., Kester, B., Mozley, L.H., Stafiniak, P. & Gur, R.C. (1994). Neuropsychological deficits in neuroleptic naive patients with first-episode schizophrenia. *Archives of General Psychiatry*, **51**, 124–31.

Schwartz, B.L., Rosse, R.B. & Deutsch, S.I. (1993). Limits of the processing view in acounting for dissociations among memory measures in a clinical population. *Memory and Cognition*, **21**, 63–72.

Schwartz, B.L., Rosse, R.B., Veazey, C. & Deutsch, S.I. (1996). Impaired motor skill learning in schizophrenia: implications for corticostriatal dysfunction. *Biological Psychiatry*, **39**, 241–8.

Shoqeirat, M.A. & Mayes, A.R. (1988). Spatiotemporal memory and rate of forgetting in acute schizophrenia. *Psychological Medicine*, **18**, 843–53.

Slater E. (1936). The inheritance of manic-depressive insanity and its relation to mental defect. *Journal of Mental Science*, **82**, 626–34.

Squire, L.R. (1987). *Memory and Brain*. Oxford: Oxford University Press.

Stevens, M., Crow, T.J., Bowman, M.J. & Coles, E.C. (1978). Age disorientation in schizophrenia: a constant prevalence of 25 per cent in a chronic mental hospital population? *British Journal of Psychiatry*, **133**, 130–6.

Stömgren, L.S. (1977). The influence of depression on memory. *Acta Psychiatrica Scandinavica*, **56**, 109–28.

Tamlyn, D., McKenna, P.J., Mortimer, A.M., Lund, C.E., Hammond, S. & Baddeley, A.D. (1992). Memory impairment in schizophrenia: its extent, affiliations and neuropsychological character. *Psychological Medicine*, **22**, 101–15.

Tarbuck, A. & Paykel, E.S. (1995). Effects of major depression on the cognitive function of younger and older adults. *Psychological Medicine*, **25**, 285–96.

Thompson, P.J. (1991). Antidepressants and memory: a review. *Human Psychopharmacology*, **6**, 79–90.

Tulving, E. (1983). *Elements of Episodic Memory*. Oxford: Oxford University Press.

Waddington, J.L. & Youssef, H.A. (1988). Tardive dyskinesia in bipolar affective disorder: aging, cognitive dysfunction, course of illness and exposure to neuroleptics and lithium. *American Journal of Psychiatry*, **145**, 613–16.

Watkins, P.C., Mathews, A., Williamson, D.A. & Fuller, R.D. (1992). Mood-congruent memory in depression: emotional priming or elaboration? *Journal of Abnormal Psychology*, **101**, 581–6.

Watts, F.N. (1995). Depression and anxiety. In *Handbook of Memory Disorders*, ed. A.D. Baddeley, B.A. Wilson & F.N. Watts. Chicester, UK: John Wiley.

Weingartner, H. & Silberman, E. (1982). Models of cognitive impairment: cognitive changes in depression. *Psychopharmacology Bulletin*, **18**, 27–42.

Willner, P. (1984). Cognitive functioning in depression: a review of theory and research. *Psychological Medicine*, **14**, 807–23.

Wilson, B.A., Cockburn, J.M. & Baddeley, A.D. (1985). *The Rivermead Behavioural Memory Test*. Bury St. Edmunds, Suffolk: Thames Valley Test Co.

Wolfe, J., Granholm, E., Butters, N., Saunders, E. & Janowsky, D. (1987). Verbal memory deficits associated with major affective disorders: a comparison of unipolar and bipolar patients. *Journal of Affective Disorders*, **13**, 83–92.

# 12

# Depressive pseudodementia

Gabriel desRosiers

## Introduction

As life expectancy steadily increases, so do the risks of medical conditions associated with advancing age (e.g. Alzheimer's disease), and more clinical services are now devoted to the physical and mental well-being of older adults (Carpenter, 1996; Grimley-Evans, 1996). With greater public awareness of Alzheimer's disease (AD), demands for better means to identify patients in their earliest stage have intensified (Cooper et al., 1996; Eastwood et al., 1996; Tierney et al., 1996); and with a steady rise in referrals from general practitioners and other agencies, specialist clinics have now been set up to help distinguish them from patients whose cognitive attenuation does not stem from AD (see Chapter 6, this volume; Philpot, 1996; Wright & Lindesay, 1995). One cardinal criterion in the diagnosis of probable AD is the presence of dementia (McKhann et al., 1984), a significant deterioration of neuropsychological functions most evident in the initial phase as memory impairment (Corey-Bloom et al., 1995). But every-day memory in aging individuals can falter for a number of reasons other than AD (e.g. major depressive illness; age-related decline), and research is now carried out to clarify the mechanisms that underlie these 'amnesic' states (see Chapter 18, this volume; desRosiers, 1999; McKenna et al., 1998).

Although referred to as pseudodementia, it is now evident the memory lapses often recorded in elderly depressed patients reflect true cognitive difficulties (Beats et al., 1996; Burt et al., 1995; King et al., 1995), but how different these are from deficits brought on by early AD remains uncharted. Sometimes associated with soft signs (Baldwin et al., 1993), and sometimes contrasted with cognitive impediments seen in patients whose 'subcortical' disease (e.g. progressive supranuclear palsy) primarily affects frontostriatal systems (Austin & Mitchell, 1995; Massman et al., 1992), this reversible dementia is thought to compromise memory primarily by disrupting accessory behaviours (e.g. attention) that are necessary to engage/maintain mnestic activity. Although depression-induced cognitive impairment is thought not to be a precursor of irreversible dementia in many of these patients (Rabins & Pearlson, 1994), findings from long-term follow-ups still produce inconsistent results (e.g. Baumgart et al., 1995; Buntinx et al., 1996; Kral & Emery, 1989;

Sachdev et al., 1990; Stoudemire et al., 1993), thus stoking the question whether remission of cognitive deficits does invariably follow, as depressive illness in many of these patients responds to treatment (Tham et al., 1997). Addonizio and Alexopoulos (1993), for example, remarked how geriatric depression with 'reversible' dementia seemed to have a yearly incidence of 'irreversible' dementia perhaps up to six times that seen in the general population. There is now a pressing need to determine whether a subset of patients labelled with pseudodementia are in the early stages of an irreversible dementia .

Research in the antecedents of cognitive difficulties in depressive illness is progressing on several fronts and, as O'Brien (1997) recently considered, one potent determinant perhaps involves pervasive biological deregulations of thyrotropin-stimulating hormones (Marangell et al., 1997), or the hypothalamic–pituitary–adrenal (HPA) hormones (Bemelmans et al., 1996; Cooney & Dinan, 1996; Rush et al., 1997) which control the production of compounds (e.g. glucocorticoids) that can disrupt the workings of neuronal systems normally activated during memory tasks (desRosiers, 1992; Ferrier & Perry, 1992; Mitchell, 1995). Whether cognitive impairments in these patients rise de novo because of such biochemical activity, or simply are the result of a goading of symptoms in preclinical conditions as yet undiagnosed is unclear (Greenwald et al., 1997). In this population, a host of contributory factors (e.g. stress, age, education, etc.) are also instrumental in bringing about a continuum of patients whose cognitive attenuations affect functional abilities (essential, but not sufficient, criterion for dementia) in varying degrees. On cognitive grounds for instance, deficits on psychometric tests sensitive to certain neuropsychological functions will apparently level off following a normalizing in emotional health in some subjects (e.g. younger ones?), while others seem to retain subtle but enduring features predictive of dementia long after remission of their depressive illness (Abas et al., 1990; Pearlson et al., 1989). As Sahakian (1991) considered, reversibility of cognitive impairments perhaps occurs in a number of well-known skills only, while deficits in less obvious areas persist. Longitudinal studies are needed to examine whether 'reversible' and 'irreversible' subsets of patients produce distinct profiles on cognitive tests used to screen for dementia in the clinic. And, if so, how is cognitive impairment in the irreversible group different from dementia in patients with preclinical AD, and not just a variant of an increasingly heterogeneous diagnostic category itself (Butters et al., 1996; Furey-Kurkjian et al., 1996; Graham & Hodges, 1997; Khachaturian, 1992; Pietrini et al., 1996).

## Depression and dementia

Current surveys suggest the occurrence of clinical depression in patients who eventually are diagnosed with probable AD may be as high as 15–20% (Allen et al., 1997;

Migliorelli et al., 1995; Ryan et al., 1995; Teri & Wagner, 1992), but research on the consistency of the affective syndrome across AD patients is limited. The characteristics of depressive illness in aging adults are complex, and often predictably associated with physical (e.g. health), psychosocial (e.g. isolation), and other (e.g. premorbid history) factors (Alexopoulos et al., 1996; Forsell et al., 1995; Murphy, 1992), but it is unclear whether the configuration of depressive symptoms in AD conform to the syndromes diagnosed in functional patients, cognitively impaired or not (e.g. Blazer et al., 1988; Buchwald & Rudick-Davis, 1993; Reischies et al., 1990). Consequently, it is still difficult to reliably apportion which, if any, clinical features of the illness are more characteristic of patients with pseudo or true dementia. Current research, for example in patients classified with 'vascular depression', in whom vegetative systems, frontal-type cognitive skills, and functional independence may be more at risk (Alexopoulos et al., 1997; Krishnan et al., 1997; Palmer et al., 1996; Salloway et al., 1996), may also become relevant in distinguishing between patients for whom reversal in cognitive decline is more/less likely.

Following Beck's (1987) model of depression in which the deepening of affective illness results from consistent distortions in the processing of information about self, future, and others, an earlier review (desRosiers, 1992) considered how one difference perhaps lay in the preponderance of physical (e.g. insomnia) or intrapsychic (e.g. guilt rationalizations, nihilistic ruminations, etc.) symptoms across the groups. Unlike in younger patients, depression in older people can take on less familiar expressions, and in some instances, with a 'masked' presentation denying dysphoric feelings (Blazer, 1989). But, in most cases with or without cognitive misgivings, evidence of intrapsychic derangement can be a major component of the syndrome. In Alzheimer patients, recent evidence suggests the presence of vegetative symptoms, more than the experience of intrapsychic distortions, plays a prominent part in the diagnosis of depression (e.g. Carpenter et al., 1995; Haupt et al., 1995; Logie et al., 1992), although such features might best be regarded as symptoms of dementia proper (Troisi et al., 1996). An early suggestion was that, with irreversible neuronal damage in AD, the cognitive apparatus may already be affected enough in the early stages of the disease to prevent the development of maladaptive mood-consistent cognitive schemata associated with intrapsychic symptoms on the scale seen in patients with pseudodementia.

A further conjecture (desRosiers & Ivison, 1988) is whether the development of such schematic symptoms covaries with the emergence of specific 'mood-congruent' patterns on a memory task that automatically highlights its emotional tone or valence (e.g. unpleasant vs. pleasant stories). Relative to control subjects for example, memory in functional patients generally seems least affected on tasks steeped in negative connotations, and most at risk when the emotional tenor of the learning material is positive; although whether this is so irrespective of how 'resource-hungry' a task is remains unsettled (Bradley et al., 1995; Dannion et al., 1995; Roediger & McDermott, 1992). Findings from recent studies (Bäckman & Forsell, 1994; Boone et al., 1995; Ilsley et al., 1995) suggest one relatively intact process in older functional patients may be their ability to profit from emphasis of a task's semantic dimensions; as this can ease learning of verbal material by facilitating the application of basic well-learned cognitive techniques of semantic organization (e.g. categorizing). The fostering of selective hedonic processing in 'depressive amnesia' may be an instance of this, although the precise neuropsychological mechanisms involved are still unclear (see below). One of AD's earliest and most pervasive cognitive effects is a gradual degradation of semantic systems (Brandt & Rich, 1995; Patterson & Hodges, 1995) which may impede the laying of semantic organizations needed to express mood-consistent intrapsychic symptoms, and congruent hedonic patterns on memory tests. The task of determining whether a patient's impoverished scores on memory tasks is symptomatic of a pseudo or true dementia therefore might become easier when including such hedonic material during diagnostic testing (desRosiers & Ivison, 1988; Watts, 1995).

## Normal cognitive aging

Directly relevant to the question of pseudodementia is the research seeking to plot normal cognitive ageing in terms of functional competence, neuropsychological performance, neuroradiological correlates, etc. (Fried et al., 1996; Masur et al., 1994; Purcell et al., 1995), and how 'non-harbiger' conditions of age-related cognitive decline (DSM4) or age-associated memory impairment (AAMI) differ from dementia. Longitudinal research to validate these conditions as separate from being prodromal/subclinical stages of AD is limited (Blass, 1996; Levy, 1995; Schmand et al., 1996). But, just as in many patients diagnosed with pseudodementia, recent findings indicate cognitive deficits on 'frontal lobe' sensitive tests may be a primary feature in many AAMI patients (Hänninen et al., 1997), several of whom eventually develop a frank dementia. Epidemiological surveys of the elderly, in general, suggest for a number of these subjects cognitive aging follows an unstable process often in the context of depressive symptoms (Ebly et al., 1995; Ritchie et al., 1993); and although formal criteria on standard AAMI protocols now stipulate the exclusion of depression as a complicating factor (Larrabee & McEntee, 1995), it is likely that a great deal of past evidence for these diagnostic categories involved patients who were also depressed (Watts, 1995). AAMI patients in Hänninen et al.'s (1997) study, for instance, significantly scored higher than controls on the Geriatric Depression Scale. Likewise, community-dwelling subjects with cognitive impairment (but not dementia) and memory complaints at baseline who then went on to develop a frank dementia one year later had scored significantly higher on the Hamilton Depression Scale (Schofield et al., 1997).

As Rabins and Pearlson (1994) considered, patients with depression-induced dementia perhaps fall in a subgroup with increased risk of age-associated difficulties, and perhaps with lifelong structural irregularities which only become manifest in the context of depression. There are no commonly accepted neuro-psychological markers that set AAMI apart from cognitive impairments in early or preclinical organic dementia (Jacobs et al., 1995; Larrabee & McEntee, 1995), and little information is available on the subset of patients who eventually develop dementia (Soininen et al., 1994). Conversely, not enough is known about AAMI patients who subsequently are diagnosed with depression, and what role this has as a predictor of organic disease. Surveys are needed to help uncover whether the cognitive effects of depression in patients already diagnosed with AAMI follow a different course to that seen in functional patients with pseudodementia, and how this differs from effects noted in depressed AD patients. As the aim is to extend the preclinical boundaries over which therapeutics (e.g. drugs) can provide benefits to Alzheimer patients (e.g. Bodick et al., 1997), our knowledge of how normal cognitive aging unfolds becomes most important (Baltes & Kliegl, 1986; Bowling & Grundy, 1997; Jonker et al., 1996; Lichtenberg et al., 1995; Powell & Whitla, 1994), particularly when emotional health is affected.

One parallel drawn by Craik and his colleagues (1995) concerned the similarity between the slowing effects of aging on the mechanisms of memory, and the mild 'dysexecutive syndrome' of patients with minimal anterior lobe injury and subtle behavioural difficulties (e.g. lack of initiation, disorganization, anergia, etc). Using Baddeley's (1988) terminology, there may be a reduction in the effectiveness of working memory components (e.g. central executive) most evident when performance is given little 'environmental support', and success must rely on self-generated activity and effort (Einstein et al., 1995). Weingartner (1986) and Hirst (1988) drew similar parallels with cognitively impaired depressed patients, while desRosiers and Ivison (1986) further suggested one way to distinguish them from patients with Alzheimer's disease might be to contrast the groups' performance on tasks standardized to highlight extremes in processing demands (e.g. automatic vs. controlled processing). Although AD patients can show difficulties in strategic/supervisory control during cognitive performance (Binetti et al., 1996), this does not seem to covary with depressive symptoms, and the benefits from easing processing demands should be less dramatic than the gains expected in patients with less neuronal damage in the regions most directly involved in memory consolidation (e.g. amygdala, hippocampus, etc.).

Studies monitoring cerebral activation during information processing (e.g.

Eustache et al., 1995; Loessner et al., 1995; Schroeder et al., 1995) suggest aging increases frontal lobe variability, with greater impact during late encoding stages; controlled stages in which the operations of working memory increasingly proceed along central executive directives (Fuster, 1995; Wheeler et al., 1995). One attentional mechanism possibly involved in this process, Craik et al. (1995) suggested, is an age-related increase in one's difficulty to inhibit task-irrelevant verbal information (Rouleau & Belleville, 1996); an onerous procedure (Fletcher et al., 1996; Knight et al., 1995) which West (1996) has likened to the maintaining of 'interference control' during cognitive performance. Recent papers suggest irrelevant processing is also a strong determinant in depression's effects on memory (Brewin et al., 1996; Gunther et al., 1996; Mialet et al., 1996). The recurrence of negative ruminations about past experiences, somatic concerns, and others, perhaps hampers the central executive's task to allocate processing resources during cognitive performance (Lemelin et al., 1996; Linville, 1996; Nolen-Hoeksema & Morrow, 1993), thus causing a drainage of resources from energy-dependent processes that normally take place during the consolidation of memory.

## Neuropsychology

A major supervisory role of the central executive is the co-ordination of several, more or less automatized, subsystems (visual scratchpad, articulatory loop), primarily drawing on the circuitry of prefrontal lobe regions (Baddeley, 1988). Prefrontal regions lie at the confluence of cortical and subcortical attentional pathways, a polymodal switchboard involved in the association of internal/external information, its organization, manipulation, and utilization in the control of behaviour (Benson, 1993; Kimberg & Farah, 1993; Milner, 1995). Unlike more posterior systems, information on the lateralization of mechanisms powering the operations of working memory is limited (Goldberg & Podell, 1995; Rueckert & Grafman, 1996; Smith et al., 1995), but a recent review by Tranel and Damasio (1995) suggested that, beside the anteroposterior axis, certain difficulties seemed to covary with lesion sites ranging along a dorsoventral axis. Findings from experimental research, for instance, show how damage to dorsolateral relays can be highly detrimental during the later stages of a memory task when spontaneous initiation of goal-oriented actions is required (Goldman-Rakic, 1990; Passingham, 1993). With damage extending to ventromedial systems, this difficulty becomes most accentuated as material increasingly promotes emotional associations (Rolls, 1990; Yamatami et al., 1990). According to Fuster (1995), dorsolateral regions mediate input from posterior systems involved in verbal semantic activity, and from 're-entrant' neuronal circuits coursing through subcortical structures most implicated in motor/motivational behaviour. This suggests some mechanisms of controlled processes in working memory, and others regulating an organism's general preparation for action, may interact in these regions during learning (Salmon et al., 1996; Zhuang et al., 1997).

One general effect of left prefrontal injury is to impede initiation (spontaneity) of behaviour, while a frequent consequence of right-sided frontal disturbances in humans is a tendency to distractibility, a failure to habituate to internal/external input from non-selected channels (Pribram, 1987). In memory, deregulated orienting mechanisms (i.e. distractibility) may come to disrupt what Squire (1992) described as the time-limited task of the hippocampus to build a permanent coherence (consolidation) between new information from selected channels, and old repositories reactivated by the learning material. On complex verbal tasks for instance (e.g. story recall), this process may rest on effort-consuming manipulations (e.g. structuring) that seem most jeopardized by instability in left anterior regions (Lang et al., 1988; Luciana et al., 1992, Sawaguchi & Goldman-Rakic, 1991). Increased vulnerability to unsolicited input during a controlled task disrupts concentration. To maintain inhibition (habituation), extra processing energies are needed, energies otherwise applied to later-stage algorithms. A primary role of the central executive during performance therefore may be to sustain inhibition in unselected channels, while counteracting habituation in selected channels (Anderson & Spellman, 1995; Cowan, 1988); and this is reflected in cerebral metabolic activity which, in major depression, often produces asymmetrical profiles.

## Neuropsychiatry

Research in affective illness indicates major depression is often associated with an asymmetry in neuroanatomical and functional patterns involving prefrontal areas and their pathways to subcortical structures (Soares & Mann, 1997). Some evidence further suggests this can also covary with fluctuations in specific elements of depression (e.g. dysphoria, psychomotor retardation, amnesia, etc.) as the disorder waxes and wanes (Austin & Mitchell, 1995; Dolan et al., 1994). Evidence from activation studies (e.g. PET) for example, suggests the dynamics of emotional processing differentially involves separate regions of the brain (Baker et al., 1997; George et al., 1995; Robinson, 1995) which, in clinical states, can become more or less polarized (Goldberg & Podell, 1995; Kinsbourne, 1989). In particular, patients with major depression often show a left, relative to right, hypofrontality. More specifically, a reduction in the normally high dorsofrontal–posterior metabolic gradient of the left hemisphere, relative to controls (Bench et al., 1993; Biver et al., 1994; Rubin et al., 1995), seem to parallel a heightened right orbitofrontal–posterior gradient. Such dynamic patterns perhaps are associated with what Klein (1974) identified as disruptions in two fundamental neurobiologic systems (Carroll, 1991;

Kinsbourne, 1989) which, according to Gray (1994), primarily engage distinct frontostriatal systems in reciprocal inhibition. First, there is a deregulation in central pain (withdrawal, no-go) mechanisms involved in the inhibition of behaviour, and this is associated with dysphoria (Healy, 1993). Overactivation of this system is reflected in heightened sensitivity to potentially aversive situations, the environment is perceived as noxious, and attention is continually disrupted by plausibly threatening events, both internal and external. Internally, chronic private consciousness is tilted towards negative characteristics of the self, and failures, and this fosters guilt feelings, pejorative attributions, and negative affect (Shaw & Katz, 1990). On cognitive tests, excessive inhibition from right frontal mechanisms perhaps results in a constant disrupting of perceptual functions carried out by ipsilateral posterior regions, as patients perform on visuospatial tasks that require little verbal activity during early processing stages.

Concurrently, Klein (1974) suggested there is an inhibition of cerebral pleasure mechanisms that normally fuel behavioural activation (go, approach) systems, and this is associated with both anhedonia (Willner, 1993) and abulia (Bhatia & Marsden, 1994), a motivational state often referred to as frontal/dysexecutive syndrome (Berrios & Gili, 1995). Disturbance in this system is reflected in a lack of reaction to normally satisfying external stimulation (e.g. work, social, personal pleasures), and in neglect of basic drives (e.g. food, sex). Mentally, anhedonia diminishes a patient's responsivity to positive internal cognitions serving self-esteem (e.g. sense of competence), and decreased experience of positive reinforcement eventually leads to loss of motivated behaviour and interest, ending in withdrawal from extrapersonal engagements (Lawton et al., 1996; Snaith, 1993; Willner, 1993). This shut-down may parallel a disrupted activation in frontostriatal dopaminergic systems, leading to an ineffectual anterior control over ipsilateral posterior verbal functions (desRosiers & Ivison, 1988). Failure to vet the products of posterior associative activity for example may lead depressed patients into what Beck (1987) described as a persistent and recurring stream of automatic negative thoughts (associations, schemata) intruding during memory performance.

Findings of asymmetrical activation in clinical depression (e.g. Bruder, 1992; Dolan et al., 1994), which may be different from those seen in patients with early Alzheimer's disease (Guze et al., 1991; Sackeim et al., 1993; Siegel et al., 1995), suggest another way to cross-reference group differences, based on specific neuropsychological deficits (e.g. delayed retention, verbal fluency, naming, etc.). However, most recent reports still specifically exclude, or fail to distinguish, AD patients who also are depressed (e.g. Franceschi et al., 1995; Meltzer et al., 1996; Welsh et al., 1994). A few reports particularly focusing on this subgroup suggested metabolic deregulation is most evident in posterior regions, but often failed to carry a comparison sample of functional patients with memory complaints

(Starkstein et al., 1995). Thus, unlike in patients with pseudodementia, it remains unclear whether depression in patients with Alzheimer's dementia is associated with specific regional metabolic deficiencies linked to recognizable cognitive failings. Here also, the question of reversibility is vexed. Is deregulation of cerebral activation associated with memory disturbances in functional patients more consistent with state markers, which then returns within bounds as depressive illness lifts? (Kinsbourne, 1989). Although this may be so in a majority of cases (Bench et al., 1995; Stoudemire et al., 1993), there is evidence that functional asymmetries in a number of patients are associated with more permanent morphological changes (O'Brien et al., 1994; Wurthmann et al., 1995). As depression gives way, there may be residual metabolic anomalies that correlate with performance on tests sensitive to frontal lobe functions, particularly those that are strongly dependent on one's inhibition of more posteriorly dependent automatic processes (Trichard et al., 1995).

## Recapitulation

A sizable number of patients with clinical depression experience memory failure, and current surveys suggest the second most common cause of 'treatable' dementia in the elderly is depressive illness (Friedland, 1993). Although considerable evidence indicates that, for most patients, this impairment results from a derailing of attentional systems, it is still unclear in what proportions failings stem from faulty selective (early-stage) and/or executive (late-stage) mechanisms (Wells & Matthews, 1994). During a depressive episode, recent findings suggest (Boone et al., 1995), disturbances in visuospatial functions initially occur in the context of relatively undiminished verbal semantic skills, while disruptions of executive functions become more prominent as the illness deepens. Dissipation of resources (distractibility) during a memory task proves most detrimental as success is made contingent on a patient's active generation (utilization) of processing strategies (Bäckman & Forsell, 1994), and metabolic studies indicate this perhaps is associated with asymmetric activation patterns interlocking fronto-subcortical structures that regulate posterior activity (Dolan et al., 1994). As depression relents, so memory impairment remits in most patients with pseudodementia, although a number of cases will deteriorate further; and these patients may coincide with AAMI patients who similarly go on to develop dementia in the context of depression. It is still unclear how profiles on cognitive diagnostics (e.g. MMSE, WAIS, CAMCOG) can be shown to reliably distinguish between reversible and irreversible patients, and whether such profiles can be used to avoid misclassifying other depressed patients in preclinical stages of AD (desRosiers et al., 1995).

## A conjecture

One overwhelming piece of evidence in Alzheimer patients is that anterograde amnesia (i.e. inability to store the product of new learning into memory) is amongst the first cognitive casualties of the disease (see Chapters 4 and 7, this volume), and perhaps the best preclinical indicator of impending dementia (Cahn et al., 1995; Devanand et al., 1997; Linn et al., 1995). In contrast to patients with pseudodementia, impairment of memory does not primarily arise from defective attentional controls that modulate the processing of information, but from disruptions in the more posterior associative mechanisms and repositories of knowledge and experience which enable the permanent processing of new information. In other words, deficits of memory in AD occur because of a gradual neuronal erosion of its semantic fabric (Chan et al., 1997; Schwartz et al., 1996; but see Johnson et al., 1995), whereas amnesia in functional patients seems to grow from an inefficient use of such repositories (Goldman-Rakic, 1990; Kimberg & Farah, 1993). This inefficiency perhaps arises as dissipation of resources (ruminations) weakens one's co-ordination of accessory operations necessary to succeed on semantic tasks. Consequently, tests psychometrically engineered to ease the application of such operations may not produce, in depressed AD patients, the predictable patterns found in functional patients whose semantic skills are not affected by AD.

One salient aspect of semantic memory is in the perceived emotional nature (e.g. pleasant vs. unpleasant) of its contents and referents; a dimension of information processing activity often found to predict, in a variety of cognitive tasks, the direction of recall (or recognition) in depressed patients not suspected of having AD (see Chapter 2, this volume). Mood-congruence findings indicate patients tend to lag behind healthy controls on memory tests whose format/contents promote positive connotations (e.g. attractive faces, pleasant associates, happy stories), while nearly matching controls on tasks with unpleasant connotations (Table 12.1). This lends support to the notion that memory impairment in pseudodementia in part originates in the patients' application of selective and/or controlled mechanisms of attention during performance. Recent conjectures (Watkins et al., 1992; Wells & Matthews, 1994) now suggest the locus of this aberration lies not in early selective processes, e.g. patients pay more (less) initial attention to negative (positive) items, but more during the operations of late-stage processing. Perhaps the need to maintain inhibition of extraneous input (ruminations) is not so crucial for success on all tests, and particularly not perhaps on tests with emotional valence that is congruent with ongoing mood. This, in turn, may free patients to more comfortably exercise normal cognitive structuring skills on material in the selected channel, and thus distance themselves from patients with true dementia (pseudo-pseudo-dementia).

Table 12.1. Success rate [computed as percentage of correct score] in selected hedonic studies of explicit memory with clinical patients

| Diagnosis | N M/F | Mean age | MS | DS | Diagnostic criterion | Pos % | Neg % | Between-groups mood-congruence | Within-subjects tone-selectivity | Comment | Reference |
|---|---|---|---|---|---|---|---|---|---|---|---|
| Depressed | 20 (20/0) | 38.4 | NS | 26.8[a] | RDC | 0.25 | 0.24 | None | None | Matched for education | Roth & Rehm (1980) Table 1 |
| Psychiatric | 20 (20/0) | 38.0 | NS | 8.1[a] | | 0.28 | 0.20 | None | None | Recall of self-relevant adjectives | |
| Depressed | 20 (20/0) | 38.4 | NS | 26.8[a] | RDC | 0.82 | 0.85 | None | None | Matched for age | Roth & Rehm (1980) Table 1 |
| Psychiatric | 20 (20/0) | 38.0 | NS | 8.1[a] | | 0.78 | 0.78 | None | None | Recognition of above adjectives | |
| Depressed | 21 (5/16) | 44.4 | NS | 28.5[b] | RDC | 0.39 | 0.56 | None | Not tested | Matched for education | Breslow et al. (1981) Table 1 |
| Healthy | 21 (5/16) | 48.9 | NS | 1.8[b] | | 0.60 | 0.61 | Positive items[e] | Not tested | Story recall | |
| Depressed | 20 (8/12) | 39.9 | NS | 26.5[a] | RDC | 0.26 | 0.45 | Not tested | Negative items[f] | Free recall. Abstract words. | McDowall (1984) Figure 1 |
| Healthy | 20 (7/13) | 44.0 | NS | 8.1[a] | | 0.60 | 0.60 | Not tested | None | Mixed lists. Not matched | |
| Depressed | 23 (9/14) | 60+ | +21[d] | +17.0[a] | RDC | 0.29 | 0.38 | Not tested | Negative items | Trigram recall. First rated for | Slife et al. (1984) Figure 1 |
| Healthy | 23 (9/14) | 60+ | +21[d] | −5.0[a] | | 0.39 | 0.35 | Not tested | Positive items | Likeability. Education matched | |
| Depressed | 30 (9/21) | 41.7 | NS | 28.3[a] | Feighner | 0.54 | 0.72 | None | Negative items | Delayed recognition hits | Dunbar & Lishman (1984) Table 3 |
| Healthy | 30 (9/21) | 40.3 | NS | 5.6[a] | | 0.73 | 0.65 | Positive items | Positive items | Hospitalized. VIQ matched | |
| Depressed | 9 (0/9) | 37.1 | NS | 22.2[c] | RDC | 0.55 | 0.67 | None | Negative items | Free recall abstract words rated | Bradley & Matthews (1988) Table 3 |
| Healthy | 12 (1/11) | 35.8 | NS | 2.3[c] | | 0.85 | 0.66 | Positive items | Positive items | for self reference. VIQ matched | |
| Depressed | 16 (0/16) | 38.4 | NS | 29.6[a] | DSM3R | 0.11 | 0.26 | None | Negative items | Free recall abstract words rated | Denny & Hunt (1992) Table 1 |
| Healthy | 16 (0/16) | 38.0 | NS | 6.0[a] | | 0.41 | 0.28 | Positive items | Positive items | for self reference. Not matched | |

| | N (M/F) | MS | DS | | Criteria | NEG | POS | | DS | Reference |
|---|---|---|---|---|---|---|---|---|---|---|
| Depressed | 17 (2/15) | NS | NS | 27.5[a] | DSM3R | 0.37 | 0.49 | Not tested | Free recall abstract words rated | Watkins et al. (1992) |
| Healthy | 17 (2/15) | NS | NS | 3.7[a] | | 0.56 | 0.41 | Not tested | for self reference. Not matched | Table 1 |
| Depressed | 19 (6/13) | 33.3 | NS | 25.1[a] | DSM3R | 0.16 | 0.33 | Negative items | Free recall. Matched for age and | Bradley et al. (1995) |
| Healthy | 18 (7/11) | 39.6 | NS | 4.2[a] | | 0.20 | 0.16 | None | verbal IQ. In/out patients | Figure 2 |
| Depressed | 30 (11/19) | 41.2 | NS | 29.5[b] | DSM3R | 0.21 | 0.19 | None | Free recall. Matched for | Danion et al. (1995) |
| Healthy | 30 (11/19) | 41.5 | NS | NS | | 0.26 | 0.19 | None | education. Medication-free | Table 1 |
| Depressed | 15 (9/6) | 47.3 | 26.9[d] | 26.4[b] | DSM3R | 0.21 | 0.18 | None | Cued-recall. Matched for age and | Ilsley et al. (1995) |
| Healthy | 15 (11/4) | 43.6 | 28.9[d] | NS | | 0.29 | 0.19 | Positive items trend | NART IQ. ECT-free for 6 months | Table 1 |

*Notes:*

DS: Depression severity. [a]Beck Depression Inventory (BDI); [b]Hamilton Depression Scale; [c]Short BDI; MS: Mental status. [d]Mini-mental state examination. POS: Positive material; NEG: Negative material. [e]Between-groups congruence: e.g., Healthy > depressed on positive). [f]Within-subjects selectivity: e.g., Negative > positive in depressed patients). RDC: Research diagnostic criteria. M: Male; F: Female. NS: Not stated.

I fear I am not in my perfect mind, methinks I should know you, and know this man, yet I am doubtful. For I am mainly ignorant, what place this is, and all the skill I have remembers not these garments. Nor I know not where I did lodge last night. (Shakespeare, King Lear)

## REFERENCES

Abas, M., Sahakian, B. & Levy, R. (1990). Neuropsychological deficits and CT scan changes in elderly depressives. *Psychological Medicine*, **20**, 507–20.

Addonizio, G., & Alexopoulos, G. (1993). Affective disorders in the elderly. *International Journal of Geriatric Psychiatry*, **8**, 41–7.

Alexopoulos, G., Vrontou, C., Kakuma, T., Meyers, B., Young, R., Klausner, E. & Clarkin, J. (1996). Disability in geriatric depression. *American Journal of Psychiatry*, **153**, 877–85.

Alexopoulos, G., Meyers, B., Young, R., Kakuma, T., Silbersweig, D. & Charlson, M. (1997). Clinically defined vascular depression. *American Journal of Psychiatry*, **154**, 562–5.

Allen, H., Jolly, D., Comish, J. & Burns, A. (1997). Depression in dementia: A study of mood in a community sample and referrals to a community service. *International Journal of Geriatric Psychiatry*, **12**, 513–18.

Anderson, M. & Spellman, B. (1995). On the status of inhibitory mechanisms in cognition: Memory retrieval as a model case. *Psychological Review*, **102**, 68–100.

Austin, M. & Mitchell, P. (1995). The anatomy of melancholia: does frontal-subcortical pathophysiology underpin its psychomotor and cognitive manifestation? *Psychological Medicine*, **25**, 665–72.

Bäckman, L. & Forsell, Y. (1994). Episodic memory functioning in a community-based sample of old adults with major depression: Utilization of cognitive support. *Journal of Abnormal Psychology*, **103**, 361–70.

Baddeley, A. (1988). Cognitive psychology and human memory. *Trends in Neurosciences*, **11**, 176–81.

Baker, S., Frith, C. & Dolan, R. (1997). The interaction between mood and cognitive function studied with PET. *Psychological Medicine*, **27**, 565–78.

Baldwin, R., Benbow, S., Marriott, A. & Tomenson, B. (1993). Depression in old age. *British Journal Psychiatry*, **163**, 82–90.

Baltes, P. & Kliegl, R. (1986). On the dynamics between growth and decline in the aging of intelligence and memory. In *Neurology*, ed. K. Poeck, H. Freund & H. Gänshirt. Heidelberg: Springer-Verlag.

Baumgart, P., Helegenberger, F., Weyerer, S., Pfeifer-Kurda, M. & Förstl, H. (1995). The course of cognition and depression in elderly patients with affective disturbances and mild cognitive impairment. *International Journal of Geriatric Psychiatry*, **10**, 420–1.

Beats, B., Sahakian, B. & Levy, R. (1996). Cognitive performance in tests sensitive to frontal lobe dysfunction in the elderly depressed. *Psychological Medicine*, **26**, 591–603.

Beck, A. (1987). Cognitive models of depression. *Journal of Cognitive Psychotherapy*, **1**, 5–37.

Bemelmans, K., Goekoop, J. & van Kempen, M. (1996). Recall performance in acutely depressed patients and plasma cortisol. *Biological Psychiatry*, **39**, 750–2.

Bench, C., Friston, K., Brown, R., Frackowiak, R. & Dolan, R. (1993). Regional cerebral blood flow in depression measured by positron emission tomography: The relationship with clinical dimensions. *Psychological Medicine*, **23**, 579–90.

Bench, C., Frackowiak, R. & Dolan, R. (1995). Changes in regional cerebral blood flow on recovery from depression. *Psychological Medicine*, **25**, 247–51.

Benson, D. (1993). Prefrontal abilities. *Behavioural Neurology*, **6**, 75–81.

Berrios, G. & Gili, M. (1995). Abulia and impulsiveness revisited: a conceptual history. *Acta Psychiatrica Scandinavica*, **92**, 161–7.

Bhatia, K. & Marsden, C. (1994). The behavioural and motor consequences of focal lesions of the basal ganglia in man. *Brain*, **117**, 859–76.

Binetti, G., Magni, E., Padovani, A., Cappa, S., Bianchetti, A. & Trabucchi, M. (1996). Executive dysfunction in early Alzheimer's disease. *Journal of Neurology, Neurosurgery, and Psychiatry*, **60**, 91–3.

Biver, F., Goldman, S., Delvenne, V., Luxen, A., De Maertelaer, V., Hubain, P., Mendlewicz, J. & Lotstra, F. (1994). Frontal and parietal metabolic disturbances in unipolar depression. *Biological Psychiatry*, **36**, 381–7.

Blass, J. (1996). Age-associated memory impairment and Alzheimer's disease. *Journal of American Geriatric Society*, **44**, 209–11.

Blazer, D. (1989). Depression in the elderly. *New England Journal of Medicine*, **320**, 164–6.

Bodick, N., Offen, W., Levey, A., Cutler, N., Gauthier, S., Satlin, A., Shannon, H., Tollefson, G., Rasmussen, K., Bymaster, F., Hurley, D., Potter, W. & Paul, S. (1997). Effects of Xanomeline, a selective muscarinic receptor agonist, on cognitive function and behavioral symptoms in Alzheimer's disease. *Archives of Neurology*, **54**, 465–73.

Boone, K., Lesser, I., Miller, B., Wohl, M., Berman, N., Lee, A., Palmer, B. & Back, C. (1995). Cognitive functioning in older depressed outpatients: Relationship of presence and severity of depression to neuropsychological test scores. *Neuropsychology*, **9**, 390–8.

Bowling, A. & Grundy, E. (1997). Activities of daily living: Changes in functional ability in three samples of elderly and very elderly people. *Age and Ageing*, **26**, 107–14.

Bradley, B. & Mathews, A. (1988). Memory bias in recovered clinical depressives. *Cognition and Emotion*, **2**, 235–45.

Bradley, B., Mogg, K. & Williams, R. (1995). Implicit and explicit memory for emotion-congruent information in clinical depression and anxiety. *Behaviour Research and Therapy*, **33**, 755–70.

Brandt, J. & Rich, J. (1995). Memory disorders in the dementias. In *Handbook of Memory Disorders*, ed. A. Baddeley, B. Wilson & F. Watts. Chichester, UK: John Wiley.

Breslow, R., Kocsis, J. & Belkin, B. (1981). Contribution of the depressive perspective to memory function in depression. *American Journal of Psychiatry*, **138**, 227–30.

Brewin, C., Hunter, E., Carroll, F. & Tata, P. (1996). Intrusive memories in depression: an index of schema activation? *Psychological Medicine*, **26**, 1271–6.

Bruder, G. (1992). P300 findings for depressive and anxiety disorders In *Psychophysiology and Experimental Psychopathology*, ed. D. Frieman & G. Bruder. New York: New York Academy Sciences.

Buntinx, F., Kester, A., Bergers, J. & Knottnerus, J. (1996). Is depression in elderly people followed by dementia? A retrospective cohort study based in general practice. *Age and Ageing*, **25**, 231–3.

Burt, D., Zembar, M. & Niederehe, G. (1995). Depression and memory impairment: a meta-analysis of the association, its pattern, and specificity. *Psychological Bulletin*, 117, 285–305.

Butters, M., Lopez, O. & Becker, J. (1996). Focal temporal lobe dysfunction in probable Alzheimer's disease predicts a slow rate of cognitive decline. *Neurology*, 46, 687–92.

Cahn, D., Salmon, D., Butters, N., Wiederholt, W, Corey-Bloom, J., Edelstein, S. & Barrett-Connor, E. (1995). Detection of dementia of the Alzheimer type in a population-based sample. *Journal of the International Neuropsychological Society*, 1, 252–60.

Carpenter, B., Strauss, M. & Kennedy, J. (1995). Personal history of depression and its appearance in Alzheimer's disease. *International Journal of Geriatric Psychiatry*, 10, 669–78.

Carpenter, I. (1996). Value of screening in old age. In *Epidemiology in Old Age*, ed. S. Ibrahim & A. Kalache. London: British Medical Journal Publications.

Carroll, B. (1991). Psychopathology and neurobiology of manic-depressive disorders. In *Psychopathology and the Brain*, ed. B. Carroll & J. Barrett. New York: Raven Press.

Chan, A., Butters, N. & Salmon, P. (1997). The deterioration of semantic networks in patients with Alzheimer's disease: A cross-sectional study. *Neuropsychologia*, 35, 241–8.

Cooney, J. & Dinan, T. (1996). Preservation of hypothalamic–pituitary–adrenal axis fast-feedback responses in depression. *Neuropsychologia*, 35, 241–8.

Cooper, B., Bickel, H. & Schäufele, M. (1996). Early development and progression of dementing illness in the elderly: a general-practice based study. *Psychological Medicine*, 26, 411–17.

Corey-Bloom, J., Thal, L, Galasko, D., Folstein, M., Drachman, D., Raskind, M. & Lanka, D. (1995). Diagnosis and evaluation of dementia. *Neurology*, 45, 211–18.

Cowan, N. (1988). Evolving conceptions of memory storage, selective attention, and their mutual constraints within the human information-processing system. *Psychological Bulletin*, 104, 163–91.

Craik, F., Anderson, N., Kerr, S. & Li, K. (1995). Memory changes in normal aging. In *Handbook of Memory Disorders*, ed. A. Baddeley, B. Wilson & F. Watts. Chichester, UK: John Wiley.

Dannion, J., Kauffmann-Muller, F., Grangé, D., Zimmermann, M. & Greth, P. (1995). Affective valence of words, explicit and implicit memory in clinical depression. *Journal of Affective Disorders*, 34, 227–34.

Denny, E. & Hunt, R. (1992). Affective valence and memory in depression: dissociation of recall and fragment completion. *Journal of Abnormal Psychology*, 101, 575–80.

desRosiers, G. (1992.) Primary or depressive dementia: clinical features. *International Journal of Geriatric Psychiatry*, 7, 629–38.

desRosiers, G. (1999). Memory assessment clinics. *Alzheimer's Disease Society Newsletter*, March, p. 4.

desRosiers, G. & Ivison, D. (1986). Paired associate learning: normative data for differences between high and low subsets of the Wechsler Memory Scale. *Journal of Clinical and Experimental Neuropsychology*, 8, 637–42.

desRosiers, G. & Ivison, D. (1988). Paired associate learning: Form 1 and Form 2 of the Wechsler Memory Scale. *Archives of Clinical Neuropsychology.*, 3, 47–67.

desRosiers, G., Hodges, J. & Berrios, G. (1995). The neuropsychological differentiation of patients with very mild Alzheimer's disease and/or major depression. *Journal of American Geriatric Society*, **43**, 1256–63.

Devanand, D., Folz, M., Gorlyn, M., Moeller, J. & Stern, Y. (1997). Questionable dementia: Clinical course and predictors of outcome. *Journal of American Geriatric Society*, **45**, 321–8.

Dolan, R., Bench, C., Brown, R., Scott, L. & Frackowiak, R. (1994). Neuropsychological dysfunction in depression: the relationship to regional cerebral blood flow. *Psychological Medicine*, **24**, 849–57.

Dunbar, G. & Lishman, W. (1984). Depression, recognition memory, and hedonic tone. *British Journal of Psychiatry*, **144**, 376–82.

Ebly, E., Hogan, D. & Parhad, I. (1995). Cognitive impairment in the non-demented elderly. *Archives of Neurology*, **52**, 612–19.

Eastwood, R. (and writing committee). (1996). The challenge of the dementias. *Lancet*, **347**, 1303–7.

Einstein, G., McDaniel, M., Richardson, S., Guynn, M. & Cunfer, A. (1995). Aging and prospective memory: Examining the influence of self-initiated retrieval processes. *Journal of Experimental Psychology: Learning, Memory, Cognition*, **21**, 996–1007.

Eustache, F., Rioux, P., Desgranges, B., Marchal, G., Petit-Taboué, M., Dary, M., LeChevalier, B. & Baron, J. (1995). Healthy aging, memory subsystems and regional cerebral oxygen consumption. *Neuropsychologia*, **33**, 867–87.

Ferrier, I. & Perry, E. (1992). Post-mortem studies in affective disorders. *Psychological Medicine*, **22**, 835–8.

Fletcher, P., Shallice, T., Frith, C., Frackowiak, R. & Dolan, R. (1996). Brain activity during memory retrieval: The influence of imagery and semantic cueing. *Brain*, **119**, 1587–96.

Forsell, Y., Jorm, A., Von Strauss, E. & Winblad, B. (1995). Prevalence and correlates of depression in a population of nonagenarians. *British Journal of Psychiatry*, **167**, 61–4.

Franceschi, M., Alberoni, M., Bressi, S., Canal, N., Comi, G., Fazio, F., Grassi, F., Perani, D. & Volonté, M. (1995). Correlations between cognitive impairment, middle cerebral artery flow velocity and cortical glucose metabolism in the early phase of Alzheimer's disease. *Dementia*, **6**, 32–8.

Fried, L., Bandeen-Roche, K., Williamson, J., Prasado-Rao, P., Chee, E., Tepper, S. & Rubin, G. (1996). Functional decline in older adults: expanding methods of ascertainment. *Journal of Gerontology: Medical Sciences*, **51**, 206–14.

Friedland, R. (1993). Alzheimer's disease: Clinical features and differential diagnosis. *Neurology*, **43**, 45–51

Furey-Kurkjian, M., Pietrini, P., Graff-Radford, N., Alexander, G., Freo, U., Szczepanik, J. & Schapiro, M. (1996). Visual variant of Alzheimer disease: distinctive neuropsychological features. *Neuropsychology*, **10**, 294–300.

Fuster, J. (1995). *Memory in the Cerebral Cortex*. Cambridge, MA: The MIT Press.

George, M., Ketter, T., Parekh, P., Horwitz, B., Herscovitch, P. & Post, R. (1995). Brain activity during transient sadness and happiness in healthy women. *American Journal of Psychiatry*, **152**, 341–51.

Goldberg, E. & Podell, K. (1995). Reciprocal lateralisation of frontal lobe functions. *Archives of General Psychiatry*, **52**, 159–60.

Goldman-Rakic, P. (1990). Cortical localization of working memory. In *Brain Organization and Memory*, ed. J. McGaugh, N. Weinberger & G. Lynch. Oxford: Oxford University Press.

Graham, K. & Hodges, J. (1997). Differentiating the roles of the hippocampal complex and the neocortex in long-term memory storage: Evidence from the study of semantic dementia and Alzheimer's disease. *Neuropsychology*, **11**, 77–89.

Gray, J. (1994). Framework for a taxonomy of psychiatric disorder. In *Emotions: Essays on Emotion Theory*, ed. S. van Goosen, N. van de Poll & J. Sergeant. New Jersey: Lawrence Erlbaum Associates.

Greenwald, B., Kramer-Ginsberg, E., Bogertz, B., Ashtari, M., Aupperle, P., Wu, H., Allen, L., Zeman, D. & Patel, M. (1997). Qualitative magnetic resonance imaging findings in geriatric depression: possible link between later-onset depression and Alzheimer's disease. *Psychological Medicine*, **27**, 421–31.

Grimley-Evans, J. (1996). Health care for older people. *Journal of the American Medical Association*, **275**, 1449–50.

Gunther, D., Ferraro, F. & Kirchner, T. (1996). Influence of emotional state on irrelevant thoughts. *Psychonomic Bulletin and Review*, **3**, 491–4.

Guze, B., Baxter, L., Schwartz, J., Szuba, M., Mazziotta, J. & Phelps, M. (1991). Changes in glucose metabolism in dementia of the Alzheimer type compared with depression. *Psychiatry Research: Neuroimaging*, **40**, 195–202.

Hänninen, T., Hallikainen, M., Koivisto, K., Partanen, K., Laakso, M., Reikkinen, P., Soininen & H. (1997). Decline of frontal lobe functions in subjects with age-associated memory impairment. *Neurology*, **48**, 148–53.

Haupt, M., Kurz, A. & Greifenhagen, A. (1995). Depression in Alzheimer's disease: Phenomenological features and association with severity and progression of cognitive and functional impairment. *International Journal of Geriatric Psychiatry*, **10**, 469–76.

Healy, D. (1993). Dysphoria. In *Symptoms of Depression*, ed. C. Costello. Chichester, UK: John Wiley.

Hirst, W. (1988). Components of memory and amnesia. In *Practical Aspects of Memory: Current Research and Issues*, vol. 2, ed. M. Gruneberg, P. Morris & R. Sykes. Chichester, UK: John Wiley.

Ilsley, J., Moffoot, A. & O'Carroll, R. (1995). An analysis of memory dysfunction in major depression. *Journal of Affective Disorders*, **35**, 1–9.

Jacobs, D., Sano, M., Dooneief, G., Marder, K., Bell, K. & Stern, Y. (1995). Neuropsychological detection and characterization of preclinical Alzheimer's disease. *Neurology*, **45**, 957–62

Johnson, M., Hermann, A. & Bonilla, J. (1995). Semantic relations and Alzheimer's disease: typicality and direction of testing. *Neuropsychology*, **9**, 529–36.

Jonker, C, Launer, L., Hooijer, C. & Lindeboom, J. (1996). Memory complaints and memory impairment in older individuals. *Journal of American Geriatric Society*, **44**, 44–9.

Khachaturian, Z. (1992). An overview of scientific issues associated with the heterogeneity of Alzheimer's disease. In *Heterogeneity of Alzheimer's Disease*. Berlin: Springer-Verlag.

Kimberg, D. & Farah, M. (1993). A unified account of cognitive impairments following frontal lobe damage: the role of working memory in complex, organized behavior. *Journal of Experimental Psychology: General*, **122**, 411–28.

King, D., Cox, C., Lyness, J. & Caine, E. (1995). Neuropsychological effects of depression and age in an elderly sample. *Neuropsychology*, **9**, 399–408.

Kinsbourne, M. (1989). A model of adaptive behavior related to cerebral participation in emotional control. In *Emotions and the Dual Brain*, ed. G. Gainotti & C. Caltagirone. Berlin: Springer-Verlag.

Klein, D. (1974). Endogenomorphic depression: a conceptual and terminologic revision. *Archives of General Psychiatry*, **31**, 447–54.

Knight, R., Grabowecky, M. & Scabini, D. (1995). Role of human prefrontal cortex in attention control. In *Epilepsy and the Functional Anatomy of the Frontal Lobe*, ed. H. Jasper, S. Riggio & P. Goldman-Rakic. New York: Raven Press.

Kral., V. & Emery, O. (1989). Long-term follow-up of depressive pseudodementia of the aged. *Canadian Journal of Psychiatry*, **34**, 445–6.

Krishnan, K., Hays, J. & Blazer, D. (1997). MRI-defined vascular depression. *American Journal Psychiatry*, **154**, 497–501.

Lang, W., Lang, M., Uhl, F., Kornhuber, A., Deecke, L. & Kornhuber, H. (1988). Left frontal lobe in verbal learning: a slow potential study. *Experimental Brain Research*, **70**, 99–108.

Larrabee, G. & McEntee, W. (1995). Age-associated memory impairment: sorting out the controversies. *Neurology*, **45**, 611–14.

Lawton, M., Parmelee, P., Katz, I. & Nesselroade, J. (1996). Affective states in normal and depressed older people. *Journal of Gerontology: Psychological Sciences*, **51**, 309–16.

Lemelin, S., Baruch, P., Vincent, A., Laplante, L., Everett, J. & Vincent, P. (1996). Attention disturbance in clinical depression. *Journal of Nervous and Mental Disease*, **184**, 114–21.

Levy, R. (1995). Report: Age-associated cognitive decline. In *Developments in Dementia and Functional Disorders in the Elderly*, ed. R. Levy & R. Howard. Bristol: Wrightson Biomedical Publishing Ltd.

Lichtenberg, P., Ross, T., Millis, S. & Manning, C. (1995). The relationship between depression and cognition in older adults: a cross-validation study. *Journal of Gerontology: Psychological Sciences*, **50**, 25–32.

Linn, R., Wolff, P., Bachman, D., Knoefel., J., Cobb, J., Bélanger, A., Kaplan, E. & D'Agostino, R. (1995). The 'preclinical phase' of probable Alzheimer's disease. *Archives of Neurology*, **52**, 485–90.

Linville, P. (1996). Attention inhibition: does it underlie ruminative thoughts. In *Ruminative Thoughts: Advances in Social Cognition*, vo.l 9, ed. R. Wyer. New Jersey: Lawrence Erlbaum Associates.

Loessner, A., Alavi, A., Lewandrowski, K., Mozley, D., Souder, E. & Gur, R. (1995). Regional cerebral function determined by FDG-PET in healthy volunteers: normal patterns and changes with age. *Journal Nuclear Medicine*, **36**, 1141–9.

Logie, S., Murphy, B., Brooks, D., Wylie, S., Barron, E. & McCulloch, J. (1992). The diagnosis of depression in patients with dementia: use of the Cambridge Mental Disorders of the Elderly Examination. (CAMDEX). *International Journal of Geriatric Psychiatry*, **7**, 363–8.

Luciana, M., Depue, R., Arbisi, P. & Leon, R. (1992). Facilitation of working memory in humans by a $D^2$ dopamine receptor agonist. *Journal of Cognitive Neurosciences*, **4**, 58–68.

McDowall, J. (1984). Recall of pleasant and unpleasant words in depressed subjects. *Journal of Abnormal Psychology*, **93**, 401–7.

McKenna, P., McKay, A. & Laws, K. (1998). Memory in functional psychoses. In: *Memory Complaints and Disorders: The Neuropsychiatric Perspective*, ed. G. Berrios & J. Hodges. Cambridge: Cambridge University Press.

McKhann, G., Drachman, D., Folstein, M., Katzman, R., Price, D. & Stadlan, E. (1984). Clinical diagnosis of Alzheimer's disease: Report of the NINCDS-ADRDA work group. *Neurology*, **34**, 939–44.

Marangell, L., Ketter, T., George, M., Pazzaglia, P., Callahan, A., Parekh, P., Andreason, P., Horwitz, B., Herscovitch, P. & Post, R. (1997). Inverse relationship of peripheral thyrotropin-stimulating hormone levels to brain activity in mood disorders. *American Journal of Psychiatry*, **154**, 224–30.

Massman, P., Delis, D., Butters, N., Dupont, R. & Gillin, J. (1992). The subcortical dysfunction hypothesis of memory deficits in depression: Neuropsychological validation in a subgroup of patients. *Journal of Experimental and Clinical Neuropsychology*, **14**, 687–706.

Masur, D., Sliwinski, M., Lipton, R., Blau, A. & Crystal, H. (1994). Neuropsychological prediction of dementia and the absence of dementia in healthy elderly persons. *Neurology*, **44**, 1427–32.

Meltzer, C., Zubieta, J., Brandt, J., Tune, L., Mayber, H. & Frost, J. (1996). Regional hypometabolism in Alzheimer's disease as measured by positron emission tomography after correction for effects of partial volume averaging. *Neurology*, **47**, 454–61.

Mialet, J., Pope, H. & Yurgelun-Todd, D. (1996). Impaired attention in depressive states: a non-specific deficit? *Psychological Medicine*, **26**, 1009–20.

Migliorelli, R., Tesón, A., Sabe, L., Petracchi, M., Leiguarda, R. & Starkstein, S. (1995). Prevalence and correlates of dysthymia and major depression among patients with Alzheimer's disease. *American Journal Psychiatry*, **152**, 37–44.

Milner, B. (1995). Aspects of human frontal lobe function. In *Epilepsy and the Functional Anatomy of the Frontal Lobe*, ed. H. Jasper, S. Riggio & P. Goldman-Rakic. New York: Raven Press.

Mitchell, A. (1995). The contribution of hypercorticolaemia to the cognitive decline of geriatric depression. *International Journal of Geriatric Psychiatry*, **10**, 401–9.

Murphy, E. (1992). Depression in the elderly. In *Depression: An Integrative Approach*, ed. K. Herbst & E. Paykel. New York: Heinemann Medical Books.

Nolen-Hoeksema, S. & Morrow, J. (1993). Effects of rumination and distraction on naturally occurring depressed mood. *Cognition and Emotion*, **7**, 561–70.

O'Brien, J. (1997). The 'glucocorticoid cascade' hypothesis in man. *British Journal of Psychiatry*, **170**, 199–201.

O'Brien, J., Desmond, P., Ames, D., Schweitzer, I., Tuckwell, V. & Tress, B. (1994). The differentiation of depression from dementia by temporal lobe magnetic resonance imaging. *Psychological Medicine*, **24**, 633–40.

Palmer, B., Boone, K., Lesser, I., Wohl, M., Berman, N. & Miller, B. (1996). Neuropsychological deficits among older depressed patients with predominantly psychological or vegetative symptoms. *Journal of Affective Disorders*, **41**, 17–24.

Passingham, R. (1993). *The Frontal Lobes and Movement*. Oxford: Oxford University Press.

Patterson, K. & Hodges, J. (1995). Disorders of semantic memory. In *Handbook of Memory Disorders*, ed. A. Baddeley, B. Wilson & F. Watts. Chichester, UK: John Wiley.

Pearlson, G., Rabins, P. & Burns, A. (1989). Structural brain CT changes and cognitive deficits in elderly depressives with and without reversible dementia (pseudodementia). *Psychological Medicine*, **19**, 573–84.

Philpot, M. (1996). The Maudsley Hospital Memory Clinic. *International Journal of Geriatric Psychiatry*, **11**, 305–8.

Pietrini, P., Furey, M., Graff-Radford, Freo, U., Alexander, G., Grady, C., Dani, A., Mentis, M. & Schapiro, M. (1996). Preferential metabolic involvement of visual cortex areas in a subtype of Alzheimer's disease: clinical implications. *American Journal of Psychiatry*, **153**, 1261–8.

Powell, D. & Whitla, D. (1994). Normal cognitive aging: toward empirical perspectives. *Current Directions in Psychological Science*, **3**, 27–31.

Pribram, K. (1987). The subdivisions of the frontal cortex revisited. In *The Frontal Lobes Revisited*, ed. E. Perecman. New York: Academic Press.

Purcell, D., Schwartz, J., Brookshire, R., Caudle, J. & Lewine, R. (1995). Neuropsychological functioning in 'normal' subjects. *Neuropsychiatry, Neuropsychology, and Behavioral Neurology*, **8**, 6–13.

Rabins, P. & Pearlson, G. (1994). Depression induced cognitive impairment. In *Dementia*, ed. A. Burns & R. Levy. London: Chapman & Hall.

Ritchie, K., LeDésert, B. & Touchon, J. (1993). The EUGERIA study of cognitive aging: who are the 'normal' elderly? *International Journal of Geriatric Psychiatry*, **8**, 969–77.

Robinson, R. (1995). Mapping brain activity associated with emotion. *American Journal of Psychiatry*. **152**, 327–9.

Roediger, H. & McDermott, K. (1992). Depression and implicit memory: a commentary. *Journal of Abnormal Psychology*, **101**, 587–90.

Rolls, E. (1990). A theory of emotion, and its implication to describing the neural basis of emotion. *Cognition and Emotion*, **4**,161–90.

Roth, D. & Rehm, L. (1980). Relationships among self-monitoring processes, memory, and depression. *Cognitive Therapy and Research*, **4**, 149–57.

Rouleau, N. & Belleville, S. (1996). Irrelevant speech effect in aging: an assessment of inhibitory processes in working memory. *Journal of Gerontology: Psychological Sciences*, **51**, 356–63.

Rubin, E., Sackeim, H., Prohovnik, I., Moeller, J., Schnur, D. & Mukherjee, S. (1995). Regional cerebral blood flow in mood disorders. *Psychiatry Research: Neuroimaging*, **61**, 1–10.

Rueckert, L. & Grafman, J. (1996). Sustained attention deficits in patients with right frontal lesions. *Neuropsychologia*, **34**, 953–63.

Rush, A., Giles, D., Schlesser, M., Orsulak, P., Parker, R., Weissenburger, J., Crowley, G., Khatami, M. & Vasavada, N. (1997). The dexamethasone suppression test in patients with mood disorders. *Journal of Clinical Psychiatry*, **57**, 470–84.

Ryan, D., Blackburn, P., Lawley, D., Ellis, A., Musil, J. & Kendrick, D. (1995). Depression and dementia in geriatric inpatients: diagnostic comparisons between psychiatrists, geriatricians, and test scores. *International Journal of Geriatric Psychiatry*, **10**, 447–56.

Sachdev, P., Smith, J., Angus-Lepan, H. & Rodriguez, P. (1990). Pseudodementia twelve years on. *Journal of Neurology, Neurosurgery, and Psychiatry*, **53**, 254–9.

Sackeim, H., Prohovnik, I., Moeller, J., Mayeux, R., Stern, Y. & Devanand, D. (1993). Regional cerebral blood flow in mood disorders. Comparison of major depression and Alzheimer's disease. *Journal of Nuclear Medicine*, **34**, 1090–101.

Sahakian, B. (1991). Depressive pseudodementia in the elderly. *International Journal of Geriatric Psychiatry*, **6**, 453–8.

Salloway, S., Malloy, P., Kohn, R., Gillard, E., Duffy, J., Rogg, J., Tung, G., Richardson, E., Thomas, C. & Westlake, R. (1996). MRI and neuropsychological differences in early- and late-life onset geriatric depression. *Neurology*, **46**, 1567–74.

Salmon, E., Van der Linden, M., Cillette, F., Delfiore, G., Maquet, P., Degueldre, C., Luxen, A. & Frank, G. (1996). Regional brain activity during working memory tasks. *Brain*, **119**, 1617–25.

Sawaguchi, T. & Goldman-Rakic, P. (1991). D1 dopamine receptors in prefrontal cortex: involvement in working memory. *Science*, **252**, 947–50.

Schmand, B., Jonker, C., Hooijer, C. & Lindeboom, J. (1996). Subjective memory complaints may announce dementia. *Neurology*, **46**, 121–5.

Schofield, P., Marder, K., Dooneief, G., Jacobs, D., Sano, M. & Stern, Y. 1997. Association of subjective memory complaints with subsequent decline in community-dwelling elderly individuals with baseline cognitive impairment. *American Journal of Psychiatry*, **154**, 609–15.

Schroeder, M., Lipton, R., Ritter, W., Giesser, B. & Vaughan, R. (1995). Event-related potential correlates of early processing in normal aging. *International Journal of Neuroscience*, **80**, 371–82.

Schwartz, T., Kutas, M., Butters, N., Paulsen, J. & Salmon, D. (1996). Electrophysiological insights into the nature of semantic deficits in Alzheimer's disease. *Neuropsychologia*, **34**, 827–41.

Shaw, B. & Katz, R. (1990). Cognitive theory of depression: where are we and where are we going? In *Contemporary Approaches to Depression*, ed. R. Ingram. New York: Plenum Press.

Siegel, B., Buchsbaum, M., Starr, A., Mohs, R. & Neto, D. (1995). Glucose metabolic rate and progression of illness in Alzheimer's disease. *International Journal of Geriatric Psychiatry*, **10**, 659–67.

Slife, B., Miura, S., Thompson, L., Shapiro, J. & Gallagher, D. (1984). Differential recall as a function of mood disorder in clinically depressed patients: between and within subjects differences. *Journal of Abnormal Psychology*, **93**, 391–400.

Smith, E., Jonides, J., Koeppe, R., Awh, E., Shumacher, E. & Minoshima, S. (1995). Spatial versus object working memory: PET investigations. *Journal of Cognitive Neuroscience*, **7**, 337–56.

Snaith, P. (1993). Anhedonia: a neglected symptom of psychopathology. *Psychological Medicine*, **23**, 957–66.

Soares, J. & Mann, J. (1997). The anatomy of mood disorders: review of structural neuroimaging studies. *Biological Psychiatry*, **41**, 86–106.

Soininen, H., Partanen, K., Pitkänen, A., Vainio, P., Hänninen, T., Hallikainen, M., Koivisto, K.

& Riekkinen, P. (1994). Volumetric MRI analysis of the amygdala and the hippocampus in subjects with age-associated memory impairment. *Neurology*, **44**, 1660–8.

Squire, L. (1992). Memory and the hippocampus: a synthesis from findings with rats, monkeys, and humans. *Psychological Review*, **99**, 195–231.

Starkstein, S., Vásquez, S., Migliorelli, R., Tesón, A., Petracca, G. & Leiguarda, R. 1995. A SPECT study of depression in Alzheimer's disease. *Neuropsychiatry, Neuropsychology, and Behavioral Neurology*, **1**, 38–43.

Stoudemire, A., Hill, C., Morris, R., Martino-Saltzman, D. & Lewison, B. (1993). Long-term affective and cognitive outcome in depressed older adults. *American Journal of Psychiatry*, **150**, 896–900.

Teri, L. & Wagner, A. (1992). Alzheimer's disease and depression. *Journal of Consulting and Clinical Psychology*, **60**, 379–91.

Tham, A., Engelbrektson, K., Mathé, A., Johnson, L., Olsson, E. & Åberg-Wistedt, A. (1997). Impaired neuropsychological performance in euthymic patients with recurring mood disorders. *Journal of Clinical Psychiatry*, **58**, 26–9.

Tierney, M., Szalai, J., Snow, W., Fisher, R., Nores, A., Nadon, G., Dunn, E. & St. George-Hyslop, P. (1996). Prediction of probable Alzheimer's disease in memory-impaired patients. *Neurology*, **46**, 661–5.

Tranel, D. & Damasio, A. (1995). Neurobiological foundations of human memory. In *Handbook of Memory Disorders*, ed. A. Baddeley, B. Wilson & F. Watts. Chichester, UK: John Wiley.

Trichard, C., Martinot, J., Alagille, M., Masure, M., Hardy, P., Ginestet, D. & Féline, A. (1995). Time course of prefrontal lobe dysfunction in severely depressed in-patients: a longitudinal neuropsychological study. *Psychological Medicine*, **25**, 79–85.

Troisi, A., Pasini, A., Gori, G., Sorbi, T., Baroni, A. & Ciani, N. (1996). Clinical predictors of somatic and psychological symptoms of depression in Alzheimer's disease. *International Journal of Geriatric Psychiatry*, **11**, 23–7.

Watkins, P., Mathews, A., Williamson, D. & Fuller, R. (1992). Mood-congruent memory in depression: emotional priming or elaboration. *Journal of Abnormal Psychology*, **101**, 581–6.

Watts, F. (1995). Depression and anxiety. In *Handbook of Memory Disorders*, ed. A. Baddeley, B. Wilson & F. Watts. Chichester, UK: John Wiley.

Weingartner, H. (1986). Automatic and effort-demanding cognitive processes in depression. In *Handbook of Clinical Memory Assessment in Older Adults*, ed. L. Poon. Washington: American Psychological Association.

Wells, A., Matthews, G. (1994). *Attention and Emotion*. Hillsdale, Lawrence Erlbaum Associates.

Welsh, K., Hoffman, J., Earl, N. & Hanson, M. (1994). Neural correlates of dementia: brain metabolism FDG-PET. and the CERAD neuropsychological battery. *Archives of Clinical Neuropsychology*, **9**, 395–409.

West, R. (1996). An application of prefrontal cortex function theory to cognitive aging. *Psychological Bulletin*, **120**, 272–92.

Willner, P. (1993). Anhedonia. In *Symptoms of Depression*, ed. C. Costello. Chichester, UK: John Wiley.

Wright, N. & Lindesay, J. (1995). A survey of memory clinics in the British Isles. *International Journal of Geriatric Psychiatry*, **10**, 379–85.

Wurthmann, C., Bogerts, B. & Falkai, P. (1995). Brain morphology assessed by computed tomography in patients with geriatric depression, patients with degenerative dementia, and normal control subjects. *Psychiatry Research: Neuroimaging*, **61**, 103–11.

Yamatami, K., Ono, T., Nishijo, J. & Takaku, A. (1990). Activity and distribution of learning-related neurons in monkey prefrontal cortex. *Behavioral Neuroscience*, **104**, 503–31.

Zhuang, P., Toro, C., Grafman, J., Manganotti, P., Leocani, L. & Hallett, M. (1997). Event-related desynchronization (ERD) in the alpha frequency during development of implicit and explicit learning. *Electroencephalography and Clinical Neurophysiology*, **102**, 374–81.

# 13

# Practical management of memory problems

Barbara A. Wilson and Jonathan J. Evans

## Introduction

Until the early 1980s there was little practical help for psychologists, therapists and others working with memory impaired people. The most widespread strategy used in memory rehabilitation in Britain (and probably elsewhere) was repeated practice on memory games and exercises (Harris & Sunderland, 1981), despite the complete lack of evidence for the success of this method. One of the classic memory experiments of the past 20 years demonstrated no effect of repeated practice for improving memory (Ericsson et al., 1980). A student was trained on a digit span task. Most people have a forward digit span of 7 plus or minus 2, i.e. a range of 5 to 9. This student was no exception. However, after almost daily practice for 20 months he managed to increase his digit span to a phenomenal 80. He did this by associating the digits with times and distances from the field of athletics which was one of the student's areas of interest. Despite this incredible performance on a forward digit span task, the student, assessed on a similar yet slightly different task, namely span for consonants, scored 6, i.e. in the normal range. In other words, there was no generalization at all of his new skill to a related task.

In the introduction to *Clinical Management of Memory Problems* (Wilson & Moffat, 1984), perhaps the first practical book for health service staff working with brain injured memory impaired people, Wilson said:

Although an enormous number of papers have been published on memory, few of these deal with the remediation or amelioration of memory deficits. Those few papers which do address this problem tend to be concerned with the teaching of lists of words or paired associates in experimental situations and are not, therefore, particularly relevant to the everyday problems which are experienced by memory impaired people (p. 1).

Conversely, the papers which might have been beneficial were largely unknown by people working in rehabilitation. For example, Lorge (1930) was interested in the learning of a difficult motor task known as mirror tracing in which the subject is required to trace a pattern (for example, a star) while only being able to see the pattern through a mirror. Lorge studied three groups, one of which was given 20 consecutive trials with no break between them, the second group was also given 20 trials but had a one minute interval between each trial, the third group was given one trial a day for each of 20 days. The outcome measure was the length of time required to trace the pattern, so the shorter the time the better the performance. Subjects who had the 20 trials without rest performed worst, subjects who had one minute intervals scored second and subjects who had a 24 hour rest between trials did best. In similar vein, Baddeley and Longman (1978) were concerned with teaching postmen to type. Like Lorge (1930) they also found that spaced or distributed practice leads to faster learning. Both these experiments are of considerable relevance to rehabilitation, yet their findings are virtually unknown in the field of rehabilitation.

Despite the dearth of practical research and publications in the early 1980s, memory rehabilitation was on the move and the intervening years have seen numerous publications which address the real life issues of people with organic memory deficits. Indeed, in the preface to the second edition of *Clinical Management of Memory Problems* (Wilson & Moffat, 1992), Wilson said:

the interest in the rehabilitation of memory problems continues to grow, and this has led to further developments in memory therapy in recent years (p. vii).

At least two other books solely concerned with memory rehabilitation have appeared since 1984: *Rehabilitation of Memory* (Wilson, 1987) and *Memory Rehabilitation for Closed Head Injured Patients* (Berg, 1993). In addition there have been numerous chapters concerned with the topic (Schacter & Glisky, 1986; Wilson, 1989, 1993) together with journal articles (Evans & Wilson, 1992; Wilson & Evans, 1996), self-help manuals (Kapur, 1991) and sections in major handbooks (Poon et al., 1989; Baddeley et al., 1995). Perhaps it is true to say then that Memory Therapy has come of age.

## Recent developments in memory rehabilitation

There have been three main strands in memory rehabilitation in recent years, namely environmental adaptations, the implementation of new technology and methods for improving learning.

## Environmental adaptations

In a recent book on brain plasticity, Kolb (1995) remarked that:

It is now clear that environmental treatments can profoundly alter the structure of the cortex (p. 26).

Kolb was talking about environmental enrichment whereby animals (and probably humans) brought up in unstimulating environments do less well at cognitive tasks than those brought up in stimulating environments. The concern in this chapter is more with modifying or restructuring environments so that people can cope without much in the way of memory functioning. This is one of the simplest ways to help people with cognitive problems. Norman (1988), discussing environments for people who are cognitively and neurologically intact, firmly believes that knowledge should be in the world rather than in the head. By this he means that the correct use of any object should be so obvious that it is almost impossible to make a mistake. Turning on cookers or showers, opening doors and boxes are just some of the examples Norman provides in his stimulating book. Norman's ideas can be extended to help people with organic memory impairment. For example, clients could be provided with kettles, cookers and electric lights which turn themselves off after a certain interval and thus avoid dangers and risks for those who are very forgetful. People who forget where things are kept, or forget which room is which, may be helped if cupboards and doors are labelled or made very distinctive. Alternatively, a line may be drawn on the floor to help someone remember the way from the kitchen to the bedroom, and a cord may lead from the dining room to the garden. Signposts appropriately positioned may achieve the same end. Positioning objects so they cannot be missed or forgotten is also worth thinking about. Examples here include clipping a notebook to a waistbelt or using a neck cord for one's spectacles so as to avoid leaving them around. It may be possible to reduce or eliminate repetitive behaviour by identifying environmental situations or verbal questions or statements which trigger the repetitions. Once the triggers have been identified, it is possible to avoid them in future.

The basic principle in the environmental adaptation model is to avoid, or bypass problems caused by memory impairment. Gross and Schutz (1986) called this the Environmental Control model, the origins of which can be found within the discipline of behaviour modification. Murphy (1987) reminds us that restructuring the environment is a useful procedure for decreasing undesirable behaviour in people with developmental learning disabilities. She says the operant view of behaviour is that it is determined both by consequences and antecedents. If it becomes clear that undesirable behaviour occurs in only one situation, it may be possible to modify the situation to prevent the behaviour occurring. This can be a very rapid and effective way of eradicating or reducing such behaviours, but it is not always possible to achieve. Even when it is achievable it may not be ethical. For example, a memory impaired person could be kept in a restrictive environment which is very structured and places no demands at all on memory, thus avoiding problems that would normally arise because of impairment. In some circumstances, however, this might be viewed as so restrictive as to be unethical let alone uneconomical. Like many psychiatric and psychological methods of management, environmental control is open to abuse. Nevertheless there is little doubt that, for many severely intellectually impaired people, environmental control is their best chance at least of some independence. For example, one patient known to us is a 66-year-old man with Korsakoff's syndrome. He lives in a psychiatric hostel where his day is structured, staff tell him when to get up, when to go to breakfast, when to go to the dayroom and so forth. He lives quite happily in these circumstances with the staff and the environment substituting for his damaged memory. Kapur (1995) also addresses the issue of environmental memory aids. Perhaps one of the most exciting developments in environmental control is the coming of 'smart' houses which use technology to provide structure designed to disable the disabling environment. This takes us on to the next section on the implementation of new technology.

## New technology

The growth in technology has benefited memory rehabilitation in several ways and this benefit is likely to increase in the future. 'Smart' houses, for example, employ computers and videos to monitor and control the living environments of people with dementia. The aim of people developing and using this technology is to increase independence and activity and to improve the quality of life for confused elderly people. If successful for this population, there is no reason why 'smart' houses cannot be adopted for other people with cognitive impairments.

Two 'smart' houses are up and running in Norway (Graeme Slaven, personal communication) addressing problems such as falls, disorientation, inadequate meals, poor hygiene, emergencies and limited home management. Examples of 'smart' house technology include the following

### Telephone

(i)   Photographs of ten people important in the client's network are pasted on to the telephone buttons. Each button is programmed to dial the number of the person in the photograph.
(ii)  A videophone link is provided between the patient's home and the care centre or main helper.
(iii) A big red HELP button is provided to call the day centre or a relative.

### Entrances and exits

(i)   A floodlight is installed by the front door that lights up when someone approaches.
(ii)  A movement detector can be connected to a verbal message that someone is approaching.

(iii)  An infrared key is provided for opening doors.

(iv)  Environmental control systems may be installed to open and close doors from a distance.

## Temperature control

(i)  A fitted control system for showers and baths can ensure the water is not too hot or too cold.

(ii)  A central control can be used to regulate the temperature of rooms.

## Alarm systems

(i)  Alarms can be fitted to sound when the cooker or other electric appliances are left on and unused for a certain length of time.

(ii)  An alarm can sound when the person leaves the house in order to prevent wandering.

(iii)  In case of fire or another emergency an alarm rings in an alarm centre and a care centre. A voice message is relayed to the client saying 'Leave the house because there is a fire'.

With the rapid development of technology, it is possible that 'smart' houses will become more important in the next decade or so, and would seem a fruitful area for psychologists, engineers, architects and computer programmers to join forces to design and evaluate new environments. Another recent and exciting tool in memory rehabilitation is NeuroPage, developed for use with brain injured memory impaired people. NeuroPage is a simple and portable paging system designed in California by the engineer father of a head injured son working together with a neuropsychologist (Hersh & Treadgold, 1994). NeuroPage uses a computer linked by modem and telephone to a paging company. The scheduling of reminders or cues for each individual is entered into the computer and, from then on, no further human interfacing is necessary. On the appropriate date and time NeuroPage automatically transmits the reminder information to the paging company who transmit the message to the individual's pager.

The system avoids most of the problems faced by memory impaired people when they try to use a compensatory aid or strategy. Employing aids or strategies involves memory, so the very people who need them most have the greatest difficulty using them. They forget to use them, may be unable to program them, may use them unsystematically and may be embarrassed by them. In contrast, NeuroPage can be controlled by one rather large button, easy to press even for those with motor difficulties. It is highly portable, it has an audible or vibratory alarm depending on the preference of the user, it has an accompanying explanatory message and is, to many people's minds, prestigious.

In a fairly recent study (Wilson et al., 1997) NeuroPage was evaluated with 15 brain injured people whose memory difficulties followed head injury, stroke or tumour. Using an ABA design whereby the first A phase was the baseline period, B the treatment and the second A phase the post-treatment baseline, we demonstrated that all 15 subjects benefited significantly from NeuroPage. The average number of problems tackled for the group as a whole was 3.86 with a range of 1–7 and a mode of 4. Typical reminders included 'take your medication'; 'feed the dog/cat'; 'pack your things for college/work' and 'check your diary'.

For the group as a whole, the mean percentage success for completing tasks in the first baseline period was 37.08, while in the treatment phase this rose to 85.56. Using an Odds Ratio Test (Everitt, 1995), which takes into account different underlying success rates for each target and calculates an average improvement factor, it was found that each subject showed a significant improvement. There were, however, wide individual differences, with some subjects changing from 0% success in the baseline period to over 90% success in the treatment period through to those with more modest changes such as 6.67% in the baseline stage to 22.93% in the treatment stage.

There were also wide variations between subjects in the post-treatment baseline phase. The mean success of the group as a whole was 74.46%, i.e. better than in the first baseline phase. The Odds Ratio Test indicated that 11 of the 15 subjects were significantly better than in the baseline phase and 4 were not. The implications here are that some subjects 'learn' to do what is expected during treatment, i.e. they learn to take their medication, feed the dog and pack their school bag, while other people will always require reminders to carry out tasks. At present, a paging service is being set up for people with everyday memory problems arising from organic amnesia and/or planning, attentional and organizational difficulties. The NeuroPage should also prove beneficial to normal elderly people and some children with everyday memory problems.

Another area where technology is likely to expand in the future is the use of computers as 'Interactive Task Guidance Systems' (Kirsch et al., 1987, 1992). In these systems the computer provides a series of cues to guide patients through the sequential steps of real life tasks, such as cooking or cleaning. The computer is a compensatory device providing step-by-step instructions. Little knowledge of computer operations is needed by the subject. One example is provided by Bergman and Kemmerer (1991). Their patient was a 54-year-old woman with a number of cognitive problems.

They taught her to use a computerized task guidance system. The patient had a left-sided neglect so only the right side of the screen was used. She also had poor visual acuity, so the colours of the screen were adjusted to make it more discriminable. An audible tone was included to enhance arousal and attentiveness. The patient learned to use the computerized system in three 1-hour training sessions. She used it for (i) writing lists of things to do or buy, (ii) writing instructions or requests to her companion helper, (iii) notes about telephone calls and letters and (iv) money management, e.g. printing out cheques to pay her electricity bill. Bergman and Kemmerer reported that the patient's self-sufficiency increased and her emotional distress decreased as a result of the computerized interactive task guidance system.

Glisky (1995) discusses the issues involved in using computers in memory re-habilitation. She says that computers are likely to play an increasingly important role as new technologies are developed and the interface between computer and user is improved. She reminds us about the problems of transfer and generalization and emphasizes the need for critical evaluation of new applications. All of Glisky's views are endorsed.

In addition to computers and new technology, there are, numerous non-electronic memory aids and strategies available; these will be discussed later in the chapter.

## New learning

Useful as external aids and environmental adaptations may be, they are rarely sufficient on their own. Memory impaired people need to learn some new infor-mation on some occasions. People's names, for example, can be written down in a notebook but in normal social interaction we need to greet people by name (at least every now and again). Referring to a notebook to retrieve the name would impair natural communication. Although learning names is difficult for many people and particularly so for those with organic memory impairment, a number of studies have shown that it is possible to teach names to amnesic people using strategies to improve learning. Wilson (1987) evaluated the strategy of visual imagery to teach names and demonstrated that it is virtually always superior to rote repetition. Thoene and Glisky (1995) also found that visual imagery was superior to other methods for teaching people's names to amnesic subjects. More recently, Linda Clare (personal communication) was able to teach a 74-year-old man in the early stages of Alzheimer's disease the names of his colleagues at a social club. She used a combination of strategies including finding a distinctive feature of the face together with backward chaining and expanding rehearsal. For example, one of the man's colleagues was called Carole. The man learned this name and others using all three methods described above. The distinctive feature for Carole was a 'curl'. The man tried to associate 'Carole with the curl on her fore-head'. At the same time backward chaining was employed. This involved giving the man written versions of her name with progressively more letters omitted such as

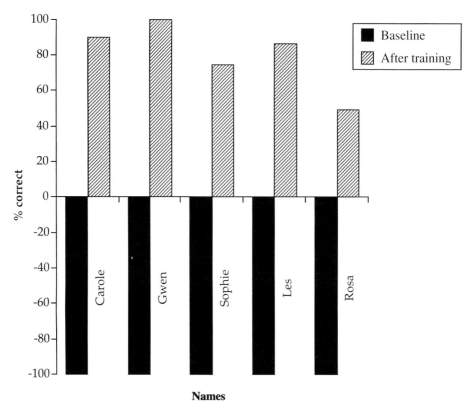

**Names**

Fig. 13.1    Name learning in a man with Alzheimer's disease: performance for each of five names during baseline testing and following intervention. Percentage of answers incorrect at baseline or correct after intervention achieved across test trials are shown.

CAROLE; CAROL_; CARO__; CAR___; and so forth. The man completed the missing letters and eventually learned the name without any letter cues. These two strategies were combined with expanding rehearsal, otherwise known as spaced retrieval, in which the information to be remembered is first presented, then tested immediately, tested after a very brief delay, tested again after a slightly longer delay and so forth. This is a form of distributed practice described in the introduction and is a fairly powerful learning strategy in memory rehabilitation (Moffat, 1989; Wilson, 1992). The method of expanding rehearsal owes much to the work of Landauer and Bjork (1978). Linda Clare's patient learned the names of his colleagues using photographs in his memory therapy sessions and demonstrated generalization by greeting his colleagues by name at the social club. The results can be seen in Fig. 13.1.

Some strategies from the field of study techniques (e.g. Robinson, 1970) and learning disability (e.g. Yule & Carr, 1987) have been applied in neuropsychological rehabilitation (Wilson, 1991a) and work continues in ways to improve learning.

One series of potentially important studies in recent years has involved errorless learning.

Errorless learning has for many years been used to teach new skills to people with learning disabilities (Sidman & Stoddard, 1967; Cullen, 1972; Jones & Eayrs, 1992) but until quite recently the principle has not been employed to any great extent with neurologically impaired adults. As the name implies, errorless learning involves learning without errors or mistakes. Most people can learn or benefit from their errors because they remember their mistakes and, therefore, avoid making the same mistake repeatedly.

People without episodic memory, however, cannot remember their mistakes so fail to correct them. Furthermore, the very fact of engaging in a behaviour may strengthen or reinforce that behaviour. Consequently, for someone with a severe memory impairment, it makes sense to ensure that any behaviour which is going to be reinforced is correct rather than incorrect.

Work on errorless learning in memory impaired adults was not only influenced by the earlier studies from the field of learning disability, but also by studies of implicit learning from the field of cognitive neuropsychology. There have been numerous studies showing that amnesic subjects can learn some things normally or nearly normally even though they may have no conscious recollection of learning anything at all (Brooks & Baddeley, 1976; Graf & Schacter, 1985; Baddeley, 1990). Glisky & Schacter (1987, 1989) tried to use the implicit learning abilities of amnesic subjects to teach them computer technology. Although some success was achieved, this was at the expense of considerable time and effort. This and other attempts to build on the relatively intact skills of memory impaired people has, on the whole, been disappointing. One reason for failures and anomalies could be that implicit learning is poor at eliminating errors. Error elimination is a function of explicit not implicit memory. Consequently, if subjects are forced to rely on implicit memory (as amnesic subjects are) trial-and-error learning becomes a slow and laborious process.

Baddeley and Wilson (1994) published the first study demonstrating that amnesic subjects learn better when they are prevented from making mistakes during the learning process. This was a theoretical study in which a stem completion task was used to teach severely memory impaired patients lists of words. Each of the 16 amnesic patients in the study showed better learning when they were prevented from making mistakes (i.e. prevented from guessing) than when they were forced to guess (i.e. forced to make mistakes). Since then several single case studies have been carried out with memory impaired patients comparing errorful and errorless learning for teaching practical, everyday, information (Wilson et al., 1994). In the majority of cases errorless learning proved to be superior to trial-and-error learning. Squires et al. (1996) and Wilson and Evans (1996) report further studies, while the latter paper discusses some of the potential problems of errorless learning.

Results from recent work (Evans et al., 1999) involving ten errorless learning experiments, suggest that tasks and situations which depend on implicit memory (such as stem completion tasks or retrieving a name from a first letter cue) are more likely to benefit from errorless learning methods than tasks which require explicit recall of new situations. Nevertheless, Wilson et al. (1994) demonstrated new explicit learning in a memory impaired head injured patient. Linda Clare (personal communication), mentioned above, also demonstrated explicit learning in a man with Alzheimer's disease. The Evans et al. (in press) studies found that the more severely amnesic patients benefited to a greater extent from errorless learning methods than those who are less severely impaired, although this may only apply when the interval between learning and recall is relatively short. One of the implications from this finding is that errorless learning should be combined with expanding rehearsal to enhance its effectiveness. This prediction is currently being tested with patients attending a memory clinic.

## Memory therapy in practice

Although some recovery of memory functioning can be expected during the early stages following head injury and other non-progressive brain injury, memory impaired people and their families should not be led to believe that significant improvement can occur once the period of natural recovery is over. This does not mean, however, that nothing can be done to help. Not only can people be taught to avoid problems, compensate for their difficulties and learn more efficiently, their distress can be reduced and their awareness and understanding can be increased. 'Memory rehabilitation does not occur in a vacuum' (Prigatano, 1995). Personality factors, awareness, motivation, anxiety, depression, lifestyle and additional cognitive problems may all affect the manifestations of memory problems in everyday life, the response to the problems, the compensations employed and the final outcome. Kopelman and Crawford (1996) found depression in over 40% of 200 consecutive referrals to a memory clinic. Evans and Wilson (1992) found anxiety common in attenders at a weekly memory group. Prigatano (1995) found the methods of treatment used in rehabilitation were influenced by social factors and the personality of patients influenced their approach to rehabilitation activities. He goes on to say that patients with low motivation and low awareness after brain injury are the most difficult to treat.

One extremely simple therapeutic strategy is to listen to what families have to say and provide information or explanations. A commonly asked question from relatives is 'why can he remember what happened 10 years ago but he can't remember what happened this morning?' or a variation on this theme. The answer is that old memories are stored differently in the brain (see Chapter 4, this volume). Some relatives like a fairly detailed anatomical or biochemical explanation, while others are happy with a more general one. Simply being reassured that this is a typical pattern found in most memory impaired people may also reduce anxiety. Written information is also appreciated by many families. *Memory Problems After Head Injury* (Wilson, 1989) written for the National Head Injuries Association, *Managing your Memory* (Kapur, 1991) a self-help manual for improving memory skills and *Coping with Memory Problems* (Clare & Wilson, 1997) are all useful booklets to have available for patients and relatives. A useful reference on the topic of self-help and support groups for memory impaired people and their carers is Wearing (1992). Wearing graphically illustrates the very limited understanding many people, including Health Service staff, have of memory impairments. To quote Wearing:

One mother in Manchester told me that her daughter, amnesic since an aneurysm at age 19, was to attend a day centre at a psychiatric hospital. She spent a couple of hours in discussion with the staff to make sure they understood her daughter's amnesia. After the first day she went to collect her but arrived to find that she was lost. 'Well' explained a staff member, 'We told her the way to lunch but she never arrived'. Naturally the poor girl had forgotten the directions almost immediately and had no idea where she was supposed to go, or why, or what she was doing there. So she found herself in the alcoholics' clinic and sat there for she knew not how long, in the expectation that somehow her mother would eventually find her. One of very many similar incidents (Wearing, 1992: 280–1).

As well as providing information, anxiety, depression, social isolation and other cognitive deficits may need to be dealt with. All of these are common in memory impaired people (Wilson, 1991a, b). Relaxation therapy may be useful in reducing anxiety. Even if memory problems are severe enough to prevent the person remembering the therapy, the beneficial effects of the relaxation are likely to remain. Relaxation audio cassette tapes can be bought or made for each patient thus avoiding the need to remember the exercises. However, if tense-and-release exercises (Bernstein & Borkovec, 1973) are employed for relaxation, therapists need to be cautious when using these with some brain-injured patients particularly those with motor difficulties. Tensing muscles may cause a spasm or increase spasticity. It is best to discuss the desirability of the tense-and-release exercises with a physiotherapist treating the patient or, alternatively, look for another form of relaxation such as that recommended by Ost (1987) or those described by Clark (1989).

Depression can impair memory functioning in those without brain injury (Watts, 1995) probably because of diminished resources available as a result of their emotional preoccupations. Depression may well exacerbate difficulties in people with organic memory impairment. It is possible that cognitive behavioural therapy approaches such as those employed by Beck (1976) would be appropriate for brain injured clients, although there do not appear to be any studies reporting this. Psychotherapy, on the other hand, is a well-established intervention with brain injured people. Prigatano et al. (1986) firmly believes in group and individual psychotherapy with brain injured patients. They use principles from the school of Jung. Jackson and Gouvier (1992) provide descriptions and guidelines for group psychotherapy with brain injured adults and their families.

Social isolation is common too (Talbot, 1989; Wilson, 1991a, b; Wearing, 1992). Wearing says some of the reasons for this isolation are because the social network often falls away because the memory impaired person forgets visits and conversations, may not be able to go out alone without getting lost, and may engage in inappropriate behaviour. One way to deal with social isolation is to run memory groups. Wilson and Moffat (1992) describe various kinds of groups for patients; Moffat (1989) reports on a relatives' memory group for people with dementia and Wearing (1992) provides suggestions on setting up self-help groups. Psychotherapy groups can achieve the same ends and guidelines for these groups can be found in Jackson and Gouvier (1992). Evans and Wilson (1992) not only point out the social value of memory groups but also the reduction in anxiety which may follow attendance at a group. Many groups have been run over the past years and the conclusion has been reached that the main value of such groups is to reduce the emotional sequelae resulting from memory impairment. Reminiscence and Reality Orientation groups may achieve the same ends.

In addition to memory and emotional factors, brain injured clients may well have additional cognitive problems which need to be addressed in rehabilitation. People with a pure amnesic syndrome (see Chapter 8, this volume) are relatively rare and most clients will present with attentional deficits, word finding problems or executive difficulties of planning and organization. The memory problems may be secondary to the other cognitive deficits or genuinely separate problems. Detailed neuropsychological assessment will probably be necessary to paint an accurate picture of cognitive strengths and weaknesses necessary for planning a coherent and sensible memory therapy programme. More detailed information on the neuropsychological assessment of memory can be found in Howieson and Lezak (1995), Mayes (1995) and Wilson (1996). In addition, this information needs to be supplemented by a behavioural assessment which identifies the real-life everyday problems that are targeted for treatment (see, for example, Wilson, 1992; Wilson & Staples, 1992; Knight & Godfrey, 1995). A number of publications address the issue of cognitive rehabilitation including memory. A recent summary can be found in Wilson (1997). Many articles in the journal *Neuropsychological Rehabilitation* are also concerned with the management and remediation of cognitive deficits.

## Other strategies for the management of memory problems

There are probably five main approaches to the management of organic memory impairment some of which have been considered earlier in this chapter. The first is to try to restore lost functioning. As was suggested earlier there is little evidence that restoration of function occurs once the period of natural recovery is over, although in a long-term follow-up study of 50 memory impaired people (Wilson, 1991a), some partial recovery appeared to occur in almost a third of patients reassessed 5 to 10 years post-injury. These were patients with non-progressive brain injury. Arkin (1991, 1992) also suggests it might be possible to slow down the rate of decline in patients with progressive conditions. Although Arkin's evidence is very tentative, her ideas would be well worth evaluating in a larger study.

A second approach to memory rehabilitation and management is to encourage anatomical reorganization. Detailed discussion is beyond the scope of this chapter. Suffice it to say here that although Kolb (1995) is very persuasive in his arguments that the brain is far more plastic than was once believed, there is no strong evidence that anatomical reorganization of the brain takes place as far as memory functioning is concerned.

A third approach is to bypass or avoid problems through restructuring or modifying the environment. This was discussed earlier.

A fourth approach is to find an alternative means to the final goal, i.e. if you cannot do something one way try to do it another way. This approach is analogous to Luria's principle of functional adaptation (Luria, 1963) or to Zangwill's principle of compensation (Zangwill, 1947). In memory rehabilitation, such compensation is often achieved through the use of external memory aids such as notebooks, lists, diaries, tape recorders and so forth. Most people use such external memory aids and they are, perhaps, the most useful strategy for people with organic memory impairment. Some patients resist using such aids, feeling that it is cheating or that any natural recovery will be slowed down by the use of aids. These feelings should be discouraged as it is very normal to use compensatory aids, and there is neither evidence nor reason to believe their use will slow down natural recovery. A bigger problem is the difficulty remembering to use these aids or to use them efficiently. This issue was addressed earlier when we discussed new technology. NeuroPage and computers are examples of external memory aids, although the majority of people use simpler non-electronic aids. Wilson (1991a) found that memory impaired people were far more likely to be using compensatory aids 5 to 10 years post-rehabilitation than they were during or at the end of rehabilitation. This was despite the fact that much of their rehabilitation emphasized the use of such aids. Furthermore, those patients using six or more aids or strategies were significantly more likely to be independent than those using five or less. The numbers of people using each kind of compensation can be found in Wilson (1995). The most popular was writing notes and the least was tying a knot in one's handkerchief (analogous to the American custom of tying a string on one's finger).

Despite general agreement that a compensatory approach is probably the most useful one to adopt, there is uncertainty about why some people use external aids efficiently and others do not. Simply providing aids and expecting them to be used appropriately is likely to lead to failure for many memory impaired people, and patience and ingenuity may be required. Kime et al. (1996) and Sohlberg and Mateer (1989) describe ways of teaching the use of aids. More recently, Wilson and Watson (1996) using a theoretical framework proposed by Bäckman and Dixon (1992) and data from a long-term follow-up (Wilson, 1991a) showed that age, severity of memory impairment and additional cognitive deficits are important variables in predicting independence and use of compensations several years post-rehabilitation.

The final approach to the management and rehabilitation of memory problems is to help people to use their residual, albeit damaged skills, more effectively. This can be done through the use of mnemonics, through rehearsal and study techniques and maybe through the use of games and exercises. Although memory games probably do not improve memory, they do enable people to:

(a)  realise they can do better if they use a strategy, and
(b)  have the opportunity of using these strategies in (hopefully) enjoyable situations.

Mnemonics are systems that enable people to organize, store and retrieve information more efficiently. Some people use the term 'mnemonics' to refer to anything that helps people remember including external aids. In memory rehabilitation, however, the term is used for methods involving mental manipulation of material. For example, in order to remember how many days there are in a month, most people use a system or mnemonic. In the United Kingdom and much of the United States of America people use a rhyme 'Thirty days hath September . . .'. In other parts of the world people use their knuckles to remember the 'long' months and the dips between the knuckles to refer to the 'short' months. Mnemonics are often used to learn the names of cranial nerves, notes of music, the colours of the rainbow and other ordered material. See Harris (1992), Moffat (1992) and Wilson (1995) for further discussion of mnemonics in memory rehabilitation and West (1995) for the use of these strategies in people with age-related memory impairment. Visual imagery or converting words or names into pictures is another well-established mnemonic for teaching names to brain injured clients (Wilson 1987).

Rehearsal strategies such as expanding rehearsal (described above) and other procedures from the field of study techniques have all been successfully employed to teach new information to memory impaired people. For a further discussion of these strategies see Robinson (1970), Moffat (1989) and Evans and Wilson (1992).

There is considerable misunderstanding about the value of mnemonics in memory therapy. Some people think that memory impaired people have been taught how to use mnemonics and how to employ them in novel situations. Although this does sometimes happen (Kime et al., 1996), most brain injured people do not spontaneously use mnemonics. If spontaneous use is considered important, this would have to be planned for and carefully incorporated into a treatment programme. The real value of mnemonics is that they are useful for teaching memory impaired people new information and, almost invariably, lead to faster learning than rote rehearsal (Evans & Wilson, 1992). When therapists, psychologists, teachers or others employ mnemonics, they should teach one piece of information at a time, take individual styles and preferences into account and plan for generalization. So, if a mnemonic is used to teach the name of a therapist in the psychologist's office by pairing the mnemonic with a photograph, one should not expect the client to spontaneously greet the therapist by name on meeting her in another place. It will be necessary to plan the generalization perhaps by having the therapist come into the room and seeing if the client can make the link between the photograph and the person. If this works, the client should be enabled to meet the therapist in other settings and other contexts and prompted (if necessary) to use her name wherever and whenever the meeting occurs. Just as generalization is incorporated into treatment programmes for people with developmental learning difficulties (Zarkowska, 1987), so it should be incorporated into programmes for people with organic memory impairments.

## Summary and conclusions

1. This chapter assumes that restoration of memory functioning is unlikely to occur in people with memory impairment following brain injury. Nevertheless, a considerable amount can be done to enable people and their relatives to understand their difficulties.

2. Environmental modifications can enable people with very severe problems to cope without adequate memory functioning. Suggestions are offered on how environmental adaptations may be carried out.

3. New technology is likely to play an increasingly important role in the future management of memory problems. Some technological aids such as pagers and computers are already proving beneficial. Others such as 'smart' houses are in the early stages of development.

4. Non-electronic external memory aids such as diaries, notebooks, tape recorders, and so forth, are widely used but are often problematic for memory impaired

people as their use involves memory. Successful use can be achieved through careful teaching methods. Successful and spontaneous use is likely to occur in people who are younger, have less severe memory problems and few additional cognitive impairments. Others may need more intensive therapy or rehabilitation to ensure efficient use of external memory aids.

5. Internal strategies such as mnemonics and rehearsal techniques can be employed to teach new information. Although these almost always lead to faster learning than rote repetition, most memory impaired people are unable to use mnemonics spontaneously. Instead relatives, carers, therapists and others employ the mnemonic to enhance learning.

6. Errorless learning, i.e. avoiding mistakes during learning, is usually to be preferred to trial-and-error learning for memory impaired people. This is because, in order to benefit from our mistakes, the mistakes need to be remembered. In the absence of episodic memory, the very fact of making an error may strengthen the erroneous response. Consequently, it is better to avoid erroneous responses in the first place.

7. In addition to poor memory, many brain injured people will have other cognitive problems which will need to be addressed.

8. The emotional sequelae of memory impairment such as anxiety, depression and loneliness can be reduced through the provision of written information, counselling, anxiety management techniques and treatment in memory groups or psychotherapy groups.

9. Although lost memory functioning cannot be restored, people can be helped to bypass problems and their difficulties compensated for. They can be helped to learn more efficiently, the effects of their problems in everyday life can be reduced, and society can be educated into what memory impairment really means.

## REFERENCES

Arkin, S.M. (1991). Memory training in early Alzheimer's disease: an optimistic look at the field. *American Journal of Alzheimer's Care and Related Disorders and Research*, July/August, 17–25.

Arkin, S.M. (1992). Audio-assisted memory training with early Alzheimer's patients: two single subject experiments. *Clinical Gerontologist*, **12**, 77–96.

Bäckman, L. & Dixon, R.A. (1992). Psychological compensation: a theoretical framework. *Psychological Bulletin*, **112**, 259–83.

Baddeley, A.D. (1990). *Human Memory: Theory and Practice*. London: Lawrence Erlbaum.

Baddeley, A.D. & Longman, D.J.A. (1978). The influence of length and frequency on training sessions on the rate of learning to type. *Ergonomics*, **21**, 627–35.

Baddeley, A.D. & Wilson, B.A. (1994). When implicit learning fails: amnesia and the problem of error elimination. *Neuropsychologia*, **32**, 53–68.

Baddeley, A.D., Wilson, B.A. & Watts, F.N. (1995). *Handbook of Memory Disorders*. Chichester, UK: John Wiley.

Beck, A.T. (1976). *Cognitive Therapy and Emotional Disorders*. New York: International Universities Press.

Berg, I. (1993). *Memory Rehabilitation for Closed Head Injured Patients*. The Hague: Koninkluke Bibliotheek.

Bergman, M.M. & Kemmerer, A.G. (1991). Computer enhanced self sufficiency: Part 2: uses and subjective benefits of a text writer for an individual with traumatic brain injury. *Neuropsychology*, **5**, 25–8.

Bernstein, D.A. & Borkovec, T.D. (1973). *Progressive Relaxation Training*. Champaign, IL: Illinois Research Press.

Brooks, D.N. & Baddeley, A. (1976). What can amnesic patients learn? *Neuropsychologia*, **14**, 111–22.

Clare, L. & Wilson, B.A. (1997). *Coping With Memory Problems*. Bury St Edmunds, UK: Thames Valley Test Company.

Clark, D.M. (1989). Anxiety states: panic and generalised anxiety. In *Cognitive Behaviour Therapy for Psychiatric Problems: A Practical Guide*, ed. K. Hawton, P.M. Salkovskis, J. Kirk & D.M. Clark, pp. 53–96. Oxford: Oxford Medical Publications.

Cullen, C.N. (1972). Errorless learning with the retarded. *Nursing Times*, **28**, 33–6.

Ericsson, K.A., Chase, W.G. & Falcon, S. (1980). Acquisition of a memory skill. *Science*, **208**, 1181–2.

Evans, J.J. & Wilson, B.A. (1992). A memory group for individuals with brain injury. *Clinical Rehabilitation*, **6**, 75–81.

Evans, J.J., Wilson, B.A., Schuri, U., Andrade, J., Baddeley, A., Bruna, O., Canavan, T., Della Sala, S., Green, R., Laaksonen, R., Lorenzi, L. & Taussik, I. (1999). A comparison of 'error' and 'trial and error' learning methods for teaching individuals with acquired memory deficits. *Neuropsychological Rehabilitation*, in press.

Everitt, B. (1995). *Cambridge Dictionary of Statistics in the Medical Sciences*. Cambridge: Cambridge University Press.

Glisky, E.L. (1995). Computers in memory rehabilitation. In *Handbook of Memory Disorders*, ed. A.D. Baddeley, B.A. Wilson & F.N. Watts, pp. 557–75. Chichester, UK: John Wiley.

Glisky, E.L. & Schacter, D.L. (1987). Acquisition of domain specific knowledge in organic amnesia: training for computer related work. *Neuropsychologia*, **25**, 893–906.

Glisky, E.L. & Schacter, D.L. (1989). Extending the limits of complex learning in organic amnesia: computer training in a vocational domain. *Neuropsychologia*, **27**, 107–20.

Graf, P. & Schacter, D.L. (1985). Implicit and explicit memory for new associations in normal and amnesic subjects. *Journal of Experimental Psychology: Learning, Memory Cognition*, **11**, 501–18.

Gross, Y. & Schutz, L.E. (1986). Intervention models in neuropsychology. In *Clinical Neuropsychology of Intervention*, ed. B. Uzzell & Y. Gross, pp. 179–205. Boston: Martinus Nijhoff Publishing.

Harris, J.E. (1992). Ways to help memory. In *Clinical Management of Memory Problems*, 2nd edn, ed. B.A. Wilson & N. Moffat, pp. 59–85. London: Chapman & Hall.

Harris, J.E. & Sunderland, A. (1981). A brief survey of the management of memory disorders in rehabilitation units in Britain. *International Rehabilitation Medicine*, **3**, 206–9.

Hersh, N. & Treadgold, L. (1994). NeuroPage: the rehabilitation of memory dysfunction by prosthetic memory and cueing. *Neurorehabilitation*, **4**, 187–97.

Howieson, D.B. & Lezak, M.D. (1995). Separating memory from other cognitive problems. In *Handbook of Memory Problems*. ed. A.D. Baddeley, B.A. Wilson & F.N. Watts, pp. 411–26. Chichester, UK: John Wiley.

Jackson, W.T. & Gouvier, W.D. (1992). Group psychotherapy with brain damaged adults and their families. In *Handbook of Head Trauma: Acute Care to Recovery*, ed. C.J. Long & L.K. Ross, pp. 309–27. New York: Plenum Press.

Jones, R.S. & Eayrs, C.B. (1992). The use of errorless learning procedures in teaching people with a learning disability: a critical review. *Mental Handicap Research*, **5**, 204–12.

Kapur, N. (1991). *Managing Your Memory: A Self Help Memory Manual for Improving Everyday Memory Skills*. Southampton General Hospital, Southampton.

Kapur, N. (1995). Memory aids in rehabilitation of memory disordered patients. In *Handbook of Memory Disorders*, ed. A.D. Baddeley, B.A. Wilson & F.N. Watts, pp. 533–56. Chichester, UK: John Wiley.

Kime, S.K., Lamb, D.G. & Wilson, B.A. (1996). Use of a comprehensive program of external cuing to enhance procedural memory in a patient with dense amnesia. *Brain Injury*, **10**, 17–25.

Kirsch, N.L., Levine, S.P., Fallon-Krueger, M. & Jaros, L.E. (1987). The microcomputer as an 'orthotic' device for patients with cognitive deficits. *Journal of Head Trauma Rehabilitation*, **2**, 77–86.

Kirsch, N.L., Levine, S.P., Lajiness O'Neill, L. & Schnyder, M. (1992). Computer assisted interactive task guidance: facilitating the performance of a simulated vocational task. *Journal of Head Trauma Rehabilitation*, **7**, 13–25.

Knight, R.G. & Godfrey, H.P.D. (1995). Behavioural and support methods. In *Handbook of Memory Disorders*, ed. A.D. Baddeley, B.A. Wilson & F.N. Watts, pp. 393–410. Chichester, UK: John Wiley.

Kolb, B. (1995). *Brain Plasticity and Behaviour*. New Jersey: Lawrence Erlbaum Associates.

Kopelman, M. & Crawford, S. (1996). Not all memory clinics are dementia clinics. *Neuropsychological Rehabilitation* , **6**, 187–202.

Landauer, T.K. & Bjork, R.A. (1978). Optimum rehearsal patterns and name learning. In *Practical Aspects of Memory*, ed. M.M. Gruneberg, P.E. Morris & R.N. Sykes, pp. 625–32. London: Academic Press.

Lorge, I. (1930). Influence of regularly interpolated time intervals upon subsequent learning. Quoted in Johnson, H.H. & Solo, R.L. (1971). *An Introduction to Experimental Design in Psychology: A Case Approach*, pp. 7–8. New York: Harper & Row.

Luria, A.R. (1963). *Restoration of Function After Brain Injury*. New York: Macmillan.

Mayes, A.R. (1995). The assessment of memory disorders. In *Handbook of Memory Disorders*, ed. A.D. Baddeley, B.A. Wilson & F.N. Watts, pp. 367–91. Chichester, UK: John Wiley.

Moffat, N. (1989). Home based cognitive rehabilitation with the elderly. In *Everyday Cognition in Adulthood and Late Life*, ed. L.W. Poon, D.C. Rubin & B.A. Wilson, pp. 659–80. Cambridge: Cambridge University Press.

Moffat, N. (1992). Strategies of memory therapy. In *Clinical Management of Memory Problems*, 2nd edn, ed. B.A. Wilson & N. Moffat, pp. 86–119. London: Chapman & Hall.

Murphy, G. (1987). Decreasing undesirable behaviours. In *Behaviour Modification for People with Mental Handicaps*, ed. W. Yule & J. Carr, pp. 102–42. London: Croom Helm.

Norman, D. (1988). *The Psychology of Everyday Things*. New York: Basic Books.

Ost, L.G. (1987). Applied relaxation: description of a coping technique and review of controlled studies. *Behaviour Research & Therapy*, **25**, 397–410.

Poon, L., Rubin, D. & Wilson, B.A. (1989). *Everyday Cognition in Adult and Late Life*. Cambridge: Cambridge University Press.

Prigatano, G. (1995). Personality and social aspects of memory rehabilitation. In *Handbook of Memory Disorders*, ed. A.D. Baddeley, B.A. Wilson & F.N. Watts, pp. 603–14. Chichester, UK: John Wiley.

Prigatano, G.P., Fordyce, D.J., Zeiner, H.K., Roueche, J.R., Pepping, M. & Wood, B.C. (1986). *Neuropsychological Rehabilitation After Brain Injury*. Baltimore: Johns Hopkins University Press.

Robinson, F.B. (1970). *Effective Study*. New York: Harper & Row.

Schacter, D.L. & Glisky, E.L. (1986). Memory remediation: restoration, alleviation and the acquisition of domain-specific knowledge. In *Clinical Neuropsychology of Intervention*, ed. B.P. Uzzell & Y. Gross, pp. 257–82. Boston: Martinus Nijhoff.

Sidman, M. & Stoddard, L.T. (1967). The effectiveness of fading in programming simultaneous form discrimination for retarded children. *Journal of Experimental Analysis of Behaviour*, **10**, 3–15.

Sohlberg, M. & Mateer, C. (1989). Training use of compensatory memory books: a three stage behavioural approach. *Journal of Clinical and Experimental Neuropsychology*, **11**, 871–91.

Squires, E.G., Hunkin, N. M. & Parkin, A.J. (1996). Memory notebook training in a case of severe amnesia: generalising from pair associate learning to real life. *Neuropsychological Rehabilitation*, **6**, 55–65.

Talbot, R. (1989). The brain injured person and the family. In *Model of Brain Injury Rehabilitation*, ed. R.Ll. Wood & P. Eames, pp. 3–16. London: Chapman & Hall.

Thoene, A.I. T. & Glisky, E.L. (1995). Learning of name face associations in memory impaired patients: a comparison of different training procedures. *Journal of International Neuropsychological Society*, **1**, 29–38.

Watts, F.N. (1995). Depression and anxiety. In *Handbook of Memory Disorders*, ed. A.D. Baddeley, B.A. Wilson & F.N. Watts, pp. 293–317. Chichester, UK: John Wiley.

Wearing, D. (1992). Self help groups. In *Clinical Management of Memory Problems*, 2nd edn, ed. B.A. Wilson & N. Moffat, pp. 271–301. London: Chapman & Hall.

West, R. (1995). Compensatory strategies for age associated memory impairment. In *Handbook of Memory Disorders*, ed. A.D. Baddeley, B.A. Wilson & F.N. Watts, pp. 481–500. Chichester, UK: John Wiley.

Wilson, B.A. (1987). *Rehabilitation of Memory*. New York: Guilford Press.

Wilson, B.A. (1989). Designing memory therapy programmes. In *Everyday Cognition in Adult and Late Life*, ed. L. Poon, D. Rubin & B. Wilson, pp. 615–38. Cambridge: Cambridge University Press.

Wilson, B.A. (1989). *Memory Problems After Head Injury*. Nottingham: National Head Injuries Association.

Wilson, B.A. (1991a). Long term prognosis of patients with severe memory disorders. *Neuropsychological Rehabilitation*, 1, 117–34.

Wilson, B. A. (1991b). Behaviour therapy in the treatment of neurologically impaired adults. In *Handbook of Behavior Therapy and Psychological Science: An Integrative Approach*, ed. P.R. Martin, pp. 277–52. New York: Pergamon Press.

Wilson, B.A. (1992). Memory therapy in practice. In *Clinical Management of Memory Problems*, 2nd edn, ed. B.A. Wilson & N. Moffat, pp. 120–52. London: Chapman & Hall.

Wilson, B.A. (1993). Coping with memory impairment. In *Memory in Everyday Life*, ed. G.M. Davies & R.H. Logie, pp. 461–81. Amsterdam: Elsevier Science Publishers B.V.

Wilson, B.A. (1995). Management and remediation of memory problems in brain injured adults. In *Handbook of Memory Disorders*, ed. A.D. Baddeley, B.A. Wilson & F.N. Watts, pp. 451–79. Chichester, UK: John Wiley.

Wilson, B.A. (1996). Assessment of memory. In *Assessment in Neuropsychology*, ed. L. Harding & J.R. Beech, pp. 135–51. London: Routledge.

Wilson, B.A. (1997). Management of acquired cognitive disorders. In *Rehabilitation Studies Handbook*, ed. B.A. Wilson & D.L. McLellan, pp. 243–61. Cambridge: Cambridge University Press.

Wilson, B.A. & Moffat, N. (1984). *Clinical Management of Memory Problems*. London: Croom Helm.

Wilson, B.A. & Moffat, N. (1992). The development of group memory therapy. In *Clinical Management of Memory Problems*, 2nd edn, ed. B.A. Wilson & N. Moffat, pp. 243–73. London: Chapman & Hall.

Wilson, B.A. & Staples, D. (1992). Working with people with physical handicap. In *What is Clinical Psychology?*, 2nd edn, ed. J. Marzillier & J. Hall, pp. 142–98. Oxford: Oxford University Press.

Wilson, B.A. & Evans, J.J. (1996). Error free learning in the rehabilitation of individuals with memory impairments. *Journal of Head Trauma Rehabilitation*, 11, 54–64.

Wilson, B.A. & Watson, P.C. (1996). A practical framework for understanding compensatory behaviour in people with organic memory impairment. *Memory*, 4, 465–86.

Wilson, B.A., Baddeley, A.D., Evans, J.J. & Shiel, A. (1994). Errorless learning in the rehabilitation of memory impaired people. *Neuropsychological Rehabilitation*, 4, 307–26.

Wilson, B.A., Evans, J.J., Emslie, H. & Malinek, V. (1997). NeuroPage: evaluation of a new memory aid. *Journal of Neurology, Neurosurgery and Psychiatry*, in press.

Yule, W. & Carr, J., (eds.) (1987). *Behaviour Modification for People with Mental Handicaps*. London: Croom Helm.

Zangwill, O. (1947). Psychological aspects of rehabilitation in cases of brain injury. *British Journal of Psychology*, 37, 60–9.

Zarkowska, E. (1987). Discrimination and generalisation. In *Behaviour Modification for People with Mental Handicaps*, ed. W. Yule & J. Carr, pp. 79–94. London: Croom Helm.

# Part III

# Paramnesias and delusions of memory

Ivana S. Marková and German E. Berrios

On occasions, patients may report memories of events that never happened in their lives, for example, they may claim with conviction to have been in a place before, or lived through a particular experience, or carried out a deed. During the second half of the nineteenth century, these clinical phenomena were conceived of as a form of memory disorder. Changes in the definition of memory occurred during the 1880s, and this, inter alia, led to their eventual neglect. But they are still met with in clinical practice and need to be discussed in a book on the neuropsychiatry of memory complaints. Since most of the interesting clinical descriptions are to be found in earlier publications, this chapter will perforce have a historical flavour.

In 1886, Emil Kraepelin[1] suggested that the term 'paramnesias' might be used to refer to the qualitative disturbances of memory whose study, as opposed to quantitative memory disturbances (general and partial amnesias and hypermnesias), had been confined to a few case reports. Such reports most commonly referred to what Walter Scott called 'sentiment of pre-existence' (and Feuchtersleben called 'phantasm of memory', and the French déjà vu) and featured prominently in the medical work of Wigan, Jensen, Jackson, Sander, Pick and Anjel. But whilst the former three writers conceived of this phenomenon as a 'disturbance of perception' (resulting from a lack of synchrony between the two hemispheres), Sander and Pick proposed that it was a disturbance of memory.

## Paramnesias as 'disturbances of perception'

### Wigan

Wigan (1844) referred to the phenomenon as:

a sudden feeling, as if the scene we have just witnessed (although, from the very nature of things it could never have been seen before) had been present to our eyes on a former occasion, when the very same speakers, seated in the very same positions, uttered the same sentiments, in the same words – the postures, the expression of countenance, the gestures, the tone of voice, all seem to be remembered, and to be now attracting attention for the second time (p. 84).

Wigan offered the following explanation:

only one brain has been used in the immediate preceding part of the scene, – the other brain has been asleep, or in an analogous state nearly approaching it. When the attention of both brains is roused to the topic, there is the same vague consciousness that the ideas have passed through the mind before, which takes place on re-perusing the page we had read while thinking on some other subject. The ideas have passed through the mind before, and as there was not sufficient consciousness to fix them in the memory without a renewal, we have no means of knowing the length of time that had elapsed between the faint impression received by the single brain, and the distinct impression received by the double brain. It may seem to have been many years (pp. 84–5).

## Jensen

Jensen (1868) was the first to draw specific clinical attention to these phenomena, calling them 'double perceptions' (*Doppelwahrnehmungen*):

occasionally, generally only fleetingly, there arises in us a vague awareness that this or other situation as it is occurring at present, has been experienced in exactly the same way before. We recall that our friend took exactly that stance, held his hands in that particular way, had the same expression, spoke the same words, etc. We are almost convinced that we can predict what he will do next, say next and how we ourselves will respond (p. 48).

Jensen believed that these phenomena were common in healthy individuals and that their study might throw light on 'similar' complaints in the mentally ill.

Like Wigan, he proposed that the experience resulted from a time disparity or lack of synchrony in the functioning of the cerebral hemispheres. According to Jensen, the cerebral hemispheres controlled the highest psychical functions, i.e. perceptions and concepts (*Vorstellungen*). Nonetheless, he observed, large sectors of a hemisphere could be 'absent' without there being a noticeable loss of function (i.e. thinking and perceiving were possible in subjects that had only one hemisphere). Like the 'paired' sense organs (eyes and ears) that received two images, the cerebral hemispheres also received two 'congruent' perceptions (i.e. normally experienced as one percept). In abnormal situations, however, there could arise a disparity in the functioning of the cerebral hemispheres akin to squinting of the eyes. The latter led to double images (double vision), and the former to double perceptions, the sole difference being that, in the case of vision, the images were projected next to each other in space and in the case of the brain the perceptions were projected one after another in time. Jensen reported four cases showing, arguably, the same phenomenon. He explained some of the differences between them on the grounds that some showed the direct expression of the phenomenon and others showed the effects of modulation by psychological factors.

## Jackson

Hughlings Jackson (1932) wrote repeatedly on the 'sensation of reminiscence'. In 1876, he also indicated that such feelings, primarily seen as the 'intellectual aura' of epilepsy, were 'not uncommon in healthy people' (Vol. 1, p. 274). At this stage, Jackson still believed that Wigan's 'double consciousness' model was a 'perfectly accurate account'.

In 1888, Jackson returned to these 'sensations of reminiscence' in relation to the case of a medical colleague who, under the pseudonym of Quærens, had reported his own temporal lobe epilepsy (Vol. 1, pp. 388–9). To describe his experience, Quærens quoted from David Copperfield:

> We have all some experience of a feeling which comes over us occasionally of what we are saying and doing having been said or done before, in a remote time – of our having been surrounded, dim ages ago, by the same faces, objects, and circumstances – of our knowing perfectly what will be said next, as if we suddenly remember it.

In 1899, Jackson repeated the view that double consciousness or 'mental diplopia' was a common accompaniment of the 'dreamy state' (pp. 467–8).

## Paramnesias as 'disturbances of memory'

### Sander

Sander (1874)[2] believed that the 'double perception' account did not explain adequately the phenomenon, and reconceptualized it as a 'memory deception' (*Erinnerungstäuschung*). The latter, Sander defined as a sudden impression, in the course of normal thinking and behaving, that a particular ongoing situation had been experienced before. Like Jensen, he believed that the phenomenon could lead to the conviction that the future could be foretold, and that it was common in the healthy, particularly in the young with a tendency to introspect. He emphasized, however, that there was an emotional component (a feeling of unease) intrinsically linked to the memory deception. On occasions this feeling, which was the result of efforts made to match memories to specific spatiotemporal experiences, could be distressing and cause marked fear.

Sander reported the case of a 25-year-old man with epilepsy who experienced this phenomenon on several occasions, each time lasting about two months. In his account, the patient stated that whilst speaking with someone, or seeing something, he would suddenly get the feeling that he had experienced the same conversation or seen a particular object in exactly the same way before. Sander highlighted two aspects of this case. First was the unusual duration of the memory deception; for, even when recalling it, the patient was still unclear as to which were real experiences and which were memories. Secondly, the memory related to all aspects of the situation including place, people, things and feelings and not just the event or object itself. This second feature Sander used to differentiate memory deceptions from phenomena such as delusions and delusional misidentifications.[3]

Sander rejected the 'double perception' hypothesis on the basis that it was not simply single objects or perceptions that were involved but the whole situation, including context and atmosphere. Consequently, memory deceptions could not be explained just on the basis of anatomical or physiological brain disturbances but a psychological explanation was needed. He proposed that memory deceptions arose from similarities to previously experienced events which could trigger the feelings and contexts associated with a previous experience and lead to the feeling that that the whole thing had taken place before. With great clinical sense, Sander placed the abnormality not on the memory itself, but on a mistaken association of ideas/feelings with the relevant memory. He conceptualized memory deceptions in the same way as sensory deceptions (*Sinnestäuschungen*): '. . . similarly [to sensory deceptions] here, it is not the memory that deceives, but memory that is being deceived through other psychological processes' (p. 253).

## Pick and Anjel

Sander's paper stimulated others to focus on 'memory deception'. For example, in an early paper Pick (1876) reported a patient who as a boy had the feeling that he had lived through particular situations in exactly the same way as before. Later in life he developed, in addition, persecutory delusions. This led to an increase in the frequency of his memory deceptions which in the event became incorporated into an elaborate delusional system involving the belief that he had a 'double life' (*Doppelleben*). Pick distinguished between simple memory deceptions (i.e. déjà vu experiences as conceptualized by Sander and – arguably – Jensen) and delusional interpretations based on these experiences – as shown by his patient. Pick propounded that the memory deception was the basic or primary phenomenon.

Although Anjel (1878) used the term 'memory deception', he returned to a version of the 'perceptual' hypothesis. Noticing an association between memory deceptions and tiredness and stress, he proposed that physiological processes were slowed down by fatigue thus leading to a prolongation of the time lapse between the sensory and the cerebral perception of an object. This led to an incongruence between the sensory system and the cerebral processes that elaborated sense data into subjective representations. Thus Anjel's hypothesis differs from the view proposed by Wigan and Jensen according to which the disparity was between the images generated by the two cerebral hemispheres.

## Other paramnesias

Apart from the déjà vu-like phenomena, other types of paramnesias were discussed in the literature prior to Kraepelin's synthesis. Of note amongst these are the so-called obsessions, hallucinations and illusions of memory, respectively.

### Eyselein

Though claiming to describe a form of memory deception in Sander's sense, Eyselein (1875) reported the case of a patient with mnestic obsessions who was persistently preoccupied with the need to recall things from her past. The patient, however, did not seem to be aware of having experienced the same things before. Eyselein focused more on the accompanying feeling of unease and distress than the feeling of recognition.

### Kahlbaum

By 'hallucinated memories' (*hallucinirte Erinnerungen*), Kahlbaum (1866) referred to hallucinations of false *past* events.[4] He reported the case of a young Catholic female inpatient who complained at a ward round that the priest (accompanying the doctors during this activity!) was confusing her with his notions. She stated that she was a Catholic and did not want to turn Protestant. It turned out that the priest had only recently started working at the institute, and had not seen her or any other patient in her ward before. Therefore, remarked Kahlbaum, the patient was either lying, which seemed unlikely, or had recently experienced hallucinations whose content related to the religious debate. Kahlbaum went on to question what sort of hallucinations might these be, i.e. were they auditory hallucinations, or facial (visual) hallucinations, or both? It had been noticed that whilst the patient frequently made such complaints, talking about conversations which she had apparently experienced in the recent past, no one had actually observed her as appearing to be experiencing hallucinations at any time.

To conceptualize her symptom as a 'hallucination of memory', Kahlbaum proposed that perception resulted from an interplay between the functional activity of peripheral and central organs of perception. The central organs of perception were of two types: (i) organs of perception proper that converted the physical stimuli into a 'psychical form', and (ii) organs of 'apperception', responsible for comparing current input to past impressions and endowing percepts with the knowledge that they had been perceived before.

In the case of his patient, Kahlbaum noted firstly that the dysfunction had to be in the central organs of perception. Consequently there were two options: one that her experiences resulted from pathology in the organs of perception proper in which case pathways subserving vision and hearing were affected. However, it was not simply the case that she was 'hearing a vision' but that the patient was involved in a dialogue and therefore would have had to have spoken to her hallucination or have hallucinated her own words. Since she had never been observed participating in imaginary dialogues, it seemed more likely that the abnormality lay in the organs of apperception, where the psychical representations were contextualized and grounded as memories. Kahlbaum thus concluded: 'we are dealing here not with a memory of a real hallucination, but with a hallucinated memory, with the hallucinatory process involving the act of remembering itself' (p. 41).

## Sully

'Illusion of memory' was defined by Sully (1895/1881)[5] as:

> a false recollection or a wrong reference of an idea to some region of the past. It might, perhaps, be roughly described as a wrong interpretation of a special kind of mental image, namely, what I have called a mnemonic image . . . Mnemonic illusion is thus distinct from mere forgetfulness or imperfect memory (pp. 241–2).

He identified three components in accurate recollections: 'When I distinctly recall an event, I am immediately sure of three things: (i) that something did really happen to me; (ii) that it happened in the way I now think; and (iii) that it happened when it appears to have happened. I cannot be said to recall a past event unless I feel sure on each of these points.' (p. 242). Based on these components, he suggested three types of illusions of memory: '(i) false recollections, to which there correspond no real events of personal history; (ii) others which misrepresent the manner of happening of the events; and (iii) others which falsify the date of the events remembered.' (p. 243). Using the analogy of 'visual illusions', Sully suggested a mechanism for each: 'Class (i) may be likened to the optical illusion known as subjective sensations of light, or ocular spectra. Here we can prove that there is nothing actually seen in the field of vision . . . similarly, we shall find that there is nothing actually recollected . . . such illusions come nearest to hallucinations in the regions of memory . . . Class (ii) has its visual analogue in those optical illusions which depend on effects of haziness and of the action of refracting media . . . in like manner we can say that the images of memory often get obscured, distorted, and otherwise altered . . . Finally, class (iii) has its visual counterpart in erroneous perceptions of distance . . . It will be found that when our memory falsifies the date of an event, the error arises much in the same way as a visual miscalculation of distance' (pp. 243–4).

Sully focused on the first group (the 'hallucinations' of memory):

> what . . . are these false and illegitimate sources of mnemonic images, these unauthorized mints which issue a spurious mental coinage, and so confuse the genuine currency?[6] They consist of two regions of our internal mental life which most closely resemble the actual

perception of real things in vividness and force, namely, dream-consciousness and waking imagination (p. 273).

Later on, Sully added a third mechanism:

Modern science suggests another possible source of these distinct spectra of memory. May it not happen that, by the law of hereditary transmission, which is now being applied to mental as well as bodily phenomena, ancestral experiences will now and then reflect in our mental life and so give rise to apparently personal recollections? (pp. 280–1).

Based on his interesting interactional model of the self, Sully went on to suggest that the notion of personal identity might, in part, be constituted by illusory or false memories.

Sully's functional classification of false memories and his emphasis on mnestic (as opposed to perceptual) function constitute an advance in regards to the old 'brain disparity' theories. However, he made little effort to test his views in the clinical field as Jensen, Sander, Pick and others had done (he does not quote their work). Nonetheless, his views were to influence Kraepelin.

## Kraepelin and the new classification

Under 'paramnesias', Kraepelin (1886) brought together the 'qualitative' memory disturbances. He expanded Sander's concept of memory deceptions by including other 'falsification of memories' (*Erinnerungsfälschungen*). Using a modified version of Sully's classification, he subdivided the entire group into 'partial' phenomena, i.e. falsifications or distortions of true memories analogous to illusions (conflating two of Sully's groups); and 'complete', i.e. 'false' experiences expressed as memories, and viewed as analogous to hallucinations. Focusing on the second group, Kraepelin believed complete falsifications of memory should be viewed as memories which did not correspond to 'real' past experiences, in the same way that hallucinations were considered as perceptions without a corresponding 'real' object. The content of such false memories or 'pseudoreminiscences' consisted of elements of past experiences, combined according to patterns other than the original ones.

Based on the clinical analysis of personal and borrowed case histories, Kraepelin subdivided pseudoreminiscences into: (i) simple (*einfachen Erinnerungsfälschung*), (ii) associating (*associirenden Erinnerungsfälschung*), and (iii) identifying (*identificirenden Erinnerungsfälschung*). The first group included any image that arose spontaneously in the mind, of whatever content, as long as it was experienced as a memory. The second type referred to apparent memories which were evoked by association with a currently perceived object, i.e. the perception of such particular object/event would trigger the false memory whose content, in turn, would involve the object in a specific role. The third type, Kraepelin identified with Sander's 'memory deceptions' (equivalent to the current definition of déjà vu), and consisted of the feeling that the current situation with all its details had been experienced in exactly the same manner at some time in the past.

## 'Simple falsification of memory'

Simple pseudoreminiscences occurred both in health and illness. Healthy subjects could fantasize about fictional characters and on occasions take on their personalities and experiences. Similarly, patients in whose minds the distinction between truth and fantasy, and even the initial intention to deceive, had become blurred could experience these phenomena. Severer forms of simple pseudoreminiscences occurred in pathological conditions, e.g. General Paralysis of the Insane (GPI) and dementia, and also in paranoid and affective psychoses. In GPI, such pseudo-reminiscences were often colourful and 'fantastic', and patients would 'recall' amazing adventures, fantastic journeys and meeting and identifying with famous people. Kraepelin's case 1 referred to a 42-year-old man with GPI who claimed that he had built, *inter alia*, beautiful ships for Russia and a castle in Nüremberg. He was 'Frederick the Great's twin brother', he 'had been with Christ on the cross', he 'was Adam in Paradise' and 'Hercules and Alexander in the battle of Gaugamela', etc., recounting such historical events as being his memories. His 'recollections' were easily guided to other areas by asking him about such new events. His memory for 'real' past experiences as well as for recent events was relatively preserved. Another patient with GPI (Case III) claimed that he had created 76618 planets, and that everything there was better, more colourful: '. . . whilst the camel here is brown, there it is a wonderful sky blue with white and gold splashes . . .' (p. 836). He had also built, in different colours, all the churches in Germany and had led all wars, etc.

Somewhat less fantastic falsification of memories occurred in other organic states such as idiocy/dementia (*Blödsinn*). Kraepelin observed that, in these cases, the immediate or recent past was also invented, and his clinical descriptions are redolent of what nowadays is termed 'confabulations'.[7] These patients would (falsely) report receiving letters or visitors and other events in a convincing manner and in full detail. In some cases, whole days might be reconstructed out of pseudo-reminiscences. Such patients tended to have relatively good memory for events in the distant past, but poor memory for recent events. Kraepelin described a 74-year-old man (Case X) with intellectual and memory deficits who had become childish and irritable, not doing anything, irresponsibly borrowing money, and eating greedily. He was disorientated in time and place and unable to recall recent events or to retain information for any length of time. In place of real memories, he reported detailed false apparent memories although on occasions he would hesitate exclaiming that he was going mad.

Less frequently than in GPI, simple falsifications of memory with fantastic content could also occur in paranoia (*Verrücktheit*).[8] Kraepelin's case V concerned a 26 year-old chronically ill patient who one day claimed that a prince was coming to fetch her. She believed herself to originate from different parents, and would no longer recognize her relatives. She then recalled having lived on earth before, recognizing coetaneous people who had lived in Spain more than 1000 years earlier. On being asked how she knew this, she would respond that this was her recollection: '. . . from memory, one doesn't forget what one has experienced in life . . .' (p. 842).

Yet another chronically psychotic patient (case VII) recounted, in detail, memories involving fantastic and impossible contents. He had taken part in duels, ended wars through his bravery, a bullet had passed through his head and 50 more through his chest – requiring several operations though the scars had all disappeared. His head had been torn off but replaced with an iron one. He believed that people around him, whom he saw for the first time, were actually known to him from earlier times. He described life on the sun, moon and Mars. He was convinced of the truth of his experiences and regarded with suspicion anyone who did not believe him. His mood was changeable but mostly pleasant and friendly. Later, he developed even more grandiose delusions, claiming that his castles and palaces were to be found on the stars, that he had placed kings in charge of these and put the Pope on the moon so that he could bless everything. He had married 1000 times but, becoming tired of his wives, he had married them off to the sovereigns of the stars. He had 100 sons. In hospital, he had been given new lungs and testicles, etc. The patient's memory for true events was intact, but quickly lapsed into his fantastical recollections. Some years later, his delusions receded and he became apathetic, neglecting his appearance, speaking little, and spending a lot of time sitting still in his room. Later on, the old grandiose and persecutory delusional ideas reappeared. These, and other such case descriptions, were grouped by Kraepelin as chronic insanities (*chronische Wahnsinns*). In some, onset was in childhood; in others as late as in their 40s. Many also had sensory deceptions (hallucinations) which tended to be unpleasant and related to persecutory delusions. In contrast, the content of grandiose delusions was considered by Kraepelin to be related to falsification of memories, not because the latter were the origin of the former but both, he believed, arose from the same pathological source.[9]

Patients thus affected were also given to misidentifying people ('Personenverkennung'). For example, new people around them would be identified with those populating their old memories, and considered as acquaintances who had shared with them journeys or experiences. In the course of one conversation, the same person could be 'identified' with any one of a number of earlier protagonists in the patient's recollections. Generally, these patients had good memory for true events, leading Kraepelin to believe that true and the false memories ran independently in their minds. Showing subjective certainty about the truth of their false memories, such patients were unaware that they clashed with their true memories.

Pseudoreminiscences also occurred in Melancholia and Mania. The melancholic mood, by affecting patients' views and perspectives of their past, gave rise to both partial and complete memory falsifications such as 'depressive delusions' of evils or sins committed; for example, one patient claimed that in her youth, she had deceived her parents and chased after men; another patient claimed that he had stolen everything, and yet another had betrayed Germany, etc.[10] Similar paramnesias also developed out of obsessional thoughts. Initially resisted, these experiences later dominated over healthy memories. Sometimes pseudoreminiscences would start with a vague feeling[11] that something terrible had been committed and then would crystallize into a specific 'recollection'. Kraepelin also observed that the content of pseudoreminiscences in Melancholia was more uniform and less colourful than that of pseudoreminiscences in GPI or chronic insanities. On the other hand, the simple pseudoreminiscences of Mania, a mixture of truth and fantasy, were similar to those seen in GPI. Rightly, Kraepelin noted that it was difficult to determine whether such experiences were true pseudoreminiscences (i.e. experienced as recollections) or the grandiose exaggerations of Mania.

In summary, simple pseudoreminiscences were heterogeneous phenomena found both in health and disease and corresponding to experiences variously classified in current terminology as delusions, delusional memories and confabulations. Kraepelin attempted to delineate them further.

(a) They had to be experienced as actual memories. This differentiated them from lying or deliberate deceptions and exaggerations, as well as from hallucinations and simple delusional ideas referring to past events. In regards to the latter, for example, a patient might infer 'information' from a hallucination concerning a past event; this was not a simple pseudoreminiscence for he would not experience it as an actual recollection with its accompanying antecedents and contexts.

(b) The 'falsification' referred to the recollecting process itself and not to the original 'memory' or experience. It was this falsification of the activity of recollecting that distinguished 'true' pseudoreminiscences from hallucinatory reminiscences and delirious reminiscences, which superficially might present in a similar way. In the latter, the reported past event was also false in the sense that it did not correspond to a 'real' event in the past; however, it could be true or 'real' in the sense that it was an actual pathological representation in the patient's mind. This would subsequently be copied by the normal recollecting processes. In other words, for Kraepelin, it was not just the discrepancy between a reported past event and an actual event that constituted a falsification of memory, but the discrepancy had to be manifested through the processes of recollection which in turn (and following the literal definition of 'hallucination' – without a corresponding object), could not be based on any object, real or pathological.

(c) Differentiating between hallucinatory or delirious reminiscences and true pseudoreminiscences might be difficult. Kraepelin suggested that it helped to focus on the content of the experience which was more constant in the case of hallucinatory and delirious reminiscences (because the memory processes were relatively intact and there was the same original representation in the mind caused by the pathology). In the case of true pseudoreminiscences, however, it was less constant as it was not based on any specific representation in the mind and could thus be triggered and/or shifted by skilful questioning.

(d) With respect to mechanisms underlying paramnesias, Kraepelin was less clear. He mentioned 'alterations of consciousness' (*Bewusstseinstrübung*) which occurred with varying severity and caused a reduced capacity to differentiate between reality and fantasy. He made analogies with the 'dream state' (also a form of altered consciousness) where fantasies and real experiences were likewise mixed and indistinguishable.

(e) It was also unclear what sort of process constituted the simple paramnesia. Although accepting that it arose from the same pathological source as the grandiose delusion, Kraepelin believed that the two phenomena were distinct. Because of their relationship to past experiences, he attached greater pathological significance to paramnesias. Following Sully, he based his reasoning on the fact that it was easier for most people (healthy or otherwise) to lose objectivity when evaluating future or present situations for this was coloured by their ongoing mood. In contrast, evaluation of past events was, he believed, less affected by such moods, wishes and biases. Hence, distortions in this sphere betrayed more serious pathology. Because Kraepelin viewed the past as a sum of all past experiences and the foundation of the personality or the self (*unseres Ich*), its pathological evaluation would also imply a significant disturbance of the person's individuality or self.

### 'Associating falsification of memory'

Kraepelin defined 'associating' pseudoreminiscences as those triggered by a current perception. The patient believed that there was a link between his (supposed) past and current perception, and constructed a false relationship between the two. Kraepelin gave the example of a 33-year-old merchant (Case XIV) who 12 years earlier had complained to the police that he was being followed. At that time, he also believed that people were looking and talking about him. He had continued to function relatively well until his psychosis became florid. He started to believe that the newspapers were publishing descriptions of his clothes, the food he ate, what he paid for things, etc. A few weeks prior to his hospital admission, he claimed that he had read in the paper that he was the Royal Pretender and that he would be enthroned within the year. Although he 'remembered' reading these things and 'knew' the exact pages on which they had appeared, he was never able to find the places again. Consequently, he became convinced that the particular articles were being deliberately removed and replaced. On closer questioning, it also emerged that at the time of reading the paper he had not been struck by any articles about him. It was only a few hours or days later that he would suddenly realize that articles were referring to him, at which point he could then recall in detail their contents.

On admission to hospital, he was calm, showed no behavioural disturbance, and his memory seemed excellent. His pseudoreminiscences became apparent when he started talking about another patient. He denied being acquainted with this person prior to his admission, but recalled having heard that he would be meeting him in hospital. Further questioning revealed that he had similar beliefs about other patients and events, for example, remembered having read about the organization of the hospital prior to admission and now knew all details concerning this. Thus, he seemed to link each pseudoreminiscence to a current impression – people, furniture, or conversation around him. News events which occurred whilst he was an inpatient, he likewise claimed to have read/heard about some months previously. Every occurrence was already known to him. He also exhibited an extensive delusional system which appeared to originate in part from sensory deceptions and in part also from simple pseudoreminiscences. He had auditory hallucinations saying that he could hear the hospital director telling another patient his whole history; such hallucinations, however, were infrequent, never hostile, and their contents were interwoven with his ideas and delusions. Kraepelin called them 'apperceptive hallucinations' (*Apperceptionshallucinationen*). As his illness progressed, the pseudoreminiscences shown by this patient became pervasive and he found that the views he had expressed earlier about other things, e.g. the Pope, social reforms etc., were now being printed in the papers, almost word for word. Similarly, jokes he had recounted were also being printed. Finally, it became clear to him that a number of thoughts he had seemingly developed whilst in hospital, he had already had earlier.

This case showed all the features Kraepelin considered as typical of associating pseudoreminiscences. First, particular objects seemed to trigger paramnesias and, as the disease progressed, more and more objects became triggers. Secondly, objects were integrated into the contents of the paramnesia. Kraepelin observed that there was a delay in time between the perception of the object and the construction of the memory which to him suggested that the object alone might not be the sole trigger. Likewise, the content of the pseudoreminiscence was far more detailed than that found in a normal recollection. In addition to real objects, hallucinations could also act as triggers of paramnesias, and, as an example, he reported the case of a patient who developed a chronic insanity following alcoholic delirium tremens and who heard the voices of his sisters talking to him, and through their 'questions', he came to realize that he had committed a number of wrong doings in the past.

The distinction between simple and associating paramnesias thus hinged on the presence in the latter of a trigger which could be a real or a pathological perception. The aetiological or prognostic significance of the trigger itself, however, is unclear. Furthermore, Kraepelin's view that the patient could be aware of the trigger 'by apperception'[12] makes it difficult to distinguish between the associating and simple forms. Nonetheless he analysed in detail the nature of the link between a current perception and a recollection in order to differentiate between associating paramnesias and other phenomena in which such a link might appear to exist, e.g. the misidentification phenomena.[13] In these clinical phenomena, however, the link between present and past impressions was, according to Kraepelin, in the opposite direction, and hence they were the converse of the paramnesias. In the latter it was the current impression that led to the construction of the recollection and was incorporated into it; on the other hand, in the misidentification the past experience gave rise to the construction and meaning attached to the current perception; hence the misidentification was not simply a perceptual disturbance but a complex process resulting from the activity of memory, imagination, judgment, etc.

## 'Identifying falsification of memory'

Kraepelin observed that this was commoner than the 'associating' type of paramnesia and corresponded to Sander's 'memory deceptions' (déjà vu experiences). Kraepelin likewise emphasized that what was perceived as 're-experienced' was the whole situation rather than some of its features. He stressed also that the situation was experienced as identical in every respect (not just similar) and, furthermore, the person was convinced of his experience even if the 'earlier' experience could not be clearly located. For Kraepelin, this 'feeling of identity' suggested an involvement of the self in the deception and was essential to the definition of the phenomenon; it therefore differentiated the identifying from the simple paramnesias. Crucially, for Kraepelin, the 'self' that was involved in the 'identifying' paramnesias related to a 'second-order' disturbance in contrast to the 'self' that was involved in the simple paramnesias which reflected a disturbance of the actual structure of the self.

These phenomena were, however, fleeting. Kraepelin argued that this made Sander's 'similarity' hypothesis implausible as this predicted a longer-lasting paramnesia. Kraepelin's views, however, seem to have been based on borrowed cases and a few reports by healthy people. Because of this he mostly iterated earlier descriptions (feelings of unease, premonition, etc.), although he suggested 'perceptual change' (environment seen as dark, shadowy) and a 'temporary halt in thought flow' as additional features. Kraepelin found all earlier explanatory theories unsatisfactory but limited himself to favouring the mechanism of 'altered consciousness' on the grounds that these paramnesias tended to be associated with fatigue (known to cause attention to shift from the outside to the self) and epilepsy.

The 'paramnesias' as a unified class encompassing Kraepelin's manifold qualitative memory disturbances did not appear to survive for long. Instead, focus on particular subgroups falling within the paramnesias resulted in the delineation of phenomena which became conceptualized as independent entities. Very broadly, this fragmentation seemed to develop along two main lines, namely: (i) paramnesias as *false recognitions* (i.e. déjà vu phenomena and subsequently jamais vu, misidentifications and reduplicative paramnesias) and, (ii) paramnesias as *false recollections* (subsequently confabulations, delusional memories).

## Paramnesias as 'false recognitions'

In France, interest in the paramnesias peaked in the 1890s as illustrated by the famous debate in the journal Revue Philosophique between Lalande, Dugas, Lapie, Le Lorrain and others where these experiences were viewed in the specific and narrow sense of false recognition, i.e. in the déjà vu sense (equivalent to Sander's memory deceptions and Kraepelin's identifying pseudoreminiscences). Lalande (1893) expressed this directly when he proposed that the term 'paramnesias' should be exclusively reserved for such experiences and reiterated the clinical characteristics described by Sander. Dugas (1894), who followed in the debate, made a distinction between the 'impression of déjà vu' and paramnesia or false memory proper. He conceived the former as a type of confusion, a partial illusion, where false 'recognition' of a situation occurred on the basis of actual similarities to previous experiences and hence was explicable by analogy. Paramnesia, by contrast, was a total illusion in that a new situation was experienced as identical to a previous one. Not based on any similarity, it was therefore inexplicable, and this resulted in the accompanying affective state. The impression of déjà vu, he noted, was commoner and involved single objects or groups of things. Paramnesia, on the other hand, related to a situation in its totality: 'a current section of life ('tranche de vie'), cut out and transported into the past' (p. 39). Dugas also differentiated between paramnesias with (complete) and paramnesias without (simple), the feeling of premonition and proposed different mechanisms for each. On the other hand, Le Lorrain (1894) argued that paramnesias with premonition should not be classed as paramnesias but as telepathic phenomena. Lapie (1894) proposed that imagination created situations that were then stored and that, on occasion, coincided with real-life perceptions and hence gave rise to false recognition.

The Revue Philosophique debate was not satisfactorily resolved. However, it narrowed and reconceptualized the paramnesias as disorders of recognition which were due to multiple disturbances involving sensory/perceptual/cognitive processes (e.g. telepathy, hypnosis, imagination, dreams, double personality) rather than memory disturbances *per se*. (Those who did concentrate on the memory model (e.g. Bourdon, 1893; Le Lorrain, 1894), tended to conceptualize the paramnesias as the false recognition of single objects or groups of objects rather than the false recognition of the total experience.) This shift in focus was made explicit by Arnaud (1896) at a meeting of the Société Médico-Psychologique: 'I believe that it would be better to abandon these words false memory and paramnesia which have the double disadvantage of being vague and inexact – since it is not certain whether the phenomenon in question is in fact associated with memory. Thus, to keep things clear and avoid theoretical assumptions, I suggest the term illusion of déjà vu' (p. 455).

After briefly referring to Wigan, Jensen, Sander, Pick, Anjel, Forel, Kraepelin, Ribot, Lalande, Dugas and Sollier, Arnaud claimed (as had earlier French authors) that the prevalence of the déjà vu illusion had been exaggerated and confused with analogous states such as vague memories. He pointed out that déjà vu had two fundamental characteristics: intensity of the feeling – which bordered on conviction, and identity of the subjective current state with the ostensible past situation. He further distinguished between a 'mild' form of déjà vu, a 'normal' experience of short duration, which ceased abruptly and was rectifiable; and a 'severe' form, a pathological phenomenon which lasted much longer and was rarely susceptible to rectification. As an example of the severe form, Arnaud (1896) reported the case of Louis, a 34-year-old graduate from Saint Cyr (the French Military Academy) who had experienced déjà vu as a child. After developing cerebral malaria, he was found, in 1891, also to be suffering from anterograde and retrograde amnesia. After 7 months, he improved from his malaria but his memory remained poor. In 1893, Louis showed 'the first symptoms characteristic of déjà vu' when he started claiming that he could recognize certain newspaper articles which he said he had read previously. He even claimed to have written many of them himself. At the marriage of his brother, he insisted that he had attended the same ceremony a year before, in identical conditions and he couldn't understand why everything was happening again. On admission to hospital, he immediately 'recognized' everything he saw, including the rooms, the park outside, the staff, their words and gestures and his own responses. He also claimed to recognize all great public events and this led him to make errors in dates saying the year was 1895 since newspapers were dated 1894. He felt that he was re-doing and re-perceiving the same things and re-experiencing the same emotions, mental states and dreams. He summarized this as 'I am living two parallel years' (p. 460).

Arnaud explored the nature of this severe form of déjà vu arguing that, although the phenomenon appeared to be experienced as a memory, it was not in fact a true disturbance of memory. First, the 'recognition' in déjà vu, in contrast to the recognition in true memories, was unstable; for example, in the case of Louis, when his environment was manipulated, his 'recognition' adapted correspondingly to the changes without apparent loss of vividness. In other words, the localization of the experience in space was in reality always that of the present perception. Similarly, the specific localization in time to one year previously was simply the result of reasoning by the patient. Secondly, a true memory consisted of a situation evoking a network of related recollections acting as its context. The illusory memory or déjà vu consisted only of the current situation: 'consisting of nothing more, nothing less than the contents of the present perception' (p. 466). For example, when Louis saw someone from behind, he claimed to 'recognize' them, but on further questioning, he could not provide any information other than the description afforded by the back view. Thus, the illusion of déjà vu was simply the current perception projected into the past or a retrospective perception (*une perception rétroactive/rétrospective*).

Arnaud's case shows singular features that differentiate it from the usual form of déjà vu: (i) it had a surprising specificity of localization in time (to one year earlier), (ii) it combined both false recognition and false recollection, e.g. Louis 'recognized' articles in newspapers but also insisted that he had written some himself, and claimed to be living parallel lives (i.e. there was a duplication of experiences), (iii) the affective component seemed at times incongruent with his experiences (e.g. smiling at his recognition of the doctor). All these features suggest alternative (current) clinical diagnoses such as a delusional state or a delusional misidentification or reduplication. Furthermore, by focusing on particular aspects of the case, Arnaud concluded that Louis had a perceptual rather than a memory disorder (hence his proposed change in terminology). Arnaud's perceptual view was touched upon by subsequent participants in the debate such as Pierre Janet, who in the main agreed, and Paul Garnier who advocated the continuous use of the term 'false memory/paramnesia' for it drew attention to the fact that the phenomenon occurred predominantly in those with memory impairment.

Arnaud's paper marks a turning point in the conceptualization of 'false recognitions'. Two years later, and based on the results of a postal survey, Bernard-Leroy (1898) tried to re-categorize false recognition/déjà vu as a memory disturbance (Berrios, 1995). Later writers, however (e.g. Dromard & Albès, 1907), continued the drift away from the 'memory' explanation.

## Dromard and Albès

These writers made a further distinction between déjà vu (or *déjà éprouvé*) and false recognition (*fausse reconnaissance*), defining the former as a simple, normal, and transient phenomenon in which the subject felt as if he were re-experiencing a section of his life, and which involved no impairment of judgment. False recognition, on the other hand, they viewed as a false, pathological and persistent belief involving an alteration of judgment (Dromard & Albès, 1907). Instead of relating to a 'section of life' or the 'totality of an experience', false recognition related to single things or groups of things or people (falsely) recognized in isolation.

Dromard and Albès introduced a new explanatory element by expanding upon Janet's idea that false recognition resulted from a loss of the 'feeling of (present) reality' (which like Janet, they conceived as a specific mental function). Patients experiencing false recognition were thus unable to distinguish the real from the unreal. As an example, Dromard and Albès (1907) reported the case of a man with a past history of hallucinations and persecutory ideas who had been admitted to hospital following arrest by the police. He was picked up outside the Ministry of the Interior where he had been demanding a full review of the birth certificates of those born after 1870. He said that people were confused and needed to know definitively who they were and where they came from. On admission to hospital, he claimed to 'recognize' amongst the patients, people he knew (e.g. a previous boss) and expressed surprise at seeing so many familiar people in the hospital.

By reconceptualizing false recognition as a misidentification of specific objects rather than as a 'false recognition' of a particular experience, Dromard and Albès came close to describing the phenomenon of delusional misidentification, specifically, the Capgras symptom, the Frégoli symptom and intermetamorphosis (Marková & Berrios, 1994); and by viewing the phenomenon of false recognition as an impairment of judgement, they reconceptualized false recognition and false non-recognition as being the positive and negative poles of a common process.

## 'Reduplicative paramnesia'

Of all the group of phenomena that originally were called paramnesias, the reduplicative paramnesia is the only one to have survived, at least in name. It is still occasionally conceived as a qualitative memory disturbance.

### Pick

After reporting at least one earlier case,[14] Arnold Pick (1903) coined the term 'reduplicative paramnesia' to refer to

a continuous series of events in the patient's remembrance, subsequently fall into manifold occurrences; the isolated events, though they remain pretty clearly in his memory, are impressed on him as repetitions thereof (p. 261).

Pick's first case had been of a patient with GPI who claimed that there were two clinics exactly alike in which he had been, two professors of the same name were at the head of these clinics, etc. Pick's second case was of a 67-year-old lady with senile dementia/presbyophrenia[15] who again showed marked memory impairment and disorientation in time. She had fluctuations in mood and various fleeting delusions changing in content and relating to numerous 'illusionary' phenomena. She also confabulated. In contrast to the first patient, her reduplicative paramnesia was more selective, i.e. she only claimed that she was in the 'same clinic' (as the one in Prague) but that this was situated elsewhere. She did not, however, duplicate the professor (and assistants) insisting instead that the same professor was head of both (identical) clinics and the assistants also worked in both clinics. In addition, the patient expressed the (false) belief that she had experienced the same situation before: 'This is already the second time that I have had the advantage of your valued treatment' (p. 264).

The 'duplication' in reduplicative paramnesia could thus relate not only to places and people but also to time. Again, this shows similarity to the false recognition/déjà vu phenomena described above. In his initial explanation for reduplicative paramnesia, Pick had suggested that the clinical phenomenon was a disturbance of the 'sense of familiarity' (*Bekanntheitsgefühl*). Subsequently, however, he proposed that the basic disturbance was a loss of continuity between consecutive mental impressions. The latter, in turn, resulted from mental and memory disturbances caused by the background disease (e.g. GPI/dementia, etc.). Thus patients 'cannot identify one situation from the other, which become duplicated and eventually divided into a multiplicity of events' (p. 267). Pick also believed that the selectivity of reduplicated 'objects' observed in his second patient was the result of a relatively greater preservation of intellect.

## Coriat

Coriat (1904) reviewed Pick's cases and reported further examples occurring in patients with Korsakov's psychosis, alcoholic deterioration and general paralysis. According to this author, reduplicative paramnesia could be explained by a combination of dissociation and disturbance of the sense of familiarity

it is the inability to bridge over the dissociated memory images, associated perhaps with a feeling of having experienced certain events . . . before, and being unable to connect or correct this sense of familiarity with previous or present experiences on account of these gaps (p. 653).

Coriat's interest in the 'sense of familiarity' biased his recognition of the disorder and it is questionable whether his second case is actually an instance of reduplicative paramnesia. It concerned a 40-year-old labourer with a long history of heavy alcohol intake. A few months prior to hospital admission, he stopped working and began accusing his wife of infidelity. His memory seemed to be deteriorating in that he failed (spontaneously) verbally to recall places he had been to before. He became increasingly flat and apathetic and was admitted to hospital whereupon he expressed his concerns about his wife's infidelity. Otherwise he was well orientated and showed no deficits in recent memory. He claimed, however, that he had been in the hospital 1 year previously and subsequently added that, at that time, he had been seen and treated by the same doctors and in the same room. Some days later, he stated that he had been in the hospital 2 years previously. Later still, he mentioned that he had been in the hospital four times in as many years, undergoing similar treatments and seeing the same people on each occasion. It is thus apparent that, in contrast to the 'classic' description, his 'reduplication' related only to time and not to places or people. Remarking on the similarity between Coriat's and Arnaud's case, Rosenberg (1912) considered that both showed pathological forms of déjà vu in the context of paranoid psychoses. He argued that since Coriat's patient remained orientated and showed no evidence of impaired memory for recent events, he did not experience any loss of continuity in his mental impressions and thus was not predisposed to reduplication of his experiences. Rosenberg went on to stress that organic memory disorder was a necessary condition for the development of reduplicative paramnesia.

During the late nineteenth century, the paramnesias conceived, in general terms, as mere 'false recognitions' became fragmented. For example, paramnesias were classified according to: (i) their object, i.e. whether the recognition related to a particular experience in its entirety ('section of life') or to a single object (persons/places/things); this favoured the differentiation between déjà vu/jamais vu phenomena and misidentification/reduplication phenomena, respectively; (ii) the duration of the false recognition, i.e. whether it was fleeting or persistent, leading to their grading as mild and severe; relevant to the latter was whether or not the underlying process was delusional; (iii) type of recognition, i.e. relationship to normal recognition processes, thus stimulating the debate on the nature of the underlying process, i.e. whether it involved memory, perception or other functions; (iv) the presence/absence of an organic-memory deficit influenced whether the phenomenon was conceptualized as 'neurological' or 'psychiatric', respectively. More recently, attempts have again been made to seek a common mechanism, particularly in respect to delusional misidentification and reduplicative paramnesia (Alexander et al., 1979; Joseph, 1986; Röhrenbach & Landis, 1995).

## Paramnesias as 'false recollections'

In general, less work has been focused on paramnesias as 'false recollections', i.e. referring to 'memories' of events that have not in reality taken place (conflation of Kraepelin's simple and associating falsification of memories). This view was sponsored by Korsakoff.

## Korsakoff

Korsakoff (1891) described two forms of memory disturbance in patients with 'polyneuritic' psychosis (*polyneurotischer Psychose*). First, patients suffered from amnesia for recent events whilst retaining relatively good memory for distant events. Secondly, patients suffered from pseudoreminiscences or falsification of memory (*gefälschten Erinnerungen*). Following earlier writers, Korsakoff sub-divided the second group (*Erinnerungstäuschungen*) into: (i) sudden feeling of having experienced a particular situation in exactly the same way before, including having the same thoughts, speech, etc. (i.e. equivalent to Kraepelin's 'identifying memory deceptions'), and (ii) real or true pseudoreminiscences (*eigentlichen Pseudoreminiscenzen*) whereby an event never experienced by the patient, simply entered his mind and was believed by him as being a true past experience. In such cases,

a patient might claim that he was Alexander of Macedonia, that he had taken the trip to India. He would claim to recall how everything happened and could relate all sorts of details about the trip as if he had actually experienced it (p. 391).

Korsakov believed that analysis of this second group revealed the kernel of the pseudoreminiscence to be a true memory; hence, they corresponded to Kraepelin's partial falsifications of memory or illusions of memory. (His case descriptions, however, are more suggestive of Kraepelin's complete falsifications of memory/hallucinations of memory.)

In addition to polyneuritic psychosis, pseudoreminiscences also occurred in paranoia, melancholia, mania, GPI, and senile dementia. He described patients with polyneuritic psychosis: 'on being questioned about how they spent their day, often gave detailed accounts of trips, meetings, etc. detailing these as if they had truly had the experiences.

. . . In most cases, the patient will change his account of such fantastic memories, e.g. one patient who had just reported that he had driven to hospital, forgot this in the next minute and subsequently gave an account of having gone hunting and shooting ducks' (p. 392).[16]

In some patients, the false content of their memories persisted and gave rise to delusional ideas.

Following some detailed case descriptions (Korsakoff, 1891), Korsakoff concluded that polyneuritic psychosis was often accompanied by memory deceptions as well as delusions based on the latter. He described such delusions as commonly relating to themes of death and funerals. With time, pseudoreminiscences became stronger and, from these, delusional ideas gained their force, resulting in a picture of partial insanity. Korsakoff claimed that in polyneuritic psychosis, pseudo-reminiscences were almost always based on a true/real memory, and likely to arise from the linking of memory traces into fairly constant associations. Such associations were, in turn, more likely to form if there was a pre-existing disorder of the mechanism involved in the association of ideas, such as was found in some psychoses.

## Wernicke

Wernicke (1906) contributed to the understanding of the paramnesias by making a further distinction between delusional misinterpretation of memories (*retrospectiven Beziehungswahn*) and falsification of memories (*Erinnerungsfälschungen*). The former consisted of real memories being delusionally misinterpreted, e.g. a patient with grandiose delusions remembered being spoken to by an Officer when he was a young boy; only later did he 'realize', on the basis of certain similarities, that this Officer, was actually Kaiser Wilhelm or Kaiser Friedrich or some equally high-ranking personality. At the same time, he had been asked at school by his teacher whether he still had a father or grandfather; this question, he also came to realize, related to this high-ranking personality and he subsequently knew where to look for his father or grandfather. The objection that this could have been a 'neutral' question was dismissed by the patient on the grounds that the teacher had given him a meaningful glance and a hand signal.

It was important, Wernicke claimed, to differentiate this delusional misinterpretation of memory from a falsification of memory which presented in a positive and a negative form. The positive form or 'confabulation' consisted of the appearance of memories of experiences which had never actually occurred; the content of these confabulations was generally in keeping with the rest of delusions (*Wahn*). For example, patients with persecutory delusions related (confabulated) adventures in which they had supposedly been followed. Wernicke believed that there was a link between confabulations and disturbances of memory and that this was further confirmed clinically by the fact that confabulations were seen particularly in mental illnesses accompanied by memory deficits such as hebephrenia, presbyophrenia and GPI. He considered that the fantastic content of some confabulations resembled that of dreams and that (once lying was excluded), such confabulations represented true memories of dreams.

On the other hand, Wernicke defined the negative form of 'falsification of memories' as consisting of the appearance of circumscribed deficits or gaps in an otherwise well-retained memory database and when there was no reason to suspect a disturbance of the senses or of attentional loss at the time of the particular experience. This was necessary since it would not be surprising to observe memory gaps in patients with meningitis, epilepsy or delirium tremens who, at the time, would have suffered from disturbed attention. In negative falsification of memories, however, single or individual events taking place in full consciousness became lost whilst attending (surrounding) events were remembered. Two elements helped explain negative falsifications of memory, namely, presence at the time of (i) a particularly strong affect, and (ii) an overvalued idea (*überwerthigen Idee*). Hence, this clinical phenomenon was common in chronic partial psychoses: for example, a patient under the influence of an overvalued idea, believed that a particular official was his personal enemy and insulted him. He subsequently denied that he had done so (i.e. he showed a memory gap for the event).

According to Wernicke, delusional interpretation of memories were to be considered as qualitative falsifications of memory whilst the positive and negative forms were quantitative falsifications of memory. The latter, he suggested, were better termed additive and subtractive forms, respectively. All three forms shared an underlying mechanism, namely a disconnection (Sejunction). For example, in confabulation (additive form) there was a disconnection between the recollected experience (whether this was real, imagined or a dream) and time. It is thus clear that Wernicke's classification was different from Kraepelin's who had considered all 'false memories' as qualitative memory disturbances. Wernicke's contribution led to a further narrowing of the falsifications of memories. Thus, he conceived qualitative memory falsification as extrinsic to the memory or recollecting process itself; in other words, memory is intact but the quality of the recollection, as manifest by the different colouring or significance, is altered by the delusional process. In contrast, quantitative memory falsifications are intrinsic to the recollection itself in the sense that there is either an increase in (false) memories or a decrease in (true) memories.

## After Wernicke

In historical terms, Wernicke's view marks the final split of the false recollections into delusions (both delusional notion and delusional perception/interpretation à la Kurt Schneider) and confabulations. Fundamental to this division is the putative link of confabulations with a real memory deficit. Indeed, this became the main criterion as for example used by Chaslin (1912) (see also Berrios 1999b). But this also means that the crucial question, namely whether delusional memories and confabulations are differentiable on phenomenological grounds alone, was left unanswered.

Jaspers' (1948/1913) classification of memory falsifications was also unclear on phenomenological grounds. He distinguished between false memories (*Trugerinnerungen*) on the one hand and other memory falsifications (*Erinnerungsfälschungen*) on the other. Conceptualizing the former as 'hallucinations of memory' (following Kahlbaum, 1866), he nevertheless did not make clear how these differed from delusional ideas (*Wahnvorstellungen*). The other memory falsifications were further divided into (i) pathological lying, (ii) attribution of new meanings to past (true) events (i.e. delusional misinterpretation) and, (iii) confabulation. Again, however, it would appear that the main distinction between false memories (*Trugerinnerungen*) and confabulation is the presence, in the latter, of an organic memory impairment. Schneider (1959) viewed memory falsification as resulting from delusional processes, either in the form of delusional perception or as sudden delusional ideas: 'qualitative disturbance of memory in schizophrenia and cyclothymia are, however, not really disturbances of memory but delusional elaboration of memory and spontaneous delusional notions' (pp. 125–6). Current textbooks (e.g. Gelder et al., 1996) and standardized interview schedules (e.g. PSE, Wing et al., 1974) continue to use the term 'delusional memories' to refer to 'false memories' reported by psychotic patients but they do not always indicate what the exact distinction is between these experiences and conventional delusional perception or delusional interpretation of memories. Lastly, others have concentrated on whether the distinction has any diagnostic significance (Buchanan, 1991).

## Conclusions

During the nineteenth century, the generic term paramnesia was used to refer to a group of clinical phenomena amongst which déjà vu, confabulations, and delusions and hallucinations of memory remain the more salient. These phenomena had been known since earlier but it was only after the work of Sander that they began to be considered as 'memory' disorders. In Kraepelin's taxonomy the paramnesias are included as 'qualitative' disorders of memory affecting either recognition or recollection. However, towards the turn of the century, the concept of memory was noticeably narrowed down and the paramnesias were set asunder. They have been neglected since. Déjà vu remains a curiosity seen in some forms of epilepsy and occasionally in the normal affected by fatigue. Delusions of memory are occasionally mentioned in the literature but hallucinations of memory have disappeared altogether.

And yet these phenomena need explanation. It has been suggested in this chapter that their study may force upon us a broader definition of memory than the one currently in play and one which may prove to be more useful to neuropsychiatry. Because these phenomena do not figure as 'symptoms' in most current nosologies, they are no longer searched for, and hence their incidence and prevalence in clinical populations (let alone their epidemiology in the community) are unknown. However, the conceptual, historical and clinical information provided in this chapter suggests that it might be clinically worthwhile to return to these phenomena not only in relation to patients explicitly complaining of memory disorders but also in subjects with functional psychosis as they might provide the clinician with new phenomenological markers.

## REFERENCES

Alexander, M.P., Stuss, D.T. & Benson, D.F. (1979). Capgras syndrome: a reduplicative phenomenon. *Neurology*, **29**, 334–9.

Anjel (no initial) (1878). Beitrag zum capitel über erinnerugstäuschungen. *Archiv für Psychiatrie und Nervenkrankheiten*, **8**, 57–64.

Arnaud, M. (1896). Un cas d'illusion de 'déjà vu' ou de 'fausse mémoire'. *Annales Médico-Psychologiques*, **54**, 455–71.

Bernard-Leroy, E. (1898). *L'Illusion de fausse reconnaissance. Contribution à l'étude des conditions psychologiques de la reconnaissance des souvenirs.* Paris: Alcan.

Berrios, G.E. (1985). Presbyophrenia: clinical aspects. *British Journal of Psychiatry*, **147**, 76–9.

Berrios, G.E. (1986). Presbyophrenia: the rise and fall of a concept. *Psychological Medicine*, **16**, 267–75.

Berrios, G.E. (1995). Déjà vu and other disorders of memory during the nineteenth century. *Comprehensive Psychiatry*, **36**, 123–9.

Berrios, G.E. (1996a). *The History of Mental Symptoms. Descriptive Psychopathology Since the 19th Century.* Cambridge: Cambridge University Press.

Berrios, G.E. (1996b). The Classification of Mental Disorders: Part III. K.L. kahlbaum. translation with an introduction. *History of Psychiatry*, 7, 167–182.

Berrios, G.E. (1999a). The History of Memory and its disorders. In *Neuropsychiatric Aspects of Memory Complaints*, ed. G.E. Berrios & J.R. Hodges. Cambridge: Cambridge University Press (in press).

Berrios, G.E. (1999b). Confabulation. In *Neuropsychiatric Aspects of Memory Complaints*, ed. G.E. Berrios & J.R. Hodges. Cambridge: Cambridge University Press (in press).

Berrios, G.E. & Luque, R. (1995). Cotard's delusion or syndrome? *Comprehensive Psychiatry*, **36**, 218–23.

Bourdon, B. (1893). La reconnaissance de phénomènes nouveaux. *Revue Philosophique*, **36**, 629–31.

Buchanan, A. (1991). Delusional memories: first rank symptoms? *British Journal of Psychiatry*, **159**, 472–4.

Chaslin, P. (1912). *Éléments de sémiologie et clinique mentales.* Paris: Asselin et Houzeau.

Coriat, I.H. (1904). Reduplicative Paramnesia. *Journal of Nervous and Mental Disease*, **31**, 571–87; 639–59.

Dromard, G. & Albès, A. (1907). Folie du doute et illusion de fausse reconnaissance. *Revue de Psychiatrie*, **11**, 12–17.

Dugas, L. (1894). Observations sur la fausse mémoire. *Revue Philosophique*, **37**, 34–45.

Eyselein, O. (1875). Ueber erinnerugstäuschungen. *Archiv für Psychiatrie und Nervenkrankheiten*, **5**, 575–7.

Feuchtersleben, von E. (1847). *The Principles of Medical Psychology.* Trans. H.E. Lloyd & B.G. Babington, London: Sydenham Society (1st German edn, 1845).

Fuentenebro, F. & Berrios, G.E. (1995). The predelusional state: a conceptual history. *Comprehensive Psychiatry*, **36**, 251–9.

Gelder, M., Gath, D., Mayou, R. & Cowen, P. (1996). *Oxford Textbook of Psychiatry*, 3rd edn. Oxford: Oxford University Press.

Hoff, P. (1995) Kraepelin. In *A History of Clinical Psychiatry*, ed. G.E. Berrios & R. Porter, pp. 261–79. London, Athlone Press.

Jackson, J.H. (1932). *Selected Writings of John Hughlings Jackson*, ed. J. Taylor, 2 vols. London: Hodder and Stoughton.

Jaspers, K. (1948). *Allgemeine Psychopathologie*, 5th edn. Berlin: Springer (1st edn 1913).

Jensen (no initial) (1868). Ueber Doppelwahrnehmungen in der gesunden, wie in der kranke Psyche. *Allgemeine Zeitschrift für Psychiatrie*, **25** (Supplement-Heft): 48–63.

Joseph, A.B. (1896). Focal central nervous abnormalities in patients with misidentification syndromes. *Bibliotheca Psychiatrica*, **164**, 68–79.

Kahlbaum, K. (1866.) Die Sinnesdelirien. *Allgemeine Zeitschrift für Psychiatrie*, **23**, 1–86.

Korsakoff, S.S. (1891). Erinnerugstäuschungen (Pseudoreminiscenzen) bei polyneuritischer psychose. *Allgemeine Zeitschrift für Psychiatrie*, **47**, 390–410.

Kraepelin, E. (1886–1887). Ueber erinnerungsfälschungen. *Archiv für Psychiatrie und Nervenkrankheiten*, **17**, 830–43, **18**, 199–239; 395–436.

Lalande, A. (1893). Des Paramnésies. *Revue Philosophique*, **36**, 485–97.

Lange, K. (1899). *Über Apperzeption*. Leipzig, R. Voigtländer.

Lapie, P. (1894). Note sur la paramnésie. *Revue Philosophique*, **37**, 351–2.

Le Lorrain, J. (1894). A propos de la paramnésie. *Revue Philosophique*, **37**, 208–10.

Marková, I.S. (1997). Sander's 'memory deceptions'. *History of Psychiatry*, **8**, 555–67.

Marková, I.S. & Berrios, G.E. (1994). Delusional misidentifications: facts and fancies. *Psychopathology*, **27**, 136–43.

Pick, A. (1876). Zur casuistik der erinnerugstäuschungen. *Archiv für Psychiatrie und Nervenkrankheiten*, **6**, 568–74.

Pick, A. (1903). Clinical studies – III. On reduplicative paramnesia. *Brain*, **26**, 260–7.

Röhrenbach, C. & Landis, T. (1995). Dream journeys: living in woven realities, the syndrome of reduplicative paramnesia. In *Broken Memories. Case Studies in Memory Impairment*, ed. R. Campbell & M.A. Conway, pp. 93–100. Oxford: Blackwell.

Sander, W. (1874). Ueber erinnerugstäuschungen. *Archiv für Psychiatrie und Nervenkrankheiten*, **4**, 244–53.

Schneider, K. (1959). *Clinical Psychopathology*. Trans. M.W. Hamilton. New York: Grune & Stratton.

Sully, J. (1895). *Illusions: a Psychological Study*, 4th edn. London: Kegan Paul (1st edn 1881).

Sully, J. (1918). *My Life and Friends. A Psychologist's Memories*. London: T. Fisher Unwin Ltd.

Wernicke, K. (1906). *Grundriss der Psychiatrie*, 2nd edn. Leipzig: Thieme.

Wigan, A.L. (1844). *The Duality of the Mind*. London: Longman, Brown, Green and Longmans.

Wing, J.K., Cooper, J.E. & Sartorius, N. (1974). *Measurement and Classification of Psychiatric Symptoms*. Cambridge, UK: Cambridge University Press.

# Déjà vu and jamais vu

Herman N. Sno

This chapter is concerned with two types of paramnesia: déjà vu and jamais vu. Paramnesia, a term which is nowadays rarely used in medical practice (Berrios, 1995), refers to a group of memory anomalies associated with both non-pathological and pathological conditions (see Chapter 14, this volume). It is to be regretted that current interest in memory disorders tends to focus on memory loss (as in the amnestic syndrome and dementia) to the detriment of the study of the paramnesias. Indeed, clinicians with little free time on their hands to keep up with the theoretical literature on memory disorders should be able to use the paramnesias as a vantage point to study the processes of memory. After discussing divergent views on, and describing some types of, 'paramnesia', this chapter will deal with the clinical features of the déjà vu and jamais vu experiences.

## Paramnesia

Paramnesia denotes false memory. The term derives from the Greek *para-*, meaning from (the side), beside near, beyond, against, and *-mnesis*, meaning memory (Campbell, 1996). The term paramnesia was coined by Emil Kraepelin (1887) in analogy of terms such as paranoia, paraphasia and paraphrenia, as a general term 'to denote pseudoreminiscences or illusions and hallucinations of memory' (Burnham, 1889). Following James Sully's book *Illusions* (1881), Kraepelin (1887) differentiated between a total (*völlige Erinnerungsfälschung*) and a partial (*'theilweise Erinnerungsverfälschung'*) form of paramnesia. The latter form is based on distortions or elaborations of real events, the former emerges independent of any real events of personal history. By comparison with perception disorders, the partial form corresponds with illusions and the total form with hallucinations. Kraepelin (1887) divided the total form of paramnesia into the *einfache* (simple), *associirende* (Berrios, 1995: 'evoked'; Burnham, 1889: 'suggested or associating') and *identificirende* (Berrios, 1995: 'identified'; Burnham, 1889: identifying) subtypes. The first subtype includes spontaneous images that appear as memories; the second includes present perceptions that evoke pseudomemories by association with something analogous or related in the past; and the third includes a new experience that appears as a photographic copy of a former one. The identifying subtype corresponds with the phenomenon that is now generally known as the déjà vu experience (Burnham, 1889; Sno & Linszen, 1990).

Since Kraepelin (1887), the international debate on paramnesia has been obscured by divergent interpretations. In France, André Lalande (1893) and Paul Lapie (1893) seemed to equate paramnesia with the déjà vu experience. More recently, Henri Ey et al. (1978) described paramnesia as falsifications of the mnemonic performance resulting in an entanglement of the present with the past, and of the perception of reality with imagination: 'Either the present is pathologically associated with the past (*fausse reconnaissances*, impression de déjà vu),' or the present is excessively dissociated from the past (*illusion de* Sosie ou de non-*reconnaissance*, impression de jamais vu). Arnold Pick (1903) coined the term reduplicative paramnesia to delineate a delusional reduplication of place. It has been recently suggested to extend Pick's concept to include the delusional reduplication of time and person (Sno, 1994).

Havelock Ellis (1911) also regarded paramnesia as 'the psychologist's name for a hallucination of memory which (. . .) is often termed by French authors "false recognition" or "sensation du déjà vu"'. This famous English physician argued that the déjà vu experience may be termed 'hypnagogic paramnesia', because it occurs in the 'ante-chamber of sleep, but not necessary before sleep' (. . .) 'when a centrally excited sensation of one order (dream image) is mistaken for a centrally excited sensation of another order (memory)'. Banister and Zangwill (1941), in turn, suggested 'restricted paramnesia' for experiences of familiarity with a genuine foundation in the past history of the individual and provoked by a less well-defined aspect of a perceptual situation. This type of paramnesia would correspond to Kraepelin's 'evoked' or 'associating' subtype. Likewise, their definition of the déjà vu experience, which Banister and Zangwill distinguished from restricted paramnesia, would correspond to Kraepelin's 'identifying' subtype. Campbell's (1996) psychiatric dictionary makes use of a definition of paramnesia very similar to Ey's: disturbance of memory in which real facts and fantasies are confused.

Reed (1979) has pointed out that a degree of distortion of recall, as opposed to forgetting, is the crucial feature of paramnesia. Influenced by Sir Frederic Bartlett (1932), the Canadian researcher sees paramnesia as illustrating well the fact that recall is never the retrieval of inert mnestic representations but involves active reconstruction. As examples, Reed (1979) reported a variety of everyday experiences such as the 'I can't quite place him', the 'know the face but not the name', the 'time-gap', the 'fleeting-thought', the 'feeling of knowing', 'tip of the tongue', cryptomnesia, 'checking', déjà vu and jamais vu phenomena. The first two correspond well to the perceptual disturbance of prosopagnosia as described by Bodamer

(1947). One form of 'time-gap' experience is also known as 'highway-hypnosis'.

In the United States, Burnham (1889) distinguished, following Kraepelin's classification, between the simple, suggested or associating, and identifying paramnesia. In 1920, Alfred Gordon also used paramnesia as a synonym for the déjà vu experience, in his own terms the illusion of 'the already seen'. In 1944, Morton Leeds described the 'illusion of déjà vu' as only one form of paramnesia. Of late, Strauss (1995) has defined paramnesia as a falsification of memory by distortion of recall, including *fausse reconnaissance*, retrospective falsification, confabulation, déjà vu and jamais vu. (Parenthetically, the term *fausse reconnaissance* is generally regarded as an alternative designation for the déjà vu experience (Sno & Linszen, 1990).) Retrospective falsification, in turn, corresponds to Kraepelin's partial paramnesia (1887). The various types of paramnesia and the corresponding descriptions are summarized in Table 15.1.

## Déjà vu experiences

Déjà vu is French for 'already seen'. Déjà vu experiences have been defined as 'any subjectively inappropriate impression of familiarity of a present experience with an undefined past' (Neppe, 1983). Their study has attracted also creative writers and accounts of déjà vu in novels and poems are consistent with clinical data (Sno et al., 1992). With a frequency ranging from 30 to 96%, and apparently uninfluenced by gender, déjà vu seems a common phenomenon (Sno & Linszen, 1990), particularly amongst the young. It also seems associated with depersonalization (Sierra & Berrios, 1997). Common features include: paroxysmal nature, accompanying feelings of tension and secondary anxiety, ability to predict the events of the next few moments (precognition) and inability to place the alleged original experience in a specific point of the past. Occurring in any sensory modality, the experiences may be viewed as positive paramnesic symptoms, involving inappropriate recognition or recollection (Reed, 1972; Sno & Linszen, 1990).

The view has also been put forward that there are pathological and non-pathological forms of déjà vu, and that they are generated by different mechanisms (Sno & Linszen 1990). Phenomenological similarities between the forms, however, suggest that the difference may only be quantitative and that it might be more appropriate to talk about a minor and a major form (Arnaud, 1896). The minor form is transient, paroxysmal and reality testing is only momentarily disturbed. Every detail of the present experience is perceived as being identical to an alleged experience in the past, while at the same time the subject is aware that this is impossible. On the other hand, the major form is of prolonged duration and reality testing is markedly impaired, though not absent as indicated by doubts about the

**Table 15.1.** Types of paramnesia

| Type of paramnesia | Description | Author |
|---|---|---|
| Partial paramnesia | Partial falsification of real memories | Kraepelin (1887) |
| Simple paramnesia | Spontaneous images that appear as memories | Kraepelin (1887) |
| Associating paramnesia | Present perceptions that evoke pseudo-memories by association with something analogous in the past | Kraepelin (1887) |
| Identifying paramnesia | A new experience that appears as a photographic copy of a former one | Kraepelin (1887) |
| Hypnagogic paramnesia | Phenomenon occurring in the hypnagogic period, when a centrally excited dream image is mistaken for a centrally excited memory | Ellis (1911) |
| Reduplicative paramnesia | Delusion of familiarity related to a reduplication of time, place or person. | Pick (1903), Sno (1994) |
| Restricted paramnesia | Experiences of familiarity with a genuine foundation in the past, provoked by a less well-defined aspect of a present perceptual situation | Banister and Zangwill (1941) |
| Fausse reconnaissance | False recognition (synonym for déjà vu experience) | Strauss (1995) |
| Retrospective falsification | Memory becomes unintentionally distorted by present emotional, cognitive and experiential state | Strauss (1995) |
| Confabulation | Unconscious filling of gaps in memory by imagined or untrue experiences | Strauss (1995) |
| Déjà vu experience | Any subjectively inappropriate impression of familiarity of a present experience with an undefined past | Neppe (1983) |
| Jamais vu experience | Any subjectively inappropriate impression of non-familiarity of a present experience with an undefined past | Neppe (1983) |
| 'I can't quite place him' – phenomenon | Inability to identify a relatively well known person | Reed (1979) |
| 'Know the face, not the name'– phenomenon | Recognition and appropriate identification of another person, without remembering the name | Reed (1979) |
| 'Time-gap'– experience | Inability to recall a series of events during the previous seconds or minutes | Reed (1979) |

**Table 15.1** (*cont.*)

| Type of paramnesia | Description | Author |
|---|---|---|
| 'Fleeting-thought' – experience | Feeling of having grasped a new idea, achieved an insight or glimpsed a problem without being able to identify it | Reed (1979) |
| Feeling of knowing | Conviction of knowing an elusive issue and the inability to demonstrate the knowing | Reed (1979) |
| 'Tip of the tongue' – experience | Feeling of knowing an unrecalled item and of being so close to recalling that it is 'on the tip of the tongue' | Reed (1979) |
| Cryptomnesia | Revival of an experience without the attributes of memory | Reed (1979) |
| Checking | Behaviour undertaken to confirm that some action or task has been completed | Reed (1979) |

appropriateness of the experience of familiarity. The present experience is perceived as identical, but not necessarily in every detail.

The cause of déjà vu has been associated with anxiety, dissociative mechanisms, mood and personality disorders, schizophrenia and organic brain syndromes. In non-psychopathological conditions, predisposing factors include emotional trauma, exhaustion, psychomimetic drugs, fatigue, severe stress, hyperventilation syndrome and illness (Sno & Linszen, 1990; Evans, 1995). Hughlings Jackson (1888) suggested a link between some forms of forced reminiscence and a particular type of complex partial seizures (CPS), and since then the relationship between déjà vu experiences and CPS has been confirmed experimentally. Electrical stimulation of both the medial and lateral temporal cortex have been shown to elicit the reporting of déjà vu experiences (Mullan & Penfield, 1959; Halgren et al., 1978; Bancaud et al., 1994). It should be stressed, however, that déjà vu experiences can solely be interpreted as an indication of epilepsy when occurring in combination with other psychiatric or neurological symptoms (Sno & Linszen, 1990).

As to psychopathogenesis, many authors have viewed déjà vu experiences primarily as a disturbance of memory (e.g. Sander, 1873; Osborn, 1884; Kraepelin, 1887; Burnham, 1889; Ribot, 1894; Ey et al., 1978; Yager & Gitlin, 1995).

Psychoanalytically oriented authors have done likewise by suggesting that déjà vu experiences have some relation to defence mechanisms, dreams and unconscious fantasies and wishes (e.g. Freud, 1901, 1914, 1936; Pötzl, 1926; Oberndorf, 1941; Marcovitz, 1952; Arlow, 1959). The parapsychological interpretation has gone much further to imply that the déjà vu experience is based on reincarnation, i.e. on memories of a past life (Chari, 1962). Given his label 'sentiment of pre-existence' it seems likely that Arthur Ladbroke Wigan (1844), the first to focus medical attention on the déjà vu experiences, also presumed such an association.

Non-mnestic hypotheses have also been put forward; for example, déjà vu experiences have been linked to a disruption in the mechanisms that integrate the functions of consciousness, identity and perception of the environment. In this regard, déjà vu experiences are classified in DSM-IV (APA, 1994) as dissociative phenomena.

## Jamais vu experiences

Jamais vu is French for 'never seen'. The jamais vu experience is generally regarded as the opposite of the déjà vu experience (Reed, 1972, 1979; Neppe, 1983). The inception of the term jamais vu is unclear. As with paramnesia, the debate on jamais vu experiences has been obscured by divergent interpretations. Yager and Gitlin (1995) assert that jamais vu experiences involve feelings that one has never seen things which, in fact, one has. Vernon Neppe (1983) in turn defines jamais vu experiences, in contrast to déjà vu experiences, as 'any subjectively inappropriate impression of non-familiarity of a present experience with an undefined past'.

Reed (1979) has viewed the jamais vu experience as the classical example of recall without recognition: 'Whereas cryptomnesia represents a failure to recognize known ideas, jamais vu represents a failure to recognize regularly experienced percepts'. Jamais vu experiences can occur in any sensory modality and may be viewed as negative paramnesic symptoms, involving inappropriate non-recognition or non-recollection (Reed, 1972; Neppe, 1983; Sno, 1994).Conceiving of jamais vu as a disturbance of perception, George Devereux (1967) called it fausse non-reconnaissance and suggested that it resulted from an immediate displacement of an initially correct perception and identification of reality by a mis- or non-identification of the observed person or object.

Isidor Silbermann (1963), in turn, called the jamais vu experience the 'jamais phenomenon' and characterized it as 'the erroneous reaction' 'I've never experienced anything like that before'. In his opinion, the jamais phenomenon is the result of fragmentation and can vary in intensity from a simple, easily correctable phenomenon to a firmly fixed and unchangeable conviction. Illustrated by two instances reported by Freud, Silbermann (1963) claims that jamais experiences appear not only during waking hours but also in dreams. Gordon (1920) cites the jamais vu experience as the 'illusion of the never seen' or 'agnosia', which he depicts as an erroneous belief of a continuous character based on a radical alteration of judgment.

Psychoanalytically oriented authors regard the jamais vu experience as a defence mechanism 'by which an event is torn out of the context of experience, removed from consciousness, and rigidly warded off' (Silbermann, 1963; Devereux, 1967). In keeping with this view, Rudolph Loewenstein (1957) referred to it as the experience of jamais raconté; and ten years later Boesky (1969) suggested that the jamais raconté experience was the reversal of déjà raconté. In the view of the latter, the reversal of déjà raconté consists of a patient saying: 'There is something I've never told you before . . .,' when in fact this particular information has already been reported. Boesky (1969) believed that the reversal of déjà raconté was a manifestation of transference analogous to depersonalization and as an expression of an effort by the ego to repudiate degraded and devalued self representations and identifications which are rooted in the pre-genital history and narcissistic precursors of castration anxiety.

As mentioned earlier, the jamais vu experience has been generally regarded as the opposite of déjà vu, namely that it is ego-alien and negative and has the finality and silence of never having happened (Silbermann, 1963). Boesky (1969) views the reversal of déjà raconté as analogous to depersonalization and Myers and Grant (1972) conceive of the jamais vu experience in general as an extreme degree of depersonalization. These notions are in keeping with Freud's view (1914), that déjà vu experiences can be considered as the 'positive' counterpart of depersonalization. Neppe (1983) has suggested that in depersonalization the emphasis is on the person itself, whereas the jamais vu experience is linked to situations or places. However, this author argues that the jamais experience and depersonalization should be regarded as distinct because of the relative specificity of the jamais vu experience in complex partial seizures.

In epidemiological terms, jamais vu appears to be far less common than déjà vu (Neppe, 1983) and according to Reed (1979) this may explain the fact that jamais vu has not been well studied in the psychiatric literature; in the opinion of this author, the phenomenon does not occur among normal individuals other than in a very fleeting manner (Reed, 1979). Others, however, have argued that the jamais vu experience is common and can be triggered by fatigue, substance abuse, complex partial seizures and other psychopathological states (Silbermann, 1963; Chari, 1964; Yager & Gitlin, 1995).

## Summary

In summary, the most common paramnesias are déjà vu and jamais vu, with the latter being the less frequent of the two. Once upon a time both were considered as disorders of memory but currently other hypotheses are being entertained, for example, these states are considered in DSM IV as being related to dissociation. Psychodynamic interpretations have also been put forward. It is safe to state that both experiences can be seen in relation to some subtypes of complex partial seizures. Beyond that, little is known about the psychopathology and neurobiology of these fascinating phenomena.

## REFERENCES

American Psychiatric Association (APA) (1994). *Diagnostic and Statistical Manual of Mental Disorders*, 4th edn (DSM-IV). Washington, DC: American Psychiatric Association.

Arlow, J.A. (1959). The structure of the déjà-vu experience. *Journal of the American Psychoanalytic Association*, 7, 611–31.

Arnaud, F.L. (1896). Un cas d'illusion du 'déjà-vu' ou de 'fausse mémoire'. *Annales Medico-Psychologignes (Paris)*, 3, 455–71.

Bancaud, J., Brunet-Bourgin, F., Chauvel, P. & Halgren, E. (1994). Anatomical origin of déjà vu and vivid 'memories' in human temporal lobe epilepsy. *Brain*, 117, 71–90.

Banister, H. & Zangwill, O.L. (1941). Experimentally induced visual paramnesias. *British Journal of Psychology*, 32, 30–51.

Bartlett, F.C. (1932). *Remembering*. Cambridge: Cambridge University Press.

Berrios, G.E. (1995). Déjà vu in France during the 19th century: a conceptual history. *Comprehensive Psychiatry*, 36, 123–9.

Bodamer, J. (1947). Die Prosopagnosie. *Archiv Psychiatrik Nervenkrankheit*, 179, 6–54.

Boesky, D. (1969). The reversal of déjà raconté. *Journal of the American Psychoanalytic Association*, 17, 1114–41.

Burnham, W.H. (1889). Memory, historically and experimentally considered. III paramnesia. *American Journal of Psychology*, 2, 431–94.

Campbell, R.J. (1996). *Psychiatric Dictionary*, 7th edn. New York/Oxford: Oxford University Press.

Chari, C.T.K. (1962). Paramnesia and reincarnation. *Proceedings of the Society of Psychical Research*, 53, 264–86.

Chari, C.T.K. (1964). On some types of déjà vu experiences. *Journal of the American Society for Psychical Research*, 58, 186–203.

Devereux, G. (1967). Fausse non-reconnaissance: clinical sidelights on the role of possibility in science. *Bulletin of the Menninger Clinic*, 31, 69–78.

Ey, H., Bernard, P. & Brisset, Ch. (1978) *Manuel de Psychiatrie*, 5th edn, pp. 102–4. Paris: Masson.

Ellis, H. (1911). Memory in dreams. In *The World of Dreams*, Chapter IX, pp. 212–60. London: Constable and Co, Ltd.

Evans, R.W. (1995). Neurologic aspects of hyperventilation syndrome. *Seminars in Neurology*, 15, 115–25.

Freud, S. (1901). The psychopathology of everyday life. In *Complete Psychological Works*, standard edn, vol. 6. pp. 265–6. London: Hogarth Press Ltd, 1960.

Freud, S. (1914). Fausse reconnaissance (déjà raconté) in psychoanalytical treatment. In *Complete Psychological Works*, standard edn, vol. 13. London: Hogarth Press, 1953.

Freud, S. (1936). A disturbance of memory on the Acropolis. In *Complete Psychological Works*, standard edn, vol. 22. London: Hogarth Press, 1964.

Gordon, A. (1920). Illusion of 'the already seen' (paramnesia) and of 'the never seen' (agnosia). *Journal of Abnormal and Social Psychology*, 15: 187–92.

Halgren, E., Walter, R.D., Cherlow, D.G. & Crandall, P.H. (1978). Mental phenomena evoked by electrical stimulation of the human hippocampal formation and amygdala. *Brain*, **101**, 83–117.

Jackson, J.H. (1888). On a particular variety of epilepsy. *Brain*, **11**, 179–207.

Kraepelin, E. (1887). Uber Erinnerungsfälschungen. *Archiv für Psychiatrie und Nervenkrankheiten*, **17**, 830–43.

Lalande, A. (1893). Des paramnésies. *Revue Philosophie*, **36**, 485–97.

Lapie, P. (1893). Note sur les paramnésies. *Revue Philosophique*, **37**, 351–2.

Leeds, M. (1944) One form of paramnesia: the illusion of déjà vu. *Journal of the American Society for Psychical Research*, **38**, 24–42.

Loewenstein, R.M. (1957). Some thoughts on interpretation in the theory and practice of psychoanalysis. In *The Psychoanalytic Study of the Child*, ed. R.S. Eissler et al., pp. 127–50. London: Imago Publishing Co. Ltd.

Marcovitz, E. (1952). The meaning of déjà vu. *Psychoanalytic Quarterly*, **21**, 481–9.

Mullan, S. & Penfield, W. (1959). Illusions of comparative interpretation and emotion. *Archives of Neurology and Psychiatry*, **81**, 269–84.

Myers, D.H. & Grant, G. (1972). A study of depersonalization in students. *British Journal of Psychiatry*, **121**, 59–65.

Neppe, V.M. (1983). *The Psychology of Déjà Vu Have I Been Here Before?* Johannesburg: Witwatersrand University Press.

Oberndorf, C.P. (1941). Erroneous recognition. *Psychiatric Quarterly*, **15**, 316–26.

Osborn, H.F. (1884). Illusions of memory. *North American Review*, **138**, 476–86.

Pick, A. (1903). Clinical studies III. On reduplicative paramnesia. *Brain*, **26**, 260–7.

Pötzl, O. (1926). Zur Metapsychologie des déjà vu. *Imago*, **12**, 393–402.

Reed, G. (1972). *The Psychology of Anomalous Experience: A Cognitive Approach.* pp. 91–111. London: Hutchinson University Library.

Reed, G. (1979). Everyday anomalies of recall and recognition. In *Functional Disorders of Memory*, ed. J.F. Kihlstrom & F.J. Evans, pp. 1–28. Hillsdale: Lawrence Erlbaum.

Ribot, Th. (1894). *Les maladies de la mémoire*, 9th edn. Paris, ed. F. Alcan, éditeur.

Sander, W. (1873). Uber Erinnerungstäuschungen. *Archiv für Psychiatrie Nervenkrankheiten*, **4**, 244.

Sierra, M. & Berrios G.E. (1997). Depersonalization: a conceptual history. *History of Psychiatry*, **8**, 213–29.

Silbermann, I. (1963). The jamais phenomenon with reference to fragmentation. *Psychoanalytic Quarterly*, 32: 181–91.

Sno, H.N. (1994). A continuum of misidentification symptoms. *Psychopathology*, **27**, 144–7.

Sno, H.N. & Linszen, D.H. (1990). The déjà vu experience: remembrance of things past? *American Journal of Psychiatry*, **147**, 1587–95.

Sno, H.N., Linszen, D.H. & de Jonghe, F. (1992). Art imitates life: déjà vu experiences in prose and poetry. *British Journal of Psychiatry*, **160**, 511–18.

Strauss, G.D. (1995). Diagnosis and psychiatry: examination of the psychiatric patient. In *Comprehensive textbook of psychiatry*, 6th edn, ed. H.I. Kaplan & B.J. Sadock, vol. 1, pp. 542–3. Baltimore: Williams & Wilkins.

Sully, J. (1881). *Illusions. A Psychological Study*. London, UK: Kegan Paul, Trubner & Co.

Yager, J. & Gitlin, M.J. (1995). Clinical manifestations of psychiatric disorders. In *Comprehensive Textbook of Psychiatry*, 6th edn. ed. H.I. Kaplan & B.J. Sadock, vol. 1, pp. 652–4. Baltimore: Williams & Wilkins.

Wigan, A.L. (1844). *The Duality of the Mind*. pp. 64–5. Malibu, CA: Joseph Simon, 1985.

# Confabulations

German E. Berrios

Confabulations are inaccurate or false narratives purporting to convey information about world or self. According to the received view, they are utterances intent on 'covering up' for a putative memory deficit. Confabulations are said to vary in terms of 'content', 'mode of production', 'duration', 'aetiology', 'form', and 'conviction'. According to content, a distinction is often made between prosaic and fantastic confabulations; and according to mode of production two types have been distinguished: 'volunteered' and 'extracted by the clinician'. Although the dearth of published case series might suggest that confabulations are a rare occurrence, this may be the result of underdiagnosis. With regard to aetiological factors, amnesia, embarrassment, 'frontal lobe' damage, a particular subtype of 'personality', a dream-like event, and a disturbance of the self have been listed.

There has been little work on the linguistic, logical, and epistemological status of confabulations although the way in which they are dealt with in the medical and neuropsychological literature suggests that confabulations are considered by most as a form of propositional attitude (i.e. a belief); if so, the problem of differentiating them from delusions remains (Berrios, 1985). Lastly, on account of the putative heterogeneity of their narratives, personalities and neurobiology, 'confabulators' (i.e. the subjects who issue confabulations) constitute a motley group.

Historical analysis shows that 'confabulation' entered psychopathology at the turn of the century as a member of a set of concepts (that included delusion, fixed idea, obsessions, overvalued idea, etc.) dedicated to capturing 'narratives' of dubious content. This means that confabulation is not an autonomous concept but part of a 'discourse formation',[1] i.e. it only has meaning within a given context. If so, it can be predicted that it will become unstable when used as if it were an independent piece of behaviour. This seems to be happening now as confabulations are being increasingly taken over by neuropsychology where they are treated without regard to the psychiatric context in which they have originated in the first place. The second inference is that, as members of a discourse formation, and before they can play a useful role in current psychiatric diagnosis, treatment and research,[2] 'confabulations' will have to be recalibrated together with the set of concepts to which they belong.

## Definitions

The definition of confabulation has changed over the years. According to Goodwin (1989), it is a 'dislocation of events in time and the fabrication of stories to fill in forgotten sequences . . . differs from lying in that the individual is not consciously attempting to deceive' (p. 65). For Moscovitch (1995) it is 'a symptom that accompanies many neurological disorders and some psychiatric ones, such as schizophrenia . . . what distinguishes confabulation from lying is that typically there is no intent to deceive and the patient is unaware of the falsehoods. It is "honest lying" . . . [When] neuronal structures involved in the reconstructive [memory] process are damaged, memory distortion becomes prominent and results in confabulation'.

These definitions move at various conceptual levels (descriptive, explanatory, etc.) and challenge some conventional wisdom, e.g. the definition of lying. Earlier definitions, on the other hand were narrower and perhaps easier to operationalize. Thus, according to Talland (1961), a confabulation is a: 'factually incorrect verbal statement or narrative, <u>exclusive</u> of intentional falsification, fantastic fabrication, random guesses, intrinsic non-sense, the chaotic themes of delirium and hallucinations, and all systematic delusions <u>other than</u> those arising from the patient's disorientation in his experienced time' [my emphasis] (p. 366). This is a good example of a definition by exclusion for which not a great deal of evidence is offered. It, however, makes some sense when linked up to Talland's aetiological views. Thus, with regard to the confabulations of Korsakoff's syndrome, he writes:

(i) . . . typically, but not exclusively, an account, more or less coherent and internally consistent, concerning the patient, (ii) this account is false in the context named and often false in details within its own context, (iii) its content is drawn fully or principally from the patient's recollection of his actual experiences, including his thoughts in the past, (iv) confabulation reconstructs this content, modifies and recombines its elements, employing the mechanisms of normal remembering, (v) this material is presented without awareness of its distortion or of its inappropriateness, and (vi) it serves no other purpose, is motivated in no other way than is factual information based on genuine data (Talland, 1961: p. 370).

Berlyne (1972) in turn defined confabulation as: 'a falsification of memory occurring in clear consciousness in association with an organically derived amnesia' (p. 38) . . . [our] study confirmed the existence of two forms of confabulation in the Korsakoff syndrome as postulated by Bonhoeffer (1904): the momentary or embarrassment confabulation[3] and the fantastic or productive confabulation' (p. 33).[4] More recent definitions are variations upon these themes;

for example, Mercer et al. (1977) defined it as 'a response that is not only false but may incorporate bizarre or fantastic features'[5] . . . [the patient appears] 'unable to utilize his own recollections or external cues in the environment to censor [it]' (p. 429) . . . a 'necessary prerequisite for confabulation is impaired memory function' (p. 433).

In his excellent review, Whitlock (1981) was right to conclude that 'although there was disagreement in the literature concerning the meaning of confabulation, there were also running themes': (i) incorrect statements were fabricated, (ii) the patient did that to cover gaps in memory; (iii) confabulation appeared to be a purposive, conscious act; (iv) the patient is aware of memory defects and wants to conceal them from his interrogator.

However, these four themes are conceptually heterogeneous and pose more problems than they solve. The first concerns the issue of the truth status of the narrative which seems to suggest that it might be necessary at some stage to ascertain the veracity of the confabulated statement. This view therefore assumes that confabulations are a form of propositional attitude, that is the patient means to convey information *oratio recta* (direct speech).

The other three themes concern the hypothesis that subjects confabulate in order to fill a memory gap. In earlier versions, it was believed that it resulted from a 'conscious' and 'deliberate' effort. More recently (like Gilbert Ryle, neuropsychology tries to conjure away the spectrum of a subjective agency), versions have appeared according to which it is a brain area that does the job: e.g. 'it is argued that in these instances, the language areas act so as to fill these "gaps" with information that, although appropriate, is linked in some manner to the fragments received' (Joseph, 1986: p. 507). It is unclear what 'the language areas act so as to' actually means. If what is meant is that the subject is not 'conscious' of his confabulated memory or becomes so only *post hoc* (and genuinely believes it to be true), then, what is the use of concepts such as 'lying' (Joseph, 1986) or 'honest lying' (Moscovitch, 1989)?

From the start, the 'gap-filling' hypothesis has also rested on the assumption that the confabulator has a memory deficit. This creates the interesting situation that the same clinical phenomenon may or may not be considered as a 'confabulation' depending on whether or not it is accompanied by such a memory deficit;[6] indeed, historically this has been used as an external criterion to differentiate confabulation from delusion (Berrios, 1985). Not everyone, however, has accepted the 'memory deficit' criterion (e.g. Weinstein et al., 1956; Weinstein, 1996).[7] To compound matters, the same memory deficit criterion has also been used as 'evidence' for the 'covering-up' hypothesis itself.[8] But then this causes further problem for the 'covering up' hypothesis cannot be used to explain the generation of spontaneous confabulations in subjects without memory impairment (e.g. as per Koehler & Jacoby, 1978; Nathaniel-James & Frith, 1996).

Most authors still consider the concept of 'confabulation' as pertaining to speech acts and discourse. Of late, however, others have started using the term to refer to visual images (e.g. Welsch et al., 1997). Swartz and Brust (1984) have also used the term to refer to hallucinations in a subject with Anton's syndrome; and Downes and Mayes (1995) have reported the case of a man whose vivid visual hallucinations seemed related to a basic confabulatory disorder. Others use confabulation to refer to the reporting of additional letters to the left end of short words in unilateral spatial-neglect (Chatterjee, 1995); and even to reporting 'touch' in 'non-touch' trials in subjects with anosognosia and hemiplegia during the Wada test (Lu et al., 1997).[9]

## Clinical aspects

As far as is known, there is no large-scale epidemiological study on the prevalence of confabulatory behaviour. So it is difficult to decide on issues such as the role of the memory deficit, on whether confabulations are 'pathological' phenomena or whether there is a putative capacity to 'confabulate' that is widely distributed in the general population and hence cases seen in Korsakoff's psychosis, presbyophrenia, brain damage, frontal lobe pathology, schizophrenia, etc. are but exaggerated presentations of this trait. Without epidemiological information, 'official' profiles obtained from few hospital cases have to be accepted faute de mieux and this creates a 'clinician's illusion'.[10]

### Subtypes

Confabulations have been classified according to content, mode of elicitation, and background disease. 'Content' is evaluated in terms of the 'true/false' and 'bizarre/fantastic' dichotomies. For example, confabulations with *plausible* content such as (the actually untrue statement by a patient that) 'Yesterday, I had porridge for breakfast' are (presumedly) judged in terms of truth values (i.e. checked against the recollection of a nurse or the fact that on that day no porridge was available in the hospital). On the other hand, confabulations with bizarre content such as 'Yesterday, I went to the other side of the moon for a walk' are (presumedly) judged *simpliciter* as *récits imaginaires*. Another classificatory criterion has been 'mode of elicitation'; in this regard, it has been claimed that 'provoked'[11] and 'spontaneous' confabulations are 'different disorders with different mechanisms' (Schnider et al., 1996a: p. 1373).

## Clinical associations

### Korsakoff's syndrome

This association is historically important for it is the source of the belief that confabulation must be related to memory failure. Based on the study of 'more than 30 cases', Korsakoff (1955) concluded that 'pseudomemories'[12] were only an occasional accompaniment[13] of 'psychosis polyneuritica' of alcoholic origin; interestingly, he found that the phenomenon did not occur in 16 cases of non-alcoholic origin (Korsakoff, 1955). Korsakoff's 'pseudomemories' were to be renamed 'confabulations' in the work of Wernicke (1906), Pick (1905) and Kraepelin (1910).

From the start, as Williams and Rupp (1938) noticed, speculation on the mechanisms of confabulation depended on what the underlying deficit was thought to be. For example, whilst Gregor and Roemer (1906) and Liepmann (1910) believed in the centrality of the amnestic disorder, van der Holst (1932) postulated a fundamental 'disturbance of time sense' leading to an inability to set experiences in a chronological frame. Consequently, for the latter author confabulation was a form of fantasy (because 'fantasy-like dreams are atemporal') but for Bonhoeffer (1904) and Pick (1905) (who believed in the memory deficit view) confabulation was a 'reactive' behaviour ('confabulation of embarrassment'). Later work, however, suggests that, after all, memory impairment may not be necessary for the formation of confabulations (Joslyn et al., 1978). This may open the gate for more aetiological speculation.

In their important monograph, Victor et al. (1971) examined 245 alcoholic subjects who presented with Wernicke's encephalopathy, Korsakoff's psychosis or both. During periods of confusion, 'transient confabulations' proved difficult to separate from delusions, misidentifications, etc. Confabulatory behaviour amongst chronic patients was infrequent (the authors provide no figures) and fluctuating, i.e. patients often replied 'I do not know' when re-examined. No embarrassment confabulations were seen, and when patients improved or gained insight they rapidly lost their tendency to confabulate (pp. 58–60).

Neither Korsakoff nor later writers on the syndrome seem to have been interested in pre-morbid personality as a risk factor in the development of confabulatory behaviour.

### Presbyophrenia

The term 'presbyophrenia'[14] was coined by Kahlbaum (1863) to provide a noun to the group of disorders he called 'paraphrenia senilis'. It was resuscitated by Wernicke (1906), who gave it clinical content and classified it as an allopsychoses (together with the Korsakoff's syndrome).[15] The clinical features of presbyophrenia included confabulations, allopsychic disorientation, hyperactivity, affective disorder (euphoria and/or irritability), and a fluctuating course. The condition was commoner amongst females and the elderly; there was an acute and a chronic form, and the latter merged with senile dementia (p. 290).

As 'a nosological concept imported from Germany', presbyophrenia was adopted by Devaux and Logre (1911); and Rouby (1911) identified four nosological views: (i) independent clinical entity, (ii) a form of acute confusion, (iii) a variety of Korsakoff's psychosis; and (iv) a form of senile dementia. Rouby (1911) concluded that presbyophrenia was a 'final common pathway' for cases suffering from Korsakoff's psychosis, senile dementia or acute confusion. Others took a 'psychiatric view' pointing out that it was not always easy to distinguish the elevated mood of the presbyophrenic from hypomania or confusional states. In the event, confabulation, disorientation and amnesia for recent events became the central features of presbyophrenia (e.g. Devaux & Logre, 1911). Not all were convinced. For example, Ziehen (1911) wrote [the cases with] 'marked confabulation described by Wernicke under the inconvenient term "presbyophrenia" are just examples of Korsakoff's psychosis'.

In-between the World Wars, hypotheses on pathogenic mechanisms began to appear. Based on 12 cases, Bostroem (1933) concluded that presbyophrenic patients tended to have cyclothymic personality and 'cerebral atherosclerosis'. Supporting the view that disinhibition, confabulations and presbyophrenic behaviour resulted from vascular pathology, Lafora (1935) reported that, in three cases with memory impairment and a relative preservation of insight, the development of aphasia led to a decline in confabulations. Ey (1950) considered presbyophrenia as a form of senile dementia with 'compensatory' confabulations (p. 47). The view that subjects with presbyophrenia showed more confabulations, confusion, and denial of illness than those with Korsakoff's psychosis was popular during this period. During the 1940s, it was suggested that this might relate to a partial occlusion of the posterior cerebral artery with involvement of occipital cortex and hippocampal–mamillary–thalamic–cingulate circuit (Berrios, 1985, 1986).

## 'Frontal lobes'

During the 1970s, the view reappeared that confabulations reflected pathological changes in the frontal lobe. For example, Stuss et al. (1978) suggested that the 'fantastic' confabulations described by Kraepelin (1886–1887) (which for some reason they attributed to Berlyne) were due to 'frontal lobe pathology'. Earlier on, Lafora (1935) had already suggested that persisting confabulatory behaviour was a form of disinhibition caused by arteriosclerotic changes affecting the anterior part of the brain. Maeda and Okawa (1974), in turn, also reported that ruptured aneurysms of the anterior communicating artery caused confabulatory behaviour.

Kapur and Coughlan (1980) and Shapiro et al. (1981) have found that confabulatory behaviour correlates with perseveration; and Kopelman (1987) has suggested that 'spontaneous confabulation' may result from the 'superimposition of frontal dysfunction'. In a later paper, the same author has gone on to state that 'frontal lobe pathology and a disorder in context memory may be necessary, but not sufficient, conditions for spontaneous confabulations to occur' . . . and he has identified three factors: confusion in the context of memories involving both time and place; a high rate of perseverations, particularly in semantic memory; and a tendency to respond indiscriminately to the immediate social and environmental context' (p. 683) (Kopelman et al., 1997).

Comparing two subjects with an 'amnestic–confabulatory' condition, Dalla Barba (1993) only found features of frontal lobe impairment in the patient whose confabulations involved episodic memory and retrieval of 'semantic information'. Baddeley and Wilson (1986), in turn, have suggested that confabulation is a consequence of a 'dysexecutive syndrome'[16]; recently Papagno and Baddeley (1997) have reported a case with normal prospective and retrospective memory, preserved autobiographical memory, dysexecutive syndrome and confabulations. Fischer et al. (1995) have reported marked attentional deficit and poor executive functions in five 'spontaneous confabulators' (caused by rupture of aneurysms in the anterior communicating artery); they were found to have extensive lesions of basal forebrain, ventral frontal lobe, and striatum.

Johnson et al. (1997), in turn, have reported a confabulator (G.S.) with a frontal lobe lesion after an anterior communicating artery aneurysm who when compared with controls showed more memory deficits for temporal duration and temporal order. More recently, Moscovitch and Melo (1997) have suggested that 'confabulation is associated with impaired strategic retrieval process resulting from damage in the region of the ventromedial frontal cortex'. The same region has been inculpated by Benson et al. (1996) who in a PET scan study found hypofusion in the orbital and medial frontal regions of a confabulator with Korsakoff's syndrome; the blood flow normalized when the patient stopped confabulating.

The frontal lobe hypothesis cannot yet account for the finding that many confabulators perform 'normally' on frontal lobe tasks (Dalla Barba et al., 1990, 1993; Delbecq-Derouesné et al., 1990) or show no damage to the frontal lobes (Dalla Barba et al., 1997).

## Other brain sites and mechanisms

The finding by Feinberg et al. (1994) that there is an association between verbal confabulation (determined as 'false positive error rates' in a visual task) and anosognosia in right sided hemiplegia suggests that lesions of other parts of the brain may also trigger this condition. Earlier on, Williams and Pennybacker (1954) had already reported a tendency to confabulate accompanied by inability to retain information, disorientation and euphoria or apathy in four subjects with tumours of the third ventricle. The same area was identified by Victor et al. (1971) as related to a tendency to memory impairment, confabulation and apathy. After finding paramedian or tuberothalamic infarcts resulting from occlusion of the posterior cerebral artery in some confabulators, Servan et al. (1994) have suggested that lesions to the dorsomedial nucleus of the thalamus may play a role in the pathogenesis of this symptom. Dalla Barba et al. (1997) have recently reported a case with rupture of the left communicating artery who exhibited confabulations, severe impairment of episodic memory, and deficits in all frontal lobe tests except cognitive estimates and no structured evidence of frontal lobe damage.

Dalla Barba (1995) suggested that 'confabulation is not just a disturbance of memory but also, if not exclusively, a disturbance of consciousness.' (p. 110); Feinberg (1997) has classified it amongst the disturbances of the self; and Hobson (1997) believes that confabulations may share mechanisms with dreams. Joseph (1986) has made the point that confabulation (or in less extreme cases, self-deception) also occurs amongst brain-injured individuals, and seems to be the byproduct of the '*normal process* via which explanations for behaviours, impulses, or other actions are provided' (p. 517). Johnson (1991), in turn, refers to 'reality monitoring' as 'a fundamental memory function that anchors us in a perceived external world' (p. 193).[17]

## A new conceptual frame

With regard to the analysis of confabulations, it would seem that confusion has arisen from mixing up levels of inquiry: phenomenology, neurobiology, disease associations, aetiological speculation and even pragmatics. At a most general level, 'confabulations' should be considered as sharing a conceptual space with delusions, mythomania (Dupré, 1925; Neyraut, 1962; Hicks & Myslobodsky, 1997), 'pseudologia fantastica' (King & Ford, 1988) and 'pathological lying'. Hence, empirical research will only help once certain decisions have been taken at a meta-level. The issue is not whether instances of behaviour redolent of what dictionaries call 'confabulation' can be found in reality, but whether they constitute an independent class. The discourse formation that provides meaning to 'confabulation' also includes related concepts such as lying, delusion, and narrative. These concepts define their meanings in relation to one other and hence their semantic extension needs to be briefly examined.

## Confabulations and (pathological) lying

Lying[18] was defined by St Augustine as 'a claim contrary to the truth, in general an intention to deceive. A liar is one who thinks something in his mind and expresses something else, whether in words or acts'.[19] In the Western tradition, the view that in some social and political situations lying was acceptable (as sponsored by a line of thinkers stretching from Plato to Machiavelli) is in stark contrast with the Christian view that lying is always an immoral act. Kant (1991) called it 'a foul spot on human nature' and considered 'internal' (as opposed to 'external') lies, such as 'dissembling a belief', as a form of self-deception (Kant, 1993). Abandoning this moralistic type of analysis (i.e. 'intention to deceive'), current research seeks to understand the ways in which lying actually coexists with the 'reality structures' of discourse (e.g. Greimas, 1983).

Whilst it might be possible to distinguish confabulation from conventional lying, it is otherwise with the clinical notion of 'pathological lying' when 'intention to deceive' is not necessarily present, i.e. it can be argued that the 'pathological liar' makes things up in a compulsive, involuntary or non-conscious manner (e.g. Koppen, 1898; Meunier, 1904; Risch, 1908). So, are confabulations just a form of lying (Joseph, 1986)? The conventional view is that they are not for: (a) the confabulator has no intention to deceive (Delay, 1942; Dalla Barba, 1993); and (b) he/she believes that the utterance is true. Things, however, are not that simple. As Whitlock (1981) noticed, confabulations are 'purposive' acts, i.e. the patient wants to 'cover up, fill gaps or deceive' about the extent of his/her memory impairment. Is this deceiving different from lying? To say that it takes place 'beyond awareness' distorts the meaning of the verb and leads to contortions of usage such as the concepts of 'non-conscious' or 'honest lying' (e.g. Moscovitch, 1995; Joseph, 1986).[20]

Related to this problem is the old chestnut of how does the clinician know that the patient is not lying? There are two stock answers: 'empirical', i.e. debriefing shows that patients at the time 'believed' in what they were saying, and had no intention to deceive; and 'meta-theoretical', i.e. that the 'intentionality' element is good enough to separate lying from confabulation. Both answers are flawed: the former because it assumes that amnestic patients can selectively recollect the status of their belief, even if they cannot remember what the belief was about; and the latter because there is no good a priori reason for not including 'intent to deceive' in the conceptual geography of confabulation. It can be concluded that, in terms of current knowledge, an absolute distinction cannot yet be made between confabulating and lying. This conclusion has important implications for its clinical definition and explanation.

## Confabulation, truth-values and delusion

Confabulations are said to bear no relationship to any ascertainable 'reality', i.e. they are considered as 'false'. The point here is how much (the content of) its 'narrative departs from the truth' rather than its insincerity, mendacity or intention to dissemble. As with delusions, the first conventional step is to determine the magnitude of such departure, and this partially depends on 'content'; for example, claims about the self involving dichotomous concepts (e.g. gender or religion) depart from the truth more precipitously than meandering narratives about continuous themes (e.g. age, weight, dates, etc.) which diverge by degrees.

But does measuring departure from the truth *always* help? In the case of confabulations with 'fantastic' (Berlyne, 1972; Kopelman, 1987) and 'extraordinary' content (Stuss et al., 1978) this seems so obvious that the issue does not arise. For example, Stuss et al. (1978) reported the case of an alcoholic who claimed that 'he was in Finland', of another who 'believed that he was in an air-conditioning plant and later in Massachusetts', and a third who, after peering out the window, 'told the examiner that his boat (the examiner's) had been stolen'; and Berlyne's (1972) case of 'fantastic confabulation' concerned a brain-damaged woman who claimed that her 'leg trouble was due to a flying accident and that she was an air hostess'.

However, the problem appears in the case of confabulations with a prosaic content or partial departure from the truth. For example, in so-called 'provoked' confabulations whose 'content is a true memory displaced in its time context' (Berlyne, 1972: p. 33) the issue is one of assessing a feature amongst many (i.e. time). This demands that the clinician undertake a decision-making task. In these cases, as it is with the assessment of disorientation (Berrios, 1982), a cut-off point is needed to determine whether the 'time displacement' warrants calling the utterer's memory a confabulation.

If truth value is not always crucial, there are cases when even a true statement may be considered as confabulatory. These cases suggest that the real issue is the evidential support on which the subject bases his claim (Berrios & Fuentenebro, 1996). On this, characteristic confabulations and delusions also show a point of contact. Reported cases of confabulations can often be reinterpreted as a combination of delusions and/or disorientation (e.g. Villiers et al., 1996; Stuss et al., 1978).

If so, rather than stating, *simpliciter*, that confabulations and delusions are utterly different (e.g. Talland, 1961), why not explore the possibility that the former may be a subset of the latter? This is the case with Johnson (1988, 1991; Johnson et al., 1993) whose model for 'reality monitoring' places confabulations, delusions, hallucinations and insight along a continuum. Over a 100 years ago, Korsakoff defined confabulatory behaviour (which he called 'pseudoreminis-cences') as experiences that occurred in subjects with memory deficit, delusions, and partial confusion:

In regard to the confusion, it must be noted that in this form of amnesia a slight degree of confusion is frequently present. This confusion does not involve that which the patient perceives at the present but affects only the recollection of the past events. Thus, when asked to tell how he has been spending his time, the patient would frequently relate a story altogether different from that which actually occurred, for example, he would tell that yesterday he took a ride in town, whereas in fact he has been in bed for two months, or he would tell of conversations which have never occurred and so forth. On occasions, such patients invent some fiction and constantly repeat it, so that a *peculiar delirium* develops, rooted in false recollections (pseudoreminiscences) (p. 399). [21]

This quotation is important for two reasons: it reflects well views on pseudo- and delusional memories reigning at the time (see Chapter 14, this volume), and shows that, before the advent of the rigid Jaspersian criteria (Berrios & Fuentenebro, 1996), the concept of 'delusion' was flexible enough to incorporate that of 'confabulation'. In other words, the problem of whether confabulations are delusions only developed after the 1910s, when the concept of delusion was arbi-trarily narrowed down.

## Confabulations and narratives

Throughout the ages, 'fabulation' and germane notions are found related to a folk psychology penchant for 'telling fables',[22] an uncommon but socially esteemed human ability. In this regard, Bergson (1959) believed that this *fonction fabula-trice* was at the basis of all human myths, superstitions, and religions. A 'subtype of the imagination, this function did not refer to either a current or a past object and hence was not represented by either a perception or a memory'. In primitive societies, this 'fabulatory function' had the important role of maintaining social cohesion. Janet (1828) wrote of confabulation:

This mental disorder has been mainly dealt with from a pathological view point . . . but in my view it is far wider as it can be found in children and in the primitive man. It represents a particular state of the evolution of memory . . . in general, confabulation presents itself as a more or less complete narrative which from certain points of view may even be called perfect but which, from the perspective of an adult observer has a major failure, namely, that it does not correspond to what we call truth (p. 275).

At the turn of the century, aspects (or disorders) of this fabulatory or narrative function seem to have been medicalized, and 'confabulation' began to mean a 'fable' that was false, insightless, and involuntary.[23] The variety of clinical observations reported suggests that these three defining 'features' were not inferred from the 'clinical facts' alone. It is far more likely that the semantic geography of 'confabulation' was determined by late nineteenth century changes in the meaning of concepts such as intentionality, lying, memory, delusion, and insight.[24] In this regard, Crisp (1995) suggested that one should go beyond a 'negative estimate' of confabulations by considering them as veritable narrative efforts.

## Confabulations and pragmatics

The view that confabulations are verbal statements conveying (as it happens to be) 'erroneous' information about world or self (e.g. Talland, 1961; Moscovitch, 1995; Myslobodsky & Hicks, 1994[25]) remains a popular one. However, at least two alternative views can be proposed: (i) that confabulations are just involuntary (mechanical, tic-like) verbal ejaculations (like those seen in Tourette's syndrome); and (ii) that they are 'utterances', i.e. 'stretches of talk' issued by a speaker within a dialogical context (usually that of 'patient and clinician').

Since the intentional component is central to the semantics of confabulation, the tic model seems inadequate. But what about the 'utterances' view? Might it be that the intention of the patient is not to convey (true or false) information but 'do something' (e.g. persuade, deceive, etc.)? Thus the old view that confabulations are generated by embarrassed amnestic patients covering up for their deficit, could be reinterpreted as meaning that confabulations are 'speech acts' through which patients try to persuade their clinical interlocutors that they have 'normal' memories. This view opens the door to the science of 'pragmatics'.[26]

The term 'pragmatics' was introduced by Charles W. Morris (1971) to 'designate the science of the relation of signs to their interpreters'; together with semantics and syntax it now constitutes one of the central sciences of linguistics. The relationship between language and speakers remains couched in terms of intentionality. For example, Green (1996) has written:

the broadest interpretation of pragmatics is that it is the study of understanding intentional human action. Thus it involves the interpretation of acts assumed to be undertaken in order to accomplish some purpose. The central notions in pragmatics must then include belief, intention (or goal), plan and act (pp. 2–3).

Before proceeding further, it is important to clarify that the concept of 'intention' is used here to refer to a component of action, and also to a pervading feature of all 'mental states'.[27]

Although central to pragmatics,[28] the meaning of 'intention' is still open to debate. For example, Schlieben-Lange (1975) wrote: 'the philosophical concept of intentionality departs from the vulgar meaning of 'doing something on purpose' . . . In the latter, however [intentionality], is marked by an ambiguity: does acting intentionally mean acting 'consciously' or acting 'with a purpose'. In the vulgar notion of purpose both meanings coincide: I 'have done something on purpose' means both 'I knew what I was doing' and 'I was pursuing a specific goal', Schlieben-Lange's analysis can be used to address the 'intentional' component of confabulations, particularly when used in the 'filling-the-gaps of memory hypothesis': Is the creation of the confabulation *conscious*, i.e. the result of 'self-conscious activity'?[29] Can degrees of self-consciousness be distinguished? Have all confabulations got the same intention to deceive? Is this intentional component explanatory in itself?

## Confabulation and 'acting with intention'

To illustrate how the *intentional* component (central to the 'covering up' hypothesis) of traditional accounts of confabulations soon gets into trouble, Davidson's (1980) analysis of intentionality will be used. According to this philosopher, the main elements of 'acting' with intention are:

(a)   the action (in the case of confabulations, and paraphrasing Davidson, this will be defined as: 'the production by patient (P) of a narrative (N) either spontaneously or in reply to a question from clinician C');

(b)   appropriate desires (pro-attitudes) and beliefs (in the case of confabulations, this would be 'the desire or pro-attitude by P to conceal his/her amnesia, and the belief that uttering a narrative is the best way of achieving that concealment'), and

(c)   an appropriate explanatory relation between (a) and (b) (in the case of confabulations, this would be 'the belief by P that providing a narrative N should suffice to satisfy C's curiosity').

Assuming that P met criteria (a), (b), and (c), could then clinician (C) 'explain' the production of confabulations (N) by patient (P) fully in terms of P's desires and beliefs (as Bonhoeffer and others purported to have explained)? In other words, can Davidson's model generate an explanation that is good enough for clinical purposes?

Central to this question is the character and quality of the narrative N. A confabulation, we are told, is by definition a narrative *manqué*[30] because it is (at least partially) false. Now, the crucial question is whether P knows that it is false. According to the received view, P must know for he is using the confabulated narrative to cover up for a loss of a 'true' narrative; for if he did not know, and believed that the narrative is relevant and true, then it would make little sense to say that he is using it instead of the truth (that is, the confabulated narrative would be his truth). Furthermore, his firm belief in the truth of the 'confabulation' would render it tantamount to a delusion. (This demarcation problem, in fact, remains unresolved.)

On the other hand, if P all the time knows that his narrative is false, how is confabulating to be differentiated from lying? And, if there is no difference, why should lying in a few subjects with amnesia be considered as an interesting phenomenon, that is, one that tells us something about the pathology of their underlying disease rather than about their personality?

It would seem therefore that the 'covering up' hypothesis is hopelessly impaled on the horns of the 'intentionality' dilemma: if it is accepted that P knows, confabulations cannot be differentiated from lying; if P does not know and firmly believes in his/her narrative then confabulations cannot be distinguished from delusions. And resorting to elements external to the confabulation itself to resolve the dilemma does not do either. Using 'presence of amnesia or frontal lobe pathology' might separate it (not necessarily from lying) but it will not demarcate it from delusions as the latter have also been reported in relation to frontal lobe pathology. Furthermore, it creates a tautological loop as the clinician may not now be able to use the presence of confabulations as a marker of frontal lobe disease.

## Summary and conclusions

Two phenomena are conventionally included under the name 'confabulation'. The first type concerns 'untrue' utterances of subjects with memory impairment; often provoked or elicited by the interviewer, these confabulations are accompanied by little conviction and are believed by most clinicians to be caused by the (conscious or unconscious) need to 'cover up' for some memory deficit. Researchers wanting to escape the 'intentionality' dilemma have made use of additional factors such as presence of frontal lobe pathology, dysexecutive syndrome, difficulty with the temporal dating of memories leading to an inability temporally to string out memory data, etc., etc.

The second type concerns confabulations with fantastic content and great conviction as seen in subjects with functional psychoses and little or no memory deficit. Less is said in the neuropsychological literature about this group although (at least in the case of a patient with schizophrenia) it has been correlated with a bad performance on frontal lobe tests. This group remains of crucial importance to psychiatrists. Little is known about the epidemiology of either type of confabulation.

In clinical practice, these two 'types' can be found in combination. It remains unclear why so many patients with Korsakoff's psychosis or frontal lobe disorder, in spite of the fact that they do meet the putative conditions for confabulation (amnesia, frontal lobe damage, difficulty with the dating of memories, etc.) do not confabulate. Furthermore, confabulations have also been reported in subjects with lesions in the non-dominant hemisphere and in the thalamus.

Under different disguises, the 'covering up' or 'gap filling' hypothesis is still going strong. Although superficially plausible, it poses a serious conceptual problem with regard to the issue of 'awareness of purpose': if full awareness is presumed, then it is difficult to differentiate confabulations from lying; if no awareness is presumed then the semantics of the concept of 'purpose' is severely stretched and confabulations cannot be differentiated from delusions.

The received view of confabulations also neglects the clinical observation that confabulations (particularly provoked ones!) do occur in dialogical situations: for example, the way in which the patient is asked questions may increases the probability of his producing a confabulation. This suggests that the view that confabulations are a disorder of a putative narrative function found in normal human subjects must be taken seriously. It is hypothesized here that this trait is normally distributed in the population. In the absence of adequate epidemiological information, research efforts should be directed at mapping the distribution of this narrative (or confabulatory) capacity in the community at large. Only then will it be possible to understand the significance of its disorders. In the long term, this approach will prove more heuristic than unwarranted speculation based on few anecdotal cases.

## REFERENCES

Arendt, H. (1972.) *Du Mensonge à la Violence. Essai de Politique Contemporaine.* Paris: Calmann-Lévy.

Baddeley, A. & Wilson, B. (1986). Amnesia, autobiographical memory and confabulation. In *Autobiographical Memory*, ed. D.C. Rubin, pp. 225–52. Cambridge: Cambridge University Press.

Benson, D.F., Djenderedjian, A., Miller, B.L., Pachana, N.A., Chang, L., Itti L.& Mena, I. (1996).Neural basis of confabulation. *Neurology*, **46**, 1239–43.

Bergson, H. (1959). Les deux sources de la morale et de la religion. In *Œuvres*, ed. A. Robinet, pp. 981–1245. Paris: Presses Universitaires de France (first published in 1932).

Berlyne, N. (1972). Confabulation. *British Journal of Psychiatry* 120: 31–39.

Berrios, G.E. (1982). Disorientation states in psychiatry. *Comprehensive Psychiatry*, **23**, 479–91.

Berrios, G.E. (1985). Presbyophrenia: clinical aspects. *British Journal of Psychiatry*, **147**, 76–9.

Berrios, G.E. (1986). Presbyophrenia: the rise and fall of a concept. *Psychological Medicine*, **16**, 267–75.

Berrios, G.E. (1996). *The History of Mental Symptoms. Descriptive Psychopathology since the 19th Century.* Cambridge: Cambridge University Press.

Berrios, G.E. & Chen, E. (1993). Symptom-recognition and neural-networks. *British Journal of Psychiatry,* **163**, 308–14.

Berrios, G.E. & Gili, M. (1995). Abulia and impulsiveness revisited. *Acta Psychiatrica Scandinavica,* **92**, 161–7.

Berrios, G.E. & Fuentenebro, F. (1996). *Delirio.* Madrid: Truetta.

Blanchet, A. (1994). Pragmatique et psychopathologie. In *Traité de Psychopathologie,* ed. D. Widlöcher, pp. 883–919. Paris: Presses Universitaires de France.

Bleuler, E. (1924). *Textbook of Psychiatry,* translated by A.A. Brill. New York: MacMillan Company.

Bonhoeffer, K. (1904). Der korsakowsche Symptomencomplex in seinen Beziehungen zu den verschieden Krankheitsformen. *Allgemeine Zeitschrift für Psychiatrie,* **61**, 744–52.

Bostroem, A. (1933). Über Presbyophrenie. *Archiv für Psychiatrie und Nervenkrankheiten,* **99**, 339–45.

Brentano, F. (1973). *Psychology from an Empirical Standpoint.* Translated by A.C. Rancurello, D.B. Terrell & L.L. McAlister. London: Routledge & Kegan Paul.

Burgess, P.W. & Shallice, T. (1996). Confabulation and the control of recollection. *Memory,* **4**, 359–412.

Chaslin, P. & Portocalis (no initial). (1908). Un cas de syphilis cérébrale avec syndrome de Korsakoff. A Forme amnésique pure. *Journal de Psychologie Normale et Pathologique,* **5**, 303–17.

Chatterjee A. (1995). Cross-over, completion and confabulation in unilateral spatial neglect. *Brain,* **118**, 455–65,

Cohen, P. & Cohen, J. (1984). The Clinician's illusion. *Archives of General Psychiatry,* **41**, 1178–242.

Crisp, J. (1995). Making sense of the stories that people with Alzheimer's tell: a journey with my mother. *Nursing Inquiry,* **2**, 133–40.

Dalla Barba, G. (1993). Different patterns of confabulation. *Cortex,* **29**, 567–81.

Dalla Barba, G. (1995) Consciousness and confabulation: remembering another past. In *Broken Memories: Case Studies in Memory Impairment,* ed. R. Campbell & M.A. Conway, pp. 101–14. Oxford, Blackwell.

Dalla Barba, G., Cipolloti, L. & Denes, G. (1990). Autobiographical memory loss and confabulation in Korsakoff's syndrome: a case report. *Cortex,* **26**, 1–10.

Dalla Barba, G., Boisse, M.F., Bartolomeo, P. & Bachoud-Levi, A.C. (1997). Confabulation following rupture of posterior communicating artery. *Cortex,* **33**, 563–70.

Danziger, K. (1997). *Naming the Mind.* London: Sage.

Davidson, D. (1980). *Essays on Actions and Events.* Oxford: Clarendon Press.

Deemter, K. & Peters, S. (1996). *Semantic Ambiguity and Underspecification.* California: CSLI Publication.

Delay, J. (1942). *Les Dissolutions de la Mémoire.* Paris: Presses Universitaires de France.

Delbecq-Derouesné, J., Beauvois, M.F. & Shallice, T. (1990). Preserved recall versus impaired recognition. A case study. *Brain,* **113**, 1045–74.

Della Sala, S., Laiacona, M., Spinnler, H. & Trivelli, C. (1993). Autobiographical recollection and frontal damage. *Neuropsychologia*, **31**, 823–39.

Devaux, A. & Logre, J.B. (1911). Amnésie et fabulation. Étude du syndrome 'presbyophrénique'. *Nouvelle Iconographie de la Salpêtrière*, **24**, 90–115.

Downes, J.J. & Mayes, A.R. (1995), How bad memories can sometimes lead to fantastic beliefs and strange visions. In *Broken Memories: Case Studies in Memory Impairment*, ed. R. Campbell & M.A. Conway, pp. 115–23. Oxford: Blackwell.

Dupré, E. (1925). La Mythomanie. In *Pathologie de l'Imagination et de l'Émotivité*, ed. E. Dupré, pp. 3–59. Paris: Payot.

Durandin, G. (1972). *Les Fondements de la Mensonge*. Paris: Flammarion.

Ekman, P. (1985). *Telling Lies*. New York: W.W. Norton.

Emmet, C.W. (1909). Fable. In *Dictionary of the Bible*, ed. J. Hastings, pp. 254–5. Edinburgh: T. & T. Clark.

Escandell-Vidal, M.V. (1993). *Introducción a la Pragmática*. Barcelona: Anthropos.

Ey, H. (1950). Étude N° 9. Les troubles de la mémoire. In *Études Psychiatriques.*, vol 2, pp. 9–68. Paris: Desclée de Brouwer.

Feinberg, T.E. (1997). Some interesting perturbations of the self in neurology. *Seminars in Neurology*, **17**, 129–35.

Feinberg, T.E., Roane, D.M., Kwan, P.C., Schindler, R.J. & Haber, L.D. (1994). Anosognosia and visuo-verbal confabulation. *Archives of Neurology*, **51**, 468–73.

Fischer, R.S., Alexander, M.P., D'Esposito, M. & Otto, R. (1995) Neuropsychological and neuroanatomical correlates of confabulation. *Journal Clinical Experimental Neuropsychology*, **17**, 20–8.

Gainotti, G. (1975). Confabulation of denial in senile dementia. *Psychiatria Clinica*, **8**, 99–108.

Gennaro, R.J. (1996). *Consciousness and Self-Consciousness*. Amsterdam: John Benjamin.

Goodwin, D.M. (1989). *A Dictionary of Neuropsychology*. Berlin: Springer.

Green, G.M. (1996) *Pragmatics and Language Understanding*, 2nd edn. London: Sage.

Gregor, A. & Roemer, H. (1906). Zur Kenntnis der Auffasung einfacher optischer Sinneseindrücke bei alkoholischen Geistesstörungen, inbesondere bei der Korsakoff'schen Psychose. *Neurologische Centralblatt*, **25**, 339–61.

Greimas, A.J. (1983). *Du Sens II. Essais Sémiotiques*. Paris: Seuil.

Hicks, L.H. & Myslobodsky, M.S. (1997). Mnemopoiesis: memories that wish themselves to be recalled. In *The Mythomanias*, ed. M.S Myslobodsky, pp. 307–26. Mahwah, NJ: Lawrence Erlbaum.

Hobson, J.A. (1997). Dreaming as delirium. *Seminars in Neurology*, **17**, 121–8.

Holst, van der (1932). Über die Psychologie des Korsakow-Syndroms. *Monatschrift der Neurologie*, **83**, 65–92.

Janet, P. (1928). *L'Évolution de la Mémoire et de la Notion du Temps*. Paris: A. Chahine.

Jaspers, K. (1948). *Allgemeine Psychopathologie*, 5th edn. Berlin: Springer.

Johnson, M.K. (1988). Discriminating the origin of information. In *Delusional Beliefs*, ed. T.F. Oltmanns & B.A. Maher, pp.34–65. New York: John Wiley.

Johnson, M.K. (1991). Reality monitoring: evidence from confabulation in organic brain disease patients. In *Awareness of Deficit after Brain Injury*, ed. G.P. Prigatano & D.L. Schacter, pp. 176–97. New York: Oxford University Press.

Johnson, M.K., Hashtroudi, S. & Lindsay, D.S. (1993). Source monitoring. *Psychological Bulletin*, **114**, 3–28.

Johnson, M.K., O'Connor, M. & Cantor, J. (1997). Confabulation, memory deficits, and frontal dysfunction. *Brain and Cognition*, **34**, 189–206.

Joseph, R. (1986). Confabulation and delusional denial: frontal lobe and lateralized influences. *Journal of Clinical Psychology*, **42**, 507–20.

Joslyn, D., Grundvig, J.K. & Chamberlain, C.J. (1978). Predicting confabulation from the Graham-Kendall Memory-for-Design Test. *Journal of Consulting and Clinical Psychology*, **46**, 181–2.

Kahlbaum, K. (1863). *Die Gruppirung der psychischen Krankheiten und die Eintheilung der Seelenstörungen*. Danzig: A.W. Kafemann (Part III, translated by G.E. Berrios, *History of Psychiatry* (1996), **7**, 167–81).

Kant, E. (1991). *The Metaphysics of Morals*. Translated by M.J. McGregor. Cambridge: Cambridge University Press. (1st edn 1797).

Kant, E. (1993). *Raising the Tone of Philosophy*. Translated by P. Fenves, Baltimore: Johns Hopkins Press (1st edn 1796).

Kapur, N. & Coughlan, A.K. (1980). Confabulation and frontal lobe dysfunction. *Journal of Neurology, Neurosurgery and Psychiatry*, **43**, 461–3.

King, B.H. & Ford, C.V. (1988). Pseudologia fantastica. *Acta Psychiatrica Scandinavica*, **77**, 1–6.

Koehler, K. & Jacoby, C. (1978). Acute confabulatory psychosis. *Acta Psychiatrica Scandinavica*, **57**, 415–25.

Kopelman, M.D. (1987). Two types of confabulation. *Journal of Neurology, Neurosurgery and Psychiatry*, **50**, 1482–7.

Kopelman, M.D., Ng, N. & Van Den Brouke, O. (1997). Confabulation extending across episodic, personal and general semantic memory. *Cognitive Neuropsychology*, **14**, 683–712.

Koppen, M. (1898). Über die pathologische Lungener. *Charité-Annalen*, **8**, 674–719.

Korsakoff, S.S. (1889). Étude médico-psychologique sur une forme des maladies de la memoire. *Revue Philosophique*, **28**, 501–30.

Korsakoff, S.S. (1891). Erinnerungsteuschungen (Pseudoreminiscenzen) bei polyneuritischer Psychose. *Allgemeine Zeitschrift der Psychiatrie*, **47**, 390–410.

Korsakoff, S.S. (1955). Psychic disorder in conjunction with multiple neuritis. Translation from the Russian by M. Victor & P.I. Yakovlev. *Neurology*, **5**, 394–406.

Kraepelin, E. (1886–1887). Über Erinnerungsfälschungen. *Archiv für Psychiatrie und Nervenkrankheiten*, **17**, 830–43; **18**, 199–239, 395–436.

Kraepelin, E. (1910). *Psychiatrie*, vol. 2, 8th edn. Leipzig: Barth.

Kraepelin, E. (1919). *Dementia Praecox*. Translated by R.M. Barclay & G.M. Robertson. Edinburgh: Livingstone.

Lafora, G.R. (1935). Sobre la presbiofrenia sin confabulaciones. *Archivos de Neurobología*, **15**, 179–211.

Levinson, S.C. (1983). *Pragmatics*. Cambridge: Cambridge University Press.

Liepmann, H. (1910). Beitrag zur Kenntnis des amnestichen Symptomenkomplexes. *Neurologische Centralblatt*, **29**, 1147–62.

Lindqvist, G. & Norlén G. (1966). Korsakoff's syndrome after operation on rupture aneurysm of the anterior communicating artery. *Acta Psychiatrica Scandinavica*, **42**, 24–34.

Lu, L.H., Barrett, A.M., Schwartz, R.L., Cibula, J.E., Gilmore, R.L., Uthman, B.M. & Heilman, K.M. (1997). Anosognosia and confabulation during the Wada test. *Neurology*, **49**, 1316–22.

Maeda, S. & Okawa, M. (1974). Psychiatric symptoms of ruptured intracraneal arterial aneurysms. *Clinical Neurology* (Japan), **14**, 1–9.

Manning, L. & Kartsounis, L.D. (1993). Confabulations related to tacit awareness in visual neglect. *Behavioural Neurology*, **6**, 211–13.

Marková, I.S. & Berrios, G.E. (1995a). Insight revisited. *Comprehensive Psychiatry*, **36**, 367–76.

Marková, I.S. & Berrios, G.E. (1995b). Insight in clinical psychiatry. A new model. *Journal of Nervous and Mental Disease*, **183**, 743–51.

Mercer, B., Wapner, W., Gardner, H. & Benson, F. (1977). A study of confabulations. *Archives of Neurology*, **34**, 429–33.

Meunier, R. (1904). Remarks on three cases of morbid lying. *Journal of Mental Pathology*, **6**, 140–2.

Morris, C.W. (1971). Foundations of the theory of signs. In *Writings on the General Theory of Signs*, pp. 17–74. The Hague: Mouton.

Moscovitch, M. (1989). Confabulation and the frontal lobe system. In *Varieties of Memory and Consciousness. Essays in Honour of Endel Tulving*, ed. H.L. Roediger & F.I. Craik. Hillsdale: Erlbaum.

Moscovitch, M. (1995). Confabulation. In *Memory Distortions*, ed. D.L. Schacter, pp. 226–51. Cambridge, MA: Harvard University Press.

Moscovitch, M. & Melo, B. (1997). Strategic retrieval and the frontal lobes: evidence from confabulation and amnesia. *Neuropsychologia*, **35**, 1017–34.

Myslobodsky, M.S. & Hicks, L.H. (1994). The rationale for confabulation: what does it take to fabricate a story. *Neurology, Psychiatry, and Brain Research*, **2**, 221–8.

Nathaniel-James, D.A. & Frith, C.D. (1996). Confabulation in schizophrenia. *Psychological Medicine*, **26**, 391–9.

Neyraut, M. (1962). La mythomanie. In *Encyclopédie Médico-Chirurgicale*. Psychiatrie, 37130 F10. Paris: Editions Techniques.

Nouët & Halberstadt (no initials) (1909). La presbyophrénie de Wernicke. *L'Encéphale*, **4**, 331–42.

Onfray, M. (1990). Mensonge. In *Les Notions Philosophiques*, vol. 2, ed. S. Auroux, pp. 1594–5. Paris: Presses Universitaires de France.

Ovsiew, F. (1992). Bedside neuropsychiatry. In *The American Psychiatric Press Textbook of Neuropsychiatry*, 2nd edn, ed. S.E. Yudofsky & R.E. Hales, pp. 89–125. Washington: American Psychiatric Press.

Papagno, C. & Baddeley, A. (1997). Confabulation in a dysexecutive syndrome. *Cortex*, **33**, 743–52.

Pick, A. (1905). Zur Psychologie der Confabulation. *Neurologische Centralblatt*, **24**, 509–16.

Potel, G. (1902). *Amnésie Continue Associée aux Polynévrites.* Paris: Asselin & Houzeau.

Régis, E. (1906). *Précis de Psychiatrie*, 3rd edn. Paris: Doin.

Rey, E. (1925). *Éloge du Mensonge.* Paris: Hachette.

Risch, B. (1908). Über die phantastische Form des degenerativen Irreseins, Pseudologia Phantastica. *Allgemeine Zeitschrift für Psychiatrie*, **65**, 576–639.

Robinson, W.P. (1996). *Deceit, Delusion and Detection.* London: Sage.

Rouby, J. (1911). *Contribution à l'Étude de la Presbyophrénie.* Thèse de Médecine. Paris, E. Nourris.

Roufineau, F.M. (1841). *Thèse sur Cette Question: Est-il Permis de Mentir dans Certains Cas?* Paris: Mautauban.

Schnider, A. Däniken, C. & Gutbrod, K. (1996). The mechanisms of spontaneous and provoked confabulations. *Brain*, 119, 1365–75.

Schlieben-Lange, B. (1975). *Linguistische Pragmatik.* Stuttgart: W. Kohlhammer.

Servan, J., Verstichel, P, Catala, M. & Rancurel, G. (1994). Syndromes amnésiques et fabulations au cours d'infarctus du territoire de l'artere cerebrale posterieure. *Revue Neurologique*, **150**, 201–208.

Shapin, S. (1994). *A Social History of Truth.* Chicago: Chicago University Press.

Shapiro, B.E., Alexander, M.P., Gardner, H. & Mercer, B. (1981). Mechanisms of confabulations. *Neurology*, **31**, 1070–6.

Sperber, D. & Wilson, D. (1995). *Relevance, Communication and Cognition*, 2nd edn. Oxford: Blackwell.

Stuss, D.T., Alexander, M.P., Lieberman, A. & Levine, H. (1978). An extraordinary form of confabulation. *Neurology*, **28**, 1166–72.

Swartz, B.E. & Brust, J.C.M. (1984). Anton's syndrome accompanying withdrawal hallucinosis in a blind alcoholic. *Neurology*, **34**, 969–73.

Talland, G.A. (1961). Confabulation in the Wernicke-Korsakoff syndrome. *Journal of Nervous and Mental Disease*, **132**, 361–81.

Victor, M., Adams, R.A. & Collins, G.H. (1971). *The Wernicke–Korsakoff Syndrome.* Philadelphia: F.A. Davies Company.

Villiers, C., Zent, R. & Swingler, D. (1996). A flight of fantasy: false memories in frontal lobe disease. *Journal of Neurology, Neursurgery and Psychiatry*, **61**, 652–3.

Weinstein, E.A. (1996). Symbolic aspects of confabulation following brain injury. *Bulletin of the Menninger Clinic*, **60**, 331–50.

Weinstein, E.A., Kahn, R.L. & Malitz, S. (1956). Confabulation as a social process. *Psychiatry*, **19**, 383–96.

Welsch, L.W., Nimmerrichter, A., Gilliland, R., King, D.E. & Martin, P.R. (1997). 'Wineglass' confabulations among brain-damaged alcoholics on the Wechsler memory Scale-Revised visual reproduction subtest. *Cortex*, **33**, 543–51.

Wernicke, K. (1906). *Grundriss der Psychiatrie*, 2nd edn. Leipzig: Thieme.

Whitlock, F.A. (1981). Some observations on the meaning of confabulation. *British Journal of Medical Psychology*, **54**, 213–18.

Williams, H.W. & Rupp, C. (1938). Observations on confabulation. *American Journal of Psychiatry*, **95**, 395–405.

Williams, M. & Pennybacker, J. (1954). Memory disturbance in third ventricle tumours. *Journal of Neurology, Neurosurgery and Psychiatry*, **15**, 115–23.

Zervas, I.M., Fliesser, J.M., Woznicki, M. & Fricchione, G.L. (1993). Presbyophrenia: a possible type of dementia. *Journal of Geriatrics, Psychiatry and Neurology*, **6**, 25–8.

Ziehen, T. (1911). Les démences. In *Traité International de Psychologie Pathologique*, vol. 2, ed. Marie, pp. 281–381. Paris: Alcan.

# Flashbulb and flashback memories

Mauricio Sierra and German E. Berrios

It is an old observation[1] that life events attended by particular emotional or cognitive relevance leave behind 'images' or 'memories' which may include vivid background detail (normally not remembered)[2] such as colour of clothes being worn at the time, weather conditions, background music, etc., etc. On account of this quality of being like a photograph such recollections have been called 'flashbulb memories' (Brown & Kulik, 1977). This metaphor has helped neither the description or understanding of this phenomenon.[3] Equally unhelpful has been the fact that the original research was carried out on parochial American events which may have introduced into the structure of flashbulb memories some social ambiguity.[4]

It is suggested in this chapter that, as far as psychiatry is concerned, 'vivid personal memories' should be studied against the wider canvas of other repetitive phenomena of the imagination such as drug flashbacks, palinopsia, palinacusis, tinnitus, post-traumatic memories, and the vivid memories of subjects suffering conditions such as phobias, panic attacks, obsessional disorder, phantom-limb phenomena, and depressive melancholia. The reason for this is twofold: first, that there is little evidence that flashbulb memories are a special phenomenon; secondly, that it is more parsimonious (and in keeping with empirical findings) to think that, like all other mnestic acts, flashbulb memories are also governed by the rules of narrative. The latter is particularly important for the very name of 'flashbulb memories' (and the fact that some have been reported as detail-perfect sensory images[5]) may have caused the misleading impression that they: (a) may be impervious to the influence of narrative templates,[6] and (b) constitute clinical evidence against a 'reconstructivist' view of memory.[7]

## Flashbulb memories

### Brown and Kulik's definition

The boundaries of a clinical phenomenon are often constrained by its original description and much of what is currently discussed on flashbulb memories remains determined by Brown and Kulik's definition (1977). According to these authors, to create a flashbulb memory an event must be 'surprising' and 'consequential'. To test their view they chose nine such events: the murders of Medgar Evers, John Kennedy, Malcolm X, Martin Luther King, and Robert Kennedy, the attempted assassination of G. Wallace and Gerald Ford, the drowning of a woman in which Ted Kennedy was allegedly involved, and the death of Franco; a tenth (control) event concerned a 'private shock'. Information from 40 Blacks and 40 Whites was scored in terms of categories such as place, ongoing event, informant, affect in others, own affect, and aftermath (some of these considered as 'canonical' categories). It was concluded that the creation of a flashbulb memory depended upon high level of 'surprise', a high level of 'consequentiality' (perceived relevance to the individual), and high level of 'arousal'.

In summary, a stimulus or event that caused (a high degree of) surprise and was re-inforced by (high) consequentiality may generate an inchoate flashbulb memory which is then strengthened by rehearsal. The memory itself was formed by a vestigial brain mechanism (like Livingston's 'now print' neurobiological device) which 'must have evolved because of the selection value of permanently retaining biologically crucial, but unexpected events' (p. 97). Brown and Kulik's views have been challenged both from the structural and phenomenological standpoint (Neisser, 1982; Winograd & Neisser, 1992) and also from an aetiological–evolutionary perspective (McCloskey et al., 1988).

Neisser (1982) criticized the 'accuracy' claim by stating that many memories were not detail-perfect and that, in many cases, 'rehearsal' may be involved. He also felt that because the 'consequentiality' criterion was post-hoc it could not be part of the explanation. Lastly, he called into question the efficiency of the high arousal condition for the 'printing of the memory' arguing that emotional situations often cause a narrowing of attention which would lead to the missing out of much background detail. In a later book, Winograd and Neisser (1992) reported data on the 1986 Challenger disaster and wondered whether: (i) memories were accurate, (ii) it was necessary to postulate a special mechanism, (iii) the phenomenon told anything about the relationship between emotion and memory, and (iv) the determinants of the flashback memory operated only at the time of putative encoding or continued shaping it for a long time after the event.

In an elegant conceptual and empirical analysis of the phenomenon, Conway (1995) has sought to explain flashbulb memories in terms of a general theory of autobiographical memories and concluded:

Brown and Kulik were correct: there is a distinct class of memories for events that are emotional and personally important, and sometimes surprising. These memories are more detailed and long-lasting than most everyday autobiographical memories, play a central role in autobiographical memory, support many different uses of memory in interpersonal relations, and facilitate cultural processes such as the expression of generational identity. Furthermore, the evidence from neurobiological studies of memory, although provisional at this stage nevertheless strongly points to the possibility of some type of preferential encoding of flashbulb memories (pp. 126–7).

## Clinical features

### Phenomenology

Whether a special visual imagery memory system is involved in the formation of flashbulb memories[8] is unclear (Wright & Gaskell, 1995). Earlier research focused on visual phenomena, e.g. particularly featural accuracy and stability of the recollection. In their study of the Challenger explosion, Neisser and Harsh (1992) found that 'visual images' were more frequent than auditory ones. In his study of the assassination attempt on President Reagan, Pillemer(1984) found that 71% of subjects reported 'visual memories'. Likewise, Rubin and Kozin (1984) found that about 58% of subjects rated visual images as 'as vivid as normal vision'. Lastly, Brewer (1988) showed that when memory episodes are experimentally singled out by the random activation of an alarm, subjects more frequently report vivid 'visual imagery'.

Accuracy (report reliability) of flashbulb memories can be assessed by comparing successive accounts of the same experience by the same individual. However, inconsistencies between two such accounts could be due to reasons other than unstable sensory features (e.g. changes in temporal tagging (Brewer, 1988), different personal context and constraints, varying testing instructions, etc.). On the whole, flashbulb memories seem more accurate and stable than ordinary memories (Bohanon & Simons, 1992; Christianson, 1989; McCloskey et al., 1988; Pillemer, 1984). However, they are *not* immune to change (Neisser & Harsh, 1992); for example, the regular finding of a change in 'visual perspective' or shift towards an 'observer's perspective' (i.e. the subject reports his memory as if he was actually watching it from the outside) suggests that flashbulb memories undergo reconstruction (Nigro & Neisser, 1983).

### The 'observer's perspective'

In a nineteenth century study of childhood memories in adults, Henri and Henri (1897) found that subjects could see themselves as external observers: 'I can see myself during an episode of illness as somebody outside myself' (p. 193). Freud (1974/1888), and more recently von Leyden (1961), have regarded this as evidence that the images for some memories are not just unchanged copies of the original experience:

I might, for example, remember falling downstairs, but when I remember it, I 'see' it, in my image, as if I were a spectator watching myself fall. This could not possibly have been my experience at the time. Clearly, then, our images in remembering are *not the original experiences produced again*, nor even present reproductions or representations of those original experiences [our emphasis] (Locke, 1971: pp. 889).

Nigro and Neisser (1983) have also reported that an important proportion of personal recollections are of this type, particularly 'old events or those associated with heightened self-awareness'. Interestingly enough, it has been recently suggested that a reduction in the affect attached to a memory may encourage this shift towards the 'observer's perspective' (Robinson & Swanson, 1993). In the literature on trauma, a similar shift is considered to be the result of a 'dissociative detachment' which is assumed to occur at the time of the traumatic event itself. For example, Spiegel (1991) reported the case of a young woman who recalled her accidental fall from a third-floor balcony 'as though she had been standing on a nearby balcony watching her falling body' (p. 261). At what stage the shift and/or reconstruction involved in these recollections takes place remains unclear.

## Mechanisms

### The role of emotions

It has been suggested that concomitant 'emotional arousal' plays a role in the vividness and accuracy of flashbulb memories (Bohanon, 1988; Brown & Kulik, 1977; Christianson & Loftus, 1990; Pillemer, 1984; Rubin & Kosin, 1984). It is unclear, however, whether emotions are *directly* involved in memory encoding (Gold, 1992)[9] or simply increase rehearsal frequency (Bohanon, 1988). However, circumstantial evidence from clinical practice supports the 'encoding hypothesis'. Thus, recollections of their first panic attack by anxious patients (Winokur & Holemon, 1963) are sometimes as detailed as flashbulb memories. On the other hand, the fact that frequency of retelling per se does not improve the quality of the memory (Brown & Kulik, 1977; Pillemer, 1984; Neisser & Harsh, 1992) suggests that rehearsal alone is sufficient.

The way in which emotions modulate memory encoding remains unclear: for example, in the short term emotional arousal seems to have a detrimental effect on memory but in the long term the effect is reversed for emotions seem to attenuate forgetting rate (Heuer & Reisberg, 1992). Vividness of memory components (regardless of 'relevance') seems also enhanced by emotional arousal: for example, memories for movies seen six months earlier (or before) were assessed and target scenes categorized into 'emotional or non-emotional'. The memories for 'emotional scenes' were found to be significantly more accurate in relation to 'plot-irrelevant details', such as colours of clothes, phrasing of dialogues, etc. (quoted in Heuer & Reisberg, 1992). According to these authors, the fact that the emotionality of the scenes did not enhance the recollection of the plot itself suggests that the effect may be specific for 'image memories'.

## Evolutionary mechanisms

The fact that flashbulb memories were originally conceived of as a 'memory picture' invited the explanatory metaphor that they were 'printed' onto the brain (Brown & Kulik, 1977). In this regard, Pillemer (1984) has written:

Walking in the tall grass, near an unfamiliar waterhole, with few companions, at dusk, these characteristics must trigger an emotional reaction and recollection of the earlier tragedy. To depend solely on purposeful, deliberate reconstruction of prior similar episodes is risky – an attack may occur before relevant information is accessed (p. 78).

Thus, a sort of 'vestigial pre-verbal memory system', available form birth, would remain operational throughout life (Pillemer & White, 1989). Supporting this view, Terr (1988) has reported that, before the age of three, traumatic events seem exclusively encoded as visual images; verbal processing only becoming available afterwards. In broader terms, 'memory recollections' are encoded as images, and 'autobiographical facts' as verbal propositional knowledge (Brewer, 1996). Clinical cases showing a 'double dissociation' suggest that these two forms of autobiographical memory have different brain locations. Patients with 'psychogenic amnesia' are reported to experience intrusive images of forgotten events without having factual knowledge for the episode (Loewenstein, 1991a); on the other hand, an amnesic patient who could remember 'autobiographical facts' such as having visited his parents' country home, claimed not to have any image recollection of having been there (Tulving, 1989).

Although mnestic images are described as less detailed and colour saturated and more blurred and unstable than those pertaining to ordinary perception (Brewer, 1996),[10] in clinical practice cases are met with of mnestic images of unusual vividness where the original event appears before the mind's eye in glorious sensory apparel.

## A psychiatric canvas: hallucinations as vivid memories

It has been suggested above that, because flashbulb memories, drug-related 'flashbacks', eidetic imagery, palinopsia, the vivid memories of a variety of psychiatric disorders, pain-hallucinations, etc. have a number of phenomenological features, they may constitute a family of mnestic events sharing similar neurobiological mechanisms. The testing of this hypothesis has not been pursued in earnest due to two main reasons: one is that it remains customary in descriptive psychopathology to consider these phenomena as independent; the other that some seem rare events. Thus, subjects with enhanced eidetic memory are now only considered to be an interesting curiosity; palinopsia is but a neurological rarity; the hallucinatory images seen in obsessional disorder are only of interest to Continental psychiatrists; pain hallucinations are more likely to be seen in the orthopaedic clinic, and flashbacks are mainly dealt with in the context of post-traumatic stress disorder and substance abuse.

## Flashbacks

### The original model

The term 'flashback' names different clinical phenomena (Frankel, 1994). It was originally introduced to describe 'returns of [visual] imagery for extended periods after the immediate effect of hallucinogens has worn off. The most symptomatic form is recurrent intrusions of the same frightening image into awareness, without volitional control' (Horowitz, 1969: p. 565). Flashbacks could also occur in the taste, smell, touch, kinaesthetic, and auditory modalities. The term was extended to include 'spontaneous recurrence of earlier drug-induced experiences' after Horowitz (1969) suggested that the imagery of these experiences was identical to (or derived from) images experienced during actual drug intoxication. For example, a patient continued having the recurrent intrusive images of a lizard: 'I see this giant iguana, all the time man. Green, in corners . . . [unlike other kinds of thought-images] it's real green' (p. 566).

This broader concept was also supported by Shick and Smith (1970) and by Matefy et al. (1978) who found that 57% of subjects rated their flashbacks as 'exact' phenomenological replicas of previous drug experiences. On the other hand, Siegel and Jarvik (1975), in an 18-month follow-up of six patients experiencing flashbacks after Ketamine anaesthesia, reported that the hallucinatory experiences changed in nature, oscillating between complex experiences and geometric patterns (pp. 132–4). This type of study is marred by the fact that retrospective ascertainment is often unreliable and may capture different clinical phenomena; furthermore, some of these experiences are 'state-dependent', namely, they are better recalled when the subject is in a similar state of intoxication as the one in which he acquired it (Eich, 1980).

### Flashbacks in psychological trauma

During the 1980s, 'flashback' was used to refer to the 're-visualization of the trauma scene that occurred with realistic intensity' in Post-Traumatic Stress Disorder

(PTSD) (Burstein, 1985). However, the indeterminatedness of the concept allowed for the inclusion of a variety of other PTSD 'symptoms' such as nightmares, illusions, and vivid imagery. The high frequency with which visual experiences are reported should not obscure the fact that subjects also experience auditory and olfactory phenomena. Whatever the sensory modality, intense emotional arousal equivalent to the levels of anxiety present in panic attacks are often present (Mellman & Davis, 1985).[11] Behavioural acting out also suggests that the subject may be 're-living the experience'.

Flashbacks are triggered by fatigue and certain moods states; and also by environmental cues assumedly related to the original situation suggesting the operation of a context-dependent retrieval mechanism (e.g. in Vietnam veterans, the sound of a helicopter or the smell of blood, etc.) (Kline & Rausch, 1985). Verbal accounts of these experiences are as detailed as the exact narratives commonly associated with flashbulb memories (Brown & Kulik, 1977). For example, a patient reported:

I was stationed in the New Hebrides. I was onshore unloading a ship, when an offshore destroyer hit a mine. I was called upon to assist in the recovery and burial of bodies. I was soaked from head to toe with ocean water, floating diesel fuel, and blood. In order to bury the sailors who had washed ashore, we had to use makeshift coffins. The best we could do for coffins was boxes we made from propeller wood. One of the boxes broke apart, exposing a body. The smell was horrendous. There were flies everywhere, millions of them. They swarmed on the body and all over me. I was covered almost instantly. I put down the box, took off all my clothes, and walked away. To this day, whenever I smell diesel fuel and salt water together, I remember that burial detail and smell those rotting bodies (Kline & Rausch, 1985: p. 384).

Such phenomenological similarities suggest a continuum of which PTSD flashbacks would just be the extreme expression. According to Pillemer (1984), 'the [evolutionary] success of the flashbulb memory system would seem to require a flashback mechanism' (p. 78).

To ascertain whether the details associated with flashbulb memories are driven by the a priori semantic network of the event or by its context, Pillemer (1984) asked a group of subjects to list their initial thoughts after hearing of the assassination attempt on President Reagan. The fact that around 25% of subjects reported thinking about their own circumstances at the time of earlier assassinations was interpreted as supporting the existence of a 'flashback mechanism'.

### Accuracy of flashbacks

The view that flashbacks are 'dissociative' traumatic experiences takes for granted their accuracy (Frankel, 1994).[12] For example, in a sample of 20 civilian patients complaining of flashbacks after accidents or assaults, Burstein (1983) only took care to ascertain the occurrence of the event assuming that the details were correct.

However, validation is of importance as it would seem that some details are better recalled than others; for example, in a recent study when verifying the content of flashback experiences in a Vietnam veteran, Spiegel (1991) found that a soldier the patient thought 'killed' was, in fact, alive.

Like personal recollections, flashbacks may also be experienced from the 'perspective of the observer'. For example, in a study of sodium lactate-induced flashbacks, Rainey et al. (1987) reported that a Vietnam veteran who had received a chest injury in combat 'saw himself' in surgery watching his own operation; and another 'saw himself falling off an armoured vehicle, and having a seizure' (p. 1318). The internal contradictions contained in other accounts suggest that reconstructions (or confabulation) may have taken place: for example, 'after passing out' one patient 'saw himself strapped down in a hospital'; another 'saw himself repeatedly killing a North Vietnamese woman: he would kill her, she would get up, and he would kill her again' (p. 1318). In their classification of flashbacks in traumatic hand injury, Grunert et al. (1988) list 'projected flashbacks', namely 'images of injuries beyond those that actually occurred' (p. 126) once again suggesting that the memory of the original experience was reconstructed.

### Electrically elicited 'flashbacks'

The vivid image recollections of past personal events elicited by Penfield and Perot (1963) in their stimulation studies are also phenomenologically redolent of PTSD flashbacks and flashbulb memories. In general, these authors found a predominance of vivid visual and auditory images, a re-experiencing of original emotions, and even inclusion of irrelevant detail. Penfield and Perot (1963) proposed the following explanation:

> Past experience, when it is recalled electrically seems to be complete including all the things of which an individual was aware at the time; also that, since the events were often unimportant, it seemed likely that the whole stream of consciousness must also be recorded somewhere, quite beyond the reach of voluntary summons (p. 289).

However, Penfield and Perot (1963) also believed that a reconstructive process was in operation whereby information from 'actual experience, from the individual's reading or from his dreaming' was also incorporated (p. 224).

Using more precise stimulation techniques, Gloor et al. (1982) have more recently concluded that, unlike the verbal narratives used by patients to report their experiences, evoked image experiences are 'fragmentary and often have the quality of a vivid 'flashback' to a specific event in the past without the full sequential re-enactment of the event. They could not be likened to the replay of a videotape' (p. 113). Importantly, these researchers also noted that the ongoing mental frame at the time of stimulation modulated the evoked memory experience.

## Post-traumatic nightmares

Victims of trauma often report 'anxious dreams' in which the traumatic event is relived in vivid multisensory images accompanied by the same intense emotions as those of the original event. Although reported as an accurate 'playback', these experiences are also subject to a 'switching of perspective'. Post-traumatic dreams seem unrelated to conventional REM sleep; thus, reporting a patient with a 'post-traumatic nightmare', Hartman (1984) commented that 'it may still make sense to consider post-traumatic nightmares as being something akin to a sub-clinical epileptic discharge'.

## Other hallucinatory phenomena

For varied lengths of time after their original occurrence, hallucinatory replicas may follow some specific events. For example, Stromeyer and Psotka (1970) ascertained this phenomenon by presenting subjects endowed with 'eidetic imagery'[13] with an image ('hidden' in a dot pattern) which only if accurately 'hallucinated' would form, in conjunction with later presentations, a three-dimensional pattern.

Palinopsia is defined as the recurrence (after varied intervals) of the image of a previously seen object (Meadows & Munro, 1977): for example, a patient: 'peeled a banana and in a few minutes saw multiple vivid images of bananas projected over the wall' (Michel & Troost, 1980, p. 887). More complex scenes can also be hallucinated such as a 'man walking in front of a window' (Cleland et al., 1981). It is usually accepted in these cases that the 'hallucinated image' is actually a replica of the original stimulus even when, in the case of moving objects, their speed may be increased. In palinacusis the patients report voices, music or random noises 'indistinguishable from the original stimulus' (Malone & Leiman, 1983, p. 1067). However, no attempt seems to have been made to verify the accuracy of these various forms of 'hallucination'. Clinical observation suggests that there are differences between these phenomena and 'normal' image-memories and other memory-dependent hallucinations (see below). For example, their vividness seems unrelated to accompanying emotions or personal relevance; furthermore, their sensory quality is at its best when the hallucination occurs shortly after the original event. These anomalies notwithstanding, the occurrence of this variety of hallucinations suggests the existence of a primitive brain mechanism that accurately processes the sensory component of memories.

### Body memories and pain hallucinations

Clinical observation suggests that a memory system for somatic images may also be in play. For example, amputees report pain with the same quality and location as the pre-amputation pain; this can happen even after cessation of their phantom limb experience (Melzack, 1971). Thus, Leriche (1947) reported a patient in whom an ill-fitting plaster cast caused painful ulcerations over the Achilles tendon and in the event he required an amputation; six years later, after an injection into the stump, the patient developed pain in the phantom limb which permanently revived the pain over the ulcerated Achilles tendon. A similar phenomenon has been reported by Nathan (1962): after having noxious stimuli applied to his stump, an amputee re-experienced the pain of an ice-skate injury he had sustained 5 years earlier when his leg was still intact. Sensations associated with the removal or de-afferentation of internal bodily organs have also been reported: for example, the feeling of passing gas and faeces after the rectum had been removed (Farley & Smith, 1968), and of labour pain and menstrual cramps after hysterectomy (Dorpat, 1971).

Relevant to the central idea of this chapter is the fact that these experiences are also accompanied by great sensory detail; for example, a report of 'blood-filled boots or blood trickling down the phantom limb' (Henderson & Smith, 1948). Likewise, the amputees (43% of 68) that reported 'somatic memories' in the retrospective study by Katz and Melzack (1990) were so detailed in their descriptions that the authors had to created 22 categories for one variety of pain 'memory' alone ('cutaneous ulcer', 'ingrown toe nail', and 'arthritis', etc.). Five patients described phantom limb sensations such as a shoe-clad phantom foot, wrapping bandages, the feeling of release of pressure after a boot was cut off to free the foot, etc. Another five patients reported visual, tactile, and motor somatosensory memories: a subject with a gangrenous big toe before the amputation reported that, upon feeling the phantom pain, he had also a mental image of his discoloured big toe. Such images were often accompanied by high levels of anxiety which again suggests a role for emotional arousal in the coding of their vividness.

The accuracy of such somatic memories has been tested. In a prospective study, Jensen et al. (1985) collected information about the general location and sensory character of pain experienced the day before the amputation, and on three different occasions afterwards. Eight days after amputation, 74% of patients reported that the location of the phantom limb pain replicated that of pre-amputation pain; two years later, this persisted in almost half of the patients. The quality of the phantom limb pain was similar in 53% and 35% of patients, at day 8 and 2 years later, respectively.

The reporting of 'somatic memories' in subjects suffering from temporary deafferentation states (e.g. spinal anaesthesia) raises the question of whether these experiences may also occur in normal individuals and be, so to speak, superimposed upon their ongoing bodily experiences. In this regard, Katz and Melzak (1990) comment 'when a missing or completely anaesthetic limb continues to be the source of pain which resembles an old injury, one of the obvious conclusions is that the pain is centrally represented. *This conclusion would not be obvious if the painful limb were present and fully functional'* (our emphasis) (p. 320). This issue raises conceptual problems akin to those discussed in relation to the inability (both by subject and observer) to tell real perceptions from hallucinations in sense modalities where the 'relevant' stimulus is not in the public domain (e.g. touch) (Berrios, 1982). It is tempting to suggest that 'somatic memories' may be one of the explanations for the bodily complaints seen in dissociative disorders when 'a traumatic event is recalled in a sensory mode without the patient's awareness of the origin of the symptom' (Loewenstein, 1991b, p. 600). Arguing along the same lines, Kluft (1991) has reported a patient who, in the absence of organic findings, complained of proctalgia and the sensation of a foreign mass in her rectum; psychiatric evaluation subsequently unravelled a history of painful anal rape for which the patient had total amnesia.

## Conclusions

'Flashbulb memory' is a recent (quasimetaphorical) name for the recollection, putatively detail – perfect both in terms of core content and background, of some specific social or personal events assumed to be of significance to the individual or the social group. Their reputed 'photographic' quality has led some to suggest that they are generated by some evolutionary mechanism for the rapid capture and storage of information. Of late, some of the assumptions on which the original description was based, have been called into question.

There has also been a tendency in the memory literature to study this phenomenon as if it were unique. To psychiatrists, however, flashbulb memories are but one of a family of experiences sharing features such as paroxysmal repetition, sensory vividness, triggering of emotions, dysphoria, and a tendency to become organized in ever more complex narratives. It has been suggested in this chapter that studying these experiences as a group is more likely to provide information on underlying neurobiological mechanism than the study of flashbulb memories alone.

## REFERENCES

Behrmann, M., Kosslyn, S.M. & Jeannerod, M. (eds.) (1995). *The Neuropsychology of Mental Imagery.* Oxford: Pergamon.

Berrios, G.E. (1982). Tactile hallucinations. *Journal of Neurology, Neurosurgery and Psychiatry,* **45,** 285–93.

Bohanon, J.N. (1988). Flashbulb memories for the Space Shuttle disaster: a tale of two theories. *Cognition*, **29**,179–96.

Bohanon, J.N. & Simons, V.L. (1992). Flashbulb memories: confidence, consistency and quantity. In *Affect and Accuracy in Recall: Studies of 'Flashbulb Memories'*, ed. E. Winograd & U. Neisser, pp. 65–91. Cambridge: Cambridge University Press.

Brewer, W.F. (1988). Memory for randomly sampled autobiographical events. In *Remembering Reconsidered: Ecological and Traditional Approaches to the Study of Memory*, ed. U. Neisser & E. Winograd, pp. 21–90. New York: Cambridge University Press.

Brewer, W.F. (1996). What is recollective memory? In *Remembering our Past*, ed. D. Rubin, pp. 19–66, Cambridge: Cambridge University Press.

Brown, B. & Kulik, J. (1977). Flashbulb memories. *Cognition*, **5**, 73–99.

Burstein, A. (1983). Risks associated with post-traumatic flashbacks. *Journal of the Medical Society of New Jersey*, **81**, 863–4.

Burstein, A. (1985). Posttraumatic flashbacks, dream disturbances, and mental imagery. *Journal of Clinical Psychiatry*, **46**, 374–8.

Christianson, S.Å. (1989). Flashbulb memories: special, but not so special. *Memory and Cognition*, **17**, 435–43.

Christianson, S. Å. & Loftus, E.F. (1990). Some characteristics of people's traumatic memories. *Bulletin of the Psychonomic Society*, **28**, 195–8.

Cleland, P.G., Saunders, M. & Rosser, R. (1981). An unusual case of visual perseveration. *Journal of Neurology, Neurosurgery, and Psychiatry*, **44**, 226–63.

Conway, M. (1995). *Flashbulb Memories*. Hove: Lawrence Erlbaum.

Cummins, R. (1989). *Meaning and Mental Representation*. Cambridge, MA: MIT Press.

Denis, M. (1979). *Les Images Mentales*. Paris: Presses Universitaires de France.

Dorpat, T.L. (1971). Phantom sensations of internal organs. *Comprehensive Psychiatry*, **12**, 27–35.

Eich, E. (1980). The cue dependent nature of state-dependent retrieval. *Memory and Cognition*, **8**, 157–73.

Farley, D. & Smith, I. (1968). Phantom rectum after complete rectal excision. *British Journal of Surgery*, **55**, 40.

Frankel, F. (1994). The concept of flashbacks in historical perspective. *The International Journal of Clinical and Experimental Hypnosis*, **42**, 321–36.

Freud, S. (1974). Screen memories. In *The Standard Edition of the Complete Psychological Works of Sigmund Freud*, vol. 3, ed. James Strachey. London: Hogarth Press (originally published 1888).

Gloor, P., Olivier, A., Quensney, L. F., Anderman, F. & Horowitz, S. (1982). The role of the limbic system in experiential phenomena of temporal lobe epilepsy. *Annals of Neurology*, **12**, 129–44.

Gold, P.E. (1992). A proposed neurobiological basis for regulating memory storage for significant events. In *Affect and Accuracy in Recall: Studies of 'Flashbulb' Memories*, ed. E. Winograd & U. Neisser, pp. 141–61. Cambridge: Cambridge University Press.

Grunert, B.K., Devine, C.A., Matloub, H.S., Sanger, J.R. & Yousif, J. (1988). Flashbacks after traumatic injuries: prognostic indicators. *The Journal of Hand Surgery*, **13A**, 125–7

Hartman, E. (1984) *The Nightmare: The Psychology and Biology of Terrifying Dreams*. New York: Basic Books.

Henderson, W.R. & Smith, G.E. (1948). Phantom limbs. *Journal of Neurology, Neurosurgery and Psychiatry*, **2**, 88–112.

Henri, V. & Henri, C. (1897). Enquête sur les premiers souvenirs de l'enfance. *L'Année Psychologique*, **3**, 184–98.

Heuer, F. & Reisberg, D. (1992) Remembering the details of emotional events. In *Affect and Accuracy in Recall: Studies of 'Flashbulb' Memories*, ed. E. Winograd & U. Neisser, pp. 162–90. Cambridge: Cambridge University Press,

Horowitz, M. (1969). Flashbacks: recurrent intrusive images after the use of LSD. *American Journal of Psychiatry*, **126**, 565–9.

Jaensch, E.R. (1930). *Eidetic Imagery*. Translation of the Second German Edition by O. Oeser. New York: Harcourt.

Jelliffe, S.E. (1928). On eidetic psychology and psychiatric problems. *Medical Journal and Record*, **28**, 80–3.

Jensen, T.S., Krebs, B., Nielsen, J. & Rasmussen, P. (1985). Immediate and long-term phantom pain in amputees: incidence, clinical characteristics and relationship to pre-amputation pain. *Pain*, **21**, 267–78.

Katz, A. (1983). What does it mean to be a high imager? In *Imagery, Memory and Cognition. Essays in Honour of Allan Paivio*, ed. J.C. Yuille, pp. 39–63. New Jersey: Erlbaum.

Katz, J. & Melzack, R. (1990) Pain 'memories' in phantom limbs: review and clinical observations. *Pain*, **43**, 319–36.

Kline, N.A. & Rausch, J.L. (1985). Olfactory precipitants of flashbacks in posttraumatic stress disorder: case reports. *Journal of Clinical Psychiatry*, **46**, 383–4

Kluft, R.P. (1991). Clinical presentations of multiple personality disorder. *Psychiatric Clinics of North America*, **14**, 605–29.

Kosslyn, S.M. (1994). *Image and the Brain*. Cambridge: MIT Press.

Krystal, J.H., Southwick, S.M. & Charney, D.S. (1995). Posttraumatic stress disorder: psychobiological mechanisms of traumatic remembrance. In *Memory Distortion*, ed. D.L. Schacter, pp. 150–72. Cambridge: Harvard University Press,

Leriche, R. (1947). A propos de la douleur des amputés. *Mémoires de l'Academie de Chirugie*, **73**, 280–4.

Locke, D. (1971). *Memory*. London: Macmillan.

Loewenstein, R.J. (1991a). Psychogenic amnesia and psychogenic fugue: a comprehensive review. In *APA Review of Psychiatry*, ed. A. Tasman & S.M. Goldfinger, Vol. 10, pp. 223–47.

Loewenstein, R.J. (1991b). An office mental status examination for complex chronic dissociative symptoms and multiple personality disorder. *Psychiatric Clinics of North America*, **14**, 567–604.

Loftus, E. F., Feldman, J. & Dashiell, R. (1995). The reality of illusory memories. In *Memory Distortion*. ed. D.L. Schacter, pp. 47–68. Cambridge, MA: Harvard University Press.

McCloskey, M., Wible, C. & Cohen, N. (1988). Is there a special flashbulb-memory mechanism? *Journal of Experimental Psychology* (General) **117**, 171–81.

Malone, G.L. & Leiman, H.I. (1983). Differential diagnosis of palinacusis in a psychiatric patient. *American Journal of Psychiatry*, **140**, 1067–8.

Matefy, R.E., Hayes, C. & Hirsch, J. (1978). Psychedelic drug flashbacks: subjective reports and biographical data. *Addictive Behaviours*, **3**, 165–78.

Meadows, J.C. & Munro, S.S.F. (1977). Palinopsia. *Journal of Neurology, Neurosurgery, and Psychiatry*, **40**, 5–8.

Mellman, T.A. & Davis, G.C. (1985). Combat-related flashbacks in posttraumatic stress disorder: phenomenology and similarity to panic attacks. *Journal of Clinical Psychiatry*, **46**, 379–82.

Melzack, R. (1971). Phantom limb pain: implications for treatment of pathological pain. *Anaesthesiology*, **35**, 409–19.

Meyerson, É. (1929). Les images. *Journal de Psychologie Normale et Pathologique*, **26**, 625–709.

Michel, E.M. & Troost, T. (1980). Palinopsia cerebral localization with computed tomography. *Neurology*, **30**, 887–9.

Mintz, S. & Alpert, M. (1972). Imagery vividness, reality testing, and schizophrenic hallucinations. *Journal of Abnormal Psychology*, **79**, 310–16.

Nathan, P.W. (1962). Pain traces left in the central nervous system. In *The Assessment of Pain in Man and Animals*, ed. C.A. Keele & R. Smith, pp. 129–34. Edinburgh: Livingstone.

Neisser, U. (1982). Snapshots or benchmarks. In *Memory Observed: Remembering in Natural Contexts*, ed. U. Neisser, pp. 43–8. San Francisco: Freeman.

Neisser, U. & Harsh, N. (1992). Phantom flashbulbs: false recollections of hearing the news about Challenger. In *Affect and Accuracy in Recall: Studies of 'Flashbulb' Memories*, ed. E. Winograd & U. Neisser, pp. 9–31. Cambridge, MA: Cambridge University Press.

Nigro, G. & Neisser, U. (1983). Point of view in personal memories. *Cognitive Psychology*, **15**, 467–82.

OED (1992). *Oxford English Dictionary*, 2nd edn. Oxford: Oxford University Press.

Penfield, W. & Perot, P. (1963). The brain's record of auditory and visual experience. *Brain*, **86**, 596–696.

Pillemer, D.B. (1984). Flashbulb memories of the assassination attempt on President Reagan. *Cognition*, **16**, 63–80.

Pillemer, D.B. (1992). Remembering personal circumstances: a functional analysis. In *Affect and Accuracy in Recall: Studies of 'Flashbulb' Memories*, ed. E. Winograd & U. Neisser, pp. 274–305. Cambridge: Cambridge University Press.

Pillemer, D.B. (1998). *Momentous Events, Vivid Memories. How Unforgettable Moments Help Us Understand the Meaning of our Lives*. Cambridge: Harvard University Press.

Pillemer, D.B. & White, S.H. (1989). Childhood events recalled by children and adults. In *Advances in Child Development and Behaviour*, Vol. 21, ed. H.W. Reese, pp. 297–340. Orlando, FL: Academic Press.

Quercy, P. (1925). Les Eidétiques. *Journal de Psychologie Normale et Pathologique*, **22**, 801–12.

Rainey, J.M., Aleem, A., Ortiz, A. et al. (1987). A laboratory procedure for the induction of flashbacks. *American Journal of Psychiatry*, **144**, 1317–19.

Ribot, T. (1882). *Diseases of Memory*. London: Kegan Paul, Trench.

Robinson, J.A. & Swanson, (1993). Field and observer modes of remembering. *Memory*, **1**, 169–84.

Rock, I. (1995). *Perception*, 2nd edn. New York: Scientific American Library.

Rubin, D.C. & Kozin, M. (1984). Vivid Memories. *Cognition*, **16**, 81–95.

Shick, J.F.E. & Smith, D.E. (1970). Analysis of the LSD flashback. *Journal of Psychedelic Drugs*, **3**, 13–19.

Siegel, R.K. & Jarvik, M.E. (1975). Drug-induced hallucinations in animals and man. In *Hallucinations*, ed. R.K. Siegel & L.J. West, pp. 81–161. London: John Wiley.

Spencer, H. (1890). *The Principles of Psychology*, vol. 1, 3rd edn. London: Williams and Norgate.

Spiegel, D. (1991). Dissociation and trauma. In *APA Review of Psychiatry*, ed. A. Tasman & S.M. Goldfinger, Vol. 10, pp. 261–73.

Stromeyer, C.F. & Psotka, J. (1970). The detailed texture of eidetic images. *Nature*, **225**, 346–9.

Terr, L. (1988). What happens to early memories of trauma? A study of twenty children under age five at the time of documented traumatic events. *Journal of the American Academy of Child and Adolescent Psychiatry*, **27**, 96–104.

Tulving, E. (1989). Remembering and knowing the past. *American Scientist*, **77**, 361–7.

Tye, M. (1991). *The Imagery Debate.* Cambridge: MIT Press.

Von Leyden, W. (1961). *Remembering.* New York: Philosophical Library.

Winograd, E. & Neisser, U. (eds.) (1992). *Affect and Accuracy in Recall. Studies of 'Flashbulb' Memories.* Cambridge: Cambridge University Press.

Winokur, G. & Holemon, E. (1963). Chronic anxiety neurosis: clinical and sexual aspects. *Acta Psychiatrica Scandinavica*, **39**, 384–412.

Wright, D.B. & Gaskell, G.D. (1995). Flashbulb memories: conceptual and methodological issues. *Memory*, **3**, 67–80.

Wright, D.B., Gaskell, G.D. & Muircheartaigh, C.A. (1998). Flashbulb memory assumptions: using national surveys to explore cognitive phenomena. *British Journal of Psychology*, **89**, 103–21.

# Functional memory complaints: hypochondria and disorganization

German E. Berrios, Ivana S. Marková and Nestor Girala

Subjects complaining of 'poor memory' (or whose 'bad' memory is complained of by others) are frequently met with in medical practice. Neuropsychological assessment will ascertain the complaint in a sizeable proportion of cases. In this group, age remains a reasonable aetiological indicator: if older than 60, some form of chronic disease of the brain (usually a form of dementia) is often found, although significant depressive illness (or combinations thereof) may play a role. Amongst the under 40s, however, functional psychiatric disorders or organic disorder of the brain other than dementia become prominent (Spiegel et al., 1993). In those falling in the range 40–60, aetiology can go either way.

In not all cases with memory complaints, however, can an objective memory deficit be demonstrated: in some doubts remain as to the reality or extent of the memory deficit; in others the team may feel that no deficit actually exists.[1] Clinical attitudes differ vis-à-vis these two groups but it is common practice to reassess the 'doubtful' group sometime in the future.[2] Attitudes towards the second group, i.e. to the persistent memory complainers with negative neurological, neuropsychological and neuropsychiatric assessments tend to be harsher, particularly in memory clinics whose objective is to collect patients for dementia drug trials.[3] But being told that 'nothing is the matter with them',[4] rarely reassures these subjects who may proceed to reject promotions, retire early or adopt some form of illness behaviour compatible with their belief that 'they are developing dementia' (Dartigues et al., 1997). Perusal of the literature also suggests that, from the therapeutic viewpoint, these patients have been neglected as 'they do not fit' into any ongoing definition of 'disorder of memory'.[5]

This was not always thus. During the nineteenth century, memory complaints of this nature were taken at face value and together with the dysnomias, déjà vu and other paramnesias (see Chapters 1, 14 and 15, this volume) were considered as yet another variety of 'memory disorder'. These clinical states were, however, cut asunder by the theoretical narrowing down of the concept of memory that took place at the turn of the century.[6] Whilst the study of the 'organic' disorders of memory[7] is likely to have benefited from these theoretical changes, memory complainers with negative investigations were disfranchised.

There is evidence that interest in the clinical disorders of memory only developed during the nineteenth century. It would be unwarranted, however, to infer from this that this reflected an increase in the incidence of memory complainers. Each historical period, however, has its own health concerns, and the one that bedevilled the latter part of the nineteenth century (at least amongst the educated classes) was neurasthenia.[8] This (now historical) ailment had as its central elements physical and mental fatigue (*surmenage*) but also included fears of cognitive failure and memory loss (i.e. concerns about 'not doing well intellectually').[9] Then as now, explanatory paradigms based on dissociative mechanisms were popular (see Chapter 19, this volume).

With regard to the group of memory complainers with negative investigations, it is the contention of this chapter that one must take a positive attitude, namely that they should be considered as having a clinical problem; and since little is known about it, their complaint should be studied in a conventional fashion: their phenomenological features should be listed first, then subtypes should be distinguished and correlated with other clinical and personality data. Only when a symptom map and a clinical taxonomy have been developed, mechanisms and management routines should be sought. This chapter will concentrate on the analysis of 'memory complainers' with no neuropsychological 'deficit', 'organicity' or 'depressive illness' ('the worried well') who, it is hypothesized, suffer from a still unknown form of memory disorder. This is based on the view that, from a psychiatric perspective, the diagnosis of 'memory disorder' should *not* be made by exclusion alone, i.e. positive psychiatric findings need to be identified.

## Epidemiology

Little is known about the incidence and prevalence of the 'worried well' in the general population, particularly those under 60.[10] Differences in the inclusion criteria used by Memory Clinics rule out reliable meta-analytic studies on the proportion of the 'worried well'. In 199 healthy subjects recruited from the community (age range 39 to 89), Bolla et al. (1991) found that memory complaints were positively correlated with depression and negatively correlated with intelligence but their project was not meant to be epidemiological in nature. In a community study of 810 adults, Spear-Bassett & Folstein (1993) found 22% of 'complainers' without objective cognitive impairment; relevant variables in this group were age, low education, depression, emotional distress, and adjustment disorder. McGlone et al. (1990) and O'Connor et al. (1990) found that depressed elderly subjects reported 'memory problems' more often than normal controls; Chandler and Gerndt (1988) described memory complaints as a 'significant marker' of depression in the elderly but not in younger (defined as <60) patients; and Plotkin et al. (1985) found that the frequency of complaints diminished after the patients were treated for their depression.

When evaluating the relationship between 'objectively measured memory functions and subjective complaints' in a subset of 403 (aged 67–78) subjects, Hanninen et al. (1994) found that 'memory loss did not correlate with the actual memory performance in the tests' and that 'subjects who most emphatically complained of memory disturbance had greater tendencies towards somatic complaining, higher feelings of anxiety about their physical health and more negative feelings of their own competence'. Weiner et al. (1991) found that 6% of 317 consecutive cases had no objective evidence of cognitive impairment, 42% of this subset, however, 'were thought to have a cognitive difficulty due to depression'; and three were thought to have 'somatization disorder'. Almeida et al. (1993) reported that 24% of their sample of 418 patients showed no obvious neuropsychiatric diagnosis and that they tended to be younger, unmarried, self-referred women, living alone and with a frequent family history of dementia. In a study of 400 consecutive cases (mean age = 58 [SD 13]; 25% < 50 years old) seen at the Cambridge Memory Clinic in a period of five years, 35 subjects (8.6%) met criteria for 'worried well' (Berrios et al., 1999).

Based on a follow-up of 64 subjects (from the Almeida et al. cohort), O'Brien et al. (1992) suggested that memory complaints may, however, be a harbinger of dementia. As against this, Flicker et al. (1993) have found that subjective dissatisfaction with memory performance did not predict cognitive deterioration after a 3-year follow-up in a sample of 54 healthy memory complainers who on first assessment had no 'clinically apparent cognitive dysfunction'.

In a sample of 200 consecutive subjects with a mean age of 63 attending a Memory Clinic, Thomas et al. (1995) did not find any 'worried well' although about 30% exhibited a 'form of psychiatric disorder'. Grut et al. (1993) did not comment upon the 'worried well' but found that, in a sample of 354 elderly subjects, depressed individuals 'tended to underestimate their own memory'. A putative association between depression and memory complaints has also been noticed in clinical populations such as diabetes, particularly amongst those over-64 (Tun et al., 1987). Lastly, Barker et al. (1994) have reported that self-referred patients complained more about memory loss and were more depressed.

Results from clinical facilities other than Memory Clinics are even more difficult to interpret. For example, based on the 'Laboratoire Lafon Study', Derouesne et al. (1992) reported that 50% of those over-50 exhibited memory complaints (*plaintes amnesiques*). It is unclear, however, how many of these subjects had neither objective memory deficit nor depression although an earlier paper by Derouesne et al. (1989) suggests that the more severe memory complaints were associated with depression. Hanninen et al. (1995) found that at a 3-year follow-up of a sample of 229 subjects (mean age 71) with 'age-associated memory impairment'[11] about nine (5%) were no longer complaining of memory impairment. Memory complainers have also been reported as having 'less enlargement of the anterior and Sylvian fissures than controls suffering from Alzheimer's disease' (Spanó et al., 1992).

## The Cambridge study

Out of a consecutive series of 500 patients (seen between 1991 and 1995) (see Chapter 6, this volume, for details pertaining to the standard assessment ) only 403 patients were included in the analysis (97 exclusions due to incomplete data).[12]

On the basis of: (a) abnormal neuropsychology, (b) other markers (e.g. neuroimages), (c) clinical interview, and (d) agreement by the three teams, the entire sample was divided into 'dementia' (277) and 'not dementia' (126) patients (without regard for the presence in either subset of any ICD-10 diagnosable psychiatric disorder). The subset 'not dementia' (126) was in turn divided into: ICD-10 depression (73), other (4); and not-ICD psychiatric diagnosis (49). The 'non-dementia, non-ICD-10 diagnosable psychiatric disorder' (49) group was studied in detail.

### Results

To recapitulate, there were 49 subjects in the group of memory complainers with negative neuropsychology, neurology, and psychiatry (Table 18.1). These patients significantly differed from the 77 cases in the ICD-10 diagnosis category on two variables: the Beck Depression Inventory ($P > 0.01$) and gender (there were more males in the ICD-10 diagnosis group) (Table 18.1).

By means of exploratory Factor and Cluster analysis, two clinically recognizable subgroups, provisionally called 'mnestic hypochondria' ($n = 13$) and 'functional cognitive disorganization' ($n = 22$), were recognized. Fourteen subjects remained unclassifiable and constituted a heterogeneous group with no identifiable psychiatric features. In what follows, only these two clinical profiles will be reported on.

## 'Mnestic hypochondria' (MnH)

### The clinical picture

Patients with this profile were predominantly male, bright, of higher education, ambitious, perfectionist and rigid, and on testing showed covert, overcontrolled anxiety; their attention was normal and occasionally overfocalized. Their complaint expressed fixed, anxious worries about a putative loss of both semantic and autobiographical memory. Only in a few cases was it possible to get the patients to

**Table 18.1.** Memory complainers without 'organic disorder' with and without ICD-10 Dx compared

| Variable | Non-ICD-10 diagnosis ($n=49$) | ICD-10 diagnosis ($n=77$)[a] | Statistics |
|---|---|---|---|
| Age | 50.7 (10)[b] | 53.6 (14) | NS |
| Gender (m/f) | 17/32 | 41/36 | $P<0.04$ ($x^2$) |
| Duration of complaints (months) | 34 (29) | 31 (26) | NS |
| Cognitive Failures Questionnaire | 70 (7) | 69 (20) | NS |
| General Health Questionnaire | 8 (7) | 10 (7) | NS |
| Dissociative Questionnaire | 9 (4) | 10 (4) | NS |
| Beck Depression Inventory | 10 (10) | 16 (9) | $P<0.01$ |
| Outward Irritability | 4.6 (2.8) | 4.6 (3.5) | NS |
| Inner Irritability | 3.4 (2.3) | 3.1 (2.9) | NS |
| Maudsley Obsessions Inventory | 7.5 (5.8) | 8 (4) | NS |
| Personality: extrapunitive | 26.8 (3.5) | 27.3 (3.6) | NS |
| Personality: intropunitive | 30.8 (3.1) | 32.3 (6.8) | NS |
| Personality: dominance | 28.5 (3.5) | 30.6 (4.1) | NS |
| Weigl | 1.28 (0.5) | 1.25 (0.4) | NS |
| Digit Span | 9.8 (3.3.) | 9.22 (2.57) | NS |
| NART | 33 (11) | 31 (10) | NS |
| Signal Detection Memory Test (d') | 2.24 (1.3) | 2.14 (1.2) | NS |

*Notes:*

[a] Depression = 73; schizophrenia = 2; chronic hallucinosis = 1; obsessive compulsive disorder = 1.

[b] Mean (standard deviation).

pinpoint the onset of their condition or to identify precipitants or magnifying factors: promotion, fears of growing older, death of a parent, and a history of an unascertained 'heart attack' were common events.

**The concept of 'MnH'**

'Hypochondriacal' symptoms are common in clinical practice and can be found either as isolated 'complaints' (in otherwise 'normal' subjects) or transiently attached to recognizable physical and psychiatric disorders (e.g. depression). Subsumed under the DSM IV (1994) concept of 'somatoform disorders',[13] 'hypochondriasis' (300.7) is defined as:

A preoccupation with fears of having, or the idea that one has, a serious disease based on a misinterpretation of one or more bodily signs or symptoms (Criterion A). A thorough medical evaluation does not identify a general medical condition that fully accounts for the person's concerns about disease or for the physical signs or symptoms (although a coexisting general medical condition may be present). The unwarranted fear or idea of having a disease persists despite medical reassurance (Criterion B). However, the belief is not of delusional intensity (i.e. the person can acknowledge the possibility that he or she may be exaggerating the extent of the feared disease, or that there may be no disease at all); the preoccupation in Hypochondriasis may be with bodily functions (e.g. heartbeat, sweating, or peristalsis); with minor physical abnormalities (e.g. a small sore or an occasional cough); or with vague and ambiguous physical sensations (e.g. 'tired heart,' 'aching veins'). The person attributes these symptoms or signs to the suspected disease and is very concerned with their meaning, authenticity, and aetiology. The concerns may involve several body systems, at different times or simultaneously. Alternatively, there may be preoccupation with a specific organ or a single disease (e.g. fear of having cardiac disease). Concern about the feared illness often becomes a central feature of the individual's self-image, a topic of social discourse, and a response to life stresses.

Three points are important in the DSM IV definition. First, two basic mechanisms are suggested: a cognitive one viewed as a 'misinterpretation' by the patient of bodily signs or symptoms (it is not specified, however, why such 'signs or symptoms' should be there in the first place), and an emotional mechanism (the hypochondriacal complaint appears in 'response to life stresses'). Secondly, there is the DSM IV view on thresholds: a 'thorough medical evaluation' is considered to be sufficient to rule out real involvement of function. Thirdly, no reason is given for not including mental experiences such as drowsiness, giddiness, fatigue, unexplained memory worries, or persistent incapacity to think or to sleep (e.g. 'Sleep State Misperception'[14]) as forms of hypochondria. Indeed, we have been unable to find any historical, conceptual or empirical reason why complaints about 'mental functions' should be excluded from the DSM IV category of 'Hypochondriasis'.

Therefore, the proposal is that any mental function can become the focus of a hypochondriacal preoccupation. Furthermore, theoretical parsimony suggests that a common mechanism should be sought in all cases, i.e. the same model should apply to complaints concerning 'sleep dissatisfaction', 'feelings of fatigue', 'inability to think', 'bad memory', etc., etc. A feature common to all these complaints is a discordance between the objective measurement of a function (by experts) and the subjective appreciation of the 'efficiency' of the said function by the subject himself (as measured by some internal, putative 'metre') (on this see more below).

## 'Functional cognitive disorganization' (FCD)

### The clinical picture

The 'functional cognitive disorganization' (FCD) subgroup included 22 subjects who were predominantly female, of low education, had had multiple marriages,

**Table 18.2.** Mnestic hypochondria vs. functional cognitive disorganization

| Variable | Mnestic hypochondria ($n=13$) | Functional cognitive disorganization ($n=22$) | Statistics |
|---|---|---|---|
| Age | 46.2 (12) | 52.8 (9) | NS |
| Gender (m/f) | 9/3 | 7/17 | $P<0.01(x^2)$ |
| Duration of complaints (months) | 31 (24) | 15 (31) | NS |
| Cognitive Failures Questionnaire | 70 (7) | 83 (27) | $P<0.025$ |
| General Health Questionnaire | 6 (8) | 7 (9) | NS |
| Dissociative Questionnaire | 5 (7) | 11 (7) | $P<0.01$ |
| Beck Depression Inventory | 9 (10) | 11 (7) | NS |
| Metamemory (anxiety) | 48.4 (8.23) | 36.2 (9) | $P<0.01$ |
| Anxiety Subscale | 7.2 (3.2) | 4.2 (2.2.) | $P<0.01$ |
| GHQ (anxiety factor) | 3.5 (2.2) | 2.1 (2) | NS |
| Outward Irritability | 6.4 (2.8) | 3.6 (3.5) | $P<0.05$ |
| Inner Irritability | 7.2 (2.8) | 3.8 (2.9) | $P<0.05$ |
| Maudsley Obsessions Inventory | 14.3 (4.8) | 7 (7) | $P<0.001$ |
| Personality: extrapunitive | 27 (2.5) | 24.3 (7) | $P<0.01$ |
| Personality: intropunitive | 29.8 (3.1) | 33 (8.5) | NS |
| Personality: dominance | 31.5 (4) | 27.6 (5) | $P<0.01$ |
| NART_IQ | 110.6 (14) | 96.2 (13) | $P<0.01$ |
| Signal Detection Memory Test (d') | 2.20 (1.3) | 2.03 (1.4) | NS |

GHG, General Health Questionnaire; NART, National Adult Reading Test.

were not very bright, and reported an important life-event (e.g. the loss of a relevant figure in their lives) as the trigger for their memory complaint. Table 18.2 shows a comparison between the FCD and MnH groups: there were significantly more females who showed much higher scores in the 'cognitive failures' and 'dissociative behaviours' questionnaires. They also showed significantly lower scores in the 'anxiety factor' of Dixon's metamemory instrument (see Chapter 3, this volume) and high scores in the anxiety factor of the 'Snaith scale' (Snaith et al., 1978). FCD subjects were less irritable and obsessional, and less 'dominant' on the 'Personality Scale' than subjects with MnH. They showed lower NART scores.

## The concept of FCD

Subjects with FCD are mostly brought by their relatives because they have become, after an identifiable event (losing a partner, moving houses, leaving a job, etc.), forgetful, distractible, vague, vacant, and on occasions unable cognitively (and emotionally) to organize themselves and their environment and unable to live on their own. Relatives understandably believe that their behaviour is an early manifestation of dementia. The patients themselves may agree with what their relatives say, although they often play down their deficits. An essential clinical feature is that they perform within range on the neuropsychological examination and are 'normal' from the neurological and psychiatric viewpoints. In other words, no memory deficits can be found and there is no evidence of depression. It is not known whether FCD patients are at a higher risk of developing dementia in the future (it will be possible to answer this question once the current follow-up project has been completed).

An important question, however, is why do these patients behave as if they had cognitive impairment when none can be found upon examination? At this stage, our hypothesis is that the central problem with these patients is one of inability to organize their autobiographical memory. They do not seem to be able to date, string together, or create meaningful narratives about their past lives. This deficit often involves their childhood from which characteristically they 'can remember next to nothing'. It is as if these patients have never carried with them efficient time frames to organize their memories and have, for this, depended upon others (whether parents or spouses). This may explain why, upon becoming disconnected from important others, they find themselves unable to do anything with their personal memories.

This explanation is based on the hypothesis that 'autobiographical memory' is a reconstructed narrative based on memory episodes organized in terms of selected and identifiable 'time' and 'meaning' frames. 'Frames', in turn, are conceived of as notional devices conceptually separable from 'memory episodes'. Frames are carried and shared by families and cultures and their usage creates a sense of identity, belongingness and meaning. Depending upon education and other personal capacities individuals will change frames throughout life, constantly recasting earlier narratives into new ones. The extent to which frames are learned, internalized and managed depends upon individual capacities best conceived as representing a 'narrative' skill. The latter, in turn, would reflect an inherited trait which (because of its adaptive value) is likely to be widely distributed in the population. It is hypothesized here that subjects with FCD suffer from an incapacity to use frames in addition to other (not yet known) deficiencies in their narrative skills (for a further discussion of these ideas see also Chapters 1 and 16, this volume).

It follows from the above that FCD subjects should belong to pedigrees with low narrative capacity and are at a higher risk of developing FCD if they have low education, intelligence, and are socially alienated. These subjects should also become 'normalized' after re-establishing supportive cognitive partnerships, i.e. social interactions where they can be helped by others to reconstruct their own past. Lastly, these subjects should not be at a higher risk of developing dementia than controls.

## The concept of 'complaint'

Research into the concept of memory complaint is beset with conceptual difficulties. In a medical context, 'complaint' refers to utterances conveying negative personal assessments with regard to the functioning and efficacy of a bodily or mental function. Measured against objective measurements (medical tests or other standard investigations), personal assessments can be concordant or discordant. If the former, the complaint will be considered as 'ascertained' and allowed to trigger a due medical process. Discordant complaints, in turn, may exaggerate or underplay the status of a function (subjects declaring as 'normal' a function that objectively is under par are dealt with in Chapter 10, this volume). This chapter focuses on discordance by 'exaggeration' or 'distortion', namely cases when a normal function is reported as being under par. There has been little work in the medical literature on whether the assessment failures that generate exaggerated complaints should be considered as related or independent from the mechanisms underlying the function involved. A model for this will be proposed below. *Mutatis mutandis*, all that is said about the concept of medical complaint will apply to that of memory complaint.

## Self-evaluation of functions

Next to nothing is known about how subjects evaluate and monitor the 'efficiency' of their physical and mental functions. One model is that there is an internal capacity to evaluate the efficacy of bodily and mental functions. This can be conceived of as a general monitoring capacity which keeps an eye on all functions or as specific functions attached to each bodily function. A second model is that such internal capacity does not exist but that individuals evaluate their functions doxastically, i.e. by using information from external observers. In this chapter it will be hypothesized that both mechanisms are important. For the effects of understanding how each may operate, however, it is worth keeping them separate.

### Internal mechanism

The idea of a dedicated 'internal mechanism' for the ongoing evaluation of bodily functions remains attractive. However, to start understanding it, a number of questions must be asked: is the operation of such a mechanism mainly implicit or non-conscious? Against what scale does it evaluate: is there, for example, an internal 'metre'? Is the evaluation modulated by mood state, age, education, culture? What determines people's capacity to tolerate dissatisfaction? Is the evaluative capacity normally distributed in the population? Can it go awry, i.e. can subjects either miss out on a malfunction or report as abnormal a good one. What determines the feeling of permanent 'dissatisfied' with a function? Is the choice of function random or determined by a *locus minor resistentiæ*? Does the latter characterize people or functions? Has such a feature evolutionary significance?

The minimum assignment for any internal mechanism to operate would have to include a monitoring of bodily functions and the issuing into the subject's consciousness of messages about what is up (both called here 'echoing'). It would be more convenient to the functional economy that the monitoring subfunction be periodic but a continuous process cannot be ruled out. In the idealized situation, one mechanism could monitor all bodily functions. However, it is more likely that the body lets the individual know about dysfunction in a number of different ways, some specific, some general. Specific mechanisms are defined here as those which convey sufficient information to the subject for him rapidly to identify the function involved; for example, pain or acute deafness or blindness. General mechanisms, on the other hand, tend to require inferential work, for example, 'feelings of fatigue' or 'not remembering' can be attributed to malfunctions in a number of bodily functions.

It is also likely that the 'periodicity' of both the monitoring and echoing routine will vary according to situation and type of function. In normal circumstances, habituation will render the echoing infrequent. However, if the subject is nursing a myocardial infarction, echoing of palpitations or other heart activity may be extremely frequent. This bias may be governed by mechanisms intrinsic to the heart or be voluntarily controlled. On the other hand, the perception by the individual of a persistent message that something is wrong does not automatically lead to the utterance of a complaint. Subjects may choose to ignore a message on a number of accounts: personality (e.g. 'stoic' so-called), context (e.g. in the midst of action in war), state of mind (e.g. manic episode), etc., etc.

Memory complaints (without an 'objective' memory deficit) can thus originate as failures at various points of a theoretical cascade, namely: (a) monitoring, (b) messaging, (c) acceptance of the messaging, and (d) utterance of the complaint. Regardless of their origin, all these complaints are currently called 'hypochondriacal' (if focusing on a 'somatic' complaint). The model described below, however, suggests that at least three subtypes should be distinguished, namely, those related to failures in: 'echoing' ((a) above), 'cœnæsthesic capacity' ((b) above), and formatting factors ((c) and (d) above). Since it is likely that each will require a different management, it is incumbent upon clinicians to develop ways of teasing them out.

## A model for the 'echoing function'

As is the case with the functions of 'insight' (Marková & Berrios, 1995a, b) or 'judgment' (Head & Berrios, 1996), discordant evaluations are relational concepts, i.e.

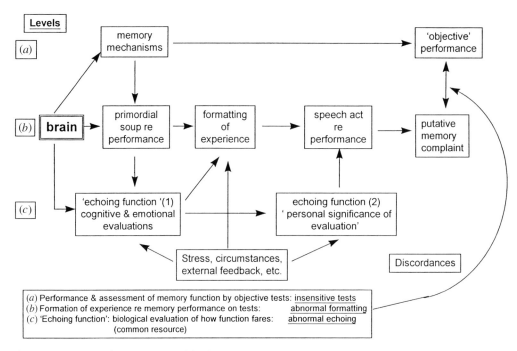

Fig. 18.1     For explanation of model, please see text section: A model for the 'echoing function'.

definable in relation to a particular and specific state. It is now time, however that the shape of the internal 'echoing' mechanism be outlined. It will be based on pathway (a) of a model of symptom-formation reported elsewhere (Marková & Berrios, 1995b) (see Fig. 18.1).

Mental symptom-formation starts with the generation of alerting signals by dysfunctional brain sites. Upon entering consciousness these signals are entertained as 'formless' experiences (called the 'primordial soup' or PS).[15] This 'inchoate', precognitive material is rapidly 'formatted' i.e. given meaning in terms of personal and cultural codes. In the state of 'normal phenomenal consciousness' an ever-changing conglomerate of PSs will also occur in response to brain signals related to environmental or internal stimuli. Formatting of such experiences normally takes place in an automatic manner determined by personal and social frames. However, when an experience generated by a dysfunctional brain site enters into consciousness, the routine formatting system may not find matching templates for the experience which may then be felt by the subject as strange, perplexing and anxiety provoking. Such 'primordial soups' may linger on and resist integration for a while but in the event the subject may force his formatting to routines to proceed or far less often seek the help of a clinical interviewer to give shape to his experiences.

At this point, a second distinction needs to be made between the actual expression of the pathological/reactional trigger (i.e. its ontological status), and awareness of the same (Marková & Berrios, 1995b). In other words, although 'awareness' is intrinsic to the notion of PS, in order to try and understand the formation of symptoms/subjective mental states in terms of the structural components, it is useful to unpack the process one step further. Thus, as seen in Fig. 18.1, this process can be envisaged as consisting of two parallel, interdependent pathways, one representing the actual formatting process, and the other, 'echoing' it as awareness of what is occurring. 'Echoing' concerns the emotional and cognitive registration (reading off) of the experience, its matching against templates of earlier experiences, and its evaluation. On this basis, a core judgment of the experience can be made. Subsequently, conceptualization processes, involving the addition and interaction of information from other sources (i.e. cultural background, environmental influences, past experiences, general outlooks, etc.), should further refine the judgment which will finally be expressed in verbal form (the reporting of the experience) as a 'symptom' or particular subjective state (the verbalization itself must be dependent on individual capacity and hence liable to further 'modify' or 'distort' the final concept).

This model thus proposes that 'symptoms or subjective states' consist of: (a) a core of neurobiological signalling which, through the echoing function, is experienced as a particular mental state, and (b) an extending multidimensional shell of multiple, interacting factors (personal, cultural, environmental, etc.) involved in the conceptualization process. The influence of such factors modifying the expression of the 'core' is likely to contribute to symptom heterogeneity. For example, what may be conceptualized and named by one patient as depression, may be conceptualized and named by another patient as fatigue.

Once a particular symptom or subjective state is formed and articulated, further conceptualization or evaluation can take place concerning its significance and impact on the subject. Again, this can be conceived of as involving both 'psychological' processes (i.e. the contribution of personal factors such as past experiences, cultural and environmental influences, current mood states, etc.) and the contribution of a putative monitoring or evaluative function.

In sum, and importantly, this model shows that mechanisms underlying the evaluations made in relation to symptoms/states/functions must be considered at two levels. First, there is the evaluation that is necessarily constitutive of the subjective state itself. Secondly, there is the evaluation, of a different order, that is made in relation to the effects of the formulated subjective state on the individual.

Returning now to the notion of discordant evaluation, it is evident that this could arise at different stages of levels (a), (b) or (c). Briefly, at (a) the subject could be making a 'correct' evaluation of a particular state, but the 'discordance' would arise from lack of appropriately sensitive tests. At level (b), the 'experience' of performing a mental function (in this case memory) could be distorted or wrongly formatted in a way which does not match the objective performance. At level (*c*), where the echoing function operates, biases of two types might originate: trait-related (as per hypochondriacal or obsessional personalities), and state-related (e.g. depression, stress, etc.). Thus, the feeling of having a 'bad memory' would not only be created by the subjective sensation 'that I cannot remember as much as I should on this test' but also by lapses in everyday tasks which are interpreted by the subject not as falling within the statistical range of forgetting but as further evidence that their memory is 'no longer what it used to be'. In contrast to the DSM IV views, the proposed model emphasizes that discordances originate not only in 'conceptualization processes' (i.e. the 'misinterpretations'), but also in (undetected) abnormalities affecting the experience caused by the operation of the function or in the echoing mechanism that monitors the presence and efficiency of the function.

## Discordant memory evaluations

For a memory complaint to start, it is necessary that the subject reads off a signal telling him that a function is performing inefficiently. However, this is not yet sufficient for at this stage the subject may decide that the drop is transient and explainable (e.g. feeling fatigued after physical exercise, or sleepy after not sleeping well or not remembering in the wake of stress or grief). For the complaint to be issued, a second factor is usually required, e.g. a lack of explanations, excessive duration of the feeling of insufficiency, particular broody moods such as depression, or manipulative intent.

Once the memory complaint has been issued, two outcomes will follow. One is confirmation by a clinician (testing instruments are now considered as providing an objective gold standard of the status of the function). The other is disconfirmation (discordance). A 'discordant evaluation' is defined here as a mismatch between the patient's and the clinician's evaluation of the same mental function (in this case of memory). Based on the view that patients are more prone to misinterpreting, misjudging or inaccurately or unreliably expressing their evaluation, it is ordinarily assumed that all discordances originate from the patient. For example, few sleep physicians will accept as true the claim by a subject with a 'normal' polysomnograph that 'his sleep is very impaired' or few memory clinic teams will believe the claim of a subject scoring in the superior range in all memory tests that 'he cannot remember anything'. However, in current practice, other 'objective' witness (usually carers or relatives) are being brought into play (for a review of such comparative assessments and the presentation of a new scale, see Chapter 10, this volume).

However, 'objectivity' of functional tests does not necessarily convey validity or sensitivity. Arguments in this area are well known. First, the tests may simply not be sensitive enough even for the functions they purport to measure, and hence the dysfunctionality perceived by the subject is warranted. Secondly, the test may not be capturing the same type of function/deficit as that experienced by the patient; for example, scores on memory tests may not necessarily represent the sort of memory deficit apparent to the patient (e.g. low narrative skill). Thirdly, tests designed to assess functions such as memory aim, by definition, to exclude subjective components and consequently no current battery assesses anything like the 'echoing function' suggested above (for this instruments such as Dixon's meta-memory questionnaire may be more useful) (see Chapter 3, this volume).

## Doxastic evaluation

According to the second or 'doxastic' view, evaluations would not be based on any privileged information or signal issued by an internal mechanism but be based on 'opinions' or 'attributions' occasionally generated by the subject in respect to his own mental functions. Such evaluations would be governed both by external cues and also by the changing cognitive and emotional status of the individual himself. Doxastic evaluation does not require positing the existence of an internal or evolutionary mechanism and can be analysed in terms of attribution theory.

## Summary and conclusions

This chapter has: (i) reviewed the clinical features of memory complaints in subjects with no objective memory deficits, (ii) reported in the said group the existence of two syndromes, (iii) suggested a model to explain the 'functional cognitive disorganization' syndrome, and (iv) proposed a new way (echoing model) to understand complaints (including memory ones).

The two syndromes are called 'mnestic hypochondria' (seen predominantly in bright, well-educated, obsessional males, with high-achievement motivation, no attentional deficit and marked anxiety) and the 'functional cognitive disorganization' syndrome (seen predominantly in females with low education and intelligence, low anxiety, and chronically dependent upon relevant others for the organization of their cognitive environment). It is emphasized that these patients require as much treatment as those suffering from organic memory disorders; and in this regard, psychiatrists and clinical psychologists should play an important role.

## REFERENCES

Almeida, O.P., Hill, K. & Howard, R. et al. (1993). Demographic and clinical features of patients attending a memory clinic. *International Journal of Geriatric Psychiatry*, **8**, 497–501.

Barker, A., Carter, C. & Jones, R. (1994). Memory performance, self-reported memory loss and depressive symptoms in attenders at a GP-referral and a self-referral memory clinic. *International Journal of Geriatric Psychiatry*, **9**, 305–11.

Bayer, A.J., Oathy, M.S.J. & Twining, C. (1987). The Memory Clinic. A new approach to the detection of dementia. *Drugs*, **33**, 84–9.

Berrios, G.E., Marková, I.S. & Girala, N. (1999). Persistent memory complaints with normal neuropsychology and neuropsychiatry. (in press).

Bolla, K.L., Lindgren, K.N., Bonaccorsy, C. & Bleecker, M.L. (1991). Memory complaints in older adults. Fact or Fiction? *Archives of Neurology*, **48**, 61–4.

Bowen, J., Teri, L. & Kukull, W. et al. (1997). Progression to dementia in patients with isolated memory loss. *Lancet*, **349**, 763–5.

Brayne, C. (1994). How common are cognitive impairment and dementia? An epidemiological viewpoint. In *Dementia and Normal Aging*, ed. F.A. Huppert, C. Brayne & D.W. O'Connor, pp. 167–207. Cambridge: Cambridge University Press.

Brown, F.H., Dodrill, C.B., Clark, T. & Zych, K. (1991). An investigation of the relationship between self-report of memory function and memory test performance. *Journal of Clinical Psychology*, **47**, 772–7.

Cammen, T.J.M. van der, Simpson, J.M. & Fraser, R.M. et al. (1987). The Memory Clinic. A new approach to the detection of dementia. *British Journal of Psychiatry*, **150**, 359–64.

Chandler, J.D. & Gerndt, J. (1988). Memory complaints and memory deficits in young and old psychiatric patients. *Journal of Geriatrics, Psychiatry and Neurology*, **1**, 84–8.

Dartigues, J.F., Fabrigoule, C., Letenneur, L., Amieva, H., Thiessard, F. & Orgogozo, J.M. (1997). Epidemiology of memory disorders. *Therapie*, **52**, 503–6.

Derouesne, C., Alperovitch, N. & Arvay, N. et al. (1989). Memory complaints in the elderly: a study of 367 community-dwelling individuals from 5o to 80 years old. *Archives of Gerontology and Geriatrics*, **8**, 151–63.

Derouesne, C., Alperovich, A. & Boyer, P. (1992). Performances cognitives objectives et plaintes amnesiques. *Psychologie Médecine*, **24**, 1075–85.

Derouesne, C., Kalafat, M. & Guez, D. et al. (1994). The age-associated memory impairment construct revisited. *International Journal of Geriatric Psychiatry*, **9**, 577–87.

Flicker, C., Ferris, S.H. & Reisberg, B. (1993). A longitudinal study of cognitive function in elderly persons with subjective memory complaints. *Journal of the American Geriatric Society*, **41**, 1029–32.

Fraser, M. (1992). Memory clinics and memory training. In *Recent Advances in Psychogeriatrics II*, ed. T. Arie, pp. 105–15. Edinburgh: Churchill and Livingstone.

Gagnon, M., Dartigués, J.F., Mazaux, J.M., Dequae, L., Lentenneur, L., Giroire, J.M. & Barberger-Gateay, P., (1994). Self-reported memory complaints and memory performance in elderly French community residents. *Neuroepidemiology*, **13**, 145–54.

Grut, M., Jorm, A.F. Fratiglioni, L. Forsell, Y., Viitanen, M. & Winblad, B. (1993). The memory complaints of elderly people in a population survey. *Journal of the American Geriatric Society*, **41**, 1295–300.

Hanninen, T., Reinikainen, K.J. & Helkala, E.L., Koivisto, K., Mykkanen, L., Laakso, M., Pyorala, K. & Reikkinen, P.J. (1994). Subjective memory complaints and personality traits in normal elderly subjects. *Journal of the American Geriatric Society*, **42**, 1–4.

Hanninen, T., Hallikainen, M., Koivisto, K., Helkala, E.L., Reinikainen, K.J., Soininen, H.,

Mykkanen, L., Laakso, M., Pyorala, K. & Reikkinen, P.J. Sr (1995). A follow up study of age associated memory impairment. *Journal of the American Geriatric Society*, 43, 1007–15.

Hauri, P. (1994). Primary insomnia. In *Principles and Practice of Sleep Medicine*, 2nd edn, ed. M.H. Kryger, T. Roth & W.C. Dement, pp. 494–9. Philadelphia: W.B. Saunders Company.

Head, L. & Berrios, G.E. (1996). 'Impaired Judgement'. A useful symptom of dementia? *International Journal of Geriatric Psychiatry*, 11, 779–85.

James, W.(1891). *The Principles of Psychology*, vol. 2. London: MacMillan.

Marková, I.S. & Berrios, G.E. (1995a). Insight in clinical psychiatry. A new model. *Journal of Nervous and Mental Disease*, 183, 743–51.

Marková, I.S. & Berrios, G.E. (1995b). Insight in clinical psychiatry revisited. *Comprehensive Psychiatry*, 36, 367–76.

McGlone, J., Gupta, S. & Humphrey, D., Oppenheimer, S., Mirsen, T. & Evans, D.R. (1990). Screening for early dementia using memory complaints from patients and relatives. *Archives of Neurology*, 47, 1189–93.

O'Brien, J.T., Beats, B. & Hill, K. et al. (1992). Do subjective memory complaints precede dementia? *International Journal of Geriatric Psychiatry*, 7, 481–6.

O'Connor, D.W., Pollit, P.A., Roth, M., Brook, P.B. & Reiss, B.B. (1990). Memory complaints and impairments in normal, depressed & demented elderly persons identified in a community survey. *Archives of General Psychiatry*, 47, 224–7.

Plotkin, D.A., Mintz, J. & Jarvik, L.K. (1985). Subjective memory complaints in depression. *American Journal of Psychiatry*, 142, 1103–5.

Ponds, E.W.H.M., Schmidt, A.J.M. & De Lugt, M. et al. (1995). De Angst om te vergeten: behandeling van functionele Geheugenklachten. *Tijdschrift voor Psychiatrie*, 37, 62–8.

Snaith, R.P., Constantopoulos, Jardine, M.Y. & McGuffin, P. (1978). A clinical scale for the self assessment of irritability. *British Journal of Psychiatry*, 132, 164–71.

Spanó, A., Förstl, H., Almeida, P. & Levy, R. (1992). Neuroimaging and the differential diagnosis of early dementia. *International Journal of Geriatric Psychiatry*, 7, 879–83.

Spear-Bassett, S. & Folstein, M.F. (1993). Memory complaint, memory performance, and psychiatric diagnosis: a community study. *Journal of Geriatrics, Psychiatry and Neurology*, 6, 105–11.

Spiegel, D., Frishholz, E.J. & Spira, J. (1993). Functional disorders of memory. In *Review of Psychiatry*, ed. J. Oldham, M. Riba & A. Tasman, Vol. 12, pp. 747–82. Washington, DC: American Psychiatric Press.

Stevens, S.J., Pitt, B.M.N. & Nicholl, C.G. et al. (1992) Language assessment in a memory clinic. *International Journal of Geriatric Psychiatry*, 7, 45–51.

Thomas-Anterion, C., Regetti, I., Lemesle, B. Foyatier-Michel, N., Laurent, B. & Michel, D. (1995). Specialized memory consultation and management of dementia. *Revue de Medecine Interne*, 16, 255–9.

Tun, P.A., Perlmuter, L.C., Russo, M. & Lott, L. (1987). Memory self-assessment and performance in aged diabetics and non-diabetics. *Experimental Ageing Research*, 13, 151–7.

Weiner, M.F., Bruhn, M., Svetlik, D., Tintner, R. & Hom, J. (1991). Experiences with depression in a dementia clinic. *Journal of Clinical Psychiatry*, 52, 234–8.

Wessely, S. (1995). Neurasthenia and fatigue syndromes. *A History of Clinical Psychiatry*, ed. G.E. Berrios & R. Porter, pp. 509–32. London: Athlone Press.

# 19

# Dissociative amnesia: re-remembering traumatic memories

Eric Vermetten and J. Douglas Bremner

## Introduction

The amnesia phenomenon in patients with dissociative disorders currently represents one of the most intriguing areas in the study of psychiatric disorders and memory processes. The hallmark of the dissociative disorders is dissociative amnesia, which involves gaps in memory for personal history, both remote and recent. Dissociative amnesia intersects with the study of normal and traumatic memory, childhood sexual abuse, and suggestibility. The recent interest in memory and delayed recall of trauma has led to lively debates regarding the accuracy of memory in traumatized individuals, the veridicality of 'recovered memories', and the profound consequences that dissociated amnesia can have on family and social relationships leading to (delayed) prosecutions and other legal complications (Loftus, 1996; see the special issue of the *International Journal of Clinical and Experimental Hypnosis*, 1994; Whitfield, 1995; see special issue of the *Journal of Psychiatry and Law*, 1996; Bremner et al., 1996; Leavitt, 1997; Bremner & Narayan, 1998). Amnesia has recently become an important issue in the courtroom as well (Spiegel & Scheflin, 1994; Koss et al., 1995; Loftus, 1996; Pezdek & Banks, 1996; Scheflin & Brown, 1996; Brown et al., 1998; Scheflin & Spiegel, 1998). This chapter focuses on dissociative amnesia as defined by the DSM-IV classification, charting a wide course from both historical and conceptual issues that are related to dissociation to what is known about neurobiological correlates of the effects of trauma on memory. This chapter also reviews assessment, diagnosis, differential diagnosis and key principles of psychotherapy in the treatment of disociative amnesia.

## Dissociated memories are traumatic in origin

Since the early 1990s there has been a revival of interest in memory processes in general and, more specifically, in the relation between trauma and memory. This interest hosted various disciplines of research, varying from neurobiological research, cognitive psychological studies to clinical aspects of trauma related psychopathology (see the special issue of the *Journal of Traumatic Stress*, 1995; *Development and Psychopathology*, 1998; Brenneis, 1996; Erdelyi, 1996; Schacter et al., 1996; Appelbaum et al., 1997; Bremner et al., 1997a, b, c; McIntosh, 1998). One of the areas of interest was the dissociative disorders of which it was hypothesized that these had their origin in traumatic childhood experiences (Putnam, 1985; Chu & Dill, 1990; Boon & Daijer, 1993; Briere & Conte, 1993; Coons, 1994; Bremner et al., 1995c). Today, there is strong evidence that traumatic events are common antecedents for dissociative phenomena and that childhood physical, sexual and emotional abuse may make one especially prone to the development of dissociative disorders. Moreover, not the trauma *per se*, but dissociation in the face of trauma is a marker for long-term psychopathology as in dissociative disorder or in Post-Traumatic Stress Disorder (PTSD) (Bremner et al., 1993b,d; Irwin, 1994; Marmar et al., 1994; Bremner & Brett, 1997; Brewin et al., 1999); e.g. after the Estonia disaster dissociative numbing, reduction of awareness, derealization, depersonalization and dissociative amnesia occurred in almost half of the survivors; all dissociative symptoms were predictive of post-traumatic reactions (Eriksson & Lundin, 1996). Recall of traumatic events in these patients often occurs in a dissociated form. The quality of their memories is suggestive of a unique type of encoding and retrieval in trauma-related dissociative memories. Empirical evidence for this is reviewed later in this chapter.

Dissociative amnesia involves the presence of information that is not available to conscious awareness for an extended period of time. Large gaps in memory, known as amnesia episodes, which occur in dissociative amnesia as well as the forgetting of identity which occurs in Dissociative Identity Disorder (DID) (formerly Multiple Personality Disorder) (Putnam, 1991) also indicates that dissociation is related to abnormal memory (Bremner et al., 1998b). Patients with a history of childhood sexual abuse have very high levels of total amnesia prior to memory retrieval. In a study by Williams it was shown that as many as 38% of abuse survivors did not remember significant episodes of abuse many years after the event (Williams, 1994a, 1995). There tends to be an age and dose relation to significant amnesia: the younger the age at the time of the trauma, the greater the likelihood of amnesia (Briere & Conte, 1993). Amnesia has also been shown to be strongly related to repetitive abuse of longer duration (Ross et al., 1991; Terr, 1991; Herman, 1992). There is currently considerable controversy about delayed recall of childhood abuse. Some authors have claimed that there is a 'false memory syndrome', in which therapists suggest to patients 'illusory' events that never actually occurred. In this heated clinical, public and legal discussion on recovered memories of childhood sexual abuse, therapists and scientists try to find evidence for pros and cons regarding the validity of the traumatic memories (Loftus, 1993, 1996; Loftus et al., 1994b; Ofshe &

Singer, 1994; Williams, 1994b; Bremner et al., 1996; Van der Hart & Nijenhuis, 1998; Kluft, 1999). Some authors claim that the forgetting of abuse that is documented in various studies is due to 'normal forgetting' and that the suggestibility of survivors is 'misused' by therapists to induce memories of abuse. They claim that recovered memories are fabricated by disturbed or vindictive adults or fostered by overzealous therapists (Wakefield & Underwager, 1992). Recent research tentatively refuted the suggestibility argument, contradicting assumptions underlying false memory creation (Scheflin & Brown, 1996; Leavitt, 1997; Brown et al., 1998).

Adding support to the delayed recall of traumatic memories is recent neurobiological evidence that special mechanisms in abuse survivors may result in a type of forgetting which is followed by recall of detailed traumatic events many years after the event first occurred; it has been shown that extreme stress has long-term effects on memory (e.g. Bremner et al., 1993d, 1997a; McEwen & Schmeck, 1994; LeDoux, 1996; Post et al., 1998).

In early history the unavailability of memory was already associated with trauma and war (Abeles & Schilder, 1935). Dramatic experiences of dissociative amnesia came from the battlefield of World War II (Torrie, 1944). The duration of this dissociative symptom of amnesia varied in the different cases described from minutes to months or years. The occurrence of the amnesia symptom itself varied from a short time after trauma to years after. Many veterans from World War II continued to suffer from 'blackouts' or loss of memory many years after their period of service (Archibald & Tuddenham, 1965). In a large sample of Danish survivors of World War II concentration camps with high levels of psychiatric symptomatology who were seeking compensation for disability, there were complaints of memory impairment ten or more years after release from internment in 87% of individuals (Thygeson et al., 1970). These phenomena have been given names like war neurosis, traumatic neurosis or psychogenic amnesia and can be described today as related to symptoms of dissociative amnesia.

Dissociative amnesia has subsequently been found to be related to factors other than war and war-related trauma. There is currently an increased focus on traumatization due to natural disasters and accidents (e.g. Madakasira & O'Brien, 1987; Cardena & Spiegel, 1993), kidnapping, rape, burns, torture and concentration camp experiences (e.g. Goldfield et al., 1988; Krystal, 1993), physical and sexual abuse (e.g. Briere & Conte, 1993; Loftus et al., 1994a; Williams, 1994a), and severe punishment (Classen et al., 1993).

## The dissociative response

Dissociation is ubiquitous, and can be viewed as being the opposite of what occurs most commonly: different stimuli, e.g. visual, acoustic or sensory, are dissociated at root, but are automatically formed to one memory piece, forming coherence and accomplishing identity. Dissociation may take the form of a physical sense, with an involuntariness to movements, as though two separate systems for interpreting somatic perception were occurring at the same time, rather than one that incorporates similar sensations from all parts of the body (Spiegel, 1990). A Vietnam combat veteran reported: 'I felt myself separating from myself and looking down at the person who was in combat, and feeling sorry for him.' He later had no immediate memory for what had happened (Bremmer et al., 1992, p. 331). Time distortion, positive and negative hallucinations and post-hypnotic amnesia can be viewed as being 'related' dissociative symptoms. The dissociative process can be associated with changes in bodily perceptions causing a feeling as if their body in total or some part was not part of themselves, leading to a kind of 'somatic estrangement'. Mental, behavioural emotional perceptions as well as perceptions of others can change (Nemiah, 1995, p. 1289). Control over different perceptual, motor and autonomic processes can be changed by involuntary mechanisms, leading to a changed physiology with an impact on different organ systems and processes: event-related potentials, blood flow, gastrointestinal changes, respiratory symptoms, neurological effects and changes in the immune system (Spiegel & Vermetten, 1994). In massive dissociative amnesia however, the patient may deal with external reality in a remarkably effective way – considering the extent of the dissociation – but he does so at the cost of losing contact with whole areas of experience that identify him as a certain social person (Cameron & Rychlak, 1985). Forms of dissociation include stupor, derealization, depersonalization, numbing and amnesia for the event.

## A historical background: from hysteria to dissociative amnesia

### Janetian influence

Recently, there has been renewed attention to the contribution that Pierre Janet made to psychiatry at the turn of the century. This attention was given impetus by contributions of Putnam (1986), Nemiah (1989), Van der Kolk and Van der Hart (1989), and Van der Hart and Spiegel (1993) and contributed to the description of the phenomenology of the multiple personality disorder (e.g. Bliss, 1984; Putnam, 1986; Spiegel, 1986; Coons et al., 1988; Ross, 1989; Kluft, 1991; Coons & Milstein, 1992). Janet described the splitting of consciousness that occurred in response to traumatic stress, and the consequences of trauma on memory and identity. Janet described a constellation of symptoms that is now categorized as Post Traumatic Stress Disorder (PTSD) or Dissociative Disorder, including dissociative amnesia and fugue, with a central assumption that different aspects of the traumatic experience are not actively available to consciousness, although they may have an influence on behaviour (Spiegel & Cardena, 1991; Loewenstein, 1993).

Except for their historical relation (Janet, 1924; Kretchmer 1926), both dissociative amnesia and hysteria share a functional psychodynamic origin. The interest in the concept of hysteria, however, decreased with the growing appraisal of cognitive and neurobiological research. Ludwig et al. described in 1972 the concept of hysteria in terms of a subtle but particular type of memory disorder. This memory disorder pertained primarily to recent memory, especially for tasks that required concentration, sustained attention, and the shifting of mental sets. It did not pertain to defects in perception and registration of information but rather to retention and/or recall functions. Further, the disorder was more marked for emotion-laden material (associated with arousal and threat) than for neutral material (Ludwig et al., 1972). Twenty-five years later, this can be regarded as the early description of dissociative amnesia. Nowadays we favour the neurobiological model of this type of memory disorder and give emphasis to special neural mechanisms that may be operative in recall of traumatic events (Bremner et al., 1993a, 1995b,c, 1997a; Charney et al., 1993; Van der Kolk, 1994; Van der Kolk et al., 1996; LeDoux, 1996). Almost a century after the contributions of Janet, the triad 'trauma, memory and dissociation' is again at the focus of psychiatric research and in clinical practice (Appelbaum et al., 1997; Bremner et al., 1998a; Brown et al., 1997). Although unusual in a classificatory sense, the development of both dissociative amnesia and dissociative fugue can be seen as a reflection of the conceptual legacy of 'classic hysteria' under which somatoform, post-traumatic and dissociative disorders were subsumed in the late nineteenth century and much of twentieth-century psychiatric nosology predating DSM.

## Other psychodynamic contributions; defence or deficit phenomenon

There has long been a controversy about whether dissociation represents a defence mechanism or is a pathological response to stress (e.g. Singer, 1990; Lerner, 1992; Cardena, 1994; Erdelyi, 1994). This controversy recalls the debate at the beginning of this century between Janet and Freud. According to Freud, dissociation was an active defence phenomenon. When the integrity of the overall system was threatened, subsystems of ideas, wishes, memories or thoughts would be forcibly repressed, dissociated or split off (Freud, 1941). In Janet's theory, dissociation was a deficit phenomenon, an insufficiency of binding energy, caused by hereditary factors, life stresses or traumas, or an interaction among them. These processes resulted in the splitting off of fragments (Janet, 1904). In his theory dissociation had to do with a lack of integration between mental processes and especially inaccessibility of mental contents or processes to phenomenological awareness in reaction to traumatic events. Repression is typically described as a reaction to 'ward off' unconscious fears and wishes, rather than a response to specific traumatic life events. In contrast to repressed memories, dissociated memories are described as consisting of discrete periods of time and lost to consciousness (Spiegel et al., 1993a).

The discussion touches the difference between conversion disorders and dissociative disorders. Both share a pathological exclusion from consciousness. The conversion symptom, however, gives unconscious symbolic expression to a conflict that may have been involved. There is a circumscribed disturbance or loss of function in some body part as far as paralysis or anæsthesia, leaving the rest of the personality little affected or sometimes even satisfied (*belle indifference*). Conversion can, in this respect, also be considered as lack of efferent signals to the central nervous system, whereas dissociation refers to the lack or blocking of afferent signals to the central nervous system. Dissociative processes usually or typically involve large segments of external or internal reality, not disposing of anxiety as in conversion disorders but of fright, phobia or panic. A psychodynamic interpretation that still holds true assumes that, in dissociation, a partial regression occurs that reactivates early and primitive ego organizations reviving processes of primitive denial and ego-splitting. These processes may lead to estrangement of the body image, depersonalization, dreamlike dissociative states and massive amnesias (Cameron & Rychlak, 1985).

## Post-Janetian conceptualization of the dissociative process

Hilgard, in his discussion of the nature of dissociation, emphasized a horizontal rather than a vertical depiction of the relation between conscious and unconscious states (Hilgard, 1977, 1986). Hilgard's theory involved the coexistence of two separate streams of consciousness, which pursue independent courses. These separate streams of consciousness are not without some mutual interference, although they operate with a large measure of independence. When two tasks are performed simultaneously, one on a conscious and one on an unconscious level, each is performed less efficiently because of the effort required for the other task and because of the effort to keep the unconscious task out of awareness. For example, when in a hypnotic state a subject's arm is made to rise in the air, the cognitive control structure for the arm has been dissociated from the main part of the central control structure. Another example of the parallel operation of two high-level information processors is the 'hidden observer' phenomenon in his neodissociation theory, in which a highly hypnotizable subject is able to produce analgesia for pain, and yet a hidden proportion of consciousness acknowledges feeling sensory pain and marks considerable discomfort (Hilgard, 1992, 1994). The hidden observer theory allows for separate non-conscious parallel processing of all perception, isolated from awareness via amnesia and retrievable via a hidden observer. New approaches have elaborated on the neodissociation theory of Hilgard. His dissociation theory seems to fit into current neural network models of psychopathology and brain function (Rumelhart & McClelland, 1986; Parks et al., 1991; Levy et al., 1995; Stein & Ludik, 1998). In Parallel Distributed Processes models (PDP) memories are not stored as discrete traces, but rather are superimposed on pre-existing memories in a composite representation (Feldman & Ballard, 1982; Schacter, 1995). State-dependent memory and consciousness provide a research model and explanation for the way in which emotional or dissociative states are modulated (LeDoux, 1996; Kahn et al., 1997). Studies have shown evidence for the fact that memory retrieval is facilitated when the mood state at the time of retrieval is the same as the mood state which was present at the time of encoding (Bower, 1981).

Some authors state that memory processes appear to be dissociated in nature (Minsky, 1986; Spiegel & Cardena, 1991). The narrowing of the (conscious) awareness affects the way in which the percepts are processed: there is reduction of cortical processing of the dissociated percept (Spiegel et al., 1985, 1989; Weiskrantz, 1987; Sigalowitz et al., 1991). Hypnotic dissociation has also been described in recent models of neural networks (Li & Spiegel, 1992; Kuzin, 1995). Discussing these developments in more detail would go beyond the scope of this chapter.

## Autobiographical memory and continuity of experience

A cognitive psychological viewpoint holds that memory formation involves encoding, storage and retrieval. In this field there is growing awareness that memory is not a unitary or monolithic entity but composed of separate yet interacting systems and subsystems (Squire & Butters, 1984; Schacter & Tulving, 1994). All interacting systems associate in the process of memory formation to bring the content together in one stream of narrative memory. The combination of autobiographical memory gaps and continued reliance on dissociation makes it hard for patients to reconstruct a precise account of either their past or their current reality (Cole & Putnam, 1992). The sense of self is in a state of continued construction. As described earlier, the continuity of experience which builds up the sense of self, however, should not be taken for granted, but be seen as an accomplishment (Spiegel, 1990). The self in this respect can nicely be considered as a centre of narrative gravity, stressing the need for giving a verbal account of experiences to promote integrative functions (Dennett, 1991). What can be forgotten and what needs to be remembered must first be consciously processed, preferably told about, before it can be stored in memory. Important in this process is the creation of a spatiotemporal track of both the immediate past and the ordinary continuity of experience. Synthesis of self-experience then occurs automatically and unconsciously. Dissociation in this respect can be considered to delete the spatiotemporal context that is normally associated with memory for events, leading to a disruption of episodic and auto-biographical memory (Kihlstom et al., 1992).

The sense of personal continuity is achieved through the maintenance of a consistent stream of memory, a kind of smoothing function under which disparate experiences under a common heading of personal integrity and identity are subsumed (Spiegel, 1990; Gergen, 1991). The accomplished integrated identity is yet subject to disruption through trauma, hypnotic influences, or disjunctions in information-processing stagies (Kihlstrom, 1987; Spiegel & Cardena, 1991). Overwhelming experiences are, in themselves, not processed in an integrated manner. The traumatic information is not 'lost' but is encoded as an emotionally supercharged and disconnected memory trace. Emotional memory traces, which are isolated in time, can lead to the disruption of identity which is seen in DID.

# Description of dissociative amnesia

## Characteristics of dissociative amnesia

Amnesia can be a manifestation of the barrier between material that is, and material that is not, integrated on a conscious level. Various differentiations by different authors have been made in the dissociative amnesia. It is commonly reported that dissociative amnesia usually involves personal events and information, rather than general knowledge or skill, and that the gaps in memory are organized according to affective rather than temporal dimensions (Spiegel & Cardena, 1991). Spiegel et al. (1993a) recognize three key issues in dissociative amnesia.

(i)     The memory loss is for a discrete period of time, a dense unavailability of memories that were clearly at one time available; explicit memory for what is wrong might be lacking,

(ii)    The dissociative amnesia is typically retrograde rather than anterograde, one or more discrete periods of past information become unavailable,

(iii)   The memories lost are generally associated with traumatic or stressful events. Dissociative amnesia tends to be age and dose related: the younger the age at the time of the trauma, and the more prolonged the traumatic event, the greater the likelihood of significant amnesia (Briere & Conte, 1993; Williams, 1995). Clinical reports contrast with the experimental studies regarding amnesia for central vs. peripheral aspects of trauma. Whereas experimental studies show that peripheral processed information might be subject to amnesia, clinical studies show that amnesia may concern the most threatening and the most central elements of a traumatic experience.

Loewenstein (1993) describes two subgroups in the disorder: one where amnesia is primarily related to traumatization, and one where amnesia develops in the context of overwhelming psychological conflict in an individual predisposed to dissociate.

A variety of disturbances in the content of memory can further characterize dissociative amnesia. Adding to the classification of amnesia along a time axis, resulting in retrograde, post-traumatic and anterograde amnesia, a distinction can be made with respect to the extent of the material forgotten. Most relevant is the distinction between partial and complete amnesia: this distinction relates to having less memory of a certain event vs. having no memory for the event. Amnesia can be localized (circumscribed to a discrete period of time), selective (failure to recall just some aspects during a certain period of time), generalized (inability to recall events after a specific time and up to the present), continuous (failure to recall successive events as they occur) or systematized (amnesia for certain categories of memory).

The criteria in the DSM-IV for dissociative amnesia are one or more episodes of inability to recall important personal information, usually of a traumatic or stressful nature, that is too extensive to be explained by ordinary forgetfulness or age. The disturbance is not due to multiple personality disorder or to an organic mental disorder (blackouts during alcoholic intoxication). Since DSM-III, the requirement that the amnesia be sudden is deleted. This means that gaps in memory may have a long history of not remembering from months to years. These gaps may be difficult to detect because the person involved may be unaware of the disturbance in recall assuming that this is a normal state of affairs (Spiegel & Cardena, 1991). This may lead to misdiagnoses and unnecessary admissions. A second change to DSM-IV involves the phrase 'usually of traumatic or stressful nature' to indicate that various stressful events are frequent precursors of dissociative amnesia (Bremner et al., 1992).

Dissociative amnesia is commonly described in DID, but amnesia is also an essential symptom among the DSM-IV diagnostic criteria for somatization disorder and PTSD (Loewenstein, 1993; Nemiah, 1993). Clinically, there is a lot of overlap with other dissociative symptoms. Increased levels of dissociation have also been found in patients with PTSD (Bremner et al., 1992). Furthermore, empirical studies have shown a high level of dissociation between different symptom areas of dissociation, including amnesia, depersonalization, derealization and identity disturbances (Bremner et al., 1993c). Using the Structured Interview for Dissociative Disorders (SCID-D, Steinberg, 1993) amnesia has been found to be the dissociative symptom area which is most elevated in Vietnam combat veterans with PTSD in comparison to Vietnam combat veterans without PTSD. However, on clinical observation all dissociative symptoms seem to be interrelated, in this systematic study, in particular, amnesia was the symptom area which best-differentiated Vietnam combat veterans with and without PTSD. The degree of amnesia in PTSD veterans was severe, and included gaps in memory lasting hours to days, with blocks of missing time that could not be accounted for, forgetting of personal information and finding oneself in new places not knowing who they were or how they got there (Bremner et al., 1992, 1993c).

## Symptomatology of dissociative amnesia

The amnesia symptoms include blackouts or time losses, fugues, reports of disremembered behaviour, unexplained possessions, inexplicable changes in relationships, chronic mistaken identity experiences, childhood amnesia and/or fragmentary recall of the entire life history, and brief (micro-)amnesias during conversations or other interactions with people (Loewenstein, 1993). DSM-IV (APA, 1994) specifies that the amnesia in dissociative amnesia must be 'too expansive to be explained by ordinary forgetfulness' (p. 229). Discriminating amnesia from forgetfulness would go beyond the scope of this review.

Amnesic symptoms can range from gaps of memory, which last from minutes to hours to days. Some patients reported driving down the highway from one place to another, suddenly realizing that they had covered two hours of the trip and had no recall of what had happened during that time. One patient said he was drinking coffee at home, and the next thing he knew he was walking in New York 700 miles away from his house, having flown overseas by plane. Another patient disappeared from an inpatient psychiatric unit, and found himself in the woods, in the middle of the night, wearing combat fatigues. A patient with a history of childhood sexual abuse reported that she was on the telephone at her day hospital programme, and the next thing she knew she was at home in bed (Bremner et al., 1996). These clinical vignettes show the wide variety and broad impact that dissociative amnesia can have in patients. Most, if not all, patients share a history of exposure to extreme psychological trauma, the existence of which has been documented in a number of studies (Loewenstein & Putnam, 1988; Carlsson & Rosser-Hogan, 1991; Bremner et al., 1992; Cardena & Spiegel, 1993; Koopman et al., 1994; Marmar et al., 1994). One needs to realize that, in most cases of dissociation, patients may report a strange feeling or attribute feelings or behaviours to things they understand or know of themselves. They don't complain of gaps in their memory but are complaining of 'distant feelings', fear, anticipation of panic attacks, differences in perception, affect, knowledge or attitude, remarks by others or social dysfunction. The complaint may come from others that the patient was unaware of certain events, had no memory for a certain period of time or could not recognize certain people or places familiar to them. It is therefore advisable, if one is suspicious of amnesic periods, to assess amnesia in as detailed a way as possible through a semistructured interview with the patient in order to guide and control the process of bridging the amnesic barrier.

There is a rather close functional resemblance between dissociative amnesia and dissociative fugue. The memory loss in fugue states is more robust and often involves the autobiographical memory in such a way that people do not remember who they are or how they got in a certain situation. In DSM-III the criterion 'assumption of new identity' (partial or complete) was deleted and, instead, 'loss of personal identity or an assumption of new identity' was added in DSM-IV. Most reported cases of fugue showed various levels of identity confusion and amnesia, rather than the clear adoption of new identity (Riether & Stoudemire, 1988).

### Post-hypnotic amnesia

The field of experimental and clinical hypnosis adds a different type of amnesia: hypnotic amnesia (Kihlstrom, 1982). Hypnosis is considered to be related to the factors absorption, suggestibility and dissociation (Spiegel, 1990). Hypnosis is well known for its sometimes striking or impressive phenomena such as catalepsy, rigidity, hallucinations, time distortion, hypermnesia, age regression and post-hypnotic amnesia. Within the domain of memory, anomalies of awareness may be noted in post-hypnotic amnesia (Kihlstrom & Evans, 1979). The narrowing of consciousness sometimes can evolve into a complete amnesia for the experience that transpired while they were hypnotized. However, the critical memories may be recovered after administration of a pre-arranged signal to cancel the suggestion or by re-hypnotizing. Rather than a failure of encoding or loss from storage, this property of reversibility shows that post-hypnotic amnesia reflects a disruption of memory retrieval. However, this retrieval disruption is selective. Amnesic subjects are affected by memories that have been adequately encoded, but are (temporarily) not accessible to conscious retrieval (Kihlstrom et al., 1994).

Most hypnotic susceptibility scales have one item on post-hypnotic amnesia: the subject is suggested not to remember an event or a sequence of items mentioned, e.g. some words or test items of the test, and that only after a cue they will all be remembered (recall amnesia). High hypnotizable subjects show amnesia prior to the cue and are able to recall the information after the cue signal has been given (e.g. tapping with a pen on the table). Amnesia for the cue (source amnesia) might still persist. Subjects responding to post-hypnotic suggestions often exhibit dual lack of awareness; although recall amnesia depends upon suggestion, source amnesia occurs spontaneously without explicit suggestion (Khan, 1986).

Hypnotizability has been described as the fundamental capacity to experience dissociation in a structured setting. The relationship between hypnotizability and dissociation continues to be a subject of empirical investigation (Vermetten et al., 1998). Both dissociative disorder patients and patients with PTSD have higher scores on classical hypnotizability scales; they also show higher levels of instructed

**Table 19.1.** Differences between dissociative and non-dissociative amnesia

|  | Dissociative amnesia | Non-dissociative amnesia |
|---|---|---|
| Due to known medical disorder or physical cause | No | Yes |
| Related to psychological trauma | Yes | No |
| Exacerbated by stress | Yes | No |
| Preferential involvement of personal information | Yes | No |
| Reversible with hypnosis | Yes | No |
| Varying extent and nature of the intrusion of the dissociated mental elements to consciousness | Yes | No |
| Reversible with amobarbital (amytal interview) | Yes (?) | No |
| Attributable to effects of psychoactive drugs | No | Some forms |

post-hypnotic amnesia (Spiegel et al., 1988; Frischholz et al., 1992). Experiments using hypnosis could provide more insight into relations between explicit and implicit memory and repressed or dissociated memories. One should always be careful extrapolating results from experimental fields to clinical settings for different mechanisms might be active in these distinct settings.

## Differentiating dissociative vs. non-dissociative amnesia

It is important to differentiate amnesia from other types of (non-dissociative) amnestic disorders (see Table 19.1). In non-dissociative amnestic disorders the key feature is an inability to learn and later recall new information (deficit in antero-grade memory). There may, or may not be, an associated impairment in recall of previously learned events (deficit in retrograde memory). The amnesia occurs despite intact attention and general intellectual function. To make the diagnosis the impairment must be sufficiently severe to compromise personal, social, or occupational functioning (Caine, 1993). The non-dissociative amnestic disorders are classified in DSM-IV in one category together with delirium, dementia and other cognitive disorders, and can be divided into amnestic disorder due to a general medical condition, substance induced persisting amnestic disorder and the amnestic disorder not otherwise specified (NOS) (APA, 1994). Pathogenic processes include neurological causes of (temporary) memory impairment. These can be related to closed-head trauma, anoxia with interruption of blood flow to the hippocampus, penetrating missile wounds, cerebrovascular disease or others (Cummings, 1993) (see Table 19.2). Examples are described in different chapters in this volume. Little is known about the effect of amytal interviews in cases of

**Table 19.2.** A list of medical conditions that must be assessed regarding non-dissociative amnesia

| | |
|---|---|
| Trauma | (Closed head) trauma, penetrating missiles |
| Vascular | CVA, ischæmia |
| Cerebral hypoxæmia | Pulmonal or cardial, CO intoxiation, post-narcotic anoxia |
| Infectious | *Cerebral*: meningitis, encephalitis; or *systemic*: HIV, syphilis, urinary tract infection |
| Neoplasma | Primary or metastatic brain tumours |
| Intoxication | Substance abuse (alcohol, drugs), medication side effects |
| Epilepsy | Temporal lobe epilepsy, absences, post-ictal phase |
| Metabolic | Uræmia, hepatic disease, electrolyte disturbances |
| Endocrine | Diabetes |
| Degenerative | Senile and presenile dementia, Parkinson's |
| Normal pressure hydrocephalus | |
| General medical condition | Nutritional, vitamin deficiency (thiamine) |

dissociative amnesia. Some older reports consider it a valid therapeutic indication in psychiatric emergency settings and in the assessment and initial management of catatonia, hysterical stupor, and unexplained muteness. It could also be used for distinguishing between depressive, schizophrenic, and organic stuporous states (Perry & Jacobs, 1982).

The dissociative disorders form a separate category in DSM-IV because they refer to symptomatic disturbances of memory, consciousness and personal identity while in the mean time sharing an underlying process of dissociation. The disorders (dissociative amnesia, dissociative fugue, dissociative identity disorder, depersonalization disorder and dissociative disorder NOS) are distinguished nosologically by phenomenological variations that are determined by the range of patient's state of awareness and the extent and the nature of the intrusion of the dissociated mental elements to consciousness (Kluft, 1988; Nemiah, 1995). Put in more cognitive terms, the essential feature can be described as a disruption of the monitoring and controlling functions of consciousness, being failures of conscious perception, memory, or motor control that are not attributable to insult, injury or disease affecting brain tissue or to the effects of psychoactive drugs. Further, the disorders are reversible, either temporarily or more permanently, by means of medication or psychotherapy (Kihlstrom, 1994). However, in patients with high levels of trauma-related pathology, dissociative responses to subsequent stressors can be chronic and persistent (Bremner & Brett, 1997).

## Assessment of dissociative amnesia

The assessment of the patient presenting with amnesia requires a differentiation of dissociative from non-dissociative amnesia. The most important information is derived from the patient history. Dissociative amnesia is always assessed through (and temporally related to) exposure to psychological trauma. Dissociative amnesia is also typically exacerbated by stress and involves trauma-related material (Bremner et al., 1993b). Assessment of early trauma can be performed through a structured interview like the Early Trauma Interview (ETI) (J.D. Bremner, E. Vermetten & C. Mazure, unpublished data). Sometimes the patient remembers and reports early trauma but does not connect it to their present difficulties; sometimes the history of early trauma is withheld in the early contacts due to feelings of shame, self-doubt or mistrust. Sometimes the history cannot be reported at all, because of persistent amnesia. After an assessment of trauma history, organic cause, substance abuse, head trauma or epilepsy should be assessed individually. Other psychiatric conditions may be associated with dissociative amnesia, such as anxiety, panic disorders, sleep disturbances or pseudoepileptic seizures (Loewenstein & Putnam, 1988; Kopelman et al., 1994; Mellman et al., 1995; Kuyk et al., 1996).

Three situations have to be elucidated: the patient may be unaware of the memory disturbance, may be aware and may pretend to have a memory disturbance. Whether a memory disorder is dissociative or non-dissociative, malingered or mixed, it must be evaluated clinically by careful assessment of the amnesic patient (Kopelman, 1995). As discussed earlier, because amnesia represents an absence of memory, patients may be unaware that something is missing from their memory. Obtaining a reliable estimate from the patients for the frequency of their amnesic episodes is often difficult for patients with the most chronic amnesias have learned to adapt to, or to compensate for, their amnesia (Kluft, 1988). Many patients meeting diagnostic criteria for dissociative amnesia or fugue will actually have a far more extensive history of amnesia, fugue-like states, and dissociation if closely questioned in the clinical interview or when they are followed up longitudinally (Kluft, 1985; Loewenstein, 1993). This can also have led to comorbidity for DSM axis II diagnoses, most likely to be found in the B cluster of DSM-IV.

Perhaps the most difficult issue concerning dissociative amnesia is determining whether the patient is truly amnesic or malingering. Since its early description of dissociative amnesia several reports on feigned amnesia cases have been published (Baker, 1901; Lennox, 1943). The predominant motivation for this behaviour can be to avoid obligation or punishment by assuming the sick role. Dissociative amnesia is thought to include confused or hysterical behaviour, unintentionally producing the symptoms and demonstrating a motivated effort for recollection in the patient, whereas feigned amnesia shows an intentional production of the amnesia, to assume the sick role. In the latter case, the diagnosis factitious disorder needs to be taken into account.

It can be a diagnostic dilemma to differentiate between amnesia and fugue-state in children. Keller and Shaywitz (1986) report of a 16-year-old boy whose presenting symptom was total retrograde amnesia. After finding no evidence for organic causes, including toxic-metabolic derangements, epilepsy, encephalitis, vasculitis, trauma, and CNS neoplasm, it was determined that the child experienced a psychogenic fugue state with a spontaneous recovery in memory over several days.

Several structured questionnaires have been developed, each focusing on slightly different aspects of dissociation, using different methodologies. Assessing dissociative amnesia can be part of a broader assessment on dissociative disorders, where the focus is more on dissociation than on amnesia, e.g. the Structured Interview for Dissociative Disorders (SCID-D, Steinberg, 1993); the Dissociative Experience Scale (DES, Bernstein & Putnam, 1986); the Dissociative Disorders Interview Schedule (DDIS, Ross et al., 1989); the Dissociative Questionnaire (DIS-Q, Vanderlinden et al., 1991; 1993); the Child Dissociation Scale (CDS, Putnam et al., 1993); the Somatoform Dissociation Questionnaire (SDQ-20, Nijenhuis et al., 1996); the Clinican Administered Dissociative States Scale (CADDS, Bremner et al., 1998a).

Non-dissociative amnesia is mostly assessed on observation in a clinical situation. Dissociation scales rely much on self-reported phenomena, reflecting one's memory, affect, behaviour, perception, knowledge, or attitude. In most of the scales the dissociative symptoms are reported, not observed (with the exception of the CADSS). However, studies have not shown a high level of association between observed dissociation and self-reported dissociation, which should be considered to be the 'gold standard' (Bremner et al., 1998a) (for an overview of the measurement of dissociation, see Vermetten et al., 1998). A pitfall is the amnesic patient who does not have a self-awareness of amnesia. The patient who complains of 'losing time', not being aware of what happened between one specific time and another is suspect for organic disease. Dissociative amnesia patients may not present themselves with such a complaint for they are not aware of, or remember, their failure to remember.

## Neurobiological theories

The neurobiology of dissociation is a rapidly expanding area of research. Based on current knowledge about the effects of stress on brain systems that play a role in memory, and on phenomenology of dissociative states with 'playback' quality of dissociative memories, mechanisms other than 'normal forgetting and remembering' are involved in the inability to remember events of, e.g. childhood abuse (Pitman, 1989; Schacter et al., 1996) or other traumatic experiences.

Individual and species survival value has been mentioned as being the psycho-biological function of the dissociative response (Ludwig, 1983). From an evolutionary standpoint, dissociation could be related to the freezing response ('Todstellreflex') of animals confronted with a predator or other life-endangering threat. Dissociation enables (or causes) detachment from anticipation or actual experience of fear, pain and helplessness in an attempt to gain psychological distance from something traumatic or from something which demands too abrupt an adaptation, resulting in a reduction of the impact of the overwhelming experience (Cameron & Rychlak, 1985; Spiegel et al., 1988; Spiegel, 1993; Marmar et al., 1994). This aspect of dissociation in response to trauma may have adaptive value for the organism (Putnam, 1985; Freyd, 1994; Bremner & Brett, 1997; Nijenhuis et al., 1998).

Modern memory research on the effects of stress on memory leads to an awareness that traumatic events are encoded and stored differently in memory than normal events, due to attentional, psychological variables and physiological factors (Cahill et al., 1994; LeDoux 1992, 1996; Southwick et al., 1994; Van der Kolk, 1994; Krystal et al., 1995; Bremner, 1999).

Different neuroendocrine systems affecting learning and memory are considered to play a role during stress: the noradrenergic (NE) system, excitatory and inhibitory amino acid systems, central dopaminergic (DA) systems and neuropeptides, such as corticotropin releasing factor (CRF), neuropeptide Y, and neurotensin (for review, see De Wied & Croiset, 1991; McGaugh et al., 1996; Bremner et al., 1997c). Limbic brain structures involved in memory, including the hippocampus and adjacent cortex, amygdala, and prefrontal cortex, are richly innervated by these neurotransmitters and neuropeptides and play an important role in the processing of experiences, both from an emotional and a cognitive standpoint. Experimental studies reveal that these brain structures help determine the individual response in terms of overt behaviour and in terms of autonomic and neuroendocrine reactions (LeDoux, 1996). Electrical stimulation of hippocampus and adjacent cortex results in symptoms similar to those seen in dissociation, including the subjective sensation of fear, complex visual hallucinations (i.e. dissociative states), memory recall, déjà vu, and emotional distress (Gloor et al., 1982). The hippocampus and adjacent perirhinal and parahippocampal cortices, through reciprocal connections with multiple neocortical areas, appeared to bind together information from multiple sensory cortices into a single memory at the time of retrieval (Squire & Zola-Morgan, 1991).

There is a variety of neurotransmitters and neuropeptides (ACTH, glucocorticoids, dopamine, acetylcholine, endogenous opiates, vasopressin, oxytocine and gamma-aminobutyric acid) which are released during stress and which modulate memory function having both strengthening and diminishing effects on memory traces, depending on the dose and on the particular type of neuromodulator. The stress hormones are affecting adrenergic, opioid peptidergic, GABA-ergic and cholinergic systems and interact with the amygdaloid complex enabling the amygdala to influence memory storage in different brain regions (McGaugh & Cahill, 1997). Emotional arousal thus activates the amygdala, which can result in the modulation of memory storage. According to state-dependent memory processes, traumatic events which are encoded in an 'abnormal' state will be expected to be retrieved in a similar 'abnormal' state. This may explain why amnesic memories emerge at certain 'triggered' times and not at others, and it explains the phenomenon of how traumatic recall often occurs in a dissociative state which is similar to the dissociative state which the individual experienced at the time of the original trauma (Spiegel, 1990; Van der Kolk et al., 1996).

It was questioned if influencing the noradrenergic system could induce the dissociative symptoms. Following administration of the alpha-2 antagonist, yohimbine, which stimulates brain norepinephrine release in the brain, PTSD patients had dissociative symptoms such as increased intrusive memories, flashbacks and anxiety in comparison to controls and had lower metabolism as measured by positron emission tomography (PET) in prefrontal, temporal (including hippocampus), parietal and orbitofrontal cortices (Southwick et al., 1993; Bremner et al., 1997b). Krystal et al. reported an increase of dissociative symptomatology, as measured on the Clinican Administered Dissociative States Scale, following administration of ketamine hydrochloride, a non-competitive antagonist of the *N*-methyl-D-aspartate (NMDA) receptor. The NMDA receptor is involved in memory function at the molecular level, through Long Term Potentiation (LTP) and is highly concentrated in the hippocampus. The subjects reported a wide range of dissociative symptomatology, including out of body experience, feeling like their arms were toothpicks, having gaps in time, feeling time stood still, disturbances in self and identity, and derealization (Krystal et al., 1994).

Gaps of memory, or amnesic episodes, seen in patients with PTSD and in patients with dissociative disorders may be also related to deficient hippocampal structure and function (Bremner et al., 1995b). We used PET and fludeoxyglucose F18 to measure brain metabolism in Vietnam combat veterans and a healthy age-matched control group following administration of yohimbine or placebo, in a randomized, double-blind fashion. A pattern of a decrease in placebo-substracted metabolism with yohimbine administration was observed in those patients who had a panic attack with dissociative symptoms, compared with those who did not have these symptoms, with the magnitude of the difference being greatest for orbitofrontal cortex and hippocampus (Bremner et al., 1997b). While this study demonstrates deficits in function of the hippocampus in challenged retrieval, deficits in function of the hippocampus and adjacent cortical areas can lead to deficits in explicit memory encoding as well. Post-mortem studies and studies utilizing neuroimaging techniques have found that stress in humans is associated with changes in brain structure, including the morphology of the hippocampus. High levels of glucocorticoids associated with stress are suggested to be responsible for hippocampal damage (McEwen et al., 1992; Sapolsky et al., 1990; Woolley et al., 1990). Monkeys exposed to extreme stress have been found to have damage in two subfields of the hippocampus (Uno et al., 1989). Comparing hippocampal volume with MRI in Vietnam combat veterans with PTSD ($n = 26$) and healthy subjects ($n = 22$) showed a decrease of 8% in right hippocampal volume in comparison to controls ($P < 0.05$) but no significant decrease in volume of comparison structures. Deficits in explicit memory as measured with the Wechsler Memory Scale-Logical Component, were associated with 8% decreased right hippocampal volume in the PTSD but not in the controls (Bremner et al., 1995a). This reduction in hippocampal volume has also been found in 17 adult survivors of childhood physical and sexual abuse in comparison to 17 matched controls. In this population there was a 12% reduction in left hippocampal volume (Bremner et al., 1997a).

There is evidence that early trauma affects the development of the limbic system (Teicher et al., 1993). Chronic corticosteroid dysregulations may occur after traumatic experience: a single episode of 24 hours maternal deprivation of the rat pup may enhance the stress system at adulthood (Rots et al., 1996). Abundant evidence exists in animal studies for abnormalities in conditioned fear responses and amygdala function with stress. Conditioned fear may lead to an unconscious avoidance of traumatic cues, in order to avoid the extreme negative emotionality associated with such cues. Failure of extinction and sensitization may lead to negative emotionality with cue exposure, which leads to avoidance behaviours (Charney et al., 1993). With behavioural sensitization and kindling as described by Post, these mechanisms may lead to increased behavioural or physiological responsivity to repeated presentation of the same inducing stimulus, involving memory-like mechanisms with long-lasting consequences for the neurobiology and behavioural reactivity of the organism (Post et al., 1995). These recent findings contribute to an understanding of processes that previously were explained by unconscious forces or defences into modern ideas of neuromodulation and encoding of traumatic or overwhelming information.

## Treatment of dissociative amnesia

Dissociative amnesia is rarely the single symptom; in the majority of cases the amnesia symptom is embedded in, and co-occurs with, other dissociative phenomena. As counts for the spectrum of dissociative disorders, in the treatment of dissociative amnesia, it is important to avoid unnecessary therapeutic manipulation and maintain a consistent and comprehensive psychotherapy. A complete assessment should be taken: the premorbid personality, premorbid social adjustment, previous conflicts and traumatic events leading to amnesia, family environment, and suicidality should be assessed. Excessive haste to recover from amnesia may lead to a clinical destabilization.

Most studies agree on treatment strategies of dissociative amnesia. There is little difference in treatment, be it in part, compared with treatment for dissociative disorder. Generally, three stages are described:

(i)     stabilization with emphasis on safety and symptom relief;
(ii)    exploration of traumatic memories with a focus on the reversal of the amnesia, e.g. using hypnotic techniques, stressing remembrance and mourning for the material that might come up; and
(iii)   reintegration with development of the self and reconnections (Herman, 1992; Kluft, 1993; Siegel, 1995).

Therapeutic psychotherapeutic strategies in dissociative amnesia therefore involve an effort to bridge the amnesia by providing emotional support and by helping the patients restructure their perspective on the information that was previously inaccessible, making it acceptable to integration into consciousness. Central issues in therapy are (Kluft, 1993; Spiegel, 1993):

(i)     enhance control over access to dissociated status;
(ii)    increase episodic memory of the traumatic experience;
(iii)   restructure traumatic episodic memory;
(iv)    enhance toleration of uncomfortable affect related to traumatic memories;
(v)     explore the significance of the new memory;
(vi)    reduce feelings of shame and guilt (Spiegel, 1993).

Clinical judgment is required to determine if the patient has strong enough personality structure to tolerate the added anxiety associated with discussing (traumatic) memories in therapy. Memory recovery can be associated with post-traumatic stress and self-difficulties. Therefore, the therapist must be prepared to treat resurgence of these symptoms and problems in the area of identity and affect regulation. When the material first is reaccessed, in clinical context, it can burst into consciousness with associated affect. Powerful and conflictual emotions of despair, grief, guilt, shame, rage, self-hatred, helplessness and terror are commonly embedded in memories for which the person is amnesic. This can reoccur when therapy is going. The affects that seem most likely to accompany abuse recollections are anxiety, depression and anger (Elliot & Briere, 1995).

The trauma may also cause profound shifts in the person's view of him or herself, significant others and the nature of the world and all human and social relations (Loewenstein, 1993). The clinician should expect the patient to use cognitive, dissociative and behavioural mechanisms to reduce his or her stress. These avoidance

strategies should be respected and not interpreted as resistance or acting out behaviour.

Hypnosis may well be used to access the memory that otherwise is unavailable
to consciousness. After assessment of the hypnotic susceptibility different techniques can be used, like age regression or a free associative screen technique
(Frankel & Covino, 1997). An effortless attention in hypnosis can be helpful in dissociated memories (Spiegel et al., 1993a, b). Because of misconceptions regarding
the malleability of memory in hypnosis, the American Society of Clinical Hypnosis
recently reviewed and evaluated findings concerning hypnosis and memory and
came up with cautious guidelines for clinicians and for forensic hypnosis
(Hammond et al., 1994).

Pharmacotherapy is an important component of treatment (i) reducing the
intensity of debilitating symptoms such as anxiety, depression, poor concentration,
insomnia, nightmares, panic states; (ii) the patient's mental state and attention focus
can be improved to be more ready to benefit from psychotherapeutic interventions;
and (iii) to treat comorbid psychiatric disorders such as major depression, bipolar
disorder, obsessive–compulsive disorder, and so forth (Torem, 1996). Specific
symptoms as occur in the treatment of dissociative identity disorder can also be
treated (Loewenstein, 1991). There are no controlled trials reported in the literature.

To treat anxiety, benzodiazepines (alprazolam, lorazepam, oxazepam, temaze-
pam, chlordiazepoxide, clorazepate, diazepam or flurazepam) and sedative anti-
histamines (hydroxizine, diphenhydramine, promethzaine hydrochloride),
buspirone or beta-blockers can be used. One should be careful prescribing benzodiazepines for they can also impair aspects of memory functions (Curran, 1991).
Some patients with severe anxiety to the point of agitation and impulsivity may
respond to small doses of sedative neuroleptics. Some patients with a comorbidity
diagnosis of a major depression, dysthymic disorder, or bipolar disorder should be
treated accordingly as indicated in the standards of practice for mood disorders.
Some relief of flashbacks and poor impulse control can be obtained from perphen-
azine, chlorprothixene, haloperidol, risperidon or eventually from intramuscular
droperidol. Agents to be considered for alleviation of hyperarousal symptoms are
also lithium, anti-convulsants and clonidine (Sutherland & Davidson, 1994). Sleep
problems should be treated with available hypnotics. (For an overview of the use
of psychopharmacology in dissociation, see Torem, 1996.)

An informed consent is considered essential for the material that can be reaccessed
and might lead to complicated matters. Legal cases have proven to be no exception.
Transference–countertransference issues in the process of therapy must be carefully
considered and supervised, preventing a patient from secondary traumatization.
Special care should be given to transference issues when medication is considered.

Therapeutic work can be done on a psychodynamic (Matthews & Chu, 1997), cognitive or cognitive–behavioural (Ross, 1997) level; no approach is more favourable than another. Many authors advocate for a complete integration of splintered aspects of memory and experience in the treatment of traumatized patients (Ross, 1989; Kluft, 1993; Nemiah, 1995). Psychotherapy can include art therapy, dance and movement therapy, and journaling and creative writing therapies. Social work can be necessary to help the patient in addressing important family issues as well as matters pertaining to work, school and aftercare treatment. This type of therapy may often be long term, since the long-term consequences of dissociative amnesia can be weakening of identity and personality structure, which makes it difficult for these patients to tolerate the intense affect that comes with the reintegration of traumatic memories.

## Concluding remarks

In diagnosing dissociative amnesia it is most important to differentiate dissociative from non-dissociative amnesia. Assessment should focus on excluding organic causes, substance abuse, head trauma, or epilepsy. Most important information assessing dissociative amnesia is derived from the patient's history for there is a strong relation to psychological (early) trauma.

Throughout the chapter a particular relationship between dissociative amnesia and psychological trauma is described, for this is recognized as a significant determinant in the development of dissociative disorders in general and dissociative amnesia in particular. There is an intimate relationship between dissociation and alterations in memory, logically suggesting that the neurobiological basis for dissociative states may be found in brain structures that mediate memory function. These perspectives, together with an understanding of the alterations in brain systems which play a role in learning and memory, give better understanding of the nature of dissociative amnesia and also help to give an answer to the current controversy about the availability of memories of abuse to consciousness, their validity and their reliability.

The clinician has to deal with controversies that are present in the public media, the scientific field and sometimes the courtroom, be cautious and, at the same time, work with the patient to reduce the symptomatology associated with the amnesia in recovering, reliving and restoring traumatic memories.

## REFERENCES

Abeles, M. & Schilder, P. (1935). Psychogenic loss of personal identity. *Archives of Neurology and Psychiatry*, **34**, 587–604.

American Psychiatric Association (APA) (1994). *Diagnostic and Statistical Manual of Mental Disorders*, 4th edn. Washington, DC: American Psychiatric Association.

Appelbaum, P.S., Uyehara, L.A. & Elin, M.R. (1997). *Trauma and Memory; Clinical and Legal Controversies*. New York: Oxford University Press Inc.

Archibald, H.C. & Tuddenham, R.D. (1965). Persistent stress reaction after combat. *Archives of General Psychiatry*, 12, 475–81.

Baker, J.J. (1901). Epilepsy and crime. *Journal of Mental Science*, 47, 260–77.

Bernstein, E.M. & Putnam, F.W. (1986). Development, reliability and validity of a dissociation scale. *Journal of Nervous and Mental Disease*, 174, 727–35.

Bliss, E. (1984). *Multiple Personality, Allied Disorders and Hypnosis*. New York: Oxford University Press.

Boon, S. & Draijer, N. (1993). Multiple personality disorder in the Netherlands: a study on reliability and validity of the diagnosis. Amsterdam: Swets and Zeitlinger.

Bower, G.H. (1981). Mood and memory. *American Psychologist*, 36, 129–48.

Bremner, J.D. (1999). Does stress damage the brain? *Biological Psychiatry*, 45, 797–805.

Bremner, J.D. & Brett, E. (1997). Trauma-related dissociative states and long-term psychopathology in posttraumatic stress disorder. *Journal of Traumatic Stress*, 10, 37–51.

Bremner, J.D. & Marmar, C. (1998). *Trauma, Memory and Dissociation*. Washington, DC: American Psychiatric Association Press.

Bremner, J.D. & Narayan, M. (1998). The effects of stress on memory and the hippocampus throughout the life cycle: implications for childhood development and aging. *Development and Psychopathology*, 10, 871–85.

Bremner, J.D., Southwick, S., Brett, E., Fontana, A., Rosenheck, R. & Charney, D.S. (1992). Dissociation and posttraumatic stress disorder in Vietnam combat veterans. *American Journal of Psychiatry*, 149, 328–33.

Bremner, J.D., Davis, M., Southwick, S.M., Krystal, J.H. & Charney, D.S. (1993a). Neurobiology of posttraumatic stress disorder. In *Review of Psychiatry*, vol. 12, ed. J.M. Oldham, M.B. Riba, & A. Tasman, pp. 183–205. Washington DC: American Psychiatric Press.

Bremner, J.D., Southwick, S.M., Johnson, D.R., Yehuda, R. & Charney, D. (1993b). Childhood physical abuse and combat related posttraumatic stress disorder in Vietnam veterans. *American Journal of Psychiatry*, 150, 235–9.

Bremner, J.D., Steinberg, M., Southwick, S.M., Johnson, D.R. & Charney, D.S. (1993c). Use of the structured clinical interview for DMS-IV Dissociative Disorders for systematic assessment of dissociative symptoms in posttraumatic stress disorder. *American Journal of Psychiatry*, 150, 1011–14.

Bremner, J.D., Scott, T.M., Delaney, R.C., Southwick, S.M., Mason, J.W., Johnson, D.R., Innis, R.B., McCarthy, G. & Charney, D.S. (1993d). Deficitis in short-term memory in posttraumatic stress disorder. *American Journal of Psychiatry*, 150, 1015–19.

Bremner, J.D., Randall, P., Scott, T.M., Bronen, R.A., Seibyl, J.P., Southwick, S.M., Delaney, R.C., McCarthy, G., Charney, D.S. & Innis, R.B. (1995a). MRI-based measurements of hippocampal volume in combat related posttraumatic stress disorder. *American Journal of Psychiatry*, 152, 973–81.

Bremner, J.D., Krystal, J.H., Southwick, S.M. & Charney, D.S. (1995b). Functional neuroanatomical correlates of the effects of stress on memory. *Journal of Traumatic Stress*, 8, 527–53.

Bremner, J.D., Randall, P., Scott, T., Capelli, S., Delaney, R., McCarthy, G. & Charney, D.S. (1995c). Deficits in short-term memory in adult survivors of childhood abuse. *Psychiatry Research*, **59**, 97–107.

Bremner, J.D., Krystal, J.H., Charney, D.S. & Southwick, S.M. (1996). Neural mechanisms in dissociative amnesia for childhood abuse: relevance to the current controversy surrounding 'false memory syndrome'. *American Journal of Psychiatry*, **8**, 71–82.

Bremner, J.D., Randall, P., Vermetten, E., Staib, L., Bronen, R.A., Mazure, C., Capelli, S., McCarthy, G., Innis, R. & Charney, D.S. (1997a). Magnetic resonance imaging-based measurement of hippocampal volume in posttraumatic stress disorder related to childhood physical and sexual abuse – a preliminary report. *Biological Psychiatry*, **41**, 23–32.

Bremner, J.D., Innis, R.B., Ng, C.K., Staib, L.H., Salomon, R.M., Bronen, R.A., Duncan, J., Southwick, S.M., Krystal, J.H., Rich, D., Zubal, G., Dey, H., Soufer, R. & Charney, D.S. (1997b). Positron emission tomography measurement of cerebral metabolic correlates of yohimbine administration in combat-related posttraumatic stress disorder. *Archives of General Psychiatry*, **54**, 246–54.

Bremner, J.D., Licino, J., Darnell, A., Krystal, J.H., Owens, M.J., Southwick, S.M., Nemeroff, C.B. & Charney, D.S. (1997c). Elevated CSF corticotropin-releasing factor concentrations in posttraumatic stress disorder. *American Journal of Psychiatry*, **154**, 624–9.

Bremner, J.D., Mazure, C.M., Putnam, F.W., Southwick, S.M., Marmar, C., Hansen, C., Lubin, H., Roach, L., Freeman, G., Krystal, J.H. & Charney, D.S. (1998a). Measurement of dissociative states with the Clinican Administered Dissociative States Scale (CADSS). *Journal of Traumatic Stress*, **11**, 125–36.

Bremner, J.D., Vermetten, E., Southwick, S.M., Krystal, J.H. & Charney, D.S. (1998b). Trauma, memory and dissociation: an integrative formulation. In *Trauma, Memory and Dissociation*, ed. J.D. Bremner & C. Marmar, pp. 365–402. Washington, DC: American Psychiatric Association Press.

Brenneis, C.B. (1996). Memory systems and the psychoanalytic retrieval of memories of trauma. *Journal of the American Psychoanalytical Association*, **44**, 1165–87.

Brewin, C.R., Andrews, B., Rose, S. & Kirk, M. (1999). Acute stress disorders and posttraumatic stress disorder in victims of violent crime. *American Journal of Psychiatry*, **156**, 360–6.

Briere, J. & Conte, J. (1993). Self-reported amnesia for abuse in adults molested as children. *Journal of Traumatic Stress*, **6**, 21–31.

Brown, D., Scheflin, A.W. & Hammond, C. (1998). *Memory, Trauma Treatment and the Law*. New York: W.W. Norton and Company.

Cahill, L., Prins, B., Weber, M. & McGaugh, J.L. (1994). B-adrenergic activation and memory for emotional events. *Nature*, **371**, 702–4.

Caine, E.D. (1993). Amnesic disorders. *Journal of Neuropsychiatry and Clinical Neuroscience*, **5**, 6–8.

Cameron, N. & Rychlak, J.F. (1985). *Personality Development and Psychopathology: A Dynamic Approach*. Boston: Houghton Mifflin Co.

Cardena, E. (1994). The domain of dissociation. In *Dissociation: Clinical and Theoretical Perspectives*, ed. S.J. Lynn & J.W. Rhue, pp. 15–32. New York: Guilford Press.

Cardena, E. & Spiegel, D. (1993). Dissociative reactions to the bay area earthquake. *Ameircan Journal of Psychiatry*, **150**, 474–8.

Carlsson, E. & Rosser-Hogan, R. (1991). Trauma experiences, posttraumatic stress, dissociation, and depression in Cambodian refugees. *American Journal of Psychiatry*, **148**, 1548–51.

Charney, D.S., Deutch, A.Y., Krystal, J.H., Southwick, S.M. & Davis, M. (1993). Psychobiologic mechanisms of posttraumatic stress disorder. *Archives of General Psychiatry*, **50**, 294–9.

Chu, J.A. & Dill, D.L. (1990). Dissociative symptoms in relation to childhood physical and sexual abuse. *American Journal of Psychiatry*, **147**, 887–92.

Classen, C. Koopman, C. & Spiegel, D. (1993). Trauma and dissociation. *Bulletin of the Menninger Clinic*, **57**, 178–94.

Cole, P. & Putnam, F.W. (1992). Effect of incest on self and social functioning: a developmental psychopathology perspective. *Journal of Consulting and Clinical Psychology*, **60**, 174–84.

Coons, P.M. (1994). Confirmation of childhood abuse in child and adolescent cases of multiple personality disorder and dissociative disorder not otherwise specified. *Journal of Nervous and Mental Disease*, **8**, 461–4.

Coons, P.M. & Milstein, V. (1992). Psychogenic amnesia: a clinical investigation of 25 cases. *Dissociation*, **5**, 73–80.

Coons, P.M., Bowman, E.S. & Milstein, V. (1988). Multiple personality disorder. A clinical investigation of 50 cases. *Journal of Nervous and Mental Diseases*, **176**, 519–27.

Cummings, J.L. (1993). Amnesia and memory disturbances in neurologic disorders. In *Review of Psychiatry*, vol. 12, ed. J.M. Oldham, M.B. Riba & A. Tasman, pp. 725–45. Washington DC: American Psychiatric Press.

Curran, H.V. (1991). Benzodiazepines, memory and mood: a review. *Psychopharmacology*, **105**, 1–8.

Dennett, D. (1991). *Consciousness Explained*. Boston: Little Brown.

Elliot, D.M. & Briere, J. (1995). Posttraumatic stress associated with delayed recall of sexual abuse: a general population study. *Journal of Traumatic Stress*, **8**, 629–49.

Erdelyi, M.H. (1994). Dissociation, defense, and the unconscious. In *Dissociation: Culture, Mind and Body*, ed. D. Spiegel, pp. 3–20. Washington, DC: American Psychiatric Press.

Erdelyi, M.H. (1996). *Recovery of Unconscious Memories; Hypermnesia and Reminiscence*. Chicago: University Chicago Press.

Eriksson, N.G. & Lundin, T. (1996). Early traumatic stress reactions among Swedish survivors of the M.S. Estonia disaster. *British Journal of Psychiatry*, **169**, 713–16.

Feldman, J.A. & Ballard, D.A. (1982). Connectionist models and their properties. *Cognitive Science*, **6**, 205–54.

Frankel, F.H. & Covino, N.A. (1997). Hypnosis and hypnotherapy. In *Trauma and Memory: Clinical and Legal Controversies*, pp. 344–60, ed. P.S. Appelbaum, L.A. Uyehara & M.R. Elin. New York: Oxford University Press.

Freud, S. (1941). Splitting of the ego in the defensive process. *International Journal of Psycho-Analysis*, **22**, 65–8.

Freyd, J. (1994). Betrayal trauma: traumatic amnesia as an adaptive response to childhood abuse. *Ethics and Behavior*, **4**, 307–29.

Frischholz, E.J., Lipman, L.S., Braun, B.G. & Sachs, R.G. (1992). Psychopathology, hypnotizability and dissociation. *American Journal of Psychiatry*, **149**, 1521–5.

Gergen, K.J. (1991). *The Saturated Self; Dilemmas of Identity in Contemporary Life*. New York: Basic Books.

Gloor, P., Olivier, A., Quesney, L.F., Andermann, R. & Horowitz, S. (1982). The role of the limbic system in experiential phenomena of temporal lobe epilepsy. *Annals of Neurology*, **12**, 129–44.

Goldfield, A.E., Mollica, R.F., Pesavento, B.H. & Faraone, S.V. (1988). The physical and psychological sequelae of torture: symptomatology and diagnosis. *Journal of the American Medical Association*, **259**, 2725–9.

Hammond, D.C., Garver, R.B., Mutter, C.B., Crasilneck, H.B., Frischholz, E., Gravitz, M.A., Hibler, N.S., Olson, J., Scheflin, A., Spiegel, H. & Wester, W. (1994). *Clinical Hypnosis and Memory: Guidelines for Clinicians and for Forensic Hypnosis*. American Society of Clinical Hypnosis Press.

Herman, J. (1992). *Trauma and Recovery*. New York: Basic Books.

Hilgard, E.R. (1977). *Divided Consciousness: Multiple Controls in Human Thought and Action*. New York: John Wiley.

Hilgard, E.R. (1986). *Divided Consciousness: Multiple Controls in Human Thought and Action*. Expanded edition. New York: John Wiley.

Hilgard, E.R. (1992). Dissociation and theories of hypnosis. In *Contemporary Hypnosis Research*, ed. E. Fromm & M.R. Nash, pp. 69–102.

Hilgard, E.R. (1994). Neodissociation theory. In *Dissociation: Clinical and Theoretical Perspectives*, ed. S.J. Lynn & J.W. Rhue, pp. 32–52. New York: Guilford Press.

Irwin, H.J. (1994). Proneness to dissociation and traumatic childhood events. *Journal of Nervous and Mental Diseases*, **8**, 456–60.

Janet, P. (1904). Amnesia and the dissociation of memories by emotion. *Journal de Psychologie*, **1**, 417–53.

Janet, P. (1924). *The Major Symptoms of Hysteria*. New York: Basic Books.

Keller, R. & Shaywitz, B.A. (1986). Amnesia or fugue state: a diagnostic dilemma. *Journal of Developmental and Behavioral Pediatrics*, **7**, 131–2.

Kahn, D., Pace-Schott, E.F. & Hobson, J.A. (1997). Consciousness in waking and dreaming: the roles of neural oscillation and neuromodulation in determining similarities and differences. *Neuroscience*, **78**, 13–38.

Khan, A.U. (1986). *Clinical Disorders of Memory*, p. 212. New York: Plenum Medical Book Co.

Kihlstrom, J.F. (1982). Hypnosis and the dissociation of memory, with special reference to post hypnotic phenomena. *Research Communications in Psychology, Psychiatry and Behavior*, **7**, 181–97.

Kihlstrom, J.F. (1987). The cognitive unconscious. *Science*, **237**, 1445–52.

Kihlstrom, J.F. (1994). One hundred years of hysteria. In *Dissociation; Clinical and Theoretical Perspectives*, ed. S.J. Lynn & J.W. Rhue, pp. 365–94. New York: Guilford Press.

Kihlstrom, J.F. & Evans, F.J. (1979). Memory retrieval processes during posthypnotic amnesia. In *Functional Disorders of Memory*, ed. Kihlstom, J.F. & Evans F.J. NJ: Erlbaum.

Kihlstrom, J.F., Barnhardt, T.M. & Tataryn, D.J. (1992). Implicit perception. In *Perception Without Awareness*, ed. R.F. Bornstein & T.S. Pittman, pp. 17–54. New York: Guilford Press.

Kihlstrom, J.F., Glisky, M.L. & Angiulo, M.J. (1994). Dissociative tendencies and dissociative disorders. *Journal of Abnormal Psychiatry*, **103**, 117–24.

Kluft, R.P. (1985). Using hypnotic inquiry protocols to monitor treatment progress and stability in multiple personality disorder. *American Journal of Clinical Hypnosis*, **28**, 63–75.

Kluft, R.P. (1988). The dissociative disorders. In *The American Psychiatric Stress Textbook of Psychiatry*, ed. J.A. Talbott, R.E. Hales & S.C. Yudofsky, pp. 557–85. Washington, DC: American Psychiatric Press.

Kluft, R.P. (1991). Multiple personality disorder. In *Review of Psychiatry*, volume 10, ed. Tasman & S.M. Goldfinger, pp. 161–88. Washington, DC: American Psychiatric Press.

Kluft, R.P. (1993). Basic principles in conducting the treatment of multiple personality disorder. In *Clinical Perspectives on Multiple Personality Disorder*, ed. R.P. Kluft & C.G. Fine, pp. 53–73. Washington, DC: American Psychiatric Press.

Kluft, R. (1999). True lies, false truths, and naturalistic raw data: applying clinical research findings to the false memory debate. In *Trauma and Memory*, ed. L.M. Williams & V. Banyard, pp. 311–17. Thousand Oaks, CA: Sage Publications.

Koopman, C., Classen, C. & Spiegel, D. (1994). Predictors of posttraumatic stress symptoms among survivors of the Oakland/Berkeley, Calif., firestorm survivors. *American Journal of Psychiatry*, **151**, 888–94.

Kopelman, M.D. (1995). The assessment of psychogenic amnesia. In *Handbook of Memory Disorders*, ed. A.D. Baddeley, B.A. Wilson & F.A. Watts, pp. 427–48. Chichester UK: John Wiley.

Kopelman, M.D., Panayiotopoulos, C.P. & Lewis, P. (1994). Transient epileptic amnesia differentiated from psychogenic 'fugue': neuropsychological, EEG, and PET findings. *Journal of Neurology, Neurosurgery and Psychiatry*, **57**, 1002–4.

Koss, M.P., Tromp, S. & Tharan, M. (1995). Traumatic memories: empirical foundations, forensic and clinical implications. *Clinical Psychology Science and Practice*, **1**, 111–32.

Kretchmer, E. (1926). *Hysteria.* New York: Nervous and Mental Disease Publishing Co.

Krystal, H.(1993). Beyond the DSM III-R; Therapeutic considerations in posttraumatic stress disorder. In *International Handbook of Traumatic Stress Syndromes* ed. J.P. Wilson & B. Raphael, pp. 841–54. New York: Plenum.

Krystal, J.H., Dkarper, L.P., Seibyl, J.P., Freeman, G.K., Delaney, R., Bremner, J.D., Heninger, G.R., Bowers, M.B. Jr & Charney, D.S. (1994). Subanesthetic effects of the noncompetitive NMDA antagonist, ketamine, in humans. *Archives of General Psychiatry*, **51**, 199–214.

Krystal, J.H., Bennett, A., Bremner, J.D., Southwick, S.M. & Charney, D.S. (1995). Toward a cognitive neuroscience of dissociation and altered memory functions in post-traumatic stress disorder. In *Neurobiological and Clinical Consequences of Stress: From Normal Adaptation to Post Traumatic Stress Disorder*, ed. M.J. Friedman, D.S. Charney & A.Y. Deutch, pp. 239–71. Philadelphia: Lippincott.

Kuyk, J., Van Dyck, R. & Spinhoven, P. (1996). The case for a dissociative interpretation of pseudoepileptic seizures. *Journal of Nervous and Mental Diseases*, **184**, 468–74.

Kuzin, I.A. (1995). Hypnosis modeling in neural networks. *Bulletin of Mathematical Biology*, **57**, 1–20.

Leavitt, F. (1997). False attribution of suggestibility to explain recovered memory of childhood sexual abuse following extended amnesia. *Child Abuse and Neglect*, **21**, 265–72.

LeDoux, J.E. (1992). Emotion as memory: anatomical systems underlying indelible neural traces. In *Handbook of Emotion and memory*, eds. A. Christianson, pp. 269–88. Hillsdale, NJ: Laurence Erlbaum.

LeDoux, J.E. (1996). *The Emotional Brain: The Mysterious Underpinnings of Emotional Life*. New York: Simon and Schuster.

Lennox, W.G. (1943). Amnesia, real and feigned. *American Journal of Psychiatry*, 732–43.

Lerner, H. (1992). Review of repression and dissociation. *International Reviews of Psychoanalysis*, **19**, 257–60.

Levy, J.P., Bavraktarin, D., Bullinaire, J.A. & Cairns, P. (eds.) (1995). *Connectionist Models of Memory and Language*. London: UCLPress.

Li, D. & Spiegel, D. (1992). A neural network model of dissociative disorders. *Psychiatric Annals*, **22**, 3.

Loewenstein, R.J. (1991). Rational psychopharmacology in the treatment of multiple personality disorder. *Psychiatry Clinics of North America*, **14**, 721–40.

Loewenstein, R.J. (1993). Dissociation, development and the psychobiology of trauma. *Journal of American Academy of Psychoanalysis*, **21**, 581–603.

Loewenstein, R.J. & Putnam, F. (1988). A comparison study of dissociative symptoms in patients with complex partial seizures, MPD, and PTSD. *Dissociation*, **1**, 17–23.

Loftus, E.F. (1993). The reality of repressed memories. *American Psychologist*, **48**, 518–37.

Loftus, E.F. (1994). The repressed memory controversy. *American Psychologist*, **49**, 443–5.

Loftus, E.F. (1996). Memory distortion and false memory creation. *Bulletin of the American Academy of Psychiatry Law*, **24**, 281–95.

Loftus, E.F., Polonski, S. & Fullilove, M.T. (1994a). Memories of childhood sexual abuse: remembering and repressing. *Psychology of Women Quarterly*, **18**, 67–84.

Loftus, E.F., Garry, M. & Feldman J. (1994b). Forgetting sexual trauma: what does it mean when 38% forget? *Journal of Consulting and Clinical Psychology*, **62**, 1177–81.

Ludwig, A.M. (1983). The psychobiological functions of dissociation. *American Journal of Clinical Hypnosis*, **26**, 93–9.

Ludwig, A.M., Brandsma, J.M., Wilbur, C.B., Bendfeldt, F. & Jameson, D.H. (1972). The objective study of a multiple personality. *Archives of General Psychiatry*, **26**, 298–310.

McEwen, B.S., Angulo, J., Cameron, H., Chao, H., Daniels, D., Gannon, M., Gould, E., Mendelson, S., Sakai, R., Spencer, R. & Woolley, C. (1992). Paradoxical effects of adrenal steroids on the brain: protection versus degeneration. *Biological Psychiatry*, **31**, 177–99.

McEwen, B.S. & Schmeck, H.M. (1994). *The Hostage Brain*. New York: Rockefeller University Press.

McGaugh, J.L. & Cahill, L. (1997). Interaction of neuromoudlatory systems in modulating memory storage. *Behavioral Brain Research*, **83**, 31–8.

McGaugh, J.L., Cahill, L. & Roozendaal, B. (1996). Involvement of the amygdala in memory storage: interaction with other brain systems. *Proceedings of the National Academy of Sciences, USA*, **93**, 13085–14.

McIntosh, A.R. (1998). Understanding neural interactions in learning and memory using functional neuroimaging. *Annals of the New York Academy of Science*, **855**, 556–71.

Madakasira, S. & O'Brien, K. (1987). Acute posttraumatic stress disorder in victims of a natural disaster. *Journal of Nervous and Mental Disease*, **175**, 286–90.

Marmar, C.R., Weiss, D.S. & Schlenger, D.S. et al. (1994). Peritraumatic dissociation and post-traumatic stress in male Vietnam Theater veterans. *American Journal of Psychiatry*, **151**, 902–7.

Matthews, J.A. & Chu, J.A. (1997). Psychodynamic therapy for patients with early childhood trauma. In *Trauma and Memory; Clinical and Legal Controversies*, ed. P.S. Appelbaum, L.A. Uyehara & M.R. Elin, pp. 316–44. New York: Oxford University Press Inc.

Mellman, T.A., Kulick-Bell, R., Ashlock, L.E. & Nolan, B. (1995). Sleep events among veterans with combat-related posttraumatic stress disorder. *American Journal of Psychiatry*, **152**, 110–15.

Minsky, M. (1986). *The Society of Mind*. New York: Simon and Schuster Inc.

Nemiah, J.C. (1989). Janet redivivus: the centenary of l'automatisme psychologique. *Am J Psychiatry*, **146**, 1527–30.

Nemiah, J.C. (1993). Dissociation, conversion and somatization. In *Dissociative Disorders, A Clinical Review*, ed. D. Spiegel, pp. 104–17. Lutherville: Sidran Press.

Nemiah, J.C. (1995). Dissociative disorders (hysterical neurosis, dissociative type). In *Comprehensive Textbook of Psychiatry*, ed. H.I. Kaplan & B.J. Sadock, Chapter 20, pp. 1281–93. Baltimore, MD: Williams & Wilkins.

Nijenhuis, E.R., Spinhoven, Ph., Van Dyck, R., Van der Hart, O. & Vanderlinden, J. (1996). The development and psychometric characteristics of the Somatoform Dissociation Questionnaire (SDQ-20). *Journal of Nervous and Mental Diseases*, **184**, 688–94.

Nijenhuis, E.R., Van der Hart, O. & Vermetten, E. (1998). From forgetting to reexperiencing trauma; from analgesia to pain. In *Images of the Body in Trauma*, ed. J. Goodwin & R. Attias.

Ofshe, R.J. & Singer, M.T. (1994). Recovered-memory therapy and robust repression: influence and pseudomemories. *International Journal of Clinical and Experimental Hypnosis*, **42**, 391–410.

Parks, R.W., Long, D.L., Levine, D.S., Crockett, D.J., McGeer, E.G., McGeer, P.L., Dalton, I.E., Zec, R.F., Becker, R.E., Coburn, K.L., Siler, G., Nelson, M.E. & Bower, J.M. (1991). Parallel distributed processing and neural networks: origins, methodology and cognitive functions. *International Journal of Neuroscience*, **60**, 195–214.

Perry, J.C. & Jacobs, D. (1982). Clinical applications of the amytal interview in psychiatric emergency settings. *American Journal of Psychiatry*, **139**, 552–9.

Pezdek, K. & Banks, W.P. (1996). *The Recovered Memory/False Memory Debate*. New York: Academic Press.

Pitman, R.K. (1989). Posttraumatic stress disorder, hormones, and memory (editorial). *Biological Psychiatry*, **26**, 221-3.

Post, R.M., Weiss, S.R.B. & Smith, M.A. (1995). Sensitization and kindling; implications for the evolving neural substrates of post-traumatic stress disorder. *In Neurobiological and Clinical Consequences of Stress: From Normal Adaptation to Post Traumatic Stress Disorder*, ed. M.J. Friedman, D.S., Charney & A.Y. Deutch, pp. 203–24. Philadelphia: Lippincot.

Post, R.M., Weiss, S.R.B., Li, H., Smith, M.A., Zhang, L.X., Xing, G., Osuch, E.A. & McCann, U.D. (1998). Neural plasticity and emotional memory. *Development and Psychopathology*, **10**, 829–55.

Putnam, F.W. (1985). Dissociation as a response to extreme trauma. In *Childhood Antecedents of Multiple Personality Disorder*, ed. R.P. Kluft, pp. 65–97. Washington, DC: American Psychiatric Press.

Putnam, F.W. (1986). Pierre Janet and modern views of dissociation. *Journal of Traumatic Stress*, 2, 413–29.

Putnam, F.W. (1991). Dissociative phenomena. In *American Psychiatric Press Review of Psychiatry*, ed. A. Tasman & S.M. Goldfinger, Vol. 10, pp. 145–60. Washington DC: American Psychiatric Press.

Putnam, F.W., Helmers, K. & Trickett, P.K. (1993). Development, reliability, and validity of a child dissociation scale. *Child Abuse and Neglect*, 17, 731–41.

Riether, A.M. & Stoudemire, A. (1988). Psychogenic fugue states: a review. *South Medical Journal*, 81, 568–71.

Ross, C.A. (1989). *Multiple Personality Disorder: Diagnosis, Clinical Features, and Treatment*. New York: John Wiley.

Ross, C.A. (1997). Cognitive therapy of dissociative identity disorder. In *Trauma and Memory; Clinical and Legal Controversies*, pp. 360–78, ed. P.S. Appelbaum, L.A. Uyehara & M.R. Elin. New York: Oxford University Press Inc.

Ross, C.A., Heber, S.& Norton, G.R. (1989). The dissociative disorders interview: a structured interview. *Dissociation*, 2, 169–89.

Ross, C.A., Joshi, S. & Currie, R.P. (1991). Dissociation in the general population: identification of three factors. *Hospital Community Psychiatry*, 42, 297–301.

Rots, N.Y., De Jong, N., Workel, J.O., Levine, S., Cools, A.R. & De Kloet, E.R. (1996). Neonatal meternally deprived rats have as adults elevated basal pituitary-adrenal activity and enhanced susceptibility to apomorphine. *Journal of Neuroendocrinology and Criminology*, 8, 501–6.

Rumelhart, D.E. & McClelland, J.L. (1986). *Parallel Distributed Processing: Explorations in the Microstructures of Cognition*, vol. 1: *Foundations*. Cambridge, MA: MIT Press.

Sapolsky, R.M., Uno, H., Rebert, C.S. & Finch, C.E. (1990). Hippocampal damage associated with prolonged glucocorticoid exposure in primates. *Journal of Neuroscience*, 10, 2897–902.

Schacter, D. (1995). Memory distortion: history and current status. In *Memory Distortion*, ed. D. Schacter, J.T. Coyle, G.D. Fishbach, M.M. Mesulam & L.E. Sullivan. Cambridge, MA: Harvard University Press.

Schacter, D. & Tulving, E. (1994). What are the memory systems of 1994? In *Memory Systems*, ed. D. Schacter & E. Tulving, E., pp. 1–38. Cambridge, MA: MIT Press.

Schacter, D., Koutstaal, W. & Norman. K.A. (1996). Can cognitive neuroscience illuminate the nature of traumatic childhood memories? *Current Opinions in Neurobiology*, 6, 207–14.

Scheflin, A.W. & Brown, D. (1996). Repressed memory or dissociative amnesia: what the science says. *Journal of Psychiatry and Law*, 2, 143–88.

Scheflin, A.W. & Spiegel, D. (1998). From courtroom to couch. Working with repressed memory and avoiding lawsuits. *Psychiatric Clinics of North America*, 21, 847–67.

Siegel, D.J. (1995). Memory, trauma and psychotherapy: a cognitive science view. *Journal of Psychotherapy Practice and Research*, 4, 93–122.

Singer, J. (1990). *Repression and Dissociation*. Chicago: University of Chicago Press.

Sigalowitz, S.J., Dywan, J. & Ismailos, L. (1991). Electrocortical evidence that hypnotically induced hallucinations are experienced. Paper presented at the Society for Clinical and Experimental Hypnosis meeting as part of a symposium entitled 'Dissociations in Conscious Experience: Electrophysical and Behavioral Evidence', New Orleans, LA, October 9–13.

Southwick, S.M., Krystal, J.H., Morgan, C.A., Johnson, D., Nagy, L.M., Nicolaou, A., Heninger, G.R. & Charney, D.S. (1993). Abnormal noradrenergic function in posttraumatic stress disorder. *Archives of General Psychiatry*, **50**, 266–74.

Southwick, S.M., Bremner, J.D., Krystal, J.H. & Charney, D.S. (1994). Psychobiologic research in posttraumatic stress disorder. *Psychiatric Clinics of North America*, **17**, 251–64.

Spiegel, D. (1986). Dissociation, double binds and posttraumatic stress in multiple personality disorder. In *Treatment of Multiple Personality Disorder*, ed. B.G. Braun, pp. 61–77. Washington, DC: American Psychiatric Press.

Spiegel, D. (1990). Hypnosis, dissociation and trauma: hidden and overt observers. In *Repression and Dissociation*, pp. 121–42. ed. J.L. Singer. Chicago: University of Chicago Press.

Spiegel, D. (1993). Dissociation and trauma. In *Dissociative Disorders, A Clinical Review*, pp. 117–31. Lutherville: Sidran Press.

Spiegel, D. & Cardena, E. (1991). The Disintegrated Experience: the dissociative disorders revisited. *Journal of Abnormal Psychology*, **100**, 366–87.

Spiegel, D. & Vermetten, E. (1994). Physiological correlates of hypnosis and dissociation. In *Dissociation: Culture, Mind and Body*, pp. 185–209. ed. D. Spiegel. Washington, DC: American Psychiatric Press.

Spiegel, D. & Scheflin, A.W. (1994). Dissociated or fabricated? Psychiatric aspects of repressed memory in criminal and evil cases. *International Journal of Clinical and Experimental Hypnosis*, **42**, 411–32.

Spiegel, D., Cutcomb, S. & Ren, C. (1985). Hypnotic hallucination alters evoked potentials. *Journal of Abnormal Psychology*, **94**, 249–55.

Spiegel, D., Hunt, T. & Dondershine, H.E. (1988). Dissociation and hypnotizability in post traumatic stress disorder. *American Journal of Psychiatry*, **145**, 301–5.

Spiegel, D., Bierre, P. & Rootenberg, J. (1989). Hypnotic alteration of somatosensory perception. *American Journal of Psychiatry*, **146**, 749–54.

Spiegel, D., Frischholz, E.J. & Spira, J. (1993a). Functional disorders of memory. In *Review of Psychiatry*, Vol 12, ed. J.M. Oldham, M.B. Riba & A. Tasman. Washington, DC: American Psychiatric Press.

Spiegel, D., Frischholz, E.J., Fleiss, J.L. & Spiegel, H. (1993b). Predictors of smoking abstinence following a single-session restructuring intervention with self-hypnosis. *American Journal of Psychiatry*, **150**, 1090–7.

Squire, L.R. & Butters, N. (eds.) (1984). *Neuropsychology of Memory*. New York: Guilford Press.

Squire, L.R. & Zola-Morgan, S. (1991). The medial tempora lobe memory system. *Science*, **253**, 1380–6.

Stein, D.J. & Ludik, J. (eds.) (1998). Neural networks and psychopathology: connectionist models in practice and research. Cambridge: Cambridge University Press.

Steinberg, M. (1993). *Structural Clinical Interview for DSM-IV Dissociative Disorders (SCIDD)*. Washington, DC: American Psychiatric Press.

Sutherland, S.M. & Davidson, J.R. (1994). Pharmacotherapy for post-traumatic stress disorder. *Pediatric Clinics of North America*, **17**, 409–23.

Teicher, M.H., Glod, C.A., Surrey, J. & Swett, C. (1993). Early childhood abuse and limbic system ratings in adult psychiatric outpatients. *Journal of Neuropsychiatry*, **5**, 301–6.

Terr, L. (1991). Childhood traumas: an outline and overview. *American Journal of Psychiatry*, 27, 96–104.

Thygesen, P., Hermann, K. & Willanger, R. (1970). Concentration camp survivors in Denmark: prosecution, disease, disability, compensation. *Danish Medical Bulletin*, 17, 65–108.

Torem, M.S. (1996). Psychopharmacology. In *Handbook of Dissociation, Theoretical, Empirical and Clinical Perspectives*, pp. 545–65, ed. L.K. Michelson & W.J. Ray. New York: Plenum Press.

Torrie, A. (1944). Psychosomatic casualties in the Middle East. *Lancet*, 29, 139–43.

Uno, H., Tarara, R., Else, J.G., Suleman, M.A. & Sapolsky, R.M. (1989). Hippocampal damage associated with prolonged and fatal stress in primates. *Journal of Neuroscience*, 9, 1705–11.

Van der Hart, O. & Spiegel, D. (1993). Hypnotic assessment and treatment of trauma-induced psychoses: the early psychotherapy of H. Breukink and modern views. *International Journal of Clinical Experimental Hypnosis*, 41, 191–209.

Van der Hart, O. & Nyenhuis, E.R.S. (1998). Recovered memories of abuse and dissociative identity disorder. *British Journal of Psychiatry*, 173, 537–8.

Van der Kolk, B.A. (1994). The body keeps the score: memory and the evolving psychobiology of posttraumatic stress. *Harvard Reviews of Psychiatry*, 253, 65.

Van der Kolk, B.A. & Van der Hart, O. (1989). Pierre Janet and the breakdown of adaptation in psychological trauma. *American Journal of Psychiatry*, 146, 1530–40.

Van der Kolk, B.A., McFarlane, A.C. & Weisaeth, L. (1996). *Traumatic Stress: The Effects of Overwhelming Experience on Mind, Body and Society*. New York: Guilford Press.

Vanderlinden, J., Van Dyck, R. & Vandereyken, W. (1991). Dissociative experiences in the general population in the Netherlands and Belgium: a study with the Dissociative Questionnaire (DIS-Q). *Dissociation*, 4, 180–4.

Vanderlinden, J., Van Dyck, R. & Vandereyken, W. (1993). The Dissociation Questionnaire: development and characteristics of a new self-reporting questionnaire. *Clinical Psychology and Psychotherapy*, 1, 21–7.

Vermetten, E., Bremner, J.D. & Spiegel, D. (1998). Dissociation and hypnotic susceptibility: a conceptual and methodological perspective on two distinct concepts. In *Trauma Memory and Dissociation*, Progress in Psychiatry, No. 54 ed. J.D. Bremner & Marmar, pp. 107–59. Ch. Washington, DC: American Psychiatric Press.

Wakefield, H. & Underwager, R. (1992). Recovered memories of alleged sexual abuse: lawsuits against parents. *Behavioral Sciences and the Law*, 10, 483–507.

Weiskrantz, L. (1987). Neuroanatomy of memory and amnesia: a case for multiple memory systems. *Human Neurobiology*, 6, 93–105.

Wied, de D. & Croiset, G. (1991). Stress modulation of learning and memory processes. *Methods of Achievement in Experimental Pathology*, 15, 167–99.

Whitfield, Ch.L. (1995). The forgotten difference: ordinary memory versus traumatic memory. *Consciousness and Cognition*, 4, 88–94.

Williams, L.M. (1994a). Adult memories of childhood abuse. *Journal of Consulting and Clinical Psychology*, 62, 1167–76.

Williams, L.M. (1994b). What does it mean to forget child sexual abuse? A reply to Loftus, Garry and Feldman. *Journal of Consulting Clinical Psychology*, 62, 1182–6.

Williams, L.M. (1995). Recovered memories of abuse in women with documented child sexual victimization histories. *Journal of Traumatic Stress*, **8**, 649–76.

Woolley, C.S., Gould, E. & McEwen, B.S. (1990). Exposure to excess glurocorticoids alters dendritic morphology of adult hippocampal pyramidal neurons. *Brain Research*, **531**, 225–31.

# 20

# Recovered and false memories

Debra A. Bekerian and Susan J. Goodrich

The question of how people remember traumatic events has recently come to the focus of international attention with the recovered memory debate. Adults claim to recover memories of being sexually abused as children after having amnesia for these events. The question of whether or not memories of childhood events can be recovered in adulthood has divided professionals. In this chapter a brief account is given of the background to the debate and some of the major issues are discussed. The impact of the debate on psychology is considered, and future directions that research on recovered memories might take are explored.

## Background

One of the first contemporary cases of recovered memories of childhood sexual abuse was reported in the United States. The accuser, a female academic, recovered memories of childhood sexual abuse by her father. In her second therapeutic session she had expressed anxiety about a forthcoming family visit; the therapist asked her if she had been sexually abused as a child. This threw her into a state of crisis, and at home a few hours after the session, she experienced intense flashbacks. Prior to this, she had no memories of actual sexual abuse, although she did have memories of years of living in a dysfunctional family with boundary violations and inappropriate sexual behaviour by her father (Freyd, 1993).

Her parents, also academics, disputed the truth of her accusations. They claimed that her 'memories' were the product of confabulation, brought about by leading and interpretative suggestions made during therapy and the general climate of abuse hysteria, generated in part by survivor 'self-help' books such as Bass and Davis' (1988) 'Courage to Heal' (Calof, 1993). A year later they started an association, The False Memory Syndrome Foundation, to support other parents similarly claiming to have been falsely accused of abusing their children. In setting up this association, the parents enlisted the expertise of other academics, as did their daughter, and extreme positions were adopted. No one could agree who was telling the truth, the press became involved, and the recovered memory debate began.

Since then, thousands of cases of recovered memories have been reported. The nature of memories of childhood sexual abuse recovered in adulthood varies: different patterns of recovery and phenomenal experience have been reported (e.g. Harvey & Herman, 1994). Much of the attention in the debate, however, has been on cases where memories of sexual abuse are recovered following a period of total amnesia for the abuse. Moreover, although cases have been reported where memories have been recovered outside therapy, the focus has been on people, mainly women, who have recovered memories subsequent to some kind of therapeutic intervention.

## The major issues

The main issues relating to the debate are as follows. First, recovery of real memories following amnesia means that information about the abuse was encoded and subsequently prevented from gaining access to consciousness. Some mechanism would have to be posited that would enable the information to be remembered later, having been preserved in memory without rehearsal during the intervening period. Whether and how this can occur has been a point of intense debate. Secondly, attention has been directed to the conditions under which memories have been recovered. Conditions of retrieval will determine, to some extent, the completeness and accuracy of the account (Bekerian & Dennett, 1993). Thirdly, and perhaps most important, there is the question of validity. How can a true account be distinguished from one that is false? Each of these issues will be addressed in turn.

### Selective forgetting of trauma

The issue of selected forgetting of childhood sexual abuse has produced very complicated and sometimes confusing arguments. Essentially, they revolve around the question of whether or not trauma can be forgotten and later remembered. The notion that people are able to repress or forget life events if they are ego-threatening was originally advanced by Freud (1915) and is still emphasized by many modern theorists (e.g. Alpert, 1991; Erdelyi, 1990; Herman & Schatzow, 1987). One argument is that memories for trauma fail to reach consciousness, but manifest themselves through alternative pathways like dreams, body language, inexplicable fears (Erdelyi, 1990). The person might later access the previously forgotten information if the environment acts as a trigger for memories of the abuse (e.g. significant life events, see Walker, 1996). The memories can then become more complete over time, with new details being added. This has been acknowledged for many years within the clinical domain as the phenomenon of reminiscence (Erdelyi, 1990).

Cognitive theories of memory similarly suggest that memory occurs on a continuum of awareness (e.g. Lindsay & Read, 1994; Morton, 1994). People can demonstrate memory for an event without any awareness of having experienced the event in the past (e.g. Jacoby & Witherspoon, 1982; Schacter, 1987). Such implicit memory is to be distinguished from explicit memory, where the person is able to retrieve information about an event and is aware that they had experienced that event in the past. Explicit memory is also known to change with time, such that memory can increase over time (see Erdelyi, 1990; Scrivener & Safer, 1988). Such arguments could be generalized to incorporate recovered memories of sexual abuse.

Early advocates of the concept of selective forgetting took the extreme view that all instances of recovered memories have historical truth (e.g. Bass & Davies, 1988). In response to such an extreme view, there were those who argued against the concept of selective forgetting. They argued that there was no empirical validation for the recovery of memories following amnesia (e.g. Gardner, 1993; Weiskrantz, 1995). Rather, it was suggested, recovered memories of childhood sexual abuse result from intense pressure placed on vulnerable clients by therapists who persuade them that their current distress is a consequence of sexual abuse suffered in childhood. This pressure from therapists could take the form of encouraging clients to 'recover' memories of abuse, telling them that this was the only cure for their distress (e.g. Loftus & Rosenwald, 1993). In addition, it was argued that the present climate of abuse hysteria was increasing the risk of people being falsely accused of child sexual abuse (Gardner, 1993; Ofshe & Watters, 1993; Weiskrantz, 1995).

This challenge to the notion of selective forgetting is consistent with evidence from patients suffering from Post-traumatic Stress Disorder (PTSD). In these cases, memories for trauma intrude into consciousness and are remembered unintentionally (e.g. Brewin et al., 1996). The individual would prefer not to remember details of the trauma; yet, thoughts and memories of the trauma cannot be controlled. For example, concentration camp victims report that images continue to intrude into consciousness, in spite of repeated attempts on the part of the individual to discard them from memory (Herman, 1992).

In conclusion, it is safe to assume that, within the context of the recovered memory debate, selective forgetting can be accommodated within most models of clinical and cognitive theories of memory (e.g. British Psychological Society (BPS) Working Party *Report on Recovered Memories*, 1995; Lindsay & Read, 1994; Morton, 1994). However, there is still disagreement over the exact conditions that lead to the selective forgetting of traumatic experiences.

## Conditions of recovery

At this time, there is little evidence regarding the conditions under which recovery of sexual abuse occurs after amnesia, although projects are under way (e.g.

Andrews et al., 1996). The conditions under which recovery occurs are likely to be as diverse as the pattern of recovery itself. There is ample experimental work that shows people can be misled into remembering details and events that never occurred through the use of leading questions (Loftus, 1979). More recently, research has examined more naturalistic conditions under which false memories of trauma are induced through suggestion. These simulations involve the experimenter falsely suggesting to an individual that s/he had experienced a traumatic event as a child. The person is then asked to recall this event over a series of sessions. The findings suggest that, not only can people be led into believing that they had experienced the trauma, they also enhance their report with confabulated details as time goes on. Some individuals maintain great confidence and certainty in the accuracy of their confabulations, even after they are debriefed and told that they had not experienced the event (see Ceci et al., 1994). However, as noted by Hyman and Pentland (1986), in order for subjects to be misled, the false event must in some way be compatible with the person's experience. Hyman et al. (1995) conclude that it is difficult to create false memories when the event is not compatible with the person's personal history.

Such data clearly illustrate the vulnerability of memory to outside influences and provide invaluable evidence regarding the conditions under which false memories can be induced. However, it is important to note that most experimental paradigms differ from real world scenarios in fundamental ways. For example, in many experiments, the person is told that X happened to them, and that the event had been verified by a significant member of the person's family (e.g. mother or older brother said it had happened). Thus, the person is led to believe that, according to family history, they had experienced the event, X. In contrast, real world scenarios involving recovered memories typically do not have the endorsement of family history. Generally, when an accuser claims to have been abused, the accused does not embrace this as truth, nor are other family members necessarily likely to do so. Furthermore, prior to memory recovery, many people report happy memories of their childhood, with loving relationships with their alleged abuser. Such total reversals in attitude have not been replicated within experimental settings.

## Reliability of recovered memories

Unfortunately, few reported cases of recovered memories document evidence that independently corroborates the accusations, or the denials. Similarly, in general, there is little experimental evidence that accurate accounts can be distinguished systematically and reliably from false or confabulated ones. Empirical studies have shown consistently that certain features of a report, like the presence of perceptual details or emotional reactions, are associated with accounts that are accurate. The literature on statement validity assessment procedures similarly suggests that accurate reports of real trauma contain certain characteristics, such as spontaneity of account, amount of perceptual and contextual detail, whereas confabulated ones do not (Steller, 1989; Bekerian & Dennett, 1993).

However, closer examination shows that indices of accuracy, or truth, are influenced by a variety of factors, and, consequently, cannot be generalized across different types of abuse and different individuals (see Bekerian & Dennett, 1993). For example, Steller (1989) has suggested that the use of certain interview techniques, such as context reinstatement, make it virtually impossible to distinguish an accurate account from one which is confabulated. The question of who is telling the truth remains elusive.

## The impact of the debate

The debate has been '. . . described as the greatest challenge currently facing applied cognitive psychology' (*Applied Cognitive Psychology*, 1994, **8**, (4)). There are some grounds for agreeing with this statement. The debate has affected a remarkable number of people. Foremost are the accusers and those accused. The estimated numbers of families who have been involved in cases of recovered memories of sexual abuse continue to grow. Even when some resolution occurs, as with retractors, the amount of suffering and damage sustained by the family continues to be substantial.

Secondly, there are the psychologists who have acted as experts in the debate. These experts have generally come from two disciplines: the experimental/cognitive and the observational/clinical. There has rarely been much sympathy between these two approaches. As a consequence of the debate, the tacit divisions in psychology have become more explicit. Characteristically, psychologists have reproached each other, criticizing each other's methodologies and challenging each other's conclusions. Some of this has resulted in promising new lines of research, which are dedicated to answering some of the more significant theoretical questions raised in the debate. However, the cost of the debate has been high. In some cases in the United States, experts have become the focus of gross intimidation tactics from both the accused and the accusers, and so have been affected personally as well as professionally.

The debate has also had a significant impact on therapy, highlighting the dangers of certain therapeutic techniques. A common assumption across most therapies is that problems present in adulthood are related to experiences from childhood. So, it is not unusual for therapists and clients to consider the effects of childhood experiences. However, the emphasis placed on childhood experiences varies across therapies. For instance, some of the humanistic approaches to therapy, such as Gestalt, place greater emphasis on the present relationship between the client and therapist.

While not disregarding that current behaviour may have its origins in the past, the focus is on what is happening in the present (Perls, 1947). Any therapy that insists on the client recovering memories of childhood experiences is likely to be dangerous.

Therapeutic techniques that encourage the individual to interpret non-verbal behaviour (e.g. body sensations), act out symbolic behaviour (e.g. engage in and enact out fantasies), or place the individual under susceptible states (e.g. hypnosis) may place both client and therapist at risk of colluding to form a false account. Evidence shows that the use of imagery can often have deleterious effects on accuracy and also can lead the person to believe that incorrect information is true (e.g. Bekerian et al., 1991; Bekerian & Dennett, 1993). Any rehearsal, particularly in the therapeutic context, of otherwise imaginary events can lead people into believing that such events were actually experienced (see Lindsay & Read, 1994). Taken together, the available evidence suggests that such techniques can promote conditions of false recovery, even though this may be done inadvertently by both the therapist and the client.

Guidelines for therapy have now been proposed by many international working parties on recovered memories of sexual abuse (e.g. see BPS Working Party *Report On Recovered Memories*, 1995). Included in these guidelines are warnings against the use of the above techniques. Further, given the adverse publicity that the recovered memory debate has had for therapy, many are now arguing for legislation on the accreditation of therapists and counsellors. The general environment is one of caution.

One of the problems here, however, is that those same therapeutic techniques, which have been deemed likely to lead to the creation of false memories, are often considered to be key elements within the therapeutic process (Bonano, 1990). People communicate information in a variety of ways; verbally, through images, non-verbal communication and through dreams. Information relating to early childhood events may not be available in verbal form and can only be expressed non-verbally (Howe et al., 1994).

The problem is that these 'memories'/body sensations are open to interpretation. An example will illustrate the point. Howe et al. (1994) describe the case of a 18-month-old, pre-verbal child (K.B.) who caught a fishbone in her throat while eating. At the time of the incident, she was not distressed but coughed and wretched so her father took her to see a family doctor who tried to remove it. The child became hysterical and was sent to the local hospital where the bone was removed. Seven months later K.B., now verbal, was unable to recount any details of the incident. She could, however, identify the physician who had removed the bone. Also, her mother reported that K.B. was refusing to eat fish and became very upset when seen by another doctor who needed to examine her throat.

Suppose, years later, K.B. goes into therapy, now a young woman of 21. During the course of therapy, she reports that, on occasions when doctors approach her and want to examine her throat, she panics. She has no memory of any event that could be the cause of this feeling.

K.B.'s symptoms of anxiety when her throat is examined are consistent with a history of abuse. It is also known that the precipitating incident could be her experience with the fishbone. The problem is that, if a client and therapist are working within a schema of abuse, then all memories that are compatible with abuse are susceptible to being interpreted as indicative of abuse.

## Future directions

In some ways, the recovered memory debate has raised more questions than it has answered. One of the most pressing questions concerns the types of memories that are recovered. Both the clinical and experimental literatures argue that a person can demonstrate memory for an event without having conscious awareness of having experienced that event. Memories can take many forms and will vary dramatically in their obvious relation to the person's past. Thus, although body reactions, fantasies and dreams may, indeed, reflect a person's experience of past abuse, the person may be unaware of their relationship. Equally, however, such dreams and fantasies, incorporating symbols that are sometimes grotesque and frightening in nature, may not '. . . derive from personal experience and (are) not a personal acquisition . . .' (Jung, 1959, p. 3). This presents problems, as some memories require interpretation if they are to be linked to specific, past experiences.

This is illustrated in Howe et al.'s example of the 18-month-old who got a fishbone stuck in her throat. On the basis of the child's behaviour alone, and due to the fact that her parents were present at the precipitating event, one could infer that her subsequent behaviour was due to her experience with the fish. However, we can only infer this causal relationship, as the child denied remembering any such experience. The extent to which the recovery of both true and false memories of child sexual abuse has relied upon the interpretation of body memories and fantasies is unknown. Future research is needed to determine the extent to which conclusions about past experiences of child abuse are based exclusively on recovery of types of memories that require interpretation.

The pattern of recovery is an equally pressing problem and is undoubtedly affected by the conditions under which recovery occurs. Clinical evidence suggests that there can be different types of recovery particularly with respect to the level of amnesia and awareness for the trauma. Harvey and Herman (1994) adamantly argue this point, citing three case studies of memory recovery which differ in terms of the awareness of the trauma, and memory for specific events. It is clear that more documentation is needed regarding the manner in which people recover memories. For example, are body sensations and dreams precursors to a person later remembering specific experiences? Are there any indications in previous sessions regarding the person's growing awareness that sexual abuse had been experienced in the past? Does awareness of past abuse come suddenly or gradually? Discourse analyses on memory for sexual assault reported in therapy indicate that the content and form of a person's report change dramatically over time, as levels of anxiety change (e.g. Wood et al., 1999). Similar analyses need to be applied to therapeutic sessions under which recovery from abuse occurs.

Critically, very little information exists regarding the conditions of recovery, including the circumstances leading up to the recovery. There are a number of projects which attempt to discover how recovery occurs in memory, and the nature of the recovery of memories over time (e.g. Andrews et al., 1996). Andrews et al. are interviewing therapists with clients who have recovered memories in order to determine both the extent to which recovery occurred in therapy and the nature of the memories recovered. These data promise to be very important, as they will also document the extent to which recovery occurs for trauma of a non-sexual nature, e.g. physical abuse.

Additionally, more detailed analyses need to be done on the dialogue between the therapist and client. The therapeutic session is a collaboration between the two. Both play an active role. Whatever the client reports in therapy will be a function of the interaction between the client and therapist. Thus, it is critical to document the contribution of the therapist. While the Andrew et al.'s data will provide some information, only detailed discourse analyses of the therapeutic sessions will ensure that the therapist's role in memory recovery is better understood.

Finally, it may be important to examine the role of culture on recovery. Experimental evidence has already been described which suggests that false memories can be created if the events and details are congruent to the individual's personal history. One would anticipate that the false memories must be consistent with the individual's culture as well. For example, Loftus (1993) reported that she could successfully convince American adolescents that they had been lost in a shopping mall as a child. Part of her success was undoubtedly due to the fact that the notion of getting lost in a shopping mall can fit quite comfortably within the cultural history of most Americans. In considering the recovery of memories of abuse, it is prudent to take note also of the culture within which they emerge, as well as reflecting on the mechanisms of memory recovery.

## Conclusions

Many people's lives have been profoundly affected by the phenomena of recovered memories: parents who have been falsely accused; retractors (people who recover memories and later retract their accounts), and people who recover memories of genuine childhood sexual abuse. While the media attention generated by the debate has certainly awakened public awareness to the reality of childhood sexual abuse, it has also had the effect of creating a climate of fear. This is particularly relevant to the therapeutic community. There is a danger that practitioners will not work with people bringing memories of sexual abuse due to the possibility of litigation.

It is likely that no one will ever be able to determine who is telling the truth in most cases of recovery of memories of abuse (Bekerian & Goodrich, 1995). Of all the points discussed in the debate, the issue of the truth is the one of which we have the least understanding. It is also the most crucial. In the light of this, practitioners have to work with the fact that they may never know the validity of a client's memories. As such, the practitioner must never take on the role of arbitrator of the truth. It is only through working in this way that the therapeutic community can safeguard its profession and provide both clients and their families with the protection they require.

# REFERENCES

Alpert, J.L. (1991). Retrospective treatment of incest victims: suggested analytic attitudes. *Psychoanalytic Review*, **78**, 425–35.

Andrews, B., Morton, J., Bekerian, D., Brewin, C., Davies, G. & Mollon, P. (1996). The recovery of memories in clinical practice: experiences and beliefs of British Psychological Society Practitioners. *The Psychologist*, **9**, 30–5.

Bass, E. & Davis, L. (1988). *The Courage to Heal: A Guide for Women Survivors of Child Sexual Abuse*. New York: Harper and Row.

Bekerian, D.A. & Dennett, J. (1993). The cognitive interview technique: reviving the issues. *Applied Cognitive Psychology*, **7**, 275–97.

Bekerian, D.A. & Goodrich, S.J. (1995). Telling the truth in the recovered memory debate. *Consciousness and Cognition*, **4**, 120–4.

Bekerian, D.A., Dennett, J.L., Hill, K. & Hitchcock, R. (1991). Effects of detailed imagery on simulated witness recall. In *Psychology and Law Facing the Nineties*, ed. F. Losel, D. Bender & T. Bleisener, 2 vols. Amsterdam: Swets and Zeitlinger.

Bonano, G. (1990). Remembering and psychotherapy. *Psychotherapy*, **27**, 175–86.

Brewin, C., Dalgleish, T. & Jacobs, S. (1996). A dual representation theory of posttraumatic stress disorder. *Psychological Review*, **103**, 670–86.

British Psychological Society (January 1995). *Recovered Memories: The Report of the Working Party of the British Psychological Society*. Leicester: British Psychological Society.

Calof, D.L.(1993). A conversation with Pamela Freyd, PhD co-founder and executive director, False Memory Syndrome Foundation, Inc., Part 1. *Treating Abuse Today*, **3**, 25–33.

Ceci, S.J., Crotteau Huffman, M.L., Smith, E. & Loftus, E. (1994). Repeatedly thinking about a non-event: Source misattributions among preschoolers. *Consciousness and Cognition*, **3**, 388–407.

Erdelyi, M.H. (1990). Repression, reconstruction and defense: history and integration of the psychoanalytic and experimental frameworks. In *Repression and Dissociation*, ed. J.L. Singer, pp. 1–32. Chicago: Chicago University Press.

Freyd, J.J. (1993). Personal perspective on the delayed memory debate. *Treating Abuse Today*, **3**, 13–20.

Freud, S. (1915/1957). Repression. In *The Standard Edition of the Complete Psychological Works of Sigmund Freud*, ed. J. Strachey, vol. 14, pp. 141–58. London: Hogarth Press.

Gardner, R. (1993). Sexual abuse hysteria: diagnosis, etiology, pathogenesis, and treatment. *Academy Forum*, **37**, 00–00.

Harvey, M.R. & Herman, J.L. (1994). Amnesia, partial amnesia and delayed recall among adult survivors of childhood trauma. *Consciousness and Cognition*, **3**, 295–326.

Herman, J.L. (1992). *Trauma and Recovered*. London, UK: Harper Collins.

Herman, J.L. & Schatzow, E. (1987). Recovery and verification of memories of childhood sexual trauma. *Psychoanalytic Psychology*, **4**, 1–14.

Howe, M.L., Courage, M.L. & Peterson, C. (1994). How can I remember when 'I' wasn't there? Long-term retention of traumatic experiences and emergence of the cognitive self. *Consciousness and Cognition*, **4**, 327–55.

Hyman, I.E. & Pentland, J. (1986). The role of mental imagery in the creation of false childhood memories. *Journal of Memory and Language*, **35**, 101–17.

Hyman, I.E., Husband, T.H. & Billings, F.J. (1995). False memories of childhood experiences. *Applied Cognitive Psychology*, **9**, 181–97.

Jacoby, L.L. & Witherspoon, L. (1982). Remembering without awareness. *Canadian Journal of Psychology*, **32**, 300–24.

Jung, C.G. (1959). *The Archetypes and the Collective Unconscious*. London, UK: Routledge, Kegan & Paul.

Lindsay, D.S. & Read, J.D. (1994). Psychotherapy and memories of childhood sexual abuse: a cognitive perspective. *Applied Cognitive Psychology*, **8**, 281–338.

Loftus, E.F. (1979). *Eyewitness Testimony*. Cambridge, MA: Harvard University Press.

Loftus, E.F. (1993). The reality of repressed memories. *American Psychologist*, **48**, 518–37.

Loftus, E. & Rosenwald, L.A. (1993). Buried memories shattered lives. *ABA Journal*, 70–3.

Morton, J. (1994). Cognitive perspectives of memory recovery. *Applied Cognitive Psychology*, **8**, 389–98.

Ofshe, R. & Watters, E. (1993). Making monsters. *Society*, **30**, 4–16.

Perls, F.S. (1947). *Ego, Hunger and Aggression: A Revision of Freud's Theory and Method*. London: Allen and Unwin.

Recovery of memories of child sexual abuse. (1994). *Applied Cognitive Psychology*, **8** (special issue).

Schacter, D.L. (1987). Implicit memory: history and current status. *Journal of Experimental Psychology: Learning, Memory and Cognition*, **13**, 501–18.

Scrivener, E & Safer, M. (1988). Eyewitnesses show hypermnesia for details about a violent event. *Journal of Applied Psychology*, **73**, 371–7.

Steller, M. (1989). Recent developments in statement analysis. In *Credibility Assessments*, ed. J. Yuille, pp. 134–54. Boston, MA: Kluwer.

Walker, M. (1996). Working with abuse survivors: the recovered memory debate. In *New Directions in Counselling*, ed. R. Bayne, I. Horton & J. Bimrose,. pp. 239–69. Routledge

Wagenaar, W.A. & Groeneweg, J. (1990). The memory of concentration camp survivors. *Applied Cognitive Psychology*, **4**, 77 – 87.

Weiskrantz, L. (1995). Comments on the report of the Working Party of the British Psychological Society on 'Recovered Memories'. *The Therapist*, **2**, 4–11.

Wood, J., Bekerian, D.A. & Foa, E. (1999). Counterfactual reasoning in traumatised individuals. *International Journal of Stress Disorders*, in press.

# 21

# The Ganser syndrome

David F. Allen, Jacques Postel and German E. Berrios

S.J.M. Ganser was born in Dresden on 24 January 1853 (Allen, 1993; Allen & Postel, 1993, 1994) and trained in Würzburg, Strasbourg, Heidelberg and Munich (Anonymous, 1901). His contribution to psychiatry has not been yet well studied (Allen, 1992). Ganser died in 1931, and only remains known for the state of 'twilight hysteria' that he observed in persons awaiting trial (Ganser, 1898).

## The 'Ganser syndrome'

The term 'Ganser syndrome' is found in use very early in the century (e.g. Soukhanoff, 1904; Cramer, 1908; Nitsche & Wilmanns, 1912). In its entirety, this clinical cluster includes the following features: (i) disorganized sense of space and time; (ii) production of 'I don't know' answers even to simple questions (which, in Ganser's opinion, implied the 'suspension of information' usually at the person's disposal); (iii) clouding of awareness; (iv) ability to understand questions matched by a psychogenic inability to give correct answers; (v) answers remain in the semantic sphere of the question (*Vorbeireden*) (Marneros, 1979) (e.g. how many ears do you have?) Three, etc. Ganser himself exemplified: 'As if a railway employee gave you a ticket at random' rather than the ticket you asked for; the point being that he did not give you a bucket of water or a cup of tea (Ganser was thus not writing *coq-à-l'âne*); (vi) the patient experiences hallucinations, and may re-enact or relive in a hallucinatory manner certain traumatic experiences; (vii) one may observe general or partial analgesia in the body (mouth area included), this may move around according to time of day or day of the week, etc.; (viii) patients are not offended by the childish nature of the questions – indeed – even questions like what is your name or what is this (watch, money, etc.) cause difficulty and stimulate 'past the point' answers (i.e. answers within the semantic area of the question showing that the general theme (identity, time, place, etc.) of the question is understood); (ix) symptoms tend to appear all at the same time, but go in a staggered manner leaving behind a 'mode of being' similar to the 'personality' before the period of twilight hysteria became established; (x) the patient is surprised when informed of his behaviour during the twilight period (Ganser specifically remarked that the period of twilight hysteria was covered by a veil of amnesia); (xi) there is no memory loss for the period of time before the appearance *en masse* of the symptoms; (xii) before onset, patients may also have suffered from physical trauma, blows to the head, accidents, etc.; (xiii) at least one confessed to imaginary crimes; (xiv) in some cases, the ability to relate reading material is disturbed under questioning; (xv) many patients were awaiting trial; (xvi) the cases cannot be simulated (Ganser argued that, to reproduce such a symptom picture, subjects would require a deep knowledge of psychopathology); (xvii) simple counting may become difficult: one of Ganser's patients, W.H., counted his fingers as follows: '1, 3, 7, 5, 10, 12, 14, 16, Yes so 14'; (xviii) answers within the semantic area or locality of the questions were common to all cases; (xix) patients put a great deal of effort in attempts to concentrate and thereby try, but often fail, to overcome their distraction (*Zerstreutheit*); (xx) the transition from the pathological to ordinary field of awareness is gradual but relatively rapid; (xxi) some complained of a difficulty in thinking (*Erschwerung im Denke*); (xxii) many were in a 'dream-like state'; (xxiii) so-called 'mistakes' are variable; (xxiv) at least one patient made a funny remark; asked how many ears he had he replied four, then when asked to explain said outside ears and with his fingers in his ears said these are the inside ears (25th Oct, 1902); (xxv) syndrome redolent of twilight hysteria.

## Historical antecedents

Reports redolent of what is now called the Ganser syndrome were made by F.M. Guazzo (pp. 168–70, 1608/1929):

Some say that they hear a voice speaking inside them, but that they know nothing of the meaning of the words. [compare to counter-will and local answers] . . . Others, when they are asked what they have done or said, confess that they remember nothing afterwards. [compare to amnesia for period of twilight state] . . . Some pretend to be stupid, and always grow even more so; but they can be detected if they refuse to recite the Psalm *Miserere mei Deus*, or *Qui habitat in auditorio Altissimi*, or the beginning of the Gospel of St John, *In principio erat Verbum*, or similar passages of Scripture. [counter-will – suspension of 'ordinary' information or hysterical negativism]. . . . Sometimes they become as if they were stupid, blind, lame, deaf, dumb, lunatic, and almost incapable of movement, whereas before they were active, could speak hear and see, and in other respects acted sensibly. [Many cases of the Ganser syndrome feature catatonia, catalepsy or vague rigidity of the body. . . .]

Likewise, Moeli (1888) had already noticed that prisoners awaiting trial might develop a sort of transitory confusional state. This writer described patients who 'forgot' well-known facts (e.g. their age, how to multiply, the coinage system), who confabulated about their lives, and whose answers, although incorrect, bore a 'certain' relationship to the question asked (p. 125).

The concept of schizophrenia was to take over some of the clinical features originally described as Ganserian, such as, for example, the language disorder which was only partially differentiated from that seen in catatonia by Henneberg (quoted in Labet, 1960). Bleuler (1911/1950) wrote of schizophrenia: 'The twilight states can show a good deal of variability. In some cases we find a consistently carried out dream-activity. The twilight state is then essentially the reaction of a mildly schizophrenic personality to a psychic trauma' (p. 220). This led in turn to a neglect of, and limited research into, Ganser's syndrome. However, a significant number of clinicians in Europe continued accepting Ganser's basic postulate that these patients showed significant memory disorder and 'answers towards the question' within the framework of traumatic or reactive hysteria. The amnesia is often seen as a form of defence or protection against the anxiety that accompanies the psychic or physical trauma. In elderly patients, Ganser type symptoms may be indicative of the onset of dementia.

## Jung and the Ganser syndrome

### The case of Godwina F.

In a lecture entitled 'Contribution to the theory of twilight hysteria' (read in Dresden in 1902 at the 8th Congress of Psychiatrists and Neurologists of Central Germany), Ganser (1904) referred to a case reported by C.G. Jung (1902/1983). Still working under E. Bleuler, Jung had, in turn, quoted Ganser's paper (Ganser, 1898) together with that by Raecke (1901) (pp. 148–9, Jung, 1902).

Jung's patient (Godwina F.) was a factory worker with a lover who provided for her and two children out of wedlock. She had a hotel bill to pay (10 000 marks) and had been (wrongly) accused of theft:

The following case of hysterical stupor in a prisoner in detention was referred to the Burghölzli Clinic for a medical opinion. Apart from the publications of Ganser and Raecke, the literature on cases of this kind is very scanty, and even their clinical status seems uncertain in view of Nissl's criticisms.

When, on the morning of 4th June 1902 the cell was opened at 6:30, the patient was standing *rigid* (. . .) came up to the warderess *quite rigid* and furiously demanded that she should 'give back the money she had stolen from her'. (. . .) She began to rage and shout, threw herself about in her cell, kept on asking for her money, saying she wanted to see the judge at once, etc. (p. 138, Jung, 1902).

The warderess called for help, and the jailer, wife and assistant held her by the hands 'shaking' her with the idea of 'calming her down'. The trio denied hitting her and she was locked up in a cell: When the cell was opened again at 11 o'clock the patient had torn the top half of her clothes to shreds. She was still very worked up, said the jailer had hit her on the head, [and that] they [the trio] had taken the money she got from her husband, 10 000 marks in gold, which she had counted on the table, etc. She showed an acute fear of the jailer. (. . .) At 6pm the District Medical Officer found her totally disoriented (Jung, 1902).

According to Jung, the following symptoms were worth noting: (i) almost complete lack of memory; (ii) easily provoked changes of mood; (iii) megalomaniac ideas; (iv) stumbling speech; (v) complete insensibility to deep pin pricks; (vi) marked tremor of the hands and head; (vii) shaky and broken writing. Godwina:

fancied that she was in a luxury hotel, eating rich food, that the prison personnel were hotel guests. Said (. . .) she had millions; that during the night a man attacked her, who felt cold. At times she was excitable, screaming and shouting gibberish. She did not know her own name and could say nothing about her past life and her family. She no longer recognised money (pp. 138–9, Jung 1902).

What Jung here chose to call 'gibberish' may well be of the same nature as the interview material of the following day (5th June). (This apparently insignificant detail must be kept in mind because it anticipates latter views on the nature of the Ganser syndrome conceived of as gibberish, hysteria (within the Freudian framework) and simulation. Indeed, Jung discussed all three possibilities.) The following day, Godwina was examined by Jung (p. 140, 1902):

Where are you? – In Munich.
Where are you staying? – In a hotel.
What time is it? – I don't know.
What's your name? – Don't know.
Christian name? – Ida. (This was the name of her second daughter.)
When were you born? – I don't know.
How long have you been here? – Don't know.
Is your name Meier or Müller? – Ida Müller.
Have you a daughter? No.
Surely you have! Yes.
Is she married – Yes.
Whom to? – To a man.
What is he? – Don't know.
Isn't he the director of a factory? – Yes he is (wrong answer).
Do you know Godwina F.? – Yes, she's in Munich.
Are you Godwina F.? – Yes.
I thought your name was Ida Müller? – Yes my name's Ida.
(. . .)
Who am I ? – The headwaiter.
What is this (a notebook)? – The menu.
(. . .)
What is three times four? – Two.
How many fingers is this (5) – Three.

No, look carefully! – Seven.
Count them. – 1, 2, 3, 5, 7.
Count up to 10. – 1, 2, 3, 4, 5, 6, 7, 10, 12.

Godwina was unable to recite the alphabet, do simple multiplications or write 'a single legible word' with her right hand because of 'strong tremor'. The following day (6th June) she recognized her Christian name but still regarded Ida to be her first name. She 'knew her age, but was otherwise totally disoriented'. The interview notes of 7th June are a carbon copy of those above and 'Ganser type' symptoms dominate the clinical picture (i.e. distractibility, answers towards the question, hallucinations, fluctuations (or dipping) in the field of awareness, conversion symptoms, etc.).

Notes from 25th June intimate that her retrograde partial amnesia and the total amnesia continue unaltered. This 'disappeared under hypnosis' but the total amnesia resisted hypnosis. Whilst under hypnosis Godwina complained that she is 'always afraid of the big fat man who beats me' (p. 146, Jung, 1902). These features of her condition imply physical and psychological trauma and are in harmony with Ganser's thinking.

## Kretschmer and the 'Bewegungssturm'

Kretschmer's clinical concept of 'instinctive flurry' or 'motor storm' is, in effect, a crude theorization of the Ganser state. According to Kretschmer (1924/1960), in the person with hysteria the perception of danger or anxiety-arousing situations will trigger 'instinctive phylogenetic mechanisms' which then dominate all his/her actions and thoughts. By making the *Bewegungssturm* a key element of hysteria, Kretschmer created a loose clinical concept linking up war neuroses (anxiety neurosis and conversion hysteria), shell-shock ('sinistrosis') (Postel, 1993) and the Ganser syndrome.

However, the German author was ambivalent vis-à- vis this concept, particularly when applied to the legal domain:

We cannot, separate fear neurosis from hysteria, yet cannot lump them together. Is the acute fear reaction a physiological reflex with an 'extraphysical' mode of operation, or is it depen- dent on hysteria-like autosuggestion? (. . .) we shall answer this question as follows: In acute fear symptoms physiological reflex mechanisms are evidenced as surely as are hysteria like elaborations of experience. An example characteristic of this first type is the vegetative–vas- omotor symptom complex which includes from the psychic viewpoint, insomnia along with lability and anxiety–depression (. . .). On the other hand, the most striking example of the direct psychic elaboration of fear through hysteria like mechanisms is the Ganser type of twi- light state (p. 28, Kretschmer 1924/1960).

In harmony with many who claim to refer to Ganser's work, Kretschmer remains characteristically 'on the fence' not only because 'reflexes can be willed to health' but also because 'perfect' hysteria (massive symptoms, reflex mechanisms, flurries, stupors, paralyses and twilight states) 'is most likely to appear in situations closely linked to basic drives, namely erotic conflicts and mortal danger' (pp. 28–9, Kretschmer 1924/1960); hysteria is simulation (fake) pure and simple and 'true' simulation – a small atypical variety of hysteria' (Kretschmer quoted in p. 340, Eissler, 1986).

It is this logic that subtends the following extraordinary statement:

(...) As strange as it may seem, the twilight state of shock, even in able-bodied, level-headed men, may assume patterns which we are accustomed to see in criminals and to look upon as indications of crude hysterical deceptive tendencies that border on simulation: the Ganser syndrome, marked by spurious, theatrical conduct (pp. 24–5, Kretschmer 1924/1960).

In this regard, it would be a pity if Ganser's concept suffered from the fact that it was first described in subjects in prison. Because it draws our attention to the complex and deep mechanisms that govern behaviour, it should rather be usefully employed to develop a veritable conception of man with which to study the nature of so-called 'mild schizophrenia' and *bouffée délirante* and other well-meaning concepts that have cluttered minds and bookshelves for much of this century.

## Clinical relationships

### Ganser and organic disorders

Ganser states have been reported in the wake of brain disease. In his important review, Whitlock (1967) suggested that it be, 'restricted to patients who, following cerebral trauma or in the course of an acute psychoses, develop clouding of consciousness . . .' (p. 28). In this regard, Heron et al. (1991) have recently reported a Ganserian state in a patient with a history of brain damage and polysubstance abuse; and Sigal et al. (1992) have concluded in their review that Ganser patients often show 'symptoms of premorbid neurological pathology'. In the same vein, McEvoy and Campbell (1977) have reported a Ganser state in the wake of carbon monoxide intoxication, and Doongaji et al. (1975) apparently related it to a tumour on the left hemisphere. Latcham et al. (1968), in turn, accept an organic aetiology but combine it with hysteria.

The appearance on the scene of the so-called pseudodementia syndrome (Bulbena & Berrios, 1986) caused the additional difficulty of making a differential diagnosis with Ganser state. Thus, cases have now been reported of patients with more or less typical pseudodementia and Ganserian features (Steinhart, 1980; Good, 1981; Gonzáles et al., 1985; Hampel et al., 1996); more surprising has been the report of a 10-year-old who, after a minor head injury, developed both syndromes (Adler, 1981).

**Table 21.1.** Ganser syndrome and schizophrenia

|  | Ganser syndrome | Schizophrenia |
| --- | --- | --- |
| Amnesia limited to period of disorder | Yes | No |
| Conversion symptoms | Yes | No |
| Return to previous personality possible | Yes | No |
| Neologisms | No | Yes |
| Answers towards the questions | Yes | (?) (not in Ganser's sense) |
| Ideas of influence | Yes[a] | Yes[b] |
| Body experienced as fragmented or in space | No | Yes |
| Breakdown of real, symbolic and imaginary (Lacan) | No | Yes |
| Visual hallucinations | Yes | Yes |
| Auditory hallucinations | Yes (rare ?) | Yes |
| Variable analgesia | Very common | Very rare |
| Condition is reversible | Yes | No |
| Time lived as infinite | No | (Melancholia[c] or schizophrenic depression) |
| Confusion regarding time and space | Yes | Yes |
| Reliving or re-enactment of trauma | Yes | No |
| Impersonal or reified ideas dominate clinical picture | No | Yes (often in structured delusions) |

*Notes:*

[a] Often erotic influences.

[b] With destruction of the sense of 'I' as in 'influence syndrome' (V. Tausk).

[c] Cotard's syndrome.

## Ganser and schizophrenia

The question of whether Ganser is or not a form of transient psychosis remains unresolved according to some. The differential diagnosis with schizophrenia, however, can be made on a number of clinical features (see Table 21.1).

## Ganser and affective disorders

Since the time of Mairet (1883), Cotard (1891) and Dumas (1894), the view has been taken that some forms of affective disorder can lead to temporal cognitive disorganization (Berrios, 1985). Tyndel (1956) suggested a connection between affectivity and the Ganser state; Grieger and Clayton (1990) have also remarked upon this relationship.

However, the mechanism of interaction and the direction of the causal arrow remain unclear: for example, whilst Arya (1997) has reported the development of a typical Ganser syndrome in a 48-year-old housewife suffering from a major depressive episode, Haddad (1993) describes the case of a patient who developed a major depressive episode after improving from a Ganser syndrome.

## Ganser and children

All the putative explanations so far suggested for the Ganser state do not necessarily predict that it should develop in children. In their review of six cases, Miller et al. (1997) referred to them as 'imperfect representations'. Apter et al. (1993) reported the syndrome in two adolescent brothers in jail, awaiting trial; Dabholkar (1987) in one 11-year-old Indian lad, and Nardi and Di Scipio (1977) in a Hispanic black girl.

More controversially, Burd and Kerbeshian (1985) reported a 15-year-old who was visually impaired, mentally retarded, and showed features of both Ganser and Tourette syndromes. The case originally reported by Adler (1981) was followed up by the same author 8 years later and found 'to remain largely unchanged' and still pursuing compensation claims (Adler, 1989).

## The forensic dimension

Perhaps because of the legal and ethical questions raised by persons pleading 'temporary insanity', forensic psychiatrists, on the whole, are reserved about the existence and/or mechanisms of the Ganser state.

For example, Gunn and Taylor (1993) hedge their bet:

[The] Ganser syndrome is advanced as an independent clinical entity . . . although one which may manifest as part of other disorders such as schizophrenia and organic brain syndromes, usually in the context of overwhelming stress. . . . The possibility that the Ganser state is a manifestation of the conscious simulation of mental disorder is considered . . . to be dismissed in favour of unconscious mechanisms, or the impact of major stress on somebody who already has a mental disorder. (. . .) Perhaps more scepticism and less acceptance of the explanatory power of the unconscious is indicated . . . but, then again, perhaps it is better to follow Scott's pragmatic advice to avoid guesses or inferences about their motivation and to concentrate on observing with greater precision, the clinical picture of these odd states (p. 426).

It is understandable, but very sad from a scientific point of view, that these authors have chosen not to see the link between the Ganser syndrome and hysteria. Even Kraepelin (1915), not a friend of the simulator or the criminal, came down in favour of Ganser:

Of (. . .) the transitory hysterical conditions, the befogged states are the most prominent. They are characterized by a marked clouding of consciousness, of varying duration, and either follow, take the place of, terminate in, or are interrupted by, a convulsion. (. . .)

Sometimes the befogged states simulates ordinary sleep. The patients become drowsy, the eyes close, the limbs become relaxed, as in a profound sleep, and the respiration deep and regular. The state is usually of short duration, and the patients awaken gradually with no recollection of the interval (. . .). This last form borders closely on somnambulism (. . .) the patients leave their beds (. . .) and perform many peculiar acts (. . .). Similar attacks may occur during the daytime (. . .). The patients then walk about muttering unintelligibly to themselves (. . .) It is very difficult to arouse them from this state, even by the application of powerful electrical currents. This last condition is perhaps related to those befogged states with inconsequential speech, which have been described by Ganser (pp. 465–8).

Likewise, Paton (1905) – an American psychiatrist follower of Kraepelin – saw a link between the Ganser state and the 'hypnoid state' (p. 504); and Enoch and Trethowan (1979) in their remarkable *Uncommon Psychiatric Syndromes* showed themselves to be far more clear-headed than the writers of DSM III and IV.

## Mechanisms

### Hysteria

Perhaps more than any other syndrome, Ganser's raises the question of the inter-action between concepts, ideology and clinical observation. For example, during the First World War, French military psychiatrists were encouraged not to use on first medical certificates words connected to hysteria and trauma. Likewise, in civil-ian life, clinical statements concerning hysteria can be rapidly called upon in litiga-tion for compensation. In other words, the issues that J.M. Charcot (1885/1984) raised concerning the concepts of railway brain and spine have not really been 'solved'. Given that the semantics of hysteria itself seems to contain the implication that it can produce an almost infinite number of symptoms, perhaps there can be no lasting solution to the problem. To make matters worse, because the dialogue between doctor and patient is not only conscious, it is likely that the gaze of the cli-nician also intensifies the production of symptoms in hysteria.

Recent work suggests that 'twilight hysteria' should be separated from simulation and psychosis (Libbrecht, 1995; Maleval, 1981, 1985). Others also have supported a hysterical aetiology (Goldin & MacDonald, 1955; Tsoi, 1973; Hoffmann & Siegel, 1982; Weller, 1988) and given a special role to stress (Weiner & Braiman, 1955).

### Dissociation

More recently, it has been pointed out that the conceptual 'instability' of the Ganser syndrome originates in changes in the definition of some background notions such as malingering and simulation (Gorman, 1982) and hysteria (Sizaret, 1989; Provence & Schlecht, 1990). Indeed, even before the Great War, both Soukhanoff

(1904) and Henri Wallon (1911) wondered about the future of the Ganser state, given that for ideological, not clinical, reasons, hysteria was beginning to disintegrate.

As the concept of 'dissociation' has come into fashion threatening to become the new overarching explanation, there have been suggestions that the Ganser state results from the action of a dissociation mechanism (e.g. Cocores et al., 1984; Feinstein & Hattersley, 1988). This view became official in DSM-IV:

> Some individuals with Dissociative Amnesia report depressive symptoms, depersonalization, trance states, analgesia, and spontaneous age regression. They may provide approximate inaccurate answers to questions (e.g. '2 plus 2 equals 5') as in Ganser syndrome. Other problems that sometimes accompany this disorder include sexual dysfunction, impairment in work and interpersonal relationships, self-mutilation, aggressive impulses, and suicidal impulses and acts. Individuals with Dissociative Amnesia may also have symptoms that meet criteria for Conversion Disorder, a Mood Disorder, or a Personality Disorder (p. 478, American Psychiatric Association, 1994).

## Conclusions

Given the above, our conclusion is that the clinical hypothesis of a Ganser syndrome should still be raised in cases of atypical amnesia with unexpected or ambiguous answers to questions and history of psychic or physical trauma. The clinician must be aware that a misdiagnosed case of Ganser-type hysteria may result in lawsuits, unnecessary surgical interventions, inappropriate use of minor and major tranquillizers, and social consequences that may be destabilizing for the patient and family. Positive results in the organic investigation should lead to a firm diagnosis and disconfirmation of Ganser syndrome. Persistent negative results and dramatic improvement should tend to confirm the diagnosis. Improvement, however, is not the end of the story. The patient has shown that he/she has in his coping mechanisms repertoire a very maladaptive form of behaviour and this needs dealing with. A period of rest is recommended, followed by psychotherapy or psychoanalysis. Medication has no specific role to play in the treatment of this condition.

## REFERENCES

Adler, R. (1981). Pseudo-dementia or Ganser syndrome in a ten year old boy. *Australian and New Zealand Journal of Psychiatry*, 15, 339–42.

Adler, R. (1989). The Ganser syndrome in a 10-year-old boy – an 8 years follow up. *Australian and New Zealand Journal of Psychiatry*, 23, 124–6.

Allen, D.F. (1992). Pour la réhabilitation de Ganser de Dresde. *Évolution Psychiatrique*, **57**, 537–46.

Allen, D.F. (1993). Petite note pour Ganser de Dresde. *Évolution Psychiatrique*, **58**, 231–5.

Allen, D.F. & Postel, J. (1993). R.D. Laing et le probléme de l'hystérie crépusculaire. *Évolution Psychiatrique*, **58**, 827–31.

Allen, D.F. & Postel, J. (1994). For S.J.M. Ganser of Dresden. *History of Psychiatry*, **5**, 289–319.

American Psychiatric Association (1994). *Diagnostic and Statistical Manual of Mental Disorders*, 4th edn. Washington, DC: American Psychiatric Association.

Anonymous (1901). *Medicinisches Deutschland, Gallerie von Zeitgenossen auf den Geschichte der medicinische Wissenschaften.* Berlin-Charlottenburg, Eckstein (unsigned and unpaginated volume containing an important biography of Ganser).

Apter, A., Ratzoni, G., Iancu, I. & Weizman, R. (1993). The Ganser syndrome in two adolescent brothers. *Journal of the American Academy of Child and Adolescent Psychiatry*, **32**, 582–4.

Arya, D. (1997). Resolution of episode of major depressive disorder with emergence of Ganser syndrome symptoms. *Irish Journal of Psychological Medicine*, **14**, 35–7.

Berrios, G.E. (1985). 'Depressive Pseudodementia' or 'Melancholic Dementia': a 19th century view. *Journal of Neurology, Neurosurgery and Psychiatry*, **48**, 393–400.

Bleuler, E. (1911/1950). *Dementia Praecox or The Group of Schizophrenias.* Madison, CT: International Universities Press.

Bulbena, A & Berrios, G.E. (1986). Pseudodementia: facts and figures. *British Journal of Psychiatry*, **148**, 87–94.

Burd, L. & Kerbeshian, J. (1985). Tourette syndrome, atypical pervasive developmental disorder and Ganser syndrome in a 15-year-old, visually impaired, mentally retarded boy. *Canadian Journal of Psychiatry*, **30**, 74–6.

Charcot, J.M. (1885–91/1984). *Leçons sur l'Hystérie Virile.* Paris: Le Sycomore.

Cocores, J.A., Santa, W.G. & Patel, M.D. (1984). The Ganser syndrome: evidence suggesting its classification as a dissociative disorder. *International Journal of Psychiatry in Medicine*, **14**, 47–56.

Cotard, J. (1891). *Études sur les maladies cérébrales et mentales.* Paris: Baillière.

Cramer, A. (1908). *Gerichtliche Psychiatrie.* Jena: Gustav Fisher.

Dabholkar, P.D (1987). Ganser syndrome. A case report and discussion. *British Journal of Psychiatry*, **151**, 256–8.

Doongaji, D.R., Apte, J.S. & Bhat, R. (1975). Ganser like state (syndrome): an unsual presentation of a space occupying lesion of the dominant hemisphere. *Neurology India*, **23**, 143–8.

Dumas, G. (1894). *Les États intellectuels dans la mélancolie.* Paris: Alcan.

Eissler, K. R. (1986). *Freud as an Expert Witness.* Madison, CT: International Universities Press.

Enoch, M.D. & Trethowan, W.H. (1979). *Uncommon Psychiatric Syndromes.* Bristol: J. Wright.

Feinstein, A. & Hattersley, A. (1988). Ganser symptoms, dissociation and dysprosody. *Journal of Nervous and Mental Disease*, **176**, 692–3.

Ganser, S.J.M. (1898). Über einen Eigenartigen Hysterischen Dämmerzustand ' [conf. of 23 Oct. 1897], *Archiv für Psychiatrie und Nervenkrankheiten*, **30**, 633–40. (Translated into French by D.F. Allen as: État particulier d'hystérie crépusculaire *L'Évolution Psychiatrique*, **58**, 237–42, and reprinted in Postel, J., *La Psychiatrie*, Paris, Larousse, 1994, pp. 373–7). (Translated into

English by Schorer C. E. as 'A peculiar hysterical state'. *British Journal of Criminology* (1965), 5, 120–31).

Ganser, S.J.M. (1904). Lehre vom hysterischen Dämmerzustande *Archiv für Psychiatrie und Nervenkrankheiten*, 38, 34–46. (Translated into French by D.F. Allen and Coll. as Contribution à la théorie de l'état crépusculaire hystérique. *L'Évolution Psychiatrique* (1992), 57, 547–55).

Goldin, S. & McDonald, J.E. (1955). The Ganser State. *Journal of Mental Science*, 101, 267–80

Gonzáles, J.C., Aranda, A., Berdullas, M & Garcia-Blanco, J. (1985). Pseudodemencia histérica o síndrome de Ganser. *Informaciones Psiquiátricas*, 100, 172–6.

Good, M.I. (1981). Pseudodementia and physical findings masking significant psychopathology. *American Journal of Psychiatry*, 138, 811–14.

Gorman, W.F. (1982). Defining malingering. *Journal of Forensic Sciences*, 27, 401–7.

Grieger, T.A. & Clayton, A.H. (1990). A possible association of Ganser's syndrome and major depression. *Journal of Clinical Psychiatry*, 51, 437–8.

Guazzo, F.M. (1608/1929). *Compendium Maleficarum*. London: John Rodker.

Gunn, J. & Taylor, P J. (1993). *Forensic Psychiatry*. Oxford: Butterworth-Heinemann.

Haddad, P.M. (1993). Ganser syndrome followed by major depressive episode. *British Journal of Psychiatry*, 162, 251–3.

Hampel, H., Berger, C. & Müller, N. (1996). A case of Ganser syndrome presenting as a dementia syndrome. *Psychopathology*, 29, 236–41.

Heron, E.A., Kritchevski, M. & Delis, D.C. (1991). The neuropsychological presentation of Ganser syndrome. *Journal of Clinical and Experimental Neuropsychology*, 13, 652–66.

Hoffmann, H & Siegel, E. (1982). Über das Ganser-Syndrom. *Psychiatry, Neurological Medicine and Psychology*, 34, 276–281.

Jung, C.G. (1902/1983). A case of hysterical stupor in a prisoner in detention. In *Psychiatric Studies*, pp. 137–58. Princeton: Princeton University Press.

Kraepelin, E. (1915). *Clinical Psychiatry* (abstracted from the 7th German revised edn). London: Macmillan.

Kretschmer, E. (1924/1960). *Hysteria, Reflex and Instinct*. New York: Philosophical Library, London: Peter Owen.

Labet, R. (1960). Le syndrome de Ganser. In *Encyclopédie Médico-Chirurgicale*. Psychiatrie, 37130 C[10]. Paris: Editions Techniques.

Latcham, R., White, A. & Sims, A. (1968). Ganser syndrome: the aetiological argument. *Journal of Neurology, Neurosurgery and Psychiatry*, 41, 851–4.

Libbrecht, K. (1995). *Hysterical Psychosis: A Historical Survey*. London: Transaction Publishers.

McEvoy, N. & Campbell, T. (1977). Ganser-like signs in carbon monoxide encephalopathy. *American Journal of Psychiatry* 134: 453–4.

Mairet, A. (1883). *De la Démence Mélancolique*. Paris: Masson.

Maleval, J.-C. (1981). *Folies Hystériques et Psychoses Dissociatives*. Paris: Payot.

Maleval, J.-C. (1985). Les hystéries crépusculaires. *Confrontation Psychiatrique*, 25, 63–97.

Marneros, A. (1979). Das Vorbeireden. *Fortschritte Neurologie und Psychiatrie*, 47, 479–89.

Miller, P., Bramble, D. & Buxton, N. (1997). Case study: Ganser syndrome in children and adolescents. *Journal of the American Academy of Child and Adolescent Psychiatry*, 36, 112–15.

Moeli, C. (1888). *Ueber irre Verbrecher*. Berlin: Fischer.

Nardi, T.J. & Di Scipio, W.J. (1977). The Ganser syndrome in an adolescent Hispanic black female. *American Journal of Psychiatry*, **134**, 453–4.

Nitsche, P. & Wilmanns, K. (1912/1970). *The History of The Prison Psychoses*, Nervous and Mental Disease Monograph Series N° 13, *The Journal of Nervous and Mental Disease Publishing Company*. New York: Johnson.

Paton, S. (1905). *Psychiatry*. Philadelphia: J.B. Lippincott.

Postel, J. (1993). *Dictionnaire de Psychiatrie*. Paris: Larousse.

Provence, M. & Schlecht, P. (1990). Syndrome de Ganser ou symptôms de Ganser? Deux cas cliniques. *Annales Médico-Psychologiques*, **148**, 876–80.

Raecke, J. (1901). Beitrag zur Kenntnis des hysterischen Dämerzustandes. *Allgemeine Zeitschrift für Psychiatrie*, **58**, 115–63.

Sigal, M., Altmark, M., Alific, S. & Gelkopf, M. (1992). Ganser syndrome: a review of 15 cases. *Comprehensive Psychiatry*, **33**, 134–8.

Sizaret, P. (1989). Le syndrome de Ganser et ses avatars. *Annales Médico-Psychologiques*, **147**, 167–79.

Soukhanoff, S. (1904). Sur le syndrome de Ganser ou le symptomo-complexus des réponses absurdes. *Revue Neurologique*, **12**, 933–6.

Steinhart, M.J. (1980). Ganser state. A case of hysterical pseudodementia. *General Hospital Psychiatry*, **3**, 226–8.

Tsoi, W.F. (1973) The Ganser syndrome in Singapore: a report of ten cases. *British Journal of Psychiatry*, **123**, 567–72.

Tyndel, M. (1956). Some aspects of the Ganser state. *Journal of Mental Science*, **102**, 324–9.

Wallon, H. (1911). Le symptome de Ganser. *Journal de Psychologie Normale et Pathologique*, **8**, 158–63.

Weiner, H. & Braiman, A. (1955). The Ganser syndrome. *American Journal of Psychiatry*, **111**, 767–73.

Weller, M.P.I. (1988). Hysterical behaviour in patriarchal communities. Four cases, one with Ganser-like symptoms. *British Journal of Psychiatry*, **152**, 687–95.

Whitlock, F.A. (1967) Ganser syndrome. *British Journal of Psychiatry*, **113**, 19–29.

# Malingering and feigned memory disorders

David G. Lamb and George P. Prigatano

That various brain injuries affect memory in predictable ways provides clinical neuropsychologists with a means by which to determine if a feigned memory disorder appears probable. The question has become progressively more important as neuropsychologists are increasingly asked to evaluate patients in civil litigation (Matarazzo, 1990).

It is important to distinguish between two types of claimed memory impairment. One is the claim of amnesia for a significant event related to a crime. This is relatively common, with Parwatiker et al. (1985) reporting 70% of accused murderers claiming such amnesia. Even in homicide cases following conviction, Kopelman's (1987) review still found an incidence rate between 25 and 45%. This chapter does not address this type of feigned memory deficit. The reader is referred to Schacter (1986) for his thorough review of simulated amnesia. The second type of claim is a reduced ability to remember new information after a known or suspected acquired brain injury. This chapter reviews studies related to the methodology and techniques available for answering this question.

Some clinicians may argue that the only tools necessary to uncover malingerers are proper training and sufficient experience. However, studies have shown that neuropsychologists essentially perform at chance levels when asked to classify malingered versus actual brain injury protocols in adults (Heaton et al., 1978), adolescents (Faust et al., 1988b), and children (Faust et al., 1988a) using only neuropsychological measures. These studies (particularly those by Faust and colleagues) have been criticized on methodological grounds (Schmidt, 1989; Bigler, 1990), but they do suggest that having confidence in one's opinion does not necessarily correspond with the accuracy of one's conclusions. In summarizing the literature on malingering, Ziskin and Faust (1988) point out '. . . that no matter what clinicians may believe about their capacity to detect malingering, lacking definitive information about who is and is not malingering, there is no objective way to determine one's actual level of success' (p. 874).

Research on the topic of malingering has expanded in the psychological literature over the last several years. For example, a search of the PsychINFO database using the keywords malingering and faking produced 23 references in 1985 and 52 references in 1990. Much of this activity has centred on the development of quantifiable methods for detecting malingering or lack of co-operation when a person is examined psychologically. These measures are likely to be useful for supplementing and enhancing clinical neuropsychological judgment when malingering is suspected.

Historical observations concerning malingering, including the development of a definition of malingering are reviewed, and then techniques currently used to detect malingering of memory deficits are discussed. Clinical examples are presented to highlight relevant points.

## Historical review of malingering

Several authors (Menninger, 1935; Brussel & Hitch, 1943) identify Grove's *Dictionary of the Vulgar Tongue*, published in 1785, as the source of the first recorded definition of the term malingering. As with most early references to malingering, Grove's definition was framed in the context of military service, 'A military term for one who under the pretense of sickness evades his duty' (Brussel & Hitch, 1943: 33). Brussel and Hitch (1943) report references to malingering as early as the ancient Greeks. The first Earl of Northumberland apparently lay 'crafty sick' to avoid the Battle of Shrewsbury in 1403 (Jones & Llewelyn, 1917). Anderson and Anderson (1984) state that soldiers attempting to avoid duty in the American Civil War attempted to simulate a variety of physical conditions, including lameness, paralysis, blindness, deafness, epilepsy, and aphonia (loss of speech).

However, not all historical cases are confined to evasion of military duty. Jones and Llewelyn (1917) cite a variety of cases in the histories of Greece, Rome, and the Middle Ages where individuals feigned insanity to escape execution. Moersch (1944) observes

> Galen in his work referred to many acts of malingering occurring in civil life. . . [and] . . . Ambroïse Paré in the sixteenth century was struck with the common occurrence of impostors about Paris attempting to gain a livelihood by feigning disease (pp. 928–9).

The external goal of malingering is shaped by the social context of the era. For example, although there has been considerable controversy in recent decades about the use of the insanity defence in criminal cases, attempts to simulate psychiatric conditions in the American Civil War were rare due to a standing order that prohibited the discharge of soldiers diagnosed as insane (Anderson & Anderson, 1984). Likewise, Miller and Cartlidge (1972) note that there was a dramatic increase in civilians claiming severe disability from minor head injury after Prussia enacted the first accident insurance laws in 1871 and 1884, a phenomenon also observed after Britain passed similar legislation (i.e. the Employers Liability Act of 1880 and the Workman's Compensation Acts of 1898 and 1906). Such external incentives still exert similar influences today.

An official diagnosis of malingering (V65.20) did not appear until the third *Diagnostic and Statistical Manual of Mental Disorders (DSM-III)* of the American Psychiatric Association (APA, 1980). The concept was not addressed at all in the first DSM (APA, 1952) and only briefly mentioned in DSM-II (APA, 1968), where it was made in conjunction with a discussion of differential diagnoses for hysterical neurosis:

This type of hysterical neurosis must be distinguished from psychophysiologic disorders, which are mediated by the autonomic nervous system; from malingering, which is done consciously; and from neurological lesions, which cause anatomically circumscribed symptoms (p. 40).

Fortunately, a more sophisticated description is now available.

## Definition of malingering

The DSM-IV defines malingering as:

... the intentional production of false or grossly exaggerated physical or psychological symptoms, motivated by external incentives such as avoiding military duty, avoiding work, obtaining financial compensation, evading criminal prosecution, or obtaining drugs (APA, 1994, p. 683).

This definition is almost unchanged from the earlier definition in DSM-III-R (APA, 1987), but the DSM-III requirement that:

the symptoms are produced in pursuit of a goal that is obviously recognizable with an understanding of the individual's circumstances rather than his or her individual psychology (APA, 1980, p. 331)

has been dropped. The two basic characteristics that distinguish malingering from the primary differential diagnoses of factitious disorders and conversion hysteria are (i) whether the incentives are external or internal, and (ii) if symptom production is conscious or unconscious.

Defining external goals is not necessarily an easy task. Malingering may be related to 'wanting to get even' with an unscrupulous supervisor or due to 'secondary gain from family' (Tager, 1985: 915). Is the desire for revenge or the need for attention and care-taking from family members internally or externally driven? While the DSM-IV indicates that 'evidence of an intrapsychic need to maintain the sick role ...' suggests factitious disorder, it flatly states '... external incentives are absent' (APA, 1994, p. 683). This implies that evidence of external incentives supersedes that of internal motivation and therefore requires the diagnosis of malingering.

The 'essential feature of malingering' (APA, 1994, p. 683) is that symptoms are intentionally produced, indicating malingerers must have self-awareness of the falseness of their symptoms. Again, making such a determination can be difficult. Cunnien (1988) observes, ' . . . most human behavior serves both conscious and unconscious goals and is undertaken with mixed intentions' (p. 15). Travin and Protter (1984) offer an interesting approach to this dilemma by suggesting a conceptualization of two intertwined continua: one representing the individual's target of deception (others or self) and the second representing the level of awareness surrounding false symptom production (conscious or unconscious). Thus, the more someone seeks to deceive others regarding their state of health, the more conscious and voluntary the production of false or exaggerated symptoms and, presumably, the easier malingering is to identify.

## Tests specifically designed to detect malingering

A number of techniques have been developed with the specific goal of helping the clinician to determine if an examinee is not exerting maximum effort on a task. Among those used to detect feigned memory disorders are Rey's 15-Item Memory Test (Rey, 1964), Rey's Word Recognition List (Rey, 1964), and various versions of symptom validity tests (Binder & Pankratz, 1987; Hiscock & Hiscock, 1989; Binder, 1993; Hanlon et al., 1996).

### Rey's 15-Item Memory Test (RFMT)

Probably the most widely cited English translation of Rey's (1964) original presentation of the 15-Item test is Lezak's presentation in her text *Neuropsychological Assessment*, currently in its third edition (Lezak, 1995). As she points out, the reader should be alert for variations on the title of this procedure, including *Rey's Memory Test* (Bernard, 1990), the *Rey Fifteen-Item Test (FIT)* (Millis & Kler, 1995), *Rey's 3 x 5 Test* (Lee et al., 1992), *Rey Dissimulation Test* (Wasyliw & Cavanaugh, 1989), *The Rey 15-Item Memory Test* (Schretlen et al., 1991), *Memorization of 15 Items* (Orsini et al., 1988), and her own *Rey Memory Test*, in which she includes the 16-item variation by Paul et al. (1992). The original test consists of the examiner emphasizing that 15 items will be exposed for only 10 seconds to create the impression that it will be a strenuous test of memory. The subject is then presented with a series of five rows of three characters (Fig. 22.1). In reality, only three concepts must be recalled.

Rey (1964) originally suggested that an inability to recall two or more series (a cut-off score of six) indicates exaggeration, but a cut-off score as high as nine (Lezak, 1983) has also been recommended. Patients with a wide variety of diagnoses typically score above nine items on the RFMT, including 100% of psychiatric patients

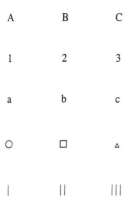

Fig. 22.1.     Items presented on Rey's 15-Item Test as shown in Lezak (1995).

(Goldberg & Miller, 1986), 89% of brain-injured patients in rehabilitation (Bernard & Fowler, 1990), 95% of temporal lobe epilepsy patients (Lee & Loring, 1994), and 95% of 'neurological' outpatients not involved in litigation (Lee et al., 1992). A recent study using well-defined clinical populations (Greiffenstein et al., 1994) found significant differences on the RFMT when comparing traumatically brain-injured (TBI) patients, individuals with post-concussive syndrome, and suspected malingerers. When a cut-off score of nine was used, sensitivity and specificity percentages were good in contrasting TBI patients with proposed malingerers (62 and 88%, respectively) as well as in contrasting post-concussive patients with malingering individuals (63 and 93%).

Lee and Loring (1994) administered the RFMT to 124 temporal lobe epilepsy inpatients and two groups of neurologic outpatients, 16 of whom were involved in litigation and 40 who were not. They examined a subset of temporal lobe patients who had scored below the fifth percentile on at least one of four standardized memory tests. The authors found that a score of seven successfully discriminated the groups. In their review of the literature, Nies and Sweet (1994) also recommended a cut-off score of seven, which provided an adequate hit rate across age, IQ score, and diagnostic category.

The clinician should apply caution, however, when using this test of memory malingering. Beetar and Williams (1995) found that, while malingerers produced significantly fewer items on the RFMT than did controls, the scores were on average considerably above the cut-off of nine suggested by Lezak (1983). Although hit rates were not reported, the means were not significantly different (malingerers = 13.07, controls = 14.70). Goldberg and Miller (1986) found that more than 37% of mildly mentally retarded adults produced scores below a cut-off of nine. Schretlen and his colleagues (1991) demonstrated that, although an analogue malingering sample performed significantly worse on the RFMT than controls, amnestic and demented patients also produced significantly lower scores than subjects instructed to feign deficits.

Greiffenstein et al. (1995) found the RFMT significantly discriminated probable malingerers (PM) from both TBI patients and persistent post-concussive subjects (PPCS) seeking only compensation for past medical bills. However, there was considerable overlap between the group means [TBI = 12.70 (3.07), PPCS = 13.26 (2.34), PM = 10.07 (3.70)], and the probable malingerer group average is above the cut-off score of nine. Finally, Millis and Kler (1995) contrasted moderate to severe TBI patients with individuals categorized as malingering via their histories and below chance performance on the Recognition Memory Test (see below). Although their sample size was small (seven in each group), they found that none of the brain-injured patients was misclassified when a cut-off of seven was used. However, almost half of the malingerers (43%) were not detected. Thus, specificity was good, but sensitivity was lacking.

### Rey's Word Recognition List (WRL)

This task, again proposed by Rey (1964) and described by Lezak (1983), requires that the examiner read a list of 15 words. After a delay of 5 seconds, the subject is presented with a list containing 15 targets and 15 foils. The score is the number of correctly cited target words. After an interval of at least 10 minutes, Rey's (1964) Auditory–Verbal Learning Test (AVLT) is administered. If the recall rate on the first trial of the AVLT equals or exceeds the WRL recognition rate, the probability of malingering is thought to increase.

Greiffenstein et al. (1994) reported that this technique significantly discriminates suspected malingerers from actual TBI and postconcussive patients. However, there was overlap of the group distributions such that a cutoff of six incorrectly identified 20% of both the TBI and post-concussive patients, while providing 81 and 86% sensitivity rates, respectively.

### Symptom validity tests (SVT)

A widely researched technique for detecting feigned memory deficits is symptom validity testing. Originally used to detect simulation of deafness (Pankratz et al., 1975) and other sensory deficits (Pankratz, 1979), Binder and Pankratz (1987) used a similar forced choice task to evaluate feigned memory complaints. The original task consisted of revealing either a yellow pencil or black pen to a patient suspected of faking memory impairment. The patient was asked to identify the object verbally before it was removed from sight. The patient was then instructed to count aloud to 20 before being asked to recall the item presented. After 100 randomly determined trials, the number of correct responses was analysed using a one-tailed normal distribution. Given the expectation of random responding in the case of true amnesia (i.e. 50% correct when guessing), it was demonstrated that the patient was responding at a worse-than-chance level.

A number of variations of the basic SVT paradigm have been developed, most of which follow the system originally presented by Hiscock and Hiscock (1989). A five-digit number is presented visually and then a distractor number is shown along side it after various time delays. The goal of this technique was to increase the perception of difficulty via the presentation of three sets of 24 trials, with each set having a greater time delay (5, 10, or 15 seconds). In their case study, the patient suspected of malingering performed at chance (50%) level on Set A, and only with additional blocks of trials using increasing delays produced an overall score of 29% correct, which was significantly below chance levels. Hiscock and Hiscock (1989) then convincingly contrasted this performance with the chance (51%) responding of a demented patient and the significantly above chance (82%) total score of a normal 5-year-old girl.

Using the Hiscock and Hiscock task, Prigatano and Amin (1993) compared a group of verified brain-injured patients and individuals with post-concussive syndrome to suspected malingerers. The brain-injured subjects produced overall scores of 99% correct, while suspected malingerers averaged only 73.8% correct. They also observed the same pattern of performance demonstrated by Hiscock and Hiscock's case study, that is, a progressive decline in accuracy as the time delay increased across sets. Although the malingering group mean is obviously above chance levels, it did discriminate such individuals from actual brain-injured patients.

Guilmette et al. (1993) reported a similar finding when they contrasted brain-injured and depressed patients with malingerers and normal controls. Using a cut-off score of 90% correct, they were able to accurately classify 90% of the subjects. Performance at or below 75% was sufficient to suggest malingering. Both studies indicate that worse-than-chance performance is not needed to identify probable malingerers.

One of the early formalized tests to evolve from the SVT paradigm was the Portland Digit Recognition Test (PDRT) by Binder (1993). Lezak (1995) notes that the PDRT differs from other SVT in that the target is presented verbally, delays are longer (5, 15, and 30 seconds), and the subject must count backwards during the delays. Lezak (1995) suggests that the PDRT is actually a stringent recognition test of working memory and has reservations about the adequacy of the original normative data. Nevertheless, an independent validation of the 27-item short form of the PDRT was conducted by Greiffenstein et al. (1994). Using a cut-off score set at 1.3 standard deviations below the mean, the authors correctly identified 89% of TBI and 94% of post-concussive patients from suspected malingerers.

The administration of these tests is often tedious. Consequently, there have been attempts to shorten the procedures (e.g. Greiffenstein et al,. 1994; Guilmette et al., 1994). Also, a number of SVT versions have been developed for presentation on a computer. Most of these utilize the basic forced two-choice paradigm with five digit target and distractor stimuli, including the Victoria Revision of Hiscock and Hiscock's forced-choice memory test (Slick et al., 1994), the Multi-Digit Memory Test (MDMT; Martin et al, 1991), the Computerized Assessment of Response Bias (Conder et al., 1992), and a computerized version of the PDMT (Rose et al., 1995). More recently, different variations on the five-digit theme have been introduced. For example, Beetar and Williams (1995) developed a symptom validity test of 100 strings of ten letters and numbers presented via a computer, with both recall and recognition responses being elicited from the subject. Their analogue study showed that the number of recognition errors on this task discriminated students instructed to malinger from controls.

Another variation uses letters as the stimuli of choice (Inman et al., 1998). However, the Letter Memory Test (LMT) does not try to introduce the perception of increasing difficulty via longer time delays, but rather presents nine blocks of five trials, crossing the number of letters (from three to five) with the number of choices (two to four) during the response phase. In a series of three studies, the authors found that analogue malingerers (both naive and those informed on how to avoid detection) had significantly lower scores on the LMT than either analogue controls or non-compensation-seeking, moderately to severely closed head-injured patients. Compensation-seeking patients with mild closed head injuries produced significantly poorer LMT scores than moderately to severely injured patients who were not trying to obtain compensation. The internal consistency reliability coefficient was 0.92 on a large sample of analogue malingerers (Hanlon et al., 1996).

## Summary

Techniques have been developed to determine whether an individual is performing below chance expectations or presents a level of impairment that is not seen in most brain dysfunctional patients. The preceding section reviewed a number of procedures that have been thought useful in detecting probable malingering. These procedures, in conjunction with traditional tests of memory, hold some clinical promise.

## Traditional tests of memory used to detect malingering

The use of standardized memory tests in detecting possible malingering have also been used. Although not formally a test, observations in the clinical interview have also been used for this purpose. How such information has been used in detecting probable or known malingerers will now be reviewed.

**Table 22.1.** Questions used in the autobiographical Interview utilized by Wiggins and Brandt (1988)

What is:
1. Your name
2. Your age
3. Your birthdate
4. Your telephone number
5. Your address
6. Your social security number
7. Mother's first name
8. Mother's maiden name
9. Father's first name
10. Brother's and/or sister's name

What did you have for:
11. Breakfast
12. Dinner last night

What is the experimenter's name: (asked on day two)
13. Recall
14. Recognition given four choices (if not recalled)

*Source:* From Wiggins, E.C. & Brandt, J., 1988.

## Generation of autobiographical information via the clinical interview

A complete neuropsychological examination requires a clinical interview that inquires into the patient's personal and medical history. Not only does this provide information about preserved memory as well as anterograde and retrograde amnesia, but it is also an opportunity to gather data about a patient's level of motivation. For example, Wasyliw and Cavanaugh (1989) note that patients with severe memory problems produced fewer complaints about memory than are observed by others (Sutherland et al., 1984) and suggest the clinicians contrast the self-report of patients with significant others. Lees-Haley (1986) offered several suggestions for modifying the clinical interview to enhance opportunities to detect malingering. They include lengthening the interview to increase opportunities for contradiction, mistakes, and losing track of the illness role; increasing the pace to give less time to think through answers; and asking about widely diverse symptoms. Reportedly, malingerers claim a long list of rare and unlikely combinations of symptoms when given the opportunity.

Unlike Lees-Haley's anecdotal evidence, Wiggins and Brandt (1988) conducted an autobiographical interview (Table 22.1) with actual amnestic patients, subjects asked to simulate amnesia, and controls. Answers were scored as incorrect if they were unambiguously wrong or the respondent insisted they had no knowledge or recall of the answer. Non-simulating controls provided correct responses for all items, except for 4% who could not recall their social security number. Incorrect responses were unusual for the four amnestic patients studied. One patient was incorrect on the social security number and recalling last night's dinner items. Two others could not recall the experimenter's name on the second day. In contrast, every question had incorrect responses in the simulator (malingering) group, with error rates ranging from 10 to 48%. Among the most frequently missed questions were age (35%), recall of the experimenter's name (37%), birth date (42%), telephone number (42%), what they had for dinner the previous night (42%), and social security number (48%).

## Wechsler Adult Intelligence Scale-Revised (WAIS-R; Wechsler, 1981) Digit Span subtest

In a study designed to determine whether personal knowledge of head injury affected the ability to simulate mild head injury symptoms, Hayes et al. (1994) administered several measures, including the Digit Span subtest of the WAIS-R (Wechsler, 1981). Instructions to malinger were a significant predictor of the total raw score on the Digit Span, while personal experience with head injury and tested knowledge of head injury symptoms were not predictive.

Iverson and Franzen (1994) cite an earlier study by Iverson (1991), where psychiatric inpatients and undergraduate college students completed the Digit Span under both normal and malingering conditions. Using an age-corrected Scale score of four as a cut-off, he was able to correctly classify 77.5% of the subjects in the malingering condition, while identifying all subjects in the normal instructions condition as well as all of an additional group of actual memory-impaired patients. In their follow-up study, Iverson and Franzen (1994) found that their student and inmate malingering groups produced significantly lower means for the Digit Span total score, Forward span, Backward span, and age-corrected Scale score.

Greiffenstein et al. (1995) examined the efficacy of the Reliable Digit Span in separating probable malingerers from TBI patients and persistent post-concussive (PPC) patients. The Reliable Digit Span score was produced by adding the longest string of digits accurately recalled on both trials in the forward and backward span conditions. This score was able to differentiate the probable malingering group from the TBI and PPC patients. The authors found good sensitivity for malingering vs. TBI (86%) and vs. post-concussive syndrome (89%), but rather modest specificity rates (57 and 68%, respectively). They recommended a cut-off of seven or less to suggest malingering.

## Wechsler Memory Scales – Revised (WMS-R; Weschler, 1987)

Mittenberg et al. (1992) cited prior research showing the Attention/Concentration Index score is higher than the global Memory Quotient score in patients suffering the acute effects of brain trauma. This finding is consistent with earlier findings that immediate attention span is preserved in TBI patients (Wechsler, 1987) and those suffering from amnestic syndromes (Strub & Black, 1977; Squire, 1987). They anticipated analogue malingerers would demonstrate the opposite pattern on the WMS-R. This proved to be the case, with actual head trauma patients scoring on average 10 points higher on the Attention/Concentration Index than the Memory Quotient, while subjects instructed to malinger produced mean scores almost 15 points below. The Attention/Concentration Index was the only WMS-R composite score that was significantly different. The two groups did not differ with regard to immediate and delayed scores on the Logical Memory (LM) and Visual Reproduction (VR) subtests.

Greiffenstein et al. (1994) compared clinical samples of TBI patients, post-concussive patients, and suspected malingerers using the immediate and delayed portions of the LM and VR subtests of both the original Wechsler Memory Scale (WMS: Wechsler, 1945, 1974) and the more recent WMS-R (Wechsler, 1987). Although the malingering group produced lower raw LM and VR subtest scores both immediately and following the delay, these scores did not prove significantly different from those generated by either the TBI or post-concussive patients.

## Auditory Verbal Learning Test (AVLT; Rey, 1964)

In the study by Greiffenstein et al. (1994) described above, a number of the scores on the AVLT proved successful in discriminating post-concussive patients from malingerers. They included total words recalled, number of words recalled on the fifth trial, both delayed free recall trials, and number of words recognized after a 30-minute delay. Although TBI patients were also distinguished from malingerers by the delayed recognition score, there were no significant group differences with regard to number of words recalled on Trial 1 or number of false positives produced during the recognition phase. In an extension of this first study, Greiffenstein et al. (1995) examined the ability of several procedures (including the AVLT) to differentiate between TBI patients, probable malingerers, and PPC patients with a reduced incentive to malinger. This reduced incentive was thought to be the case with the PPC patient group because they were only involved in first-party lawsuits (seeking payment of past medical bills by insurance), unlike the probable malingerers involved in litigation to obtain third-party jury awards. Using Rey's original recognition paragraph along with the 15 foils presented by Lezak (1983), the authors subtracted the number of false positive errors from the total number correct and found this score was significantly different for all three groups: PPC patients had higher scores than the TBI patients, who were higher than the probable malingering group.

**Table 22.2.** Classification percentages for separate scores on the CVLT as reported by Millis et al. (1995)

|                            | Sensitivity (%) | Specificity (%) | Overall (%) |
| -------------------------- | --------------- | --------------- | ----------- |
| Total words (Trials 1–5)   | 74              | 91              | 83          |
| Recognition discrimination | 96              | 91              | 93          |
| Recognition hits           | 83              | 96              | 89          |
| Long-delay cued recall     | 83              | 91              | 87          |

*Note:*
CVLT = California Verbal Learning Test.
*Source:* From Millis et al., 1995.

### California Verbal Learning Test (CVLT; Delis et al., 1987)

Along with other neuropsychological measures, Trueblood and Schmidt (1993) examined the effectiveness of the CVLT in detecting individuals undergoing out-patient neuropsychological examinations who were determined to be malingering by below chance performance on the Digit Memory Test (DMT) or who had questionable validity due to highly improbable test findings. Both the malingering and questionable validity groups were matched to controls and their CVLT Total T, Primacy, Recency, and Recognition scores were compared. Those in the malingering group showed a significantly greater recency effect, while significant differences on Recognition and Total T scores were observed between the questionable validity group and their matched controls. While seeking to minimize false positives, Trueblood and Schmidt (1993) found that a cut-off of less than 13 Recognition errors identified 63% of the malingerers and 50% of the questionable validity group, without producing any false positive errors.

Millis et al. (1995) also examined the ability of the CVLT to discriminate mild head-injury patients actively seeking compensation through personal injury or worker's compensation litigation from matched severe head-injury patients not involved in such litigation. The mild head-injury group produced significantly lower scores on the Total words recalled across Trials 1–5 (List A), Recognition discrimination, Long-delay cued recall, and Recognitions hits. Excellent sensitivity, specificity, and overall classification rates were observed using the first three scores in linear and quadratic discriminant function analyses (91 and 96%, respectively, for all three classification rates). However, cut-off scores derived from the individual measures also produced good classification rates (Table 22.2). Due to an ethical concern about the possible misuse of exact cut-off scores in coaching individuals to malinger, such cut-off scores are available only from the senior author of this study (Scott R. Millis, Rehabilitation Institute of Michigan, 261 Mack Blvd, Detroit, MI 48201-2417, USA).

**Rey-Osterrieth Complex Figure (ROCF; Osterrieth, 1944)**

Knight and Meyers (1994) determined a priori patterns of performance on the ROCF (copy, immediate recall, and delayed recall) based upon a conceptual memory theory presented by Sohlberg and Mateer (1989). They then categorized the profiles of brain-injured patients' performance on the ROCF and contrasted them with those of community volunteers, college students, and rehabilitation staff instructed to malinger. The combined malingering sample tended to produce either an Attention Error or Storage Error pattern, while the brain-injured sample had a predominately Retrieval Error pattern. Also, they observed that an Attention Error or Storage Error pattern rarely occurred in patients with a Ranchos Los Amigos level VIII rating. A discriminant function analysis utilizing their memory pattern designation and Ranchos Los Amigos level produced an 89% correct classification rate. Although this study had large samples ($n = 100$ for both the patient and analogue malingerers), it uses a new method of scoring and the resultant profiles lack evidence for construct validity.

**Benton Visual Retention Test (BVRT; Benton, 1955)**

Among the earliest authors to study the simulation of memory impairment, Benton and Spreen (1961) instructed college students to perform on the BVRT as if they were brain injured. These performances were compared to those of an actual brain-injured sample. Both quantitative and qualitative differences were found. Simulators produced a mean of only 2.16 correct compared to a mean of 3.73 correct by the patient group. When qualitative differences in the type of errors made by the two groups on the BVRT were examined, brain-damaged patients made more errors of perseveration and omission (particularly the small peripheral figure). Simulators produced drawings with more distortions and fewer size errors.

In a follow-up study, Spreen and Benton (1963) asked 26 hospitalized patients with other than neurological or psychiatric conditions and 49 college students to simulate mental deficiency on the BVRT. They contrasted these drawings with those produced by patients classified as mentally defective (i.e. an IQ between 58 and 75). Interestingly, the two simulating groups did not differ significantly with regard to the number of correct reproductions, errors, or specific classification of errors and were therefore combined for subsequent analyses. Due to atypical distributions, the median number of correct reproductions (simulators = 1.04, actual patients = 3.00) and errors (simulators = 14.00, actual patients = 10.67) were analysed by Chi-square tests and found to be significantly different. The authors note that the simulators produced significantly more unusual responses, as defined by seven specific scoring rules. Unfortunately, neither variance data nor cutting scores were presented in these studies.

### Recognition Memory Test (RMT; Warrington, 1984)

The RMT consists of two sections, recognition memory for words (RMW) and recognition memory for faces (RMF). The subject is presented with either 50 consecutive words or faces one every three seconds and then immediately tested via a forced-choice two-alternative recognition task. In essence, this procedure is a SVT and has been used as such to detect malingering via below chance performance (Millis & Kler, 1995). Iverson and Franzen (1994) contrasted the utility of the RMT, Knox Cube Test (Stone & Wright, 1980) and the Digit Span. Students and volunteer federal inmates instructed to malinger had significantly fewer correct responses than normal student and inmate groups as well as a head-injury patient group. Using a RMW cut-off of 32 or less words correct, 90% of the malingerers, 100% of the normal controls, and 100% of the patients were identified correctly with no false positives. A RMF cut-off score of less than 30 faces recognized produced 80, 100, and 100% classification rates, respectively, also without false positives. Moreover, a discriminant function analysis using scores from the RMT, Knox Cube Test, and Digit Span on the first half of the sample yielded a 98% correct classification rate (one non-malingerer was misclassified), while a cross-validation of the function on the second half of the sample proved 100% correct in its classification.

### Memory Assessment Scales (MAS; Williams, 1991)

Beetar and Williams (1995) randomly assigned 60 paid ($5) student volunteers to either malingering or control conditions. They administered the 12 subtests of the MAS via computer, as well as Rey's Dot Counting task (Rey, 1941 as cited in Lezak, 1995), Memorization of 15-Items Test (Rey, 1964), and a symptom validity test using letters and numbers (the last two procedures are described above). On the MAS, subjects instructed to malinger performed significantly lower than controls on all 12 subtests. However, as a group, their composite memory scores were in the low average range, leading the authors to conclude the subjects were able to fake a poor performance on the MAS effectively without being obvious. None the less, several measures discriminated malingering subjects from controls. First, subjects demonstrated their lack of knowledge about memory disorders by performing equally poorly on both recall and recognition tasks. They also recalled significantly fewer items on both the Verbal and Visual Span subtests, although persons with true amnesia usually fall in the lower end of the normal range for attention and concentration relative to immediate auditory recall (Black, 1986).

### Implicit memory tasks

Wiggins and Brandt (1988) assumed malingerers would not be aware of the specific aspects of neuropsychological test performance found among true amnestic patients. They predicted that simulators would do poorly on both explicit and implicit memory tasks, which would contrast with the performance of actual amnestic patients who have difficulty with explicit memory but perform normally on tests of implicit memory.

On a word stem completion task, simulators produced fewer words than controls but had a similar serial position profile, demonstrating both primacy and recency effects. Amnestics did not show a primacy effect, only a recency effect. Although simulators presented fewer words, the pattern across the two days of testing between presented and unpresented words was similar for both controls and true amnestics. Simulators were statistically less likely to give the same responses on both days. An almost identical pattern of results was found on the word-association task. Contrary to the authors' prediction, simulators performed similarly to controls and amnestics by showing priming effects on implicit memory tasks.

In a second study, Wiggins and Brandt (1988) administered two 20-item word lists, followed by a free recall test and then a two alternative, forced-choice test. Simulators demonstrated better recall performance and worse recognition scores than the actual amnestic patients. As in Study 1, simulators resembled controls in that they showed both a primacy and recency effect, whereas amnestic patients again demonstrated only a recency effect.

## Summary

Individuals instructed to simulate memory impairment on standardized memory tests often perform worse than patients with known brain dysfunction, particularly on recognition tasks. Use of such data from established clinical tests provides the additional benefits of diagnostically relevant information without the time and expense of administering procedures specifically designed to detect malingering. Recently, Dikmen et al.(1995) demonstrated a dose–response relationship between severity of brain injury and level of cognitive dysfunction, such that mild brain injury should produce mild sequelae and severe impairment would only be expected in conjunction with evidence of severe brain injury. Thus, when an individual performs at a level considerably worse than would be expected given their medical history, the potential for malingering has to be considered. Case examples that highlight this problem when patients with and without brain injury are now reviewed as well as evaluations for patients with and without psychiatric symptomatology.

## Clinical manifestations of probable malingering

Patients with and without brain injury can feign memory impairments. The same is true of psychiatric patients. Given these realities, the major question facing the clinician who is examining memory function is as follows: am I getting a co-operative performance in which the individual is not intentionally exaggerating their memory disturbance?

As noted earlier, suspicion of probable malingering arises when (i) the patients' subjective complaints of neuropsychological impairment far exceed what would normally be expected given their medical history, and (ii) the level and pattern of neuropsychological test performance are highly unusual given the patients' history. Typically, these two events occur in the context of an examination where the patient will benefit financially if the test scores are interpreted as reflecting significant brain dysfunction. It is important to note here, however, that suspicion of probable malingering is seldom raised if patients clearly demonstrate emotional difficulties that would explain poor performance on memory and other related tests. Here is such a scenario.

## Case example 1

A 36-year-old woman suffered a superior sagittal sinus thrombosis. She was not involved in litigation, but when seen for follow-up was receiving financial benefits for her medical disability. The patient was first examined 3 weeks post-stroke and her performance on the Barrow Neurological Institute Screen for Higher Cerebral Functions (BNI Screen; Prigatano et al., 1995) was within normal limits (i.e. 47 of 50 points, producing an age-corrected T score of 48). On the CVLT (Delis et al., 1987), she was able to recall 62 words across five trials for a T score of 64. Long-term free recall on this test was within the average range (T score of 50). Recognition memory was perfect (16 of 16).

During the next year, this woman was unable to receive adequate rehabilitative help. She developed a severe depressive disorder. Neuropsychological examination 1 year later revealed a BNI Screen score of 42 of 50 points (T score = 22) and a total of 41 words on the CVLT (T score = 20). Long-term free recall was now 7 of 16 words (T score = 20), and recognition memory was only 12 of 16 words (T score = 20).

Malingering was not considered probable in this case for two reasons. First, her depression was straightforward and appeared to account for the observed decline in memory and cognitive functioning. Secondly, she appeared fully co-operative with the examination procedures. To check on this latter clinical impression, she was administered the DMT a few days after her second examination. Her performance was within the normal range at 97.7% correct. She made only two errors over 72 trials. The errors appeared to be the result of concentration difficulties and she immediately identified her own errors.

## Case example 2

In contrast, a 36-year-old male who had suffered a rupture of a posterior communicating artery aneurysm 8 years before his neuropsychological examination reported a level of disability incompatible with his history. The patient's internist noted that the patient could drive a car, easily care for his children, perform a variety of fairly complicated tasks at home, and spend several hours playing bingo during the course of a week. Yet the patient reported to his physician a complete inability to return to work. On the BNI Screen, the man obtained a total score of 37 of a possible 50 points (T score = 6). On the CVLT, he could recall only 21 words over five trials (T score = 5). Given that his lesion was on the right side of the brain, one would not expect this degree of verbal memory impairment. He demonstrated a degree of memory impairment that was worse than what would be expected on the basis of his medical history. It was also incompatible with his reported day-to-day functioning. Malingering was therefore suspected. The patient was given Set C of the DMT. He obtained a score of only 62.5% correct, which suggested failure to be fully co-operative (using the previous research findings of Prigatano & Amin, 1993).

The patient was confronted with these suspicions. He was told of the consequences of not being fully co-operative and testing was terminated that day. The patient agreed to return for repeat testing. Although he did not state that he was frankly feigning memory deficits, he did admit that perhaps he was not 'trying very hard' on some tests. He was re-examined 1 week later, and his recognition memory was now completely in the normal range. The difference in test scores was so substantial that it could not be explained on the basis of practice effects or measurement error. Thus, DMT findings were helpful in identifying probable feigning of memory deficit in a patient with actual brain dysfunction.

## Case example 3

A 24-year-old man suffered a 'mild' brain injury while at work and was evaluated 9 months after injury. Previous examiners believed that he had recovered adequately to return to work. The patient, however, continued to complain of significant problems with memory and controlling his temper. On the BNI Screen, he obtained a score of 30 of 50 points, (T score < 1). On the CVLT, he could recall only 32 words (T score = 7). Recognition memory was also five standard deviations below average. This degree of memory impairment is incompatible with a history of mild TBI, and it raised the suspicion of malingering.

Set C of the DMT was administered and the patient obtained a score of 79.1% correct. During a subsequent testing session, he completed the remainder of the DMT. He made four errors on Set A of the DMT (83.3% correct) and six errors on Set B (75% correct). It was concluded that the patient was not fully co-operative with testing procedures.

## Case example 4

A 50-year-old man developed a psychotic depression approximately 4 years after a head injury of mild to possibly moderate severity. The patient was also diagnosed by a psychiatrist as having an organic amnestic disorder. He was referred to help determine whether a mild head injury could cause not only a psychotic depression but this degree of amnestic impairment.

His neuropsychological test scores were universally very poor, including extremely poor performance on memory tests. For example, his performance on the CVLT was five standard deviations below average on learning (total words recalled), delayed recall, and recognition. Despite his poor performance on all tests, he never demonstrated any difficulty understanding instructions nor any evidence of language impairment. For example, he read and answered a series of questions concerning functioning on a scale called the Patient Competency Rating Scale (Prigatano et al., 1986). He never once asked for help in understanding the items or in reading the questions. He was given the Minnesota Multiphasic Personality Inventory-2 (Regents of the University of Minnesota, 1989). He proceeded for approximately one hour and then refused to continue. He stated that the test was giving him headaches. Despite offering him multiple breaks to complete the test, he refused to do so.

The patient was given the DMT. He performed at near chance level over the three sets (a total value of 54% correct). Unlike demented patients tested with the DMT (Prigatano et al., 1997), he never once appeared confused about the DMT task or asked that instructions be repeated. His DMT scores, coupled with his failure to show any language impairment, raised serious concerns that he was not fully co-operative with testing procedures despite clear evidence of a psychotic depression. Parenthetically, it was the second author's opinion that a history of mild-to-moderate head injury in and of itself could not produce a psychotic depression 4 years later or an organic amnestic syndrome without other confirming evidence based on neurological or neuropsychological test findings. Other factors would have to be considered as most likely contributing to such a psychotic reaction.

## Conclusions

The detection of feigned memory impairments for patients with known or suspected brain disorders has attracted increasing interest in the field of clinical neuropsychology. Psychologists have developed new methods for assessing subtle indications of an unco-operative attitude while taking various neuropsychological tests. This methodology can be coupled with suspicious performances on standard neuropsychological memory tests to provide more objective evidence of reduced effort. Also, knowledge of how memory disorders reveal themselves in psychiatric and neurologic patients can be very helpful to experienced clinical neuropsychologists who must draw conclusions about whether an individual is feigning or exaggerating a memory disorder.

Literature that highlights how this problem has been approached using various tests has been reviewed. Also, specific case examples have been presented to highlight the fact that an unco-operative attitude and/or malingering can often be detected in the presence of either brain dysfunction or psychiatric disability. It is important to emphasize, however, that there are no 'foolproof' methods for detecting feigned memory impairments. Suspicions of malingering evolve from clinical judgment. That clinical judgment must be based on objective, scientifically derived measures and interpreted by experienced clinical neuropsychologists.

Unfortunately, in this day of litigation, it becomes extremely important that clinical neuropsychologists not be naive about the notion that some patients will in fact exaggerate memory impairments to obtain secondary (typically financial) gain. This chapter attempts to summarize some of the literature that might help clinicians who face this problem in their clinical practice.

## ACKNOWLEDGEMENT

The authors thank the Neuroscience Publications Office of the Barrow Neurological Institute for their assistance in editing and preparing this manuscript.

## REFERENCES

American Psychiatric Association (APA) (1952). *Diagnostic and Statistical Manual: Mental Disorders,* Washington, DC.

American Psychiatric Association (APA) (1968). *Diagnostic and Statistical Manual of Mental Disorders,* (DSM-II) 2nd edn. Washington, DC.

American Psychiatric Association (APA) (1980). *Diagnostic and Statistical Manual of Mental Disorders,* 3rd edn. Washington, DC.

American Psychiatric Association (1987). *Diagnostic and Statistical Manual of Mental Disorders,* 3rd edn. revised. Washington, DC.

American Psychiatric Association (1994). *Diagnostic and Statistical Manual of Mental Disorders,* 4th edn. Washington, DC.

Anderson, D.L. & Anderson, G.T. (1984). Nostalgia and malingering in the military during the Civil War. *Perspectives in Biology and Medicine,* **28,** 156–66.

Beetar, J.T. & Williams, J.M. (1995). Malingering response styles on the Memory Assessment Scales and symptom validity tests. *Archives of Clinical Neuropsychology,* **10,** 57–72.

Benton, A.L. (1955). *The Revised Visual Retention Test: Clinical and Experimental Applications.* New York: Psychological Corporation.

Benton, A.L. & Spreen, O. (1961). Visual memory test: the simulation of mental incompetence. *Archives of General Psychiatry,* **4,** 79–83.

Bernard, L.C. (1990). Prospects for faking believable deficits on neuropsychological tests and the use of incentives in simulation research. *Journal of Clinical and Experimental Neuropsychology,* **12,** 715–28.

Bernard, L.C. & Fowler, W. (1990). Assessing the validity of memory complaints: performance of brain-damaged and normal individuals on Rey's task to detect malingering. *Journal of Clinical Psychology,* **42,** 770–82.

Bigler, E.D. (1990). Neuropsychology and malingering: comment on Faust, Hart, & Guilmette (1988). *Journal of Consulting and Clinical Psychology,* **58,** 244–7.

Binder, L.M. (1993). Assessment of malingering after mild head trauma with the Portland Digit Recognition Test. *Journal of Clinical and Experimental Neuropsychology,* **15,** 170–82.

Binder, L.M. & Pankratz, L. (1987). Neuropsychological evidence of a factitious memory complaint. *Journal of Clinical and Experimental Neuropsychology*, **9**, 167–71.

Black, W.F. (1986). Digit repetition in brain-damaged adults: clinical and theoretical implications. *Journal of Clinical Psychology*, **42**, 770–82.

Brussel, J.A. & Hitch, K.S. (1943). The military malingerer. *The Military Surgeon*, **93**, 33–44.

Conder, R.L., Allen, L.M. & Cox, D.R. (1992). CARB: Computerized Assessment of Response Bias. Paper presented at the 12th Annual Meeting of the National Academy of Neuropsychology, Pittsburgh, PA.

Cunnien, A.J. (1988). Psychiatric and medical syndromes associated with deception. In *Clinical Assessment of Malingering and Deception*, ed. R. Rogers. New York: The Guilford Press.

Delis, D.C., Kramer, J.H., Kaplan, E. & Ober, B.A. (1987). *California Verbal Learning Test-Adult Version Manual: Research Edition.* San Antonio, Texas: The Psychological Corporation.

Dikmen, S.S., Machamer, J.E., Winn, H.R. & Temkin, N.R. (1995). Neuropsychological outcome at 1-year post head injury. *Neuropsychology*, **9**, 80–90.

Faust, D., Hart, K. & Guilmette, T.J. (1988a). Pediatric malingering: the capacity of children to fake believable deficits on neuropsychological testing. *Journal of Consulting and Clinical Psychology*, **56**, 578–82.

Faust, D., Hart, K., Guilmette, T.J. & Arkes, H.R. (1988b). Neuropsychologists capacity to detect adolescent malingerers. *Professional Psychology: Research and Practice*, **19**, 508–15.

Goldberg, J.O. & Miller, H.R. (1986). Performance of psychiatric inpatients and intellectually deficient individuals on a task that assesses the validity of memory complaints. *Journal of Clinical Psychology*, **42**, 792–5.

Greiffenstein, M.F., Baker, W.J. & Gola, T. (1994). Validation of malingered amnesia measures with a large clinical sample. *Psychological Assessment*, **6**, 218–24.

Greiffenstein, M.F., Gola, T. & Baker, W.J. (1995). MMPI-2 Validity scales versus domain specific measures in detection of factitious traumatic brain injury. *The Clinical Neuropsychologist*, **9**, 230–40.

Guilmette, T.J., Hart, K.J. & Giuliano, A.J. (1993). Malingering detection: the use of a forced-choice method in identifying organic versus simulated memory impairment. *The Clinical Neuropsychologist*, **7**, 59–69.

Guilmette, T.J., Sparadeo, F.R., Whelihan, W. & Buongiorno, G. (1994). Validity of neuropsychological test results in disability evaluations. *Perceptual and Motor Skills*, **78**, 1179–86.

Hanlon, T., Berry, D., Lamb, D., Patel, R. & Edwards, C. (1996). Preliminary validity and reliability data on a new motivational procedure: The Letter Memory Test. Paper presented at the 24th Annual Meeting of the International Neuropsychological Society, Chicago, IL.

Hayes, J.S., Martin, R., Smiroldo, B.B., Stafford, C. & Gouvier, W.D. (1994). Influence of prior knowledge on the ability to feign mild head injury symptoms in head injured and non head injured college students. Paper presented at the 14th Annual Meeting of the National Academy of Neuropsychology, Orlando, FL.

Heaton, R.K., Smith, H.H., Lehman, R.A.W. & Vogt, A.T. (1978). Prospects for faking believable deficits on neuropsychological testing. *Journal of Consulting and Clinical Psychology*, **46**, 892–900.

Hiscock, M. & Hiscock, C.K. (1989). Refining the forced-choice method for the detection of malingering. *Journal of Clinical and Experimental Neuropsychology*, **11**, 967–74.

Inman, T.H., Vickery, C.D., Berry, D.T.R., Lamb, D.G., Edwards, C.L. & Smith, G.T. (1998). Development and initial validation of a new procedure for evaluating adequacy of effort given during neuropsychological testing: The Letter Memory Test. *Psychological Assessment*, **10**, 128–39.

Iverson, G.L. (1991). Detecting malingered memory deficits through the use of multiple objective methods: a preliminary investigation. Unpublished master's thesis, West Virginia University, Morgantown.

Iverson, G.L. & Franzen, M.D. (1994). The Recognition Memory Test, Digit Span, and Knox Cube Test as markers of malingered memory impairment. *Psychological Assessment*, **1**, 323–34.

Jones, A.B. & Llewelyn, J.L. (1917). *Malingering*. London: Heinemann.

Knight, J.A. & Meyers, J.E. (1994). Malingered memory performance patterns on the Rey–Osterrieth Complex Figure test. Paper presented at the 14th Annual Meeting of the National Academy of Neuropsychology, Orlando, FL.

Kopelman, M.D. (1987). Crime and amnesia: a review. *Behavioral Sciences and the Law*, **5**, 323–42.

Lee, G.P. & Loring, D.W. (1994). Normative data on Rey's $3 \times 5$ memory test for the detection of malingering. Paper presented at the 14th Annual Meeting of the National Academy of Neuropsychology, Orlando, FL.

Lee, G.P., Loring, D.W. & Martin, R.C. (1992). Rey's 15 item visual memory test for the detection of malingering: Normative observations on patients with neurological disorders. *Psychological Assessment*, **4**, 43–6.

Lees-Haley, P.R. (1986). How to detect malingerers in the workplace. *Personnel Journal*, **65**, 108, 110, 196.

Lezak, M. (1983). *Neuropsychological Assessment*, 2nd edn. New York: Oxford University Press.

Lezak, M. (1995). *Neuropsychological Assessment*, 3rd edn. New York: Oxford University Press.

Martin, R., Bolter, J., Todd, M. & Gouvier, W.D. (1991). Effects of sophistication and motivation on the detection of malingered memory performance using a computerized force-choice task. Paper presented at the 11th Annual Meeting of the National Academy of Neuropsychology, Dallas, Texas.

Matarazzo, J.D. (1990). Psychological assessment versus psychological testing: Validation from Binet to the school, clinics, and courtroom. *American Psychologist*, **45**, 999–1017.

Menninger, K.A. (1935). Psychology of a certain type of malingering. *Archives of Neurology and Psychiatry*, **33**, 507–15.

Miller, H. & Cartlidge, N. (1972). Simulation and malingering after injuries to the brain and spinal cord. *Lancet*, **i**, 580–6.

Millis, S.R. & Kler, S. (1995). Limitations of the Rey Fifteen-Item Test in the detection of malingering. *The Clinical Neuropsychologist*, **9**, 241–4.

Millis, S.R., Putman, S.H., Adams, K.M. & Ricker, J.H. (1995). The California Verbal Learning Test in the detection of incomplete effort in neuropsychological evaluation. *Psychological Assessment*, **7**, 463–71.

Mittenberg, W., Azrin, R., Millsaps, C. & Heilbronner, R. (1992). Identification of malingered head injury on the Wechsler Memory Scale-Revised. Paper presented at the 20th Annual Meeting of the International Neuropsychological Society, San Diego, CA.

Moersch, F.P. (1944). Malingering; with reference to its neuropsychiatric aspects in civil and in military practice. *Medical Clinics of North America*, pp. 928–44. (Mayo Clinic Number 928)

Nies, K.J. & Sweet, J.J. (1994). Neuropsychological assessment and malingering: a critical review of past and present strategies. *Archives of Clinical Neuropsychology*, 9, 501–52.

Orsini, D.L., Van Gorp, W.G. & Boone, K.B. (1988). *The Neuropsychology Casebook.* New York: Springer-Verlag.

Osterrieth, P.A. (1944). Le test de copie d'une figure complexe. *Archives de Psychologie*, 30, 206–356; translated by J. Corwin & F.W. Bylsma (1993), *The Clinical Neuropsychologist*, 7, 9–15.

Pankratz, L. (1979). Symptom validity testing and symptom retraining: Procedures for the assessment and treatment of functional sensory deficits. *Journal of Consulting and Clinical Psychology*, 47, 409–10.

Pankratz, L., Fausti, S.A. & Peed, S. (1975). A forced-choice technique to evaluate deafness in the hysterical and malingering patient [Case Study]. *Journal of Consulting and Clinical Psychology*, 43, 421–2.

Parwatikar, S.D., Holcomb, W.R. & Menninger, K.A. (1985). The detection of malingered amnesia in accused murderers. *Bulletin of the American Academy of Psychiatry and Law*, 13, 97–103.

Paul, D.S., Franzen, M.D., Cohen, S.H. & Fremouw, W. (1992). An investigation into the reliability and validity of two tests used in the detection of dissimulation. *International Journal of Clinical Neuropsychology*, 14, 1–9.

Prigatano, G.P. & Amin, K. (1993). Digit Memory Test: unequivocal cerebral dysfunction and suspected malingering. *Journal of Clinical and Experimental Neuropsychology*, 15, 537–46.

Prigatano, G.P., Fordyce, D.J., Zeiner, H.K., Roueche, J.R., Pepping, M. & Wood, B.C. (1986). *Neuropsychological Rehabilitation after Brain Injury.* Baltimore, MD: Johns Hopkins Press.

Prigatano, G.P., Amin, K. & Rosenstein, B.A. (1995). *Administration and Scoring Manual for the BNI Screen for Higher Cerebral Functions.* Phoenix, Arizona: Barrow Neurological Institute.

Prigatano, G.P., Smason, I., Lamb, D.G. & Bortz, J.J. (1997). Suspected malingering and the Digit Memory Test: A replication and extension. *Archives of Clinical Neuropsychology*, 12, 609–19.

Regents of the University of Minnesota (1989). *Minnesota Multiphasic Personality Inventory-2.* Minneapolis: University of Minnesota Press.

Rey, A. (1941). L'examen psychologique dans le cas d'encephalopathie traumatique. *Archive de Psychologie*, 37, 126–39.

Rey, A. (1964). *L'examen Clinique en Psychologique.* Paris: Presses Universitaires de France.

Rose, F.E., Hall, S. & Szalda-Petree, A.D. (1995). Portland Digit Memory Test – computerized: measuring response latency improves the detection of malingering. *The Clinical Neuropsychologist*, 9, 124–34.

Schacter, D.L. (1986). On the relation between genuine and simulated amnesia. *Behavioral Sciences and the Law*, 4, 47–64.

Schmidt, J.(1989). Why recent researchers have not assessed the capacity of neuropsychologists to detect malingering. *Professional Psychology: Research and Practice*, 20, 140–1.

Schretlen, D., Brandt, J., Krafft, L. & Van Gorp, W. (1991). Some caveats in using the Rey 15-item memory test to detect malingered amnesia. *Psychological Assessment*, 3, 667–72.

Slick, D., Hopp, G., Strauss, E., Hunter, M. & Pinch, D. (1994). Detecting dissimulation: profiles of simulated malingerers, traumatic brain-injury patients, and normal controls on a revised version of Hiscock and Hiscock's Forced-Choice Memory Test. *Journal of Clinical and Experimental Neuropsychology*, **16**, 472–81.

Sohlberg, M. & Mateer, C. (1989). *Introduction to Cognitive Rehabilitation: Theory and Practice.* New York: Guilford Press.

Spreen, O. & Benton, A.L. (1963). Simulation of mental deficiency on a visual memory test. *American Journal of Mental Deficiency*, **67**, 909–13.

Squire, L.R. (1987). *Memory and Brain.* New York: Oxford University Press.

Stone, M.H. & Wright, B.D. (1980). *Knox's Cube Test (manual).* Chicago: Stoelting.

Strub, R.L. & Black, W.F. (1977). *The Mental Status Examination in Neurology.* Philadelphia: F.A. Davis.

Sutherland, A., Harris, J.E. & Gleave, J. (1984). Memory failure in everyday life following severe head injury. *Journal of Clinical Neuropsychology*, **6**, 127–42.

Tager, R.M. (1985). Simulated disability. *Journal of Occupational Medicine*, **27**, 915–16.

Travin, S. & Protter, B. (1984). Malingering and malingering-like behavior: some clinical and conceptual issues. *Psychiatric Quarterly*, **56**, 189–97.

Trueblood, W. & Schmidt, M. (1993). Malingering and other validity considerations in the neuropsychological evaluation of mild brain injury. *Journal of Clinical and Experimental Neuropsychology*, **15**, 578–90.

Warrington, E.K. (1984). *Recognition Memory Test Manual.* Windsor, Berkshire: NFER-Nelson.

Wasyliw, O.E. & Cavanaugh, J.L. (1989). Simulation of brain damage: assessment and decision rules. *Bulletin of the American Academy of Psychiatry and Law*, **17**, 373–86.

Wechsler, D. (1945). A standardized memory scale for clinical use. *Journal of Psychology*, **19**, 87–95.

Wechsler, D. (1974). *Wechsler Memory Scale Manual.* San Antonio, TX: The Psychological Corporation.

Wechsler, D. (1981). *Wechsler Adult Intelligence Scale-Revised Manual.* New York: The Psychological Corporation.

Wechsler, D. (1987). *Wechsler Memory Scale-Revised Manual.* San Antonio, TX: The Psychological Corporation.

Wiggins, E.C. & Brandt, J. (1988). The detection of simulated amnesia. *Law and Human Behavior*, **12**, 57–78.

Williams, J.M. (1991). *Memory Assessment Scales.* Odessa, FL: Psychological Assessment Resources.

Ziskin, J. & Faust, D. (1988). *Coping with Psychiatric and Psychological Testimony*, vols. 1–3, 4th edn. Marina del Rey, CA: Law and Psychology Press.

# Legal aspects of memory disorders

Bohdan Solomka and Adrian Grounds

## Introduction

Disorders of memory may be relevant to a wide variety of legal issues. In the context of criminal proceedings memory disorders may affect, for example, the reliability of witness evidence, fitness to stand trial and criminal responsibility. In the civil context memory disorders may affect an individual's mental capacity to make decisions in relation to medical treatment and other matters concerning their welfare, property and financial affairs. Such individuals may need forms of legal protection and safeguards. Memory disorders may also feature in claims for compensation. More generally, an understanding of normal and abnormal memory functioning may be important in assessing the accounts of victims of trauma. The chapter concludes with a brief note about the preparation of court reports.

## Police custody and interviewing

Disorders of memory will obviously be important when individuals are being interviewed by the police for the purpose of obtaining evidence in the investigation of crime. Disorders of memory may affect the ability of a suspect to exercise his or her rights, fitness to be interviewed, and reliability of testimony.

In England and Wales the Police and Criminal Evidence Act 1984 sets out arrangements and safeguards for interviewing suspects in police custody, and police practice has to conform with the Codes of Practice issued under the Act. Zander (1995) provides an excellent guide to this legislation.

If a police officer suspects or is told that a person in police custody may be mentally disordered, handicapped, or incapable of understanding the significance of questions or his answers, an 'appropriate adult' should be called. This may be a relative or other person responsible for the individual's care, or someone who has experience in dealing with mentally disordered people. The suspect must not be interviewed, nor be asked to provide or sign a written statement, in the absence of an 'appropriate adult'. Suspects have a right of access to a solicitor, and this is particularly important for mentally disordered or vulnerable suspects. A custody officer must also obtain a medical assessment if a person brought to a police station or already detained there appears to be suffering from a mental disorder, or fails to respond normally to questions or conversation, or otherwise appears to need medical attention. The police may have to be advised that the individual is not medically fit to be interviewed. If a mentally disordered suspect is interviewed, the role of the 'appropriate adult' is not simply to act as a passive observer, but to advise the interviewee, to observe whether or not the interview is being conducted properly and to facilitate communication with the person being interviewed.

A person detained in police custody must be informed of the three basic rights he has, namely to have someone informed of the arrest, to obtain legal advice, and to consult the Codes of Practice of the Police and Criminal Evidence Act 1984. The individual is usually given a written 'Notice to Detained Persons' describing these rights. The suspect must also be cautioned before being interviewed. At present, the caution is expressed in the following terms:

You do not have to say anything. But it may harm your defence if you do not mention when questioned something which you later rely on in court. Anything you do say may be given in evidence.

Suspects in police custody need to be able to recall the information given about their rights in order to be able to exercise those rights. Clare and Gudjonnson (1992) found that poor levels of understanding and recall of the 'Notice to Detained Persons' are common amongst people of average intellectual ability, and more so amongst people with mild mental handicap. The authors argued for the introduction of a simplified version of the 'Notice'. Since then, two useful booklets have been written by Hollins et al. (1996a, b) for people with learning disabilities providing information and advice in pictorial form about being in police custody and a criminal court.

## Eyewitness memory

The law of evidence has always been concerned with processes of human perception and memory. The area of witness memory has received research attention since the 1970s. Much has focused on errors that interfere with the normal functioning of witness memory (Loftus, 1979). Unless witnesses are able to remember and accurately discuss events they have witnessed, they will probably be of little value on the witness stand. In order to give credit to witness testimony, a jury should have assurances that the witness' memory is functioning properly – that he or she is remembering the event as it actually happened. In the legal arena, errors in remembering have been attributed to the process of questioning a witness about the event (Loftus, 1979). The reasons suggested include:

(i)     A witness exposed to the atmosphere of the court may want to emphasize that his story is important.

(ii)    Once a witness is committed to a version of events by testifying, it is unlikely that he will change that version even when a change may be necessary for accuracy.

(iii)   The questioning process can give cues which a witness may seek in order to fill gaps in the memory, or in order to please the questioner.

A number of studies have shown that mistaken eyewitness testimony is a common reason for miscarriages of justice (Gudjonsson, 1992).


## Mentally disordered witnesses

Mentally disordered witnesses, suspects and victims are vulnerable in different ways to giving unreliable testimony, and each will be dealt with separately in relation to impairments of memory.

A considerable amount of work has been carried out on the psychological vulnerabilities of suspects detained at police stations. For a detailed review of this area, the reader should consult Gudjonsson's book (1992). Briefly, Gudjonsson divides false confessions into:


### Voluntary false confessions

These are given by individuals without external pressure from the questioner. Four reasons are put forward for voluntary false confessions: first, a pathological need to be infamous; secondly, a need to relieve guilt about matters unrelated to the confessed crime; thirdly, an inability to distinguish between fantasy and reality, as may be found in people with impaired 'reality monitoring' associated usually with severe mental illness; and, fourthly, an attempt to protect the real culprit.


### Coerced–compliant false confession

Here it is suggested that the suspect does not confess voluntarily, but acquiesces to pressure from the questioner for some immediate instrumental gain. The perceived gain may include being allowed to go home, ending the questioning, avoiding continuing detention in police custody, and as a way of coping with perceived pressure.


### Coerced–internalized false confessions

Sometimes a suspect accepts and believes that he committed the crime he is accused of, even though he has no memory of it.

Gudjonsson and Mackeith (1982) describe two types of 'memory distrust syndrome'. In the first type, the suspect has no memory at all for the time of the offence whether or not they actually committed it. They may then come to believe that they must have committed the offence. In the second type, the suspect has a clear recollection that he did not carry out the offence, but by the end of the interviewing process, that memory is doubted. The real concern is that coerced–internalized false confessors may experience permanent distortion of memory relating to a criminal offence. Gudjonsson and Lebegue (1989) did not find evidence to support permanently altered original memory, and Ofshe (1991) suggests that such distortions are unstable, being reversed by removal from the social environment supporting the distortion.

Gudjonsson and Mackeith (1988) note that those who internalize erroneous information during police interview have a tendency to become confused when placed under pressure, lack confidence in their memory and reconstruction of events, and display marked suggestibility. It is important in this regard to distinguish between 'belief' and 'memory' of committing a criminal act. Some critics of the 'witness memory' studies (Zaragoza & Koshmider, 1989) suggest that the 'subjects in the typical misinformation experiment are not encouraged to distinguish what they believe happened in the original event and what they specifically remember seeing in the original event'. Weingardt et al. (1994), argue that, although 'misled' subjects may report misinformation with confidence in a range of experimental settings, it does not conclusively prove that they base their response on a 'true belief'.

Gudjonsson (1992) cites a number of studies demonstrating an association between memory and suggestibility where the poorer the memory, the more suggestible the subject (Gudjonsson, 1987, 1988; Singh & Gudjonsson, 1984; Sharrock & Gudjonsson, 1993).

In order to give evidence in a criminal case in court, a witness must be competent to do so, which means, in this context, that the witness understands the nature and importance of the oath to tell the truth in open court. Competence will be assumed unless the person's disability is evident to the court, or the issue is raised by the prosecution or defence. A recent guide to criminal procedure in the English courts is given by Seabrooke and Sprack (1996).

## Recovered memory

'Recovered memory' refers to reported memories of childhood events by adults who were previously amnesic about them (British Psychological Society, 1995). This is an area that has aroused controversy and counter claims about a 'false memory syndrome'. There appear to be more legal case reports from the US than from the UK.

Winbolt (1995) finds it 'alarming' that the testimony of one person supported by a therapist or investigator can lead to prosecution. Many States in the US have statutes of limitation which prevent civil actions being brought on the basis of memories of molestation, where the events purportedly occurred many years ago. In the UK, courts have blocked attempts to prosecute allegations of child abuse that are many years old as an abuse of 'due process' (*R* v *Telford* 1991). Attempts to sue civilly were blocked by the House of Lords through strict interpretation of the six year rule in the Limitations Act 1980 (*Stubbings* v *Webb* 1993). Also, the distance in time and the loss of factual evidence deter prosecutors from filing charges. Boland et al. (1994) argue that techniques of questioning can contaminate and even create false memories in vulnerable minds. They note that the concept of recovered memory requires better scientific support, and that 'repressed memory' evidence should only be allowed in the rarest circumstances. The American Psychiatric Association (1993) in their 'Statement on Memories of Sexual Abuse' state:

[all stages of memory] can be influenced by a variety of factors including developmental stage, expectations, and knowledge base prior to an event; stress and bodily sensations experienced during an event; and the experience and context of the recounting of the event. In addition, the retrieval and recounting of a memory can modify the form of the memory, which may influence the content and the conviction about the veracity of the memory in the future. Scientific knowledge is not yet precise enough to predict how a certain experience or factor will influence a memory in the future.

The Australian Psychological Society (1995) published guidelines with similar warnings, underlining the dangers of evaluating recovered memories in the forensic context by stating that 'available scientific and clinical evidence does not allow accurate, inaccurate and fabricated memories to be distinguished in the absence of independent corroboration'. A report by the British Psychological Society (1995) follows similar cautious lines.

However, Boland et al. (1994) argue that research supports the existence of amnesia of childhood sexual abuse. They cite a case where a 39-year-old man began to have memories of sexual abuse by a priest. At the time of reporting, 130 other victims had filed legal action against this priest who was sentenced to 18–20 years' imprisonment. Without reforms of the law, prosecuting such cases is difficult. The risk is that courts are closed to adult survivors of sexual abuse and persistent offenders are unpunished and continue to harm others.

Guidance from case law is sparse in this area, and what little there is comes from US, Canadian, or Australian cases. Freckelton (1996) reviews case law in relation to admissibility of evidence that has been assisted or recovered by psychotherapeutic intervention. Two categories of evidence have been distinguished in North American cases where the complainant recovers 'repressed memories':

(i)    where the complainant concedes that he or she has always known and remembered the sexual assaults, but says that he or she was unaware that other physical or psychological problems were caused by the abuse;

(ii)   where the plaintiff claims that, for a long while, because of the traumatic experience, he or she had no recollection of the abuse (*Mary D* v *John D* 1989; *KM* v *HM* 1992).

In *Longman* v *The Queen* (1989, High Court of Australia) an 'imperative' warning was given concerning a long delay in reporting a sexual assault:

As the evidence of the complainant could not be adequately tested after the passage of more than twenty years, it would be dangerous to convict on that evidence alone unless the jury, scrutinizing the evidence with great care, considering the circumstances relevant to its evaluation and paying heed to the warnings, were satisfied of its truth and accuracy.

In *R.* v *Norman* (1993) the Court of Appeal of Ontario expressed grave concerns that a therapeutically orientated memory retrieval process may not elicit, 'real memories of what actually occurred. In either case the patient is convinced of the truth of what he or she is recalling. Honesty of recall is not a factor; the concern is instead the reliability of the recall'. Where a witness has the appearance of honesty and integrity this may lead to undue weight being placed on this testimony. The court in this case held that such a situation may lead to an error in verdict.

Guidelines have been given on the admissibility of memories (of sexual abuse as well as other situations) recovered whilst under hypnosis, and these will be discussed in a separate section below.

From a clinical point of view, the management of a patient who discloses sexual abuse many years ago can be difficult if the revelations in therapy become the basis on which to press charges. Winbolt (1995) warns against two types of circumstances which may lead to unreliable evidence:

(i)    where the client says they think they might have been abused and the therapist or investigator accepts this as a fact without question;

(ii)   where a therapist suggests memories of abuse with no prior mention of the fact by the client.

Winbolt advises against any systematic attempts to persuade, and urges that psychotherapists do not encourage clients to engage in legal action. Even answering questions posed by the client about possible legal action should take into account the warnings about the accuracy of uncorroborated recovered memories. Comprehensive records (as ever) are invaluable, as is an awareness of the different demands and processes of the therapeutic and legal contexts in dealing with such allegations.

## Hypnotically refreshed memories

In a recent Californian case reported by Katz (1996), a 57-year-old man was convicted of murder and sentenced to life imprisonment in 1990. One of his daughters
testified that she remembered her father molesting and killing her friend 20 years
earlier, that this memory had become suppressed, and had only been recovered
recently. The Appellate Court quashed the conviction on the grounds that both
daughters were hypnotised prior to giving evidence. Under Californian law, such
evidence is considered unreliable, and therefore inadmissible. This case perhaps
illustrates the difficulties faced by legal systems in dealing with recovered memories. As with memories recovered during psychotherapy, the risk is that episodes of
abuse are not believed and that perpetrators go unpunished. On the other hand,
the effects on the accused of ill founded allegations can be devastating, leading on
occasions to suicide.

A defendant's right to testify on his own behalf may at times involve the use of
hypnotically refreshed memory. In some States of the US, rules prohibit the use of
such testimony on the grounds that it is unreliable. In *Rock* v *Arkansas* (1987), the
Supreme Court acknowledged that hypnosis may produce 'inaccurate memories
because the subject becomes suggestible and may try to please the hypnotist with
answers he thinks will meet with approval, and because the subject is likely to confabulate or fill the memory gaps with imagined details in order to make an answer
more coherent and complete'. The trial court also noted that the subject may experience 'memory hardening', which gives him great confidence in both true and false
memories. This makes the testing of evidence difficult in cross-examination.

However, it was held that hypnotically refreshed testimony is not inadmissible
per se. The Supreme Court stated that hypnosis had gained credit as a valid means
of retrieving memories in investigations. It also added the proviso that, with safeguards, the artefactual inaccuracies may be reduced. Further, all the traditional
means of testing the evidence would still apply, including cross-examination and
seeking corroborating evidence. It was also advised that the jury be educated to
the risks of hypnosis, and that where the trier of fact is a jury, a cautionary instruction should be given regarding potential unreliability of such testimony. With all
this in mind, it is for the courts dealing with individual cases to decide on the
admissibility of hypnotically refreshed memory, rather than a matter for general
exclusion.

The procedural safeguards designed to reduce inaccuracies include:
(i)     preservation of the defendant's prehypnotic recollection;
(ii)    recording the hypnotic session;
(iii)   conduct of the procedure by a qualified and independent practitioner;
(iv)    a neutral setting with no one else present.

Following these guidelines the court is in a position to decide on whether any undue suggestion took place, and to what extent the testimony is reliable.

At the time of writing, English courts have not yet dealt with this issue. It is possible however, that they would be aware of the ruling in the Canadian case, *R. v Pitt* (1968). The accused was charged with the attempted murder of her husband. It was accepted that the defendant had been heard to say 'Call the police, call an ambulance,' at the material time. The prosecution claimed that the accused had struck her husband with a hammer. The defendant testified on her own behalf, but could remember little. Her counsel applied for her to be hypnotized, in order to help her recollect events surrounding this incident. The court heard evidence from two psychiatrists that the defendant had a 'functional amnesia' relating to the material time, and that, 'to the medical profession, hypnosis is regarded as a useful and efficacious way to bring back to conscious recollection those events which had been forgotten'. In ruling on this case, the British Columbia Supreme Court stated that the accused should be allowed to give testimony following hypnosis. The exact procedure was approved: a psychiatrist would hypnotize the defendant in front of the jury. He would then ask her, while in the hypnotic trance, to remember everything she could about the period in question. She would then be brought out of the trance and testify to the jury. It was made clear that she should not testify whilst under hypnotic trance.

## Fitness to stand trial

A factor of basic importance in determining a defendant's capacity to stand trial is the defendant's mental ability to render to his counsel such assistance as is necessary to form a proper defence. All cases to date recognize that a defendant's amnesia does not in itself render him incapable of standing trial, of receiving a fair trial, or of assisting his counsel in the defence of his case. If the defendant is mentally alert enough, despite the amnesia, to advise his counsel whether the 'broad outline' of the defence was, or was not correct, then he is fit, in this regard.

In itself, amnesia does not raise the issue of fitness to stand trial. Arguments were put forward in the report of the Butler Committee that where a person has no recollection of the events charged against him, he is seriously handicapped in instructing counsel (Home Office/Department of Health and Social Security, 1975). Against this, it is recognized that other situations give rise to missing evidence or testimony, for example, failure to trace an essential witness, or loss of documents or a diary recording relevant information. In this sense, the defendant's memory is considered as another witness, a useful area of evidence, but not one without which the trial cannot proceed.

The Butler Committee explored the further possibility of bringing amnesia within the meaning of 'mental disorder', and thus allowing memory loss in itself to become a reason for being under disability. The majority conclusion was that:

The lack of memory can be caused by forgetfulness, by hysterical dissociation, or by concussion (whether or not connected with the circumstances of the offence). This has not hitherto been within the concept underlying the tests of unfitness to stand trial, and ought not to be brought within it by giving too literal a meaning to the criteria . . . (para 10.6).

In the minority argument against this approach, it was acknowledged that 'mere forgetfulness' should indeed never entitle someone to be regarded as 'under disability'. The view was that only amnesia caused by severe mental disorder (excluding hysterical dissociation where it is the only evidence of mental disorder) should qualify as a criterion for unfitness to plead. It was also held by the minority, that:

it is inconsistent to concede on the one hand, that conditions such as severe subnormality, deaf mutism, psychosis, or depression may render a person unable to conduct a proper defence, and on the other to maintain that complete loss of memory can *never* render anyone unable to conduct a proper defence (para. 10.8).

The prevailing lines of reasoning maintained to the present time have excluded memory loss for the offence as a sole reason to be found under disability. People found to be under disability are usually suffering from a severe mental disorder, and since the enactment of the Criminal Procedure (Insanity and Unfitness to Plead) Act 1991, courts in England and Wales have had a flexibility in dealing with people found unfit to plead that was not available at the time of the 'Butler report'.

A common objection to the claim that amnesia should be a to bar to trial is the perception by the courts that memory loss can be easily feigned. Although in some cases medical history, examination, investigations and psychometry may support the defendant's claim to amnesia, it is usually the case that a psychologist or psychiatrist will be unable to give a definitive conclusion. There is concern that allowing amnesia to bar trial would result in an 'opening of floodgates' to such cases, where there might be an easy route to avoid justice by malingering memory loss.

In any discussion of fitness to plead and amnesia, the case of *R* v *Podola* (1959) is central. It remains the authority in this area and to date, has not been successfully challenged in an English court. Gunther Podola was charged with murdering a police officer. At the time of trial he claimed complete amnesia for the time in question and his defence counsel argued that as a result, he could not give instructions to his counsel and was therefore unfit to plead. All the psychiatric reports excluded an organic cause of amnesia, and concluded that he suffered a hysterical amnesia. The jury were asked to decide whether they believed the amnesia to be genuine, and they decided it was not. The trial proceeded and Podola was convicted. He did not appeal but the Court of Criminal Appeal heard the case after it was referred by the Home Secretary. The rulings of the Court of Appeal can be summarized as follows.

(i)    Whenever the court is faced with a defendant whose fitness to plead is raised as an issue, the jury must be directed to consider the whole of the evidence and answer the question 'Are you satisfied on that evidence that the accused is insane so that he cannot be tried on the indictment?'. The jury would, in the case of amnesia, have to conclude that memory loss amounted to insanity. According to the criteria laid down in *R v Pritchard* (1836), amnesia would have to amount to a deficit that would make the accused not of 'sufficient intellect to comprehend the course and proceedings of the trial so as to make a proper defence'. In *Podola*, both the 'insanity' and 'intellect' arguments for amnesia were rejected.

(ii)   The burden of proof in a case of fitness to plead, if it is contested, is on the defence if they raised it ('on balance of probabilities'), or on the prosecution if they raised it ('beyond reasonable doubt').

(iii)  Although amnesia does not render the accused unfit to stand trial, a trial judge should 'point out to the jury that they must take into consideration carefully the fact that the accused cannot remember the events'.

Amnesia can be an indicator of underlying mental disorder. Where such a mental disorder is of a degree that would fulfil the legal criteria for being under disability, it is the mental disorder rather than the amnesia alone which allows the court to find the defendant unfit to plead.

## Memory loss and criminal responsibility

Legal mental capacity to commit a crime is an essential requisite to criminal responsibility. The general rule has been that amnesia, in itself, is no defence to a criminal charge. The fact that a defendant is subsequently unable to remember the crime is in itself no proof of his mental condition when the crime was carried out.

It is common in forensic psychiatry to come across individuals facing serious charges for which they have little or no memory of the alleged events. North American studies have found reports of amnesia in 10 to 70% of homicide cases (Bradford & Smith, 1979; Schachter, 1986; Parwatikar et al., 1985), whilst UK studies have found amnesia in between half and a third of defendants facing serious charges (Taylor & Kopelman, 1984; Kopelman, 1987). Factors involved included alcohol intoxication and high emotional arousal at the time of the crime (Bradford & Smith, 1979), depressed mood (Parwatikar et al., 1985) and the violent nature of the offence (Taylor & Kopelman, 1984).

## Automatism

Amnesia can be an indicator of an episode of automatic functioning. The legal significance of automatism is that it can lead to the acquittal of a sane defendant.

An example of sane automatism with amnesia is the case of *R.* v *Quick* (1973). The defendant, a nurse in a mental hospital, faced charges of assaulting a patient. The defendant claimed that he was suffering from hypoglycaemia at the time for which there was medical evidence. Whilst experiencing the effects of hypoglycaemia, it would be argued that his behaviour was automatic, and that he therefore lacked the necessary *mens rea*. The defence argued that an acquittal should be the outcome.

However, the defendant pleaded guilty when the trial judge ruled that he may be found insane, for which the only disposal at the time was a hospital order with restrictions without limit of time. After pleading guilty he appealed. The Appeal Court ruled that the trial judge should have allowed a defence of sane automatism to be open to the appellant, and his conviction was quashed.

## Intoxication

Amnesia for a criminal act may be as a result of intoxication, but again, the memory loss in itself does not amount to a defence. The rules on intoxication are complex but in essence centre on the issue of voluntary and involuntary intoxication. The general principle has been held that voluntary drunkenness is no excuse for crime.

In the case of *R* v *Kingston* (1993), the appellant had been convicted of indecent assault on a 15-year-old boy. He admitted to paedophilic homosexual tendencies, and together with another man P, lured the victim to P's flat. The boy was given cannabis and a seemingly innocuous drink which was in fact laced with a sedative. The boy fell asleep and whilst in this condition the appellant was invited to sexually abuse him. This activity was audiotaped by P for the purposes of blackmailing the appellant. The appellant's defence was that his drink had also been laced with a sedative. His evidence for this was that he had seen the boy lying asleep, but had no further recollection for any events that night until waking up at home the following morning. The trial judge directed the jury to acquit the appellant if they found that due to intoxication with drugs he did not intend or may not have intended to commit an indecent assault. The appellant was convicted. On appeal it was held that, although there was no doubt that the appellant committed the *actus reus* of an indecent assault, there was evidence that could allow a defence of involuntary intoxication. The trial judge had withdrawn this issue from the jury, which amounted to a misdirection, and the conviction was therefore quashed. This case illustrates that although amnesia did not form the central focus of legal debate, its presence was a crucial sign of involuntary intoxication that allowed the appeal to succeed.

## Absent-mindedness

A situation of memory failure that may amount to a lack of intent to carry out the offence is the 'absent-minded' shoplifter. Harper (1994) describes a case report where the defendant claimed to have no memory of taking the items found in her possession. The psychological formulation concluded that the defendant was preoccupied with stressful events, had depressive symptoms and was concentrating poorly. Similar cases have been allowed as a defence, where the cognitive deficit was believed to be genuine, and the absent-mindedness clearly related to the act in question (R v Clarke, 1972; R v Ingram, 1975).

### Forgotten possession

Most crimes are committed over a relatively short period of time. Criminal possession is an example of a continuing offence – so that the illegal action may continue for days or years without abatement. This would mean that, although the defendant would have at some stage knowingly commenced this offence, if he subsequently experienced loss of memory for the continuing offence, his *mens rea* could arguably be affected. Mahoney (1989) debates this issue in an 'unashamedly academic' context. Three cases highlight the legal thinking in this area.

In R v Russell (1984) the appellant was convicted of possession of an offensive weapon following discovery of a knife and a cosh in his car during a police search. He was acquitted of possession of the knife but convicted on the count involving the cosh. His claim at trial was that although he admitted to placing the cosh in his car, he had completely forgotten about it. On appeal, it was ruled that the judge had failed to direct the jury that the onus was on the prosecution that the appellant had the cosh on him 'knowingly'. The Appeal Court stated that 'it would be wrong to hold that a man knowingly has a weapon with him if his forgetfulness of its existence is so complete as to amount to ignorance that it is there at all'. The conviction was quashed but it was recognized by the court that juries would rarely accept such a defence. Indeed, this 'gosh a cosh!' defence was criticized and has not been generally followed.

The ruling in R v Buswell (1972) is more usually followed. In R. v Martindale (1986) an application for appeal against a conviction of unlawful possession of cannabis was made. The applicant's claim was that he had forgotten about the cannabis and therefore possession did not exist in the absence of knowledge of its presence. In turning down his leave to appeal it was stated that 'possession did not depend on the powers of memory of the alleged possessor and did not come and go as memory revived and faded'.

### Forgotten knowledge

A similar ruling was held in different circumstances in R v Bello (1978). In this case a Nigerian man was convicted with overstaying his 6 months' limited leave under the 1971 Immigration Act. Whilst in England he received a letter from Nigeria notifying him of his mother's death. His defence was to be that as a result of his mother's death his memory had been 'destroyed', so that he could not deal with business affairs for a long period. It was contended that having forgotten that he was in this country beyond the expiry of his permit he did not knowingly remain. The trial judge acceded to the prosecution's claim that this was no defence. In dismissing his application for leave to appeal, the Court of Appeal ruled that:

A man cannot plead that he did something unknowingly if he had the capacity for reviving the recollection of that event from his memory. A man can do an act knowingly even though at the moment he does it the relevant fact is not in his mind. If he has the capacity to restore that fact to his mind, then on the face of it we have thought that the requirement of 'knowingly' is satisfied.

The ruling quoted Glanville Williams' discussion of 'forgotten knowledge' (Williams, 1961) which surmised that: 'to have knowledge of an event is not the same as to be thinking about it. Probably the test is: Was the defendant capable of recalling the fact at the moment in question, if he had addressed his mind to it?' (p. 170). This, on the face of it would allow any genuine amnesia to qualify as 'lack of knowledge'.

## Competence in decision making

Criminal proceedings involving people with memory disorders are likely to be relatively uncommon. The legal issues that are more likely to arise are those that concern decision making about personal, civil matters in everyday life. The Law Commission, which is responsible for reviewing, and proposing changes to, complex areas of the law, has conducted a thorough appraisal of this field and published four consultation papers and a subsequent report (Law Commission 1991, 1993a, b, c, 1995). A wide variety of conditions may lead to mental incapacity in relation to decision making. Most commonly those concerned will be the elderly and those with learning disabilities, but other specific disorders leading to memory impairment may also be important.

As noted in the most recent of these documents, the Law Commission's report *Mental Incapacity* (1995), there is a need to specify clearly how decisions may lawfully be made on behalf of those who cannot make decisions for themselves. Public authorities may also need legal powers to intervene and protect people at risk of abuse or neglect.

The review by the Law Commission arose out of a recognition that existing law is deficient, and in particular, the case of *Re F* demonstrated how English law had no procedure enabling another person or a court to take a medical decision on behalf of an adult incapacitated patient.

The Law Commission proposed the introduction of a single piece of new legislation to make provision for people lacking mental capacity, and to give new functions to local authorities in relation to those needing care or protection. The Commission suggested a new definition and specific criteria of mental incapacity, relating to decision making abilities. One of the proposed criteria is as follows:

> . . . A person should be regarded as unable to make a decision by reason of mental disability if the disability is such that, at the time when the decision needs to be made, he or she is unable to understand or retain the information relevant to the decision, including information about the reasonably foreseeable consequences of deciding one way or another, or failing to make the decision (Draft Bill, clause 2(2)(a)).

At present those who are incapable of managing their property and financial affairs may have authority for substitute decision making transferred to members of their family, other individuals, or the Court of Protection. Before the onset of the incapacity it is also possible to delegate authority for financial decision making by using an enduring power of attorney. The Law Commission has argued for a clearer and more extended jurisdiction to enable decisions and orders to be made relating to the welfare of incapacitated adults and the management of their finances (Law Commission, 1993a). It also proposed the extension of this new jurisdiction to enable substitute decisions to be made about medical treatment (Law Commission, 1993b).

## Assessments for court reports

Clinical reports prepared for legal proceedings need to be written with meticulous care in order to be credible and effective. A good general guide to writing court reports and giving evidence in court is given by Bluglass (1995).

In cases where the evaluation involves a disorder of memory it will normally be appropriate for the party requesting the assessment to instruct both a clinical psychologist and a psychiatrist to provide individual reports. Clinicians preparing reports should expect clear instructions that outline the relevant legal matters, and should also expect to receive a full set of documentation about the case.

A report should list the sources on which it is based, and the account of the patient's background history should be clear, concise and objective. The description of the investigations and tests that have been carried out should summarize their purpose and the results in a way that is understandable to lay people. Technical terms, where used, should be explained. It is particularly important to describe psychological impairments and disabilities in a way that enables the lay reader to grasp their nature, their practical effects, and how they compare with the normal range of ability and functioning. Where the report is prepared to assist in determining claims for damages in personal injury cases, the effects of the impairments on personal functioning and prognosis are especially relevant. In such cases, factors taken into account in assessing psychiatric damage include: the individual's ability to cope with work, effects on family relationships, the prospects for successful treatment, future vulnerability, the extent of associated physical injuries and whether medical help has been sought (Judicial Studies Board, 1992).

Inferences drawn from clinical findings must be soundly substantiated, and the reasons for all conclusions – both positive and negative – in the report must be given. The clinician may reach firm opinions on some questions, but more qualified and uncertain opinions on others. It is therefore important to convey the degree of confidence with which an opinion on a particular matter is expressed. In both written and oral evidence, the professional or expert witness should not allow him or herself to be pushed into expressing a view with more certainty than is warranted, nor an opinion that goes beyond what is clinically accurate, however strong the pressure to do so from the court or lawyer.

Finally, it should be noted that, at the time of writing (May 1999), new 'Civil Procedure Rules' for the conduct of civil litigation cases in England and Wales are being introduced, and clinicians who are engaged as Expert Witnesses should ensure that they are fully appraised of the new arrangements.

## REFERENCES

American Psychiatric Association (1993). *Statement on Memories of Sexual Abuse*, adopted by the Board of Trustees of the APA, 12 December 1993, p.2.

Australian Psychological Society (1995). *Guidelines Relating to the Reporting of Recovered Memories*. Bulletin of the Australian Psychological Society. February 1995, 20–1.

Boland, P.L., Quirk, S.A. & Loftus, E.F. (1994). Repressed memories. *American Bar Association Journal* (Sep): 42–3.

Bluglass, R. (1995). Writing reports and giving evidence. In *Seminars in Practical Forensic Psychiatry*, ed. D. Chiswick & R. Cope. London: Gaskell (Royal College of Psychiatrists).

Bradford, J.McD.W. & Smith, S.M. (1979). Amnesia and homicide: the Podola case and a study of thirty cases. *Bulletin of the American Academy of Psychiatry and the Law*, 7, 219–31.

British Psychological Society (1995). *Recovered Memories: The Report of the Working Party of the British Psychological Society*. Leicester: The British Psychological Society.

Clare, I.C.H. & Gudjonnson, G.H. (1992). *Devising and Piloting an Experimental Version of the 'Notice to Detained Persons'*. The Royal Commission on Criminal Justice: Research Study No. 7. London: HMSO.

Freckleton, I. (1996). Repressed memory syndrome: counterintuitive or counterproductive? *Criminal Law Journal*, **20**, 7–34.

Gudjonsson, G.H. (1987). A parallel form of the Gudjonsson suggestibility scale. *British Journal of Clinical Psychology*, **26**, 215–21.

Gudjonsson, G.H. (1988). The relationship of intelligence and memory to interrogative suggestibility: the importance of range effects. *British Journal of Clinical Psychology*, 27, 185–7.

Gudjonsson, G.H. (1992). *The Psychology of Interrogations, Confessions and Testimony.* Chichester, UK: John Wiley.

Gudjonsson, G.H. & Mackeith, J.A.C. (1982). False confessions. Psychological effects of interrogation: a discussion paper. In *Reconstructing The Past: The Role of the Psychologist in Criminal Trials*, ed. A. Trankell, pp. 253–69. Stockholm: P.A. Norstedt and Söners Förlag.

Gudjonsson, G.H. & Mackeith, J.A.C. (1988). Retracted confessions: legal psychological and psychiatric aspects. *Medicine, Science and the Law*, **28**, 187–94.

Gudjonsson, G.H. & Lebegue, B. (1989). Psychological and psychiatric aspects of a coerced-internalised false confession. *Journal of the Forensic Science Society*, **29**, 261–9.

Harper, D.J. (1994). Absent-mindedness and shoplifting – a case study. *Medicine, Science and the Law*, **34**, 74–7.

Hollins, S., Clare, I.C.H. & Webb, B. (1996a). *You're under Arrest.* London: Gaskell (Royal College of Psychiatrists).

Hollins, S., Clare, I.C.H. & Webb, B. (1996b). *You're on Trial.* London: Gaskell (Royal College of Psychiatrists).

Home Office/Department of Health and Social Security (1975). *Report of the Committee on Mentally Abnormal Offenders.* Cmnd.6244. London: HMSO.

Judicial Studies Board (1992). *Guidelines for the Assessment of General Damages in Personal Injury Cases.* London: Blackstone Press.

Katz, I. (1996). Recovered memory evidence dealt a blow as father is released. *The Guardian*, p.14, Saturday July 6.

Kopelman, M.D. (1987). Crime and amnesia: a review. *Behavioural Sciences and the Law*, **5**, 323–42.

Law Commission (1991). *Mentally Incapacitated Adults and Decision-Making: An Overview.* Consultation Paper No. 119. London: HMSO.

Law Commission (1993a). *Mentally Incapacitated Adults and Decision-Making: A New Jurisdiction.* Consultation Paper No. 128. London: HMSO.

Law Commission (1993b). *Mentally Incapacitated Adults and Decision-Making: Medical Treatment and Research.* Consultation Paper No. 129. London: HMSO.

Law Commission (1993c). *Mentally Incapacitated Adults and Other Vulnerable Adults: Public Law Protection.* Consultation Paper No. 130. London: HMSO.

Law Commission (1995). *Mental Incapacity*, Law Com No. 231. London: HMSO.

Loftus, E.F. (1979). *Eyewitness Testimony.* Cambridge, MA: Harvard University Press.

Mahoney, R. (1989). Memory and mens rea: the defence of forgotten possession. *Criminal Law Quarterly*, **32**,16–69.

Ofshe, R. (1991). Coercive persuasion and attitude change. In *The Encyclopaedia of Sociology*, vol. 1, ed. E. Borgatta and M. Borgalla, pp. 212–24. Macmillan: New York.

Parwatikar, S.D., Holcomb, W.R. & Menninger, K.A. (1985). The detection of malingered amnesia in accused murderers. *Bulletin of the American Academy of Psychiatry and the Law*, **13**, 97–103.

Schachter, D.L. (1986). On the relation between genuine and simulated amnesia. *Behavioural Sciences and the Law*, **4**, 47–64.

Seabrooke, S. & Sprack, J. (1996). *Criminal Evidence and Procedure: The Statutory Framework.* London: Blackstone Press.

Sharrock, R. & Gudjonsson, G.H. (1993). Intelligence, previous convictions and interrogative suggestibility: a path analysis of alleged false-confession cases. *British Journal of Clinical Psychology*, **32**, 169–75.

Singh, K.K. & Gudjonsson, G.H. (1984). Interrogative suggestibility, delayed memory and self-concept. *Personality and Individual Differences*, **5**, 203–9.

Taylor, P.J. & Kopelman, M.D. (1984). Amnesia for criminal offences. *Psychological Medicine*, **14**, 581–8.

Weingardt, K.R., Toland, H.K. & Loftus, E.F (1994). Reports of suggested memories: do people truly believe them? In *Adult Eyewitness Testimony. Current Trends and Developments*, ed. D.F. Ross, J.D. Read & M.P. Toglia. Cambridge: Cambridge University Press.

Williams, G. (1961). *Criminal Law, The General Part*, 2nd edn. London: Stevens & Sons.

Winbolt, B. (1995). False memory syndrome – an issue clouded by emotion. *Medicine, Science and the Law*, **36**, 100–9.

Zander, M. (1995). *The Police and Criminal Evidence Act 1984*, 3rd edn. London: Sweet & Maxwell.

Zaragoza, M.S. & Koshmider, J.W.III. (1989). Misled subjects may know more than their performance implies. *Journal of Experimental Psychology, Learning, Memory and Cognition*, **15**, 246–55.

# Appendix

## Legal cases
*KM* v *HM* [1992] 96 DLR (4th) 289
*Longman* v *The Queen* [1989] 168 CLR 79
*Mary D* v *John D* [1989] 264 Cal Rptr 633
*Pearson's case* [1835] 2 Lew CC 144
*R* v *Bello* [1978] 67 Cr App R 288, CA
*R* v *Buswell* [1972] 1 WLR 64
*R* v *Clarke* [1972] Crim App 56, 225
*R* v *Ingram* [1975] Crim Law Rev 457
*R* v *Kingston* [1993] 4 All ER 373
*R* v *Martindale* [1986] 1 WLR 1042
*R* v *Norman* [1993] 87 CCC (3rd) 153
*R* v *Pitt* [1967] 68 DLR (2nd) 513
*R* v *Podola* [1959] 3 All ER 418
*R* v *Pritchard* [1836] 173 ER 135
*R* v *Quick* [1973] 3 WLR 26
*R* v *Russell* [1984] 81 Cr App R 315, CA
*R* v *Telford JJ, ex parte Badham* [1991] 2 QB 78
*Re F (mental patient sterilization)* [1990] II AC I
*Rock* v *Arkansas* 97 L Ed 2nd 37 [1987], cited in 77 ALR 4th 927
*Stubbings* v *Webb* [1993] AC 498

## Key to legal references
2 Lew CC      *Lewin's Crown Cases Reserved* (168 ER) 1822–38
AC            *Law Reports, Appeal Cases*

| | |
|---|---|
| All ER | *The All England Law Reports* |
| ALR 4th | *American Law Reports Annotated, 4th series* |
| DLR (4th) | *Dominion Law Reports, 4th series* |
| Cal Reptr | *California Reporter (West)* |
| CCC (3rd) | *Canadian Criminal Cases, 3rd series* |
| CLR | *Comonwealth Law Reports* |
| Cr App R (CA) | *Criminal Appeal Reports (Court of Appeal)* |
| Crim App | *Criminal Appeal Reports* |
| Crim Law Rev | *Criminal Law Review* |
| DLR | *Dominion Law Reports* |
| ER | *English Reports* |
| L Ed (2nd) | *Lawyers Edition, United States Supreme Court Reports, 2nd series* |
| QB | *Law Reports, Queen's Bench Division* |
| WLR | *Weekly Law Reports* |

# Notes

## Chapter 1

1 Equally anachronistic and/or inaccurate are claims that it was the 'English surgeon Robert Dunn' who started it all (Levin et al., 1983) or that 'autobiographical memory' was not discussed before Galton and Freud (Robinson, 1986).

2 Complex discussions on memory can be found, for example, in the 'faculty of the mind' literature (Janet & Sailles, 1902; Mill, 1869; Hamilton, 1859; Bain, 1864; Garnier, 1852; Spencer, 1890).

3 In spite of this, 'organic' accounts of memory deficits were not altogether neglected; see, for example, nineteenth-century work attempting to explain amnesia (retrograde and anterograde), dysmnesia, and paramnesia (Louyer-Willermay, 1819; Bouillaud, 1829; Falret, 1865. During the second half of the nineteenth century these terms also named all manner of memory disorders including 'confabulation', 'déjà vu', 'delusions of memory' (Berrios, 1995), and memory disorders in the insanities (Baret, 1887).

4 There is a large primary and secondary literature on the history of memory (e.g. Young, 1961; Herrmann & Chaffin, 1988). This includes work on the 'Art of memory' or 'Mnemonics' which 'in the not too distant past held pride of place in the councils of learning . . .' (Hutton, 1987: p. 371). Mnemonics, of great relevance to clinical practice, have been superbly studied by the late Francis Yates (1966) and will not be mentioned further here.

5 For example, Aristotle claimed that memory 'is always accompanied by the notion of time' (Sorabji, 1972).

6 On this see, for example, Callinicos, 1995; Neisser and Fivush, 1994; Tannen, 1993; Bruner, 1990; White, 1987.

7 in *Theogony* 54, 15, for example, is mentioned Mnemosyne (memory) a daughter of Uranus and one of the *Titanides*. In her, Zeus fathered all the muses (for further information see Smith, 1870: p. 1106).

8 'First we must comprehend what sort of things are objects of memory; for mistakes are frequent on this point. It is impossible to remember the future, which is object of conjecture or expectation; nor is there memory of the present, but only conception; for it is neither the future nor the past that we cognize by perception, but only the present. But memory is of the past; no one could claim to remember the present while it is present' (Aristotle, 1908: p. 289) . . . 'memory is neither sensation nor judgement, but is a state or affection of one of these, when time has elapsed' . . . 'all memory, then implies a lapse of time' . . . 'hence only these

living creatures which are conscious of time can be said to remember . . .' (Aristotle, 1908: p. 291).

9  'Recollecting (anamnesis) differs from remembering (*mneme*) not merely in the matter of time, but also because while other animals share in memory (*mneme*), one may say that none of the known animals can recollect (*anamnesis*) except man. This is because recollecting is, as it were, a kind of inference (*sylogismos*) . . .' (Aristotle, 1908: p. 311).

10 see, for example, the explanation of the 'sentiment of pre-existence' (déjà vu) in Wigan, 1844: p. 84).

11 'Moreover, the memory contains the innumerable principles and laws of numbers and dimensions. None of them has been impressed on memory through any bodily sense-perception . . .' (Saint Augustine, 1992: p. 190); 'Note also that I am drawing on my memory when I say there are four perturbations of the mind – cupidity, gladness, fear, sadness and from memory I produce whatever I say in discussing them . . . Yet none of these perturbations disturbs me when by act of recollection I remember them. And even before I recalled and reconsidered them, *they were there*' (Saint Augustine, 1992: pp. 191–192).

12 'Attention and repetition help much to the fixing any ideas in the memory. But those which naturally at first make the deepest and most lasting impressions, are those which are accompanied with pleasure or pain' (Locke, 1959: p. 194, Book II, Chapter X) . . . 'The pictures drawn in our minds are laid in fading colours; and if not sometimes refreshed, vanish and disappear. How much the constitution of our bodies (and the make of our animal spirits) are concerned in this; and whether the temper of the brain makes this difference . . . I shall not inquire here' (Locke, 1959: p. 196, Book II, Chapter X).

13 Pierre Laromiguière (1756–1837) provided the transition between Condillac, the Idéologues, and nineteenth-century French philosophy. A fine teacher, it is said that he counted Esquirol amongst his disciples. As opposed to his teacher Condillac, he conceived of the subject as an active entity.

14 Pierre-Paul Royer-Collard (1763–1845), brother of Athanasius Royer-Collard, the great French physician and alienist, was a politician, historian and one time philosopher considered as an important divulgator of the views of Thomas Reid.

15 in Louyer-Willermay, 1819: p. 321. Around the time of Ribot, authors also commented on the fact that his 'law of regression' only applied to cases of progressive dementia and not to post-traumatic 'retrograde' amnesia (Mairet & Piéron, 1915).

16 for example, Jackson stated: 'we would usually say that in failing memory old events (or strictly the most organised) are remembered, and recent (the least organized) are forgotten. This is not without a very obvious qualification: it would be better to say that recent events are soon forgotten.', in Jackson, 1931: p. 305 (footnote), Vol 1. A follower of Jackson, at the very end of the century, however, was still emphasizing that memory was 'a mode of consciousness' and that 'our primary knowledge of memory is obtained by means of introspection' (Ross, 1891: p. 35).

17 Ribot pre-published most of these ideas in *Revue Philosophique*, his own journal (e.g. Ribot, 1880) (see also Gasser, 1988).

18 On Semon's theory, see the classical dissertation by Schatzmann (1968) and Schacter et al. (1978).

19  There was also the question of whether such emotion would be the same or a different one. For an excellent historical analysis of this problem, and of the contribution of Ribot and his group see: Meletti, 1991: pp. 387–454.

20  An active writer in the early twentieth century, he fought for the use of the notion of time (duration) as a category of understanding in the natural and social sciences and in subjectivity itself (Bergson, 1914) (see also Chevalier, 1928).

21  For a good analysis, see: Sollier, 1892; Kay, 1902. Jackson's concept of 'dissolution' was influential at the time: Ross, 1891; Delay, 1942; Ey, 1950; Walser, 1974.

22  On the quantification of psychological events see Boring, 1942; 1950; 1961; Zupan, 1976; Cattell, 1890; on the measurement of dementia see Jaspers, 1910.

23  His notion of 'understanding' (*Verstehen*) influenced Jaspers (Berrios, 1992a; Walker, 1988) and is very important in psychiatry.

24  Born in Lyon on 10th October 1876, Blondel had a brilliant academic career. He studied at *l'École Normale Supérieure* becoming *agrége* in philosophy in 1900, *pensionnaire* de la Fondation Thiers in 1901, doctor of medicine in 1906 and of letters in 1914. He trained as a psychiatrist under G. Deny (one of the most imaginative alienists of the period) and J. Dejerine, taking from the former his independent and heterodox attitude. A follower of Durkheim, Bergson, and Levi-Bruhl, he wrote on psychopathology, schizophrenia, suicide, intelligence, history of psychiatry (e.g. Gall), etc. (for more biographical details see Courbon, 1939; Gilson, 1940)

25  Maurice Halbwachs was born at Reims in 1877 and brought up in Paris. After schooling at the Lycée Henri IV, (where Bergson was teaching at the time!) he attended *l'École Normale Supérieure* and started a career in philosophy spending some years in Germany working on the Leibniz archives. He then retrained as a sociologist and became a follower of Durkheim. In 1919 he became a professor at Strasbourg, then la Sorbonne and the Collège de France. In 1944 he was taken to a concentration camp and it is unclear whether he died in 1944 or 1945. Halbwachs wrote on suicide, the social frames of memory, and technical work on social class, social morphology, etc. (for more information see Coser, 1992; Anonymous, 1946)

26  Indeed, this was acknowledged by Bloch (1925) in a review, and Blondel in his South America Lectures of 1926 (Blondel, 1928a) and also in an unstinting review (Blondel, 1926).

27  On the deep question of 'social memory in history' see Burke (1989); Le Goff (1992); Hutton (1993).

28  This concept has been attacked in Anglo-Saxon social thought, where questions have been asked as to the nature, survival, model of transmission, etc. of such 'external frames' (e.g. Lloyd, 1990; Turner, 1994); for a classical account see Cassirer (1945), also Vovelle (1990); and for a promising model for the 'transmission' of social practices see Sperber (1996).

29  Blondel (1928b) believed that, starting from diverging points, Durkheim, Lévy-Bruhl and Bergson had reached the same conclusion: 'As a result, [Durkheim reached the view that] psychology is, by itself, unable to give a complete account of the development of individual minds. Mental life in its highest form belongs to the realm of sociology'. . . . '[Lévy-Bruhl] had shown that it is impossible to reproduce in our own minds the thoughts of primitive races because the whole life of these people is scored from one end to the other by collective influences' . . . '[According to Bergson], the light of clear consciousness does not enable us to

grasp immediate psychological reality. The latter underlies the former. Clear consciousness only presents to us psychological reality fundamentally modified in its structure by practical necessities, by intelligence, language, and by society' (pp. 27–30).

30  Very much the view researched upon by Treadway et al., 1992 who, however, do not mention Blondel.

31  Situations such as those recently analyzed by Bruner (1994) who neither in this chapter nor in his elegant 'Acts of Meaning' (Bruner, 1990) refers to Blondel or Halbwachs. With few exceptions (e.g. Schachtel, 1947), the reconstructive dimension of self-narratives and 'autobiographical memory' was neglected up to the 1970s when many publications have marked its rediscovery in the Anglo-Saxon literature (e.g. Neisser & Winograd, 1988; Neisser & Fivush, 1994; Rubin, 1986; 1996; Ross, 1991; Conway et al., 1992; Schuman & Scott, 1989; Loftus, 1979). On the historical & conceptual aspects of the reconstructive hypothesis see: Kelley & Jacoby, 1990; Garzón, 1992; Coady, 1992; (also Chapter 18 on 'Functional memory complaints', this volume).

32  On this see Chapter 18 on 'Functional memory complaints', this volume.

33  *L'Évolution de la mémoire et de la notion du temps* has three sections; the second, dedicated to memory, includes ten chapters on memory, narratives, confabulation, déjà vu, anterograde and retrograde amnesia, etc.

34  Lieury (1975) has suggested that on this Janet was influenced by Darwin and Spencer. See also Chapter 16, 'Confabulations', this volume.

35  Before Feuchtersleben, this clinical phenomenon had been described by Dickens (in David Copperfield) and by Wigan (1844). After him, it was increasingly described as a phantom of memory, double perception, diplopie (seeing double in time), error of identification, déjà vécu, déjà éprouvé, false recognition. Dugas (1894b) called it déjà vu at the end of the century (see Berrios, 1995).

36  It is important to remark here that during this period the aphasic disorders were considered by most as a form of memory impairment: see for example, Edridge-Green, 1897: Chapter XII.

37  In English, amnesia can be found in use as early as 1674 (OED, 2nd Edition). Gradual changes in the meaning of amnesia can be traced in successive dictionary entries: e.g. Louyer-Willermay, 1819; Andral, 1829; Fabre, 1840; Bernutz, 1865; Falret, 1865; see also Rouillard, 1888.

38  see, for example, p. 640, in Régis, 1906; p. 52, Claude, 1922; Galtier-Boissière, 1929. The word 'rétroactive', however, is already found in 1865 to refer to loss of information acquired before a brain insult: p. 739, in Falret, 1865. The earliest usage of the word 'anterograde' I have found is Arnaud, 1896: p. 457.

39  On the case Félida see Azam, 1876; also Bourgeois & Geraud, 1990.

40  For example, see Sollier, 1892; Edridge-Green, 1897; Biervliet, 1902; Paulhan, 1904; Piéron, 1910; Offner, 1911; Dugas, 1917.

41  Behr et al. (1985) have suggested that three stages should be distinguished in the history of 'fugue': (a) psychiatric, including the earliest descriptions up to the 1910s, (b) psychopathological, extending up to the Second World War – during which fugues were often considered as 'disorders of psychomotility', and (c) clinico-psychological, stretching to the present and

exploring multifactorial and psychosocial explanations for fugue behaviour. Although these three approaches can be identified, they run parallel and do not constitute successive stages in the evolution of the concept of fugue.

42  See, for example, Bergeron, 1956; Rice & Fisher, 1976; Akhtar & Brenner, 1979; Behr et al., 1985; Riether & Stoudemire, 1988; Loewenstein, 1996; and Chapter 19, 'Dissociative amnesia', this volume.

43  By 'historical convergence' is meant here the process by which word, behaviours and concepts *come together* (in the work of one author or as a result of a collective effort) and a mental symptom is formed. Some convergences prove more stable and it is incumbent upon historians to identify the rules guaranteeing stability. The three components have usually different histories and origins and may have been involved in earlier convergences. *Words* may be neologisms or recycled old terms; *behaviours*, often biologically conditioned, may be surprisingly invariant (and recognizable) across times and cultures; and *concepts*, efforts *to explain* the said behaviours in terms of some medical theory, are changeable elements and hence help *to date* the origin of a convergence unless, as it occasionally happens, the convergence is updated.

44  For a review of cases and ideas before Charcot see Benon and Froissart, 1909.

45  This is well described by Meige (1993). Charcot considered these cases as suffering from neurosis, neurasthenia and degeneration and even identified their physical stigmata. It was said that all spoke German but were polyglots, wore beards, were pale and had high cheekbones, etc. Charcot's stereotyped descriptions can only be understood in the context of the anti-Semitic and anti-German feelings that pervaded France at the time (see Goldstein, 1985). For a good analysis of current French views on *le clochard* and vagabondage in general see Mouren et al., 1978; and for Spanish views on *el vagabundeo* see Vega and Palomo, 1995).

## Chapter 14

1  On Kraepelin's ideas see: Hoff (1995); on the historiographical reasons for differentiating the history of terms, concepts and behaviours see Berrios (1996a).

2  On Sander see: Marková (1997).

3  On this, see Marková and Berrios (1994).

4  On Kahlbaum, see Berrios (1996b).

5  Although James Sully (1842–1923) was well acquainted with the German psychological literature (he spent the year 1867 in Göttingen, and 1871 in Berlin), the only German sources he quotes in his book on illusions are Wundt and Goethe. He based his study on British sources claiming that it was 'Carpenter who first set me seriously to consider the subject of mnemonic error' (p. 230; Sully, 1895). At the time his book appeared, Sully had unsuccessfully applied for a chair in psychology 'to support himself' as his father 'had lost his fortune' and his allowance had been stopped: 'My volume on Illusions appeared just after the futile academic experiments. Amongst others, Wundt wrote to me expressing satisfaction with the book, more especially with the treatment of illusions in the narrower sense along with analogous errors of memory, etc.' (p. 189; Sully, 1918).

6  Sully's assumption was that normal memories were photographic in their accuracy and that spurious ones could be told both on the basis of their phenomenology and mechanisms.

   7  For further details on this behaviour see Berrios (1999b).

   8  In 1886, *Verrücktheit* referred both to mental disorder in general and to 'paranoia' (this latter usage had been just introduced by Krafft Ebing). In this latter meaning, paranoia included those insanities resulting from a primary lesion of the intellect (i.e. delusional disorder by also what nowadays would be called paranoid schizophrenia).

   9  This contrasts with Pick's conceptualisation of memory deceptions as forming the basis of delusions – though the actual phenomena were still clearly different.

  10  This comes close to the type of delusional syndrome that Cotard was reporting around the same time in France (see Berrios & Luque, 1995).

  11  On the important issue of the pre-delusional state and the crystallization of delusions and other symptoms (see Fuentenebro & Berrios, 1995).

  12  The concept of 'apperception', introduced by Leibnitz, became popular in late 19th century psychology and education (see Lange, 1899).

  13  i.e. misidentifying people, places, objects from the present as known in different guises from the past; for a conceptual analysis of these complex phenomena (see Marková & Berrios, 1994).

  14  Röhrenbach and Landis (1995) have suggested that Bonnet (1788) and Kahlbaum (1866) had already reported this type of phenomenon but we have been unable to ascertain this claim.

  15  At the turn of the century, 'presbyophrenia' was a central descriptive and explanatory term for some forms of dementia. For a full account of its current clinical applicability and history (see Berrios 1985, 1986, respectively).

  16  Once again, these descriptions are redolent of what was later to be known as confabulation (see Chapter 16, this volume).

## Chapter 16

   1  On the view that psychological concepts do not have epistemological autonomy and hence cannot be used independently of the frames within which they were first constructed, see Danziger (1997). A good example of a 'discourse formation' can be found in the system of concepts created by Wernicke (1906) to link delusion and confabulation. According to this author, there were *qualitative* (*delusional* interpretation of memories) and *quantitative* falsifications of memory; and the latter were divided into positive or additive (confabulations) and negative or subtractive falsifications. All three forms were related to a pathology of associations (of Sejunction): for example, in confabulation (additive form) there was a disconnection between the recollected experience (whether this was real, imagined or a dream) and time (for more detail on Wernicke's views see Chapter 14, this volume).

   2  This can only be undertaken on the basis of a theory of mental-symptom formation and construction. Such a theory has not been available until recently (see Berrios, 1996).

   3  Translation of Bonhoeffer's term *Verlegenheitskonfabulation*.

   4  Two points are important here. One is, what is the evidence that an 'organically derived amnesia' constitutes a *condition* for the development of the disorder? The other, why should the two 'types' of phenomena described (clinically so different) be considered as members of the *same* class of phenomena (i.e. 'confabulation')? Is there any evidence that they are

generated by the same mechanisms? Burgess and Shallice (1996) seem to believe that they are not: 'we will be concerned primarily with developing a theory to explain the less fantastic type of confabulations: those that are apparently sensible but untrue . . . we will consider the possibility that they correspond to the memory lapses shown in normal people.' (p. 360). Likewise, Schnider et al. (1996a) have suggested that the two types are 'different disorders' rather than 'different degrees of the same disorder'. But if this is confirmed, the clinician may well ask what is the point in keeping a *general* class of confabulations?

5  This runs counter to Talland's stricture that 'fantastic themes' should not be considered.

6  This threatens the conventional rule that mental symptoms are recognized on their specified *intrinsic* features, and that surface ambiguity is resolved by looking for more intrinsic features. In fact the reliability and validity of clinical categories are undermined by the fact that symptom-disambiguation often requires external criteria such as a diagnostic hypothesis! (Berrios & Chen, 1993; for a study of the general problem of semantic ambiguity and underspecification see Deemter & Peters, 1996).

7  Weinstein et al. (1956) defined confabulation as 'a false narrative of an event or series of events' which differed from delusion 'in that it is limited in respect to time, place, and person, while delusion in this sense is timeless and limitless.' 'Generalizability of belief' is, however, a weak criterion. To be fair, Weinstein et al. have recognized that the 'distinction was admittedly arbitrary . . . for most of the principles involved in the understanding of confabulation apply to delusions as well' (p. 384).

8  Why should memory deficit have to be a criterion is, in itself, an interesting question. The historical answer is that 'pseudo-memories' (confabulations) were described by Korsakoff in the context of subjects with an 'amnestic' syndrome.

9  Bleuler (1924) noticed and complained about this: 'Unfortunately the term confabulation is also used for vivid memory hallucinations and for half-conscious fantasy manifestations of schizophrenia. We must, however, adhere to the concept in the above given sense of the confabulation, for thus conceived it is a sign of organic psychoses, when observed in non-delirious states' (p. 107). Jaspers (1948) considered confabulations as a subtype of 'falsifications of memory' which were characterized by being weak experiences: (a) 'memories without background and lacking in connection with the temporal and causal context of other memories'; and (b) because they were easily understandable as 'fillers' of memory gaps (p. 150).

10  This useful concept describes a tendency to define the profile of a disease on the basis of few severe or anomalous hospital exemplars, and to the fallacy of generalizing from such biased profile (Cohen & Cohen 1984). Most cases of confabulations reported in the literature are related to Korsakoff's or 'frontal lobe' patients (in both cases, confabulations are extremely rare).

11  The 'operational' definition of 'provoked' confabulation is unclear. In some cases, it refers to patients issuing wrong accounts in reply to specific *questions*. In others, the provocation is carried out by means of tests. For example, Lindqvist & Norlén's (1966) called confabulators subjects who made a high number of false identifications in the Cronholm-Molander Figure Test (p. 32). Likewise, the interview method of Mercer et al. (1977) (also used by Shapiro et al., 1981), and the 'burning house test' (Manning & Kartsounis, 1993) constitute yet different ways of 'provoking' confabulations.

12 There is no evidence that Korsakoff ever used the term 'confabulation', not even in the full paper he dedicated to 'false recollections' in polyneuritic psychosis (Korsakoff, 1891).

13 Indeed, Potel (1902) in his important book on the subject did not even refer to confabulations; nor do Chaslin & Portocalis (1908).

14 For a full study of presbyophrenia see Berrios, 1985; 1986; and Zervas et al., 1993.

15 Wernicke (1906) classified the insanities into three groups: allo-, somato- and autopychoses. There were five allopsychoses: delirium tremens, Korsakoff's psychosis, presbyophrenia, acute and chronic hallucinoses and pathological drunkenness.

16 This concept has come to replace the older and nobler one of volitional disorder (see Berrios & Gili, 1995). The 'frontal lobe view' has been taken up in earnest; based on it, Ovsiew (1992) has, for example, classified confabulations as a form of thought disorder: 'severe and elaborate confabulation betokens disease outside memory systems, particularly the failure of self-monitoring characteristic of frontal lobe disease' (p. 111).

17 This is the function more recently referred to as 'insight' by Marková and Berrios (1995a, b). For more detail see Chapter 10, this volume.

18 A full analysis of the linguistic, semantic, pragmatic, political and moral aspects of lying is well beyond the scope of this chapter (see Roufineau, 1841; Rey, 1925; Arendt, 1972; Durandin, 1972; Ekman, 1985; Castilla de Pino, 1988; Shapin, 1994; Robinson, 1996).

19 St Augustine *Du Mensonge* I,III,3 (quoted in Onfray, 1990).

20 In this sense Delay's (1942) analysis remains the most sensible one: 'The liar knows that he is lying, he knows that there is a truth; the fabulator does not tell the truth but he does not lie because he does not know that he is lying. The liar offers a falsehood instead of the truth, the fabulator is outwith truth and falsehood and within error and truth. The liar deceives, the fabulator is deceived' (pp. 101–102).

21 By 'delirium' Korsakoff (1955) is likely to have meant 'delusion'. Elsewhere, when writing about a patient with false recollections, he states: 'In this way, the patient had populated of fantasies the obscure regions of his past, in other words, he was in a delusional state (*délire*)' (Korsakoff, 1889: pp. 514–515). On difficulties to translate *délire* into English see Berrios (1996). Emil Régis (1906: pp. 640–642) was the main sponsor of the delusional interpretation of confabulations in French psychiatry.

22 For example, comparing the Old and New Testaments, Emmet (1909) noticed a change in the usage of 'fable': whilst in the OT it was still used for moral instruction, in the NT, 'fable' occurs in a different sense. It is used to translate the Greek 'myth,' which has lost its better sense as an allegorical vehicle for the truth whether growing naturally or deliberately invented . . . and has come to mean a deluding fiction of a more or less extravagant character' (pp. 254–255).

23 See, for example, the use and definition of *Confabulationen* by Wernicke (1906), in relation both to Korsakoff (p. 269) and presbyophrenia (p. 302). The German author believed confabulations to be tantamount to 'pseudo-memories' (*Erinnerungsfälschung*) (p. 297): in the case of Korsakoff's they were related to the memory deficit, and in presbyophrenia seemed to be 'based on misreported experiences and hypochondriacal sensations' (p. 302). Nouët & Halberstadt (1909), in their summary of Wernicke's concepts, called confabulations 'récits imaginaires' (p. 333).

24  Being conscious of one's own motivation for 'covering up' and of the 'falsehood of the narrative' can also be approached from the perspective of 'insight'. Research into this area is progressing rapidly and 'insightlessness' can no longer be considered as just another 'mental symptom' to be 'correlated' with other 'symptoms'. It has been recently suggested that insightlessness reflects a pervading failure in the quality and organization of self-knowledge (Marková & Berrios, 1995a, 1995b) (see Chapter 10, this volume).

25  I came across the imaginative paper by Myslobodsky & Hicks (1994) after I had completed writing this chapter. These authors define confabulations as 'verbalizations containing various degrees of distortions of the target material (submitted in the course of a trial or implied), propelled by a handicapping situation (deficient mnemonic functions, a state of discomfort or anxiety with a reduced level of self-monitoring) and unusual avidity to irrelevant associations in the realm of memory akin to environmental dependency syndrome' (p. 226).

26  The application of pragmatics to psychopathology has not yet started in earnest; for some examples see Blanchet (1994).

27  Intentionality ('aboutness'), the abstract noun, has been in use since the Medieval period and derives from the Latin *intendo*: 'to aim at'. Brentano (1973) used it to differentiate mental (intentional) from physical phenomena: 'What positive criterion shall we now be able to provide? . . . every mental phenomenon is characterized by what the Scholastics of the Middle Ages called the intentional (or mental) in-existence of an object . . . every mental phenomenon includes something as object within itself . . .' (p. 88). This latter sense of intentionality has less relevance to confabulations and will not be pursued further.

28  For example see: Escandell-Vidal, 1993: pp. 40–44; Sperber & Wilson, 1995: p. 58; Levinson, 1983: p. 15.

29  Following Gennaro's (1996) lead, the terms 'self-conscious' and 'self-consciousness' are used here to refer to a state of consciousness accompanied by a *meta-psychological thought*. This author has also argued that 'being a conscious system entails having episodic memory' (p. 183).

30  Some authors might argue that even if the narrative is shown to be false, it is not necessarily *manqué* for it *still fulfils* an important function. For example, Weinstein et al. (1956) have argued that confabulations are composed to 'minimise the impact of the disease'; and Gainotti (1975) has suggested that 'confabulations of denial' (claims of normality) 'play the function of avoiding catastrophic reaction' (p. 100).

## Chapter 17

1  For example, Herbert Spencer (1890) described it fully: 'at times when strong emotion has excited the circulation to an exceptional degree, the clustered sensations yielded by surrounding objects are revivable with great clearness, often throughout life, a fact noticed by writers of fiction as a trait of human nature' (p. 235); the chapter from which this quotation is taken 'The Revivability of Feelings' can be said to be dedicated to behaviours akin to what is now named 'flashbulb memories'. Ribot (1882) discussed similar phenomena in the chapter entitled 'Exaltations of Memory, or Hypermnesia'.

2 On account of these features, these memories have also been called 'personal event memories' (Pillemer, 1998).

3 Flashbulbs came into wide use no more than 100 years ago. Transposing its features onto a memory phenomenon imposes upon it wrong analogical characteristics by suggesting some sort of one-trial mechanism, and effectively disconnects it from its history. In a way, Brown and Kulik (1977) themselves acknowledged this: 'an actual photograph, taken by flashbulb, preserves everything within its scope; it is altogether indiscriminate. Our flashbulb memories are not . . .' (p. 75).

4 In other words, it suggests that 'collective' flashbulb memories may be different from the private and humdrum memories of ordinary people which on occasions may also have a flashbulb quality (for an analysis of this assumption see Wright et al., 1998). Brown and Kulik (1977) seem to have made their choice on the basis that the assassination of some political figures was *surprising* and would have personal relevance to a large number of people (consequentiality). Whilst the former reason may be relevant to the triggering of the encoding mechanism, the latter seems to have been dictated by research expediency.

5 It goes without saying that accepting such reports implies the assumption, on the part of the clinician, of the 'conventional' view of visual image. A 'visual image' is defined here as an evocation (by a given subject) of the *sensory aspects* of an object when this is not within his/her perceptual purview. The visual image is believed to be a representation (on the concept of representation see: Cummins, 1989) 'projected onto' some inner screen and available to an 'inner eye'. These two elements are constitutive parts of the 'perceptual metaphor' which up to the late nineteenth century provided the basis of 'introspection'. The 'conventional' view of visual images, predominant since the time of Democritus and Aristotle, reigned supreme until the early twentieth century when, in the Anglo-Saxon world, it was challenged by behaviourism (on this see the important historical book by Denis, 1979). The view that images have a symbolic and codificatory function never quite disappeared from continental philosophy of mind (see, for example, the superb paper by Meyerson, 1929). Interest in visual images has re-appeared in Anglo-Saxon psychology in the wake of the new 'cognitive psychology'; however, the new sponsors rarely acknowledge Continental work. (For a good account of the conceptual problems, see Tye, 1991. For the neuropsychological perspective, see Behrmann et al., 1995; Kosslyn, 1994. For a recent general account of perception, see Rock, 1995.)

6 In spite of the fact that there is evidence that memory images for personal events also undergo reconstruction (see Nigro & Neisser, 1983).

7 i.e. the view that memories are *always* stories constituted by morsels of information selected and edited according to social and personal frames (Pillemer, 1992; Loftus et al., 1995; etc.).

8 As mentioned above, the term flashbulb memory names particularly vivid, long-lasting recollections of the personal circumstances in which the subject first learned of a shocking public or private event. Such memories are said to contain 'irrelevant details', e.g. the brand of cigarettes being smoked at the time of the event. Such sensory richness is considered as evidence in favour of the alleged accuracy and stability of flashbulb memories (Brown & Kulik, 1977).

9 In this regard it has been postulated that: (a) emotional memories may increase the levels of hormones and glucose thereby promoting efficient consolidation; (b) the participation of the amygdala in emotionally-charged memories adds attributes to final memory processing

including important cognitive links with the frontal lobes; and (c) flashbulb memories may be multi-represented in terms of Kesner's model (see Conway, 1995).

10  Such distinction has, of course, been made at least since the time of Aristotle. See this volume, Chapter 1 on the 'History of memory and its disorders'.

11  The nature of this emotional accompaniment led, between the 1880s to the first World War, to a famous debate in clinical psychology. Known as the 'affective memory' debate it revolved around the issue of whether there was a memory for emotions or whether each time the cognitive component or the image of the memory was remembered it would trigger a fresh token of the emotion in question (see Berrios, 1999, in press).

12  Indeed, such assumption is implicit in the therapeutic usage of abreaction (Krystal et al., 1995).

13  Eidetic refers to 'an image that revives an optical impression with hallucinatory clearness, or to the faculty of seeing such images, or to a person having this faculty' (OED, 2nd edition). The locus classicus for the study of 'eidetics' remains Jaensch (1930); there are also excellent papers on the traditional approach by Quercy (1925) and Jelliffe (1928); more recently, the concept has been included into the wider definition of 'high imager' (Katz, 1983). The concept of eidetic imagery has not been used as frequently as it might in the context of the psychopathology of perception. It has been suggested, however, that 'vivid auditory imagery may be a necessary (although not sufficient) pre-requisite for hallucinations in schizophrenics' (Mintz & Alpert, 1972: p. 311).

# Chapter 18

1  Because full memory assessments remain expensive, it would be ideal if analysis of the 'phenomenology' of the memory *complaint* or a discriminant function constituted by some crucial variables could be worked out that may tell the team what the likely cause and outcome of the memory complaint might be.

2  This procedure is to be commended as evidence is accumulating that, at least in the *older* age groups, a so-called 'isolated memory loss' may herald an organic memory disorder (Bowen et al., 1997).

3  For this emphasis on dementia to the detriment of other conditions related to memory complaints see, for example Bayer et al., 1987; Cammen et al., 1987; Stevens et al., 1992.

4  For example, Fraser (1992) writes: 'a memory clinic is essentially a facility for the diagnosis and management of early dementia'. After listing three objectives which pertain to dementia or other organic disorders; a fourth is included: 'to *re-assure* those who are worried that they are losing their memory, when in fact no morbid deficits are found'. [our italics] (p. 105).

5  As earlier on was shown by Brown et al. (1991) in younger complainers there was no correlation between the level of the complaint and the results of memory tests.

6  Why were these patients excluded from the class of 'memory disorders' in the first place? It would seem that central to this decision was the implausible clinical inference that performing 'within a normal range' in some tests actually determined normality of function. There are at least two problems with this: one that there is no good evidence that memory tests, originally developed to measure function in some subjects, should apply to all cases; another, that

there is no evidence that the *concept of memory* built into such tests included putative 'feelings of satisfaction with one's own memory' function. In other words, the assumption that feelings of dissatisfaction with one's mental and bodily functions are external (and/or irrelevant) to the performing of those functions is groundless and originated during a period in the history of medicine when behaviourism was rampant. Evidence is accumulating that such feelings might be, in fact, sensitive predictors of current or future dysfunction (Bowen et al., 1997).

7   Indeed, a similar refashioning has taken place in other areas of medicine (e.g. sleep, gastro-intestinal complaints, cœnæsthesia, etc.).

8   There seems to have been a social class effect on the prevalence of this condition now replaced by the chronic fatigue syndrome (on its history, see Wessely, 1995).

9   The sort of problem that Ponds et al. (1995) have deal with in their paper on 'the fear of forgetting'.

10  Cohort studies dedicated to 'early dementia' include as a rule subjects over 50 (see Brayne, 1994). It has been suggested that amongst the over 65s there may be a dissociation between self-evaluation and objective performance and that this may be due to 'anosognosia of mild memory deficit' (Gagnon et al., 1994).

11  There is a debate on the validity of this construct (see Derouesne et al., 1994).

12  The most common reason for data missing was inability by patients to complete the computerized psychiatric instruments; and this was almost always due to severe dementia. In few cases, computer files had been overwritten or lost. The bias introduced by either reason is unlikely to affect the matter of this chapter.

13  DSM-IV Somatoform disorders are defined as 'the presence of physical symptoms that suggest a general medical condition (hence, the term *somatoform*) and are not fully explained by a general medical condition, by the direct effects of a substance, or by another mental disorder (e.g. Panic Disorder). . . . In contrast to Factitious Disorders and Malingering, the physical symptoms are not intentional (i.e. under voluntary control).

14  SSM is defined as 'a disorder in which a complaint of insomnia or excessive sleepiness occurs without objective evidence of any sleep disturbance' (p. 498; Hauri, 1994).

15  At this initial stage, this 'formless experience' refers to conglomerates of 'elements' or 'sensations' in consciousness whose main feature is raw immediacy (James, 1891).

## Chapter 22

1   Scott R. Millis, Rehabilitation Institute of Michigan, 261 Mack Boulevard, Detroit, MI 48201, USA.

# Index

absent-mindedness, as legal defence 489–90
abulia 275
acetylcholine 76–7, 83
acetylcholinesterase inhibitors (CAT I) 83
Addison's disease 150
affect, *see* mood
affective disorders 247–59
    comorbid, in dissociative amnesia 419
    Ganser syndrome and 449–50
    general intellectual impairment 247–51
    insight 204, 205
    memory impairment 251–5, 256–8
    *see also* depression
age
    disorientation, in schizophrenia 237
    dissociative amnesia and 407
    functional memory complaints and 384
    memory problems in depression and 36
    *see also* elderly
age-associated memory impairment (AAMI)
    271–3, 276
    animal studies 82
    depression and 271–2
    therapeutic interventions 51
agnosia
    progressive 179
    topographical 170–1
    visual apperceptual 138
aids, external memory 53, 303–4
AIDS, opportunistic infections 151
AIDS-dementia complex 151
alcohol abuse, chronic 151, 180, 352
alien hand sign 131, 149
alienists, nineteenth century 7, 17–18
α-receptor agonists 79–80, 82, 86–7
α2 adrenoceptor system 82, 86–7
α2-receptor antagonists 82, 86–7, 416
Alzheimer's disease (AD, DAT) 132–9
    animal models 80
    atypical 138–9
    cholinergic hypothesis 82–3
    clinical features 135–9
    depression in 138, 270, 275–6
    diagnosis 115, 130, 131, 132–5
        clinical guidelines 135
        early disease 136, 139

differential diagnosis 131–2
    early amnestic prodrome 136
    implicit memory 128–9, 227
    insight 138, 209, 215–16
        brain mechanisms 226–7
        depression and 225–6
        stage of illness and 218–25
    memory impairment 126–7, 128–9, 135–8,
        178–9
    neuropathology 132, 178–9
    pharmacological strategies 83–4, 85
    rehabilitation of memory 297, 298
    scopolamine model 76, 77
    subcortical pathology 125
    vs. cortical Lewy body disease 148
    vs. dementia of frontal type 138, 139, 143
    vs. depressive pseudodementia 258, 269–71,
        277
    vs. normal cognitive aging 272
    vs. vascular dementia 148
amnesia (amnesic syndrome) 164–75
    aetiology 178–80
    anatomical correlates 175–8
    awareness 206–9
    defendants claiming 456, 486–8
    for faces and people 170
    history of concept 17–18, 500
    ictal 187, 197
    organic, *see* organic amnesia
    post-traumatic 180
    retrograde, *see* retrograde amnesia
    semantic 171–3
    slowly progressive 179
    topographical 170–1
    transient, *see* transient amnesia
    vs. dementia 125
    vs. functional psychosis 258
    *see also other specific types of amnesia*
amputees, body memories 377–9
amygdala 175, 176
    lesions involving 179
amytal injection 174, 411–12
anamnesis 4, 498
anhedonia 275
animal models 80–2
    Alzheimer's disease 80

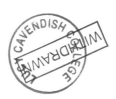